Cardiac Arrhythmias and Mapping Techniques

Peter W. Macfarlane · Adriaan van Oosterom · Michiel Janse · Paul Kligfield · John Camm · Olle Pahlm (Eds.)

Cardiac Arrhythmias and Mapping Techniques

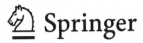

Editors
Peter W. Macfarlane
University of Glasgow
Glasgow
UK

Adriaan van Oosterom
Radboud University Nijmegen
Nijmegen
The Netherlands

Olle Pahlm
Lund University
Lund
Sweden

Paul Kligfield
Weill Cornell Medical College
New York, NY
USA

Michiel Janse
University of Amsterdam
Amsterdam
The Netherlands

John Camm
St. George's, University of London
London
UK

ISBN 978-0-85729-876-8
DOI 10.1007/978-0-85729-877-5

Library of Congress Control Number: 2011943335

First published in 2010 as part of Comprehensive Electrocardiology, 2nd Edition (ISBN 978-1-84882-045-6)

Printed on acid-free paper

Springer is part of Springer Science+Business Media (www.springer.com)

Editors-in-Chief

Peter W. Macfarlane
University of Glasgow
Glasgow
UK

Paul Kligfield
Weill Cornell Medical College
New York, NY
USA

Adriaan van Oosterom
Radboud University Nijmegen
Nijmegen
The Netherlands

Michiel Janse
University of Amsterdam
Amsterdam
The Netherlands

Olle Pahlm
Lund University
Lund
Sweden

John Camm
St. George's, University of London
London
UK

Preface

The first edition of *Comprehensive Electrocardiology* was published in 1989, when e-mail was still in its infancy (!!), and it was never envisaged at that time that a new edition would be prepared. It is probably fair to say that the majority of physicians would have regarded electrocardiography in particular as having reached its maximum usefulness with little additional information to be obtained therefrom. The intervening 20 years have shown how untrue this was.

An update to the book is long overdue. Sadly, some of our former contributors have died since the first edition was published and it is with regret that I note the passing of Philippe Coumel, Rudolph van Dam, Karel den Dulk, Ramesh Gulrajani, Kenici Harumi, John Milliken, Jos Willems and Christoph Zywietz. Where relevant, their contributions continue to be acknowledged but in some cases, chapters have been completely rewritten by new contributors. On the other hand, eight completely new chapters have been added and the appendices restructured.

The publisher felt it would be opportune to produce separate paperback versions of each of the four volumes of the second edition of *Comprehensive Electrocardiology* – hence this book entitled. *Cardiac Arrhythmias and Mapping Techniques.*

In some ways, it is inconceivable what has taken place in the field of electrocardiology since the first edition. New ECG patterns have been recognised and linked with sudden death, new prognostic indices have been developed and evaluated, the ECG has assumed a pivotal role in the treatment of an acute coronary syndrome and among many other things, automated ECG interpretation is now commonplace. Significant advances have been made in the field of mathematical modeling and a solution to the inverse problem is now applied in routine clinical use. Electrophysiological studies have taken giant steps over the past 20 years and biventricular pacing is a relatively recent innovation. Electrocardiology has certainly not stood still in the last 20 years. Of course there have been parallel advances in imaging techniques but the ECG still retains a unique position in the armamentarium of the physician, let alone the cardiologist.

For this edition, my previous co editor, Professor T.D. Veitch Lawrie, decided to step aside and I wish to congratulate him on reaching his 91st birthday in September 2011. However, I am pleased that other very eminent individuals agreed to assist with the editing of the book, namely Adriaan van Oosterom, Olle Pahlm, Paul Kligfield, Michiel Janse and John Camm. In the nature of things, some of these co editors undertook much more work than others. For this book, I particularly have to acknowledge the support of Olle Pahlm and John Camm. Without their support, this revised version of the material in the first edition would not have been possible.

Locally, I am very much indebted to my secretary Pamela Armstrong for a huge contribution in checking and subediting every chapter which went out from my office to the publisher. This was a Herculean task carried out with great aplomb. I would also like to thank Ms. Julie Kennedy for her contribution to a variety of tasks associated with preparing selected chapters, including enhancements to the English presentation on occasions.

I also wish to thank the publishers Springer for their considerable support throughout. Grant Weston initially commissioned the book and I am grateful to him for his confidence in supporting the preparation of a new edition. Jennifer Carlson and her team in New York also assisted significantly. I am also indebted to Mr. R. Samuel Devanand and his team at SPi Global, in India, for production of the paperback edition.

I again must thank my long suffering wife Irene who has had to fight to gain access to our home PC every night over these past few years!

Comprehensive Electrocardiology aims to bring together truly comprehensive information about the field and *Basic Electrocardiology* provides a strong theoretical foundation to the principles of electrocardiography. A book can never be completely up to date given the speed of publication of research findings over the internet these days but hopefully this publication will continue to be of significant use to readers for many years to come. *Basic Electrocardiology*, together with the other three paperback versions of the other volumes of *Comprehensive Electrocardiology*, contains much information that should be of use both to the practising clinician and the experienced researcher.

Now that this huge effort has been completed and the book is available electronically, it should be much easier to produce the next edition...!!

Peter Macfarlane
Glasgow
Autumn

Table of Contents

List of Contributors

Luigi De Ambroggi
University of Milan
Milan
Italy

Frits W. Bär
University of Maastricht
Maastricht
The Netherlands

A. John Camm
St. George's, University of London
London
UK

Alexandru D. Corlan
University Emergency Hospital of Bucharest
Bucharest
Romania

Alain Coulomb
Hopital Pitie-Salpetriere
Paris
France

D. Wyn Davies
Imperial College London
London
UK

Parvin C. Dorostkar
University of Minnesota
Minneapolis, MN
USA

Karel Den Dulk
University of Maastricht
Maastricht
The Netherlands

Guy Fontaine
Hopital Pitie-Salpetriere
Paris
France

Robert Frank
Hopital Pitie-Salpetriere
Paris
France

Anton P.M. Gorgels
University of Maastricht
Maastricht
The Netherlands

Julian Jarman
Imperial College London
London
UK

Demosthenes G. Katritsis
Athens Euroclinic
Athens
Greece

Michael Koa-Wing
Imperial College London
London
UK

Jèrôme Lacotte
Hopital Pitie-Salpetriere
Paris
France

Jerome Liebman
Case Western Reserve University School of Medicine
Cleveland, OH
USA

Robert L. Lux
University of Utah
Salt Lake City, UT
USA

Vias Markides
Imperial College London
London
UK

Andrew D. Mcgavigan
Royal Melbourne Hospital
Melbourne, VIC
Australia

Nicholas Peters
Imperial College London
London
UK

F. Russell Quinn
Glasgow Royal Infirmary
Glasgow
UK

Alan P. Rae
Royal Infirmary Glasgow
Glasgow
UK

Andrew C. Rankin
University of Glasgow
Glasgow
UK

Michael R. Rosen
Columbia University
New York, NY
USA

Oliver R. Segal
University College London
London
UK

Hein J.J. Wellens
University of Maastricht
Maastricht
The Netherlands

Andrew L. Wit
Columbia University
New York, NY
USA

Part I

Cardiac Arrhythmias

1 Cellular Electrophysiological and Genetic Mechanisms of Cardiac Arrhythmias

Andrew L. Wit · Michael R. Rosen

P. W. Macfarlane et al. (eds.), *Cardiac Arrhythmias and Mapping Techniques*, DOI 10.1007/978-0-85729-877-5_1,

© Springer-Verlag London Limited 2012

1.1   Introduction

Cardiac arrhythmias result from abnormalities in the rate, regularity or site of origin of the cardiac impulse or disturbance in the conduction of that impulse such that the normal sequence of activation of atria and ventricles is altered [1]. Thus, arrhythmias result from abnormalities in the initiation of impulses or in conduction of these impulses through the heart [2, 3]. Such alterations in impulse initiation or conduction are readily apparent in recordings of extracellular signals from the heart, in the form of either the electrocardiogram or more direct electrographic recordings from the atria and ventricles. However, the recording of the transmembrane electrical events of the individual myocardial cells with microelectrodes has provided the information necessary for understanding the mechanisms that are responsible for the arrhythmias. The importance of this approach was recognized in the 1960s by Hoffman and Cranefield [2]. Although arrhythmias may have many different pathological causes, in the final analysis all arrhythmias are the consequence of critical alterations in the cellular electrophysiology. How these changes in cellular electrophysiology occur, what they are, and how they cause arrhythmias are the subject of this chapter.

Much of the discussion is focused on abnormalities in the membrane currents that flow across the sarcolemma and that determine the transmembrane resting and action potential. The reader is therefore advised to consult ❷ Chap. 3, which describes the normal properties of the membrane channels and currents, before reading this chapter.

1.2   Arrhythmias Caused by Abnormal Impulse Initiation

The term "impulse initiation" is used to indicate that an electrical impulse can arise in a single cell or group of closely coupled cells through depolarization of the cell membrane, and once initiated, spread through the rest of the heart (impulse conduction). Impulse initiation occurs because of localized changes in the ionic currents, which flow across the membranes of individual cells. There are two major causes for the impulse initiation that may result in arrhythmias: automaticity and triggered activity. Each has its own unique cellular mechanisms resulting in membrane depolarization. Automaticity is the result of spontaneous (diastolic) phase 4 depolarization (see ❷ Fig. 1.1) that can occur *de novo*, whereas triggered activity is caused by afterdepolarizations, which require a preceding action potential for their induction. These different cellular mechanisms result in arrhythmias that have very different characteristics in their mode of onset, their rate, and their response to interventions such as external pacemakers and drugs.

1.2.1   Automaticity

It is convenient to subdivide automaticity into two categories, normal and abnormal. Normal automaticity is found in the primary pacemaker of the heart –the sinus node – as well as certain subsidiary or latent pacemakers which can become the pacemaker if the function of the sinus node is compromised. Impulse initiation is a normal function of these latent pacemakers. Abnormal automaticity, whether the result of experimental interventions or pathology, only occurs in cardiac cells when major changes occur in their transmembrane potentials. This property is not confined to any specific latent pacemaker but may occur anywhere in the heart. Arrhythmias characterized by abnormalities in the rate, regularity or site of origin of the cardiac impulse can result from either normal or abnormal automaticity.

1.2.1.1   Normal Automaticity

The cause of normal automaticity in the sinus node is a spontaneous decline in the transmembrane potential during diastole, referred to as phase 4 or diastolic depolarization (❷ Fig. 1.1). When the depolarization reaches threshold potential, a spontaneous action potential (impulse) is initiated. The fall in membrane potential during phase 4 reflects a gradual shift in the balance between inward and outward membrane currents in the direction of the net inward (depolarizing) current.

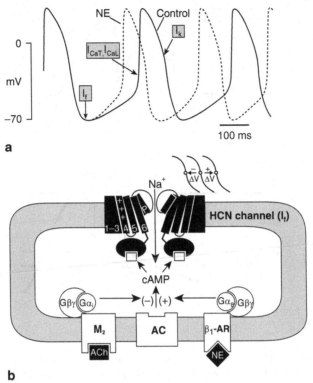

◻ Fig. 1.1

Panel A: Representation of sinoatrial node action potential (Control: *solid lines*) and some of the ion channels that contribute to it. I_f is activated on hyperpolarization and provides inward current during phase 4. T- and L-type Ca currents are initiated towards the end of phase 4: the latter also contributes the major current to the upstroke of the action potential. Delayed rectifier current (I_K) is responsible for repolarization. The acceleratory effects of norepinephrine (NE) are shown as *broken lines*. Note the prominent increase in phase 4, reflecting the actions of NE on I_f. *Panel B*: Cartoon of the pacemaker channel. There are six transmembrane spanning domains: when the channel in the open position, Na is the major ion transmitted. Cyclic AMP binding sites are present near the amino terminus. Also depicted are β_1-adrenergic (B1-AR) and M2-muscarinic receptors, providing, respectively, norepinephrine and acetylcholine binding sites. Via G-protein coupling these regulate adenylyl cyclase (AC) activity which in turn regulates intracellular cAMP levels, determining availability of the second messenger for binding and for channel modulation (Reproduced with permission from Biel et al. (2002))

The specific properties of the pacemaker current which causes phase 4 depolarization have been studied with voltage-clamp techniques. These investigations have shown that diastolic depolarization results from the initiation on of an inward current, I_f, that is activated after repolarization of the action potential is complete [4, 5]. As shown in ❷ Fig. 1.1 several currents contribute to phase 4 depolarization and to the sinus node action potential, but the process is initiated by the pacemaker current I_f [5]. The channel carrying I_f, which is an inward sodium current, activates as the membrane hyperpolarizes. For this reason, it was designated "funny current" or I_f [4, 5]. The cartoon in ❷ Fig. 1.1 also depicts the α subunit of the HCN (hyperpolarization-activated, cyclic nucleotide gated) channel that carries I_f [5]. HCN has four isoforms, designated as HCN1–4. The predominant isoform in sinus node is HCN4 and in ventricle, HCN2. HCN3 is not found in heart. A cyclic-AMP binding site on the HCN channel permits catecholamines to modulate activation. It is largely this property that regulates the autonomic responsiveness of the cardiac pacemaker. ❷ Figure 1.1 also demonstrates that other channels contribute to the voltage-time course of the pacemaker potential, including inward calcium current [6] and outward potassium current.

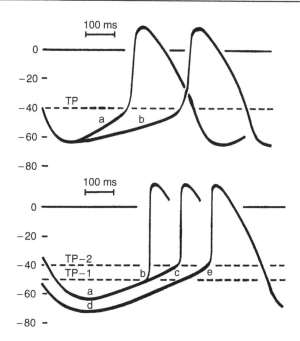

◻ Fig. 1.2
Transmembrane action potential recorded from a sinus node fiber showing the mechanism responsible for impulse initiation and its change in frequency. In the upper diagram, trace "a" shows phase 4 depolarization (normal automaticity) that carries membrane potential to the threshold potential TP, after which action potential upstroke occurs. Trace "b" shows how a decrease in the slope or rate of phase 4 depolarization increases the time required for the transmembrane potential to reach threshold, and thereby slows the rate. The lower diagram shows how changes in maximum diastolic potential or threshold potential affects rate when the slope of phase 4 depolarization remains unchanged. Changing threshold potential from TP-1 to TP-2 increases the time required for phase 4 depolarization to bring membrane potential to the TP (trace "b" to "c") and slows the rate. Increasing maximum diastolic potential from "a" to "d" has a similar effect (Reproduced with permission after Hoffman and Cranefield (1960) © McGraw Hill, New York)

The intrinsic rate at which sinus node pacemaker cells initiate impulses is determined by three factors:

(a) The maximum diastolic potential which is maintained by the outward potassium current, I_{k1} and the Na/K pump:
(b) The threshold potential, at which the action potential upstroke is initiated; and
(c) The rate or slope of phase 4 depolarization (❯ Fig. 1.2), which is determined by the properties of the pacemaker current [7].

A change in any one of these three factors will alter the time required for phase 4 depolarization to carry the membrane potential from its maximum diastolic level to threshold, and thereby alter the rate of impulse initiation. For example, if the maximum diastolic potential increases (becomes more negative), as may be induced by vagal nerve stimulation, spontaneous depolarization to threshold potential will take longer and the rate of impulse initiation will fall. Conversely, a decrease in the maximum diastolic potential will tend to increase the rate of impulse initiation. Similarly, changes in threshold potential or changes in the slope of phase 4 depolarization will alter the rate of impulse initiation (❯ Fig. 1.2) [7]. Such alterations in the rate of impulse initiation in the sinus node may lead to arrhythmias as discussed below.

In addition to the sinus node, normal cardiac cells with pacemaking capability are located in parts of the atria (plateau fibers along the crista terminalis and interatrial septum [8]), in the atrioventricular (AV) junctional region [9–11] and in the His-Purkinje system [7]. Yet, there is a hierarchy of a pacemaker activities in the heart such that the sinus nodes initiate impulses most rapidly and the distal Purkinje system most slowly [12–14]. The membrane currents causing spontaneous diastolic depolarization at ectopic sites have been studied most thoroughly in Purkinje fibers also, using voltage-clamp techniques [15, 16]. We can best understand the hierarchy of pacemaker function by contrasting pacemaker current (I_f) and the sinus node and in the ventricles. We stress that I_f is present throughout the heart, although it activates at the most positive potentials in sinus node while in myocardium it activates at levels negative to the physiologic range of membrane potentials(N-150 mL). These differences in activation are in part determined by HCN isoforms (HCN$_4$ predominates in sinus node, HCN$_2$ in ventricle and in part by other properties. For example in the neonatal ventricle activation is more positive than in adult, and a shift to more negative activation voltages occurs with growth and development [17].

In the normal heart, the intrinsic rate of impulse initiation by the sinus node is higher than that of other potentially automatic cells. Hence, latent pacemakers are excited by impulses propagated from the sinus node before they can depolarize spontaneously to threshold potential. Not only are latent pacemakers prevented from initiating an impulse because they are depolarized before they have a chance to fire, but also the diastolic (phase 4) depolarization of the latent pacemaker cells is actually inhibited because they are repeatedly depolarized by the impulses from the sinus node [12, 18]. This inhibition can be demonstrated easily by suddenly stopping the sinus by, for example, vagal stimulation. Impulses then usually arise from a subsidiary pacemaker, but that impulse initiation is generally preceded by a long period of quiescence [19]. Impulse initiation by subsidiary pacemakers begins at a low rate and only gradually speeds up to a final steady rate which is, however, still slower than the rate of the original sinus rhythm.

The quiescent period following termination of the sinus rhythm reflects the inhibitory influence exerted on the subsidiary pacemaker by the dominant sinus node pacemaker. This inhibition is called overdrive suppression. Overdrive suppression has been best characterized in microelectrode studies on isolated Purkinje fiber bundles exhibiting pacemaker activity (❷ Fig. 1.3) [18]; it is the result of driving a pacemaker cell faster than its intrinsic spontaneous rate and is mediated by enhanced activity of the Na$^+$ K$^+$ exchange pump. During normal sinus rhythm, the sinus node drives the latent pacemakers at a faster rate than their normal automatic rate. As a result, the intracellular sodium concentration of the latent pacemakers is increased to a higher steady-state level than would be the case were the pacemaker firing at its own intrinsic rate. This is the result of sodium ions entering the cell during each action-potential upstroke. The rate of activity of the sodium pump is largely determined by the intracellular sodium concentration [20], so that pump activity is enhanced during high rates of stimulation [18]. Since the sodium pump usually moves more Na$^+$ outward than K$^+$ inward,

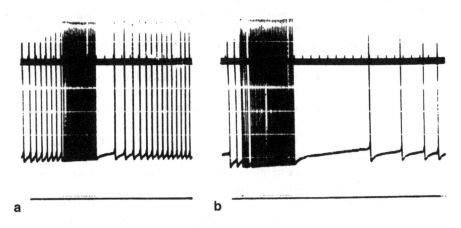

a   b

❏ Fig. 1.3

Overdrive suppression of normal automaticity in a Purkinje fiber. The first eight action potentials in (a) occur spontaneously at the intrinsic firing rate of the Purkinje fiber. Note the phase 4 depolarization preceding the upstroke or the action potential. A period of rapid stimulation is then imposed for 25 s at the end of which there is a short quiescent period followed by the reappearance of the spontaneous rhythm with gradually increases to the control rate. In (b) a longer period of overdrive is followed by prolonged quiescence and a far slower rate than the control rate. Stimulus pulses are shown in the bottom traces and the time marks in the top traces occur at 5 ms intervals (Reproduced with permission after Cranefield (1975) © Futura, Mount Kisco, New York)

it generates a net outward (hyperpolarizing) current across the cell membrane [21]. When subsidiary pacemaker cells are driven faster than their intrinsic rate (such as by the sinus node), the enhanced outward pump current suppresses spontaneous impulse initiation in these cells, which, as described above is dependent on the net inward current (❷ Fig. 1.3). When the dominant (overdrive) pacemaker is stopped, this suppression is responsible for the period of quiescence which lasts until the intracellular Na^+ concentration, and hence the pump current becomes small enough to allow subsidiary pacemaker cells to depolarize spontaneously to threshold. Intracellular sodium concentration decreases during the quiescent period, because sodium is constantly being pumped out of the cell and little is entering [22]. Intracellular Na^+ and pump current continue to decline after the first spontaneous impulse, resulting in gradual increases in the discharge rate of the subsidiary pacemaker. The higher the rate, or the longer the duration of overdrive, the greater is the enhancement of pump activity, so that the period of quiescence following the cessation of overdrive is directly related to the rate and duration of overdrive (❷ Fig. 1.3) [18].

The sinus node, itself, can also be overdrive-suppressed if it is driven at a rate more rapid than its intrinsic rate [23, 24]. Thus, there may be a quiescent period after termination of a rapid ectopic tachycardia before the sinus rhythm resumes [25]. However, when overdrive suppression of the normal sinus node occurs, it is of lesser magnitude than that of subsidiary pacemakers overdriven at comparable rates [23]. As described above, overdrive suppression of pacemaker fibers depends on sodium entering the fibers during phase 0 of the action potential, stimulating sodium pump activity. In the sinus node, the action-potential upstroke is largely dependent on slow inward current carried by calcium, and far less sodium enters the fiber during the upstroke than occurs in latent pacemaker cells such as Purkinje fibers. As a result, the activity of the sodium pump is probably not increased to the same extent in sinus node cells after a period of overdrive and, therefore, there is less overdrive suppression. The relative resistance of the normal sinus node to overdrive suppression may be important in enabling it to remain as the dominant pacemaker even when its rhythm is transiently perturbed by external influences (such as transient shifts of the pacemaker to an ectopic site). The diseased sinus node, however, may be much more easily overdrive-suppressed [26].

Another mechanism that may suppress subsidiary pacemakers, in addition to overdrive suppression, is the electronic interaction among pacemaker cells and the nonpacemaker cells in the surrounding myocardium [27] (❷ Fig. 1.4). This mechanism may be particularly important in suppressing AV nodal automaticity [28]. AV nodal cells have intrinsic pacemaker activity that may be nearly as rapid as that in the sinus node. This can be demonstrated in small pieces of the AV node superfused in a tissue chamber [9]. Such pacemaker activity is not easily overdrive-suppressed, probably for the same reasons discussed above for the sinus node. However, the pacemaker activity of the AV node may be suppressed by axial current flowing through the connections between the node and the surrounding atrial cells (❷ Fig. 1.4). The atrial cells have resting potentials which are more negative that those of the nodal cells and are not latent pacemakers. As a result of the more negative potentials of the atrial cells, current flow between them and the nodal cells should be in a direction which prevents spontaneous phase 4 depolarization of the latter. This current flow is apparently sufficient to prevent nodal automaticity despite the paucity of the intercellular junctions in the nodal region. The same mechanisms might be operative in the other regions of the atria where latent pacemaker cells may be surrounded by nonpacemaker cells, or in the distal Purkinje system where the Purkinje fibers are in contact with working ventricular muscle [27].

Arrhythmias caused by the normal automaticity of the cardiac fibers may occur for several different reasons. Such arrhythmias might result simply from an alteration in the rate of impulse initiation by the normal sinus node pacemaker without the shift of impulse origin to an ectopic site; sinus bradycardia and tachycardia are such arrhythmias. The cellular mechanisms which can change the rate of impulse initiation have been described above.

A shift in the site of impulse initiation to one of the regions where subsidiary pacemakers are located is another factor which results in arrhythmias caused by a normal automatic mechanism. This would be expected to happen when any of the following occurs:

(a) The rate of the sinus node pacemaker falls considerably below the intrinsic rates of the subsidiary pacemakers;
(b) Inhibitory electrotonic influences between nonpacemaker and pacemaker cells are interrupted;
(c) Impulse initiation in subsidiary pacemaker cells is enhanced.

The rate at which the sinus node activates subsidiary pacemakers may be decreased in a number of situations. Impulse initiation by the sinus node may be slowed or completely inhibited by heightened activity in the parasympathetic nervous

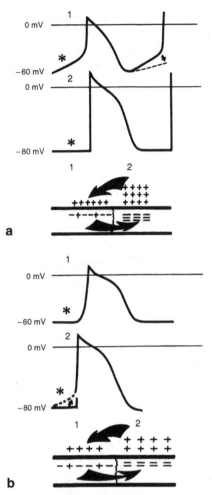

◘ Fig. 1.4

Part (a) is a diagrammatic representation of the effects of current flow from a cell with a high resting potential on the spontaneous diastolic depolarization of a cell with a lower resting potential; *1*, the transmembrane potential of a cell with a maximum diastolic potential of −60 mV and spontaneous diastolic depolarization (*); *2*, the transmembrane potential of an adjacent cell with a steady maximum diastolic potential −80 mV (*). Below it is a schematic representation of the membrane during the diastolic period. Since 1 has a lower potential across the membrane than 2, there is a flow of positive charge from 2 to 1 in extracellular space and from 1 to 2 in intracellular space, tending to oppose the decrease in membrane potential. Part (b) shows the interaction between: *1*, a cell with a steady low membrane potential of −60 mV and *2*, a cell with a higher membrane potential but spontaneous diastolic depolarization. Below is a schematic representation of the membrane during the diastolic period. Current (positive charge) flows from the cell with the higher membrane potential 1 in extracellular space and from 1 to 2 in intracellular space. This has a depolarizing effect on 2 and accelerates spontaneous diastolic depolarization while having some hyperpolarizing effects on 1

system [29], or as a result of sinus node disease [13]. Alternatively, there may be block of impulse conduction from the sinus node to the atria or block of conduction from the atria to the ventricles. Under any of the above conditions there may be "escape" of a subsidiary pacemaker as a result of the removal of overdrive suppression by the sinus pacemaker. As stated earlier, there is a natural hierarchy of intrinsic rates of subsidiary pacemakers, with atrial pacemakers having faster intrinsic rates than ventricular pacemakers [12–14, 30]. Once overdrive suppression is removed, the pacemaker with the faster rate becomes the site of impulse origin after sinus node inhibition [12]. As a result, there is a tendency for ectopic rhythms to arise in the atria or the AV junction when the sinus node impulse initiation is impaired or when there is sinus exit block. During AV block, the pacemaker will be in the AV junction or ventricular specialized conducting system, depending on the site of the block. The His bundle has a faster intrinsic rate than the more distally located Purkinje fibers [14]. Sometimes, however, pathologic processes that are responsible for the suppression of impulse initiation in the sinus node also suppress pacemaking in the atria and AV junction, so ectopic impulses may occur in the ventricular conducting system. This may occur during the sick sinus syndrome where ectopic ventricular beats, rather than junctional beats sometimes occur during the period of sinus bradycardia or arrest [31].

Any event which decreases intercellular coupling among latent pacemaker cells and surrounding nonpacemaker cells also removes inhibitory influences on the latent pacemakers [27]. Coupling might be reduced by fibrosis which can separate myocardial fibers. For example, fibrosis in the atrial aspect of the AV junctional region that results in heart block might release nodal pacemakers from electrotonic suppression by surrounding atrial cells and permit them to become the dominant pacemakers of the ventricle. Uncoupling might also be caused by factors which increase the intracellular Ca^{2+} [32] since intracellular calcium levels control coupling resistance among myocardial cells. This might result, for example, from treatment with digitalis [33], which inhibits the Na/K pump and sodium extrusion, and thus increases calcium levels in the cell [34].

Subsidiary pacemaker activity also may be enhanced, causing impulse initiation to shift to ectopic sites, even when sinus node function is normal. Norepinephrine released locally from sympathetic nerves steepens the slope of diastolic depolarization of latent pacemaker cells [10, 35], and diminishes the inhibitory effects of overdrive [36]. Localized effects may occur in the absence of sinus node stimulation [37]. Therefore, sympathetic stimulation may enable membrane potential of ectopic pacemakers to reach threshold before they are activated by an impulse from the sinus node, resulting in ectopic premature impulses or automatic rhythms. From studies of isolated tissues superfused with catecholamines and from studies on sympathetic stimulation in dogs, it appears that the limit for automatic rates generated by subsidiary pacemakers in the atria is close to $200\,min^{-1}$ [38], and in the Purkinje fibers of the ventricles around $120\,min^{-1}$ [39]. Normal automaticity enhanced by sympathetic stimulation, therefore, probably does not cause very rapid ventricular rhythms although it might cause atrial tachycardia.

The flow of current between partially depolarized myocardium and normally polarized latent pacemaker cells, also might enhance automaticity [40]. The mechanism has been proposed to be a cause of the ectopic beats that arise in the ventricle [41]. Ischemia causes a reduction in membrane potential of the affected cells. Thus, at the border of an ischemic area there is a transition, which might be quite abrupt, between depolarized and normal tissue. As a result of the differences in membrane potential, depolarizing current is expected to flow into the normal area and if cells in this area have some spontaneous diastolic depolarization (Purkinje fibers adjacent to the infarct) it would be enhanced, possibly to an extent sufficient to cause spontaneous impulse initiation (❥ Fig. 1.4).

Inhibition of the electrogenic sodium-potassium pump results in a net increase in inward current during diastole because of the decrease in outward current normally generated by the pump and, therefore, increases automaticity in subsidiary pacemakers. This might occur after adenosine triphosphate (ATP) is depleted during prolonged hypoxia or ischemia or in the presence of toxic concentrations of digitalis [42]. A decrease in the extracellular potassium level also enhances normal automaticity [43], as does acute stretch [44].

Working atrial and ventricular myocardial cells do not normally show spontaneous diastolic depolarization. However, if left unstimulated for long intervals atrial myocardium can depolarized to lower membrane potentials at which abnormal automaticity (see below) is initiated [45]. This membrane depolarization is attributed to two causes: (1) in the absence of frequent stimulation the hyperpolarizing effect of the Na/K pump is lost; (2) The inward rectifying current I_{k1} which is responsible for maintaining a high membrane potential is weak in atrium [46]. In contrast, ventricular myocardium does not initiate spontaneous impulses even when it is not excited for long periods of time by propagated impulses. Although, Na/K pump function is minimal in this setting, there is a prominent I_{k1} in ventricle which maintains cells at a high membrane potential.

Neither atrial nor ventricular myocardium expresses pacemaker currents at the normal range of membrane potentials, although the pacemaker current, I_f, is present in myocardium, activating at membrane potentials around -150 mV, far outside the physiologic range [47]. Interestingly, in settings of myocardial hypertrophy [48] and failure [49] the activation of I_f shifts to more positive voltages, within the physiologic range. This has led to the suggestion [50] that some arrhythmias occurring in clinical disease may in fact result from an I_f-based automatic mechanism.

1.2.1.2   Abnormal Automaticity

In some instances of cardiac disease, the resting potentials of the atrial or ventricular myocardial cells are reduced. The same reduction can be achieved experimentally. When membrane potential is less than about −60 mV, spontaneous diastolic depolarization may occur and cause repetitive impulse initiation [51–53]. This is called "abnormal automaticity." Likewise, cells such as those in the Purkinje system which are normally automatic at high levels of membrane potential also show abnormal automaticity when the membrane potential is reduced (❷ Fig. 1.5) [54, 55]. However, if a low level of membrane potential is the only criterion used to identify abnormal automaticity, the automaticity of the sinus node would have to be considered abnormal. Therefore, an important distinction for abnormal automaticity is that the membrane potentials of fibers showing this type of activity are markedly reduced from their own normal level.

At the low level of membrane potential at which abnormal automaticity occurs, it is likely that at least some of the ionic currents causing the automatic activity are not the same as those causing normal automatic activity. A likely cause of automaticity at membrane potentials of around −50 mV is deactivation of K^+ current I_{k1} [56]. This current under normal control conditions produces repolarization of the membrane after the upstroke of an action potential. In addition, the spontaneously occurring action potentials usually have upstrokes dependant on slow inward Ca^{2+} current [55] because the fast inward Na^+ current is inactivated at the low levels of membrane potential.

The decrease in membrane potential of cardiac cells required for abnormal automaticity to occur may be induced by a variety of factors related to cardiac disease. The causes of a low resting potential are best considered in terms of the Goldman-Hodgkin-Katz equation [57] which closely approximates the resting potential V_r of working myocardial cells over a wide range of extra cellular K^+ concentrations.

$$V_r = \frac{RT}{F} \ln \left(\frac{[K]_o + P_{Na}/P_K[Na]_o}{[K]_i + P_{Na}/P_K[Na]_i} \right)$$

❐ Fig. 1.5
Normal and abnormal automaticity in a canine Purkinje fiber. Part (a) shows automatic firing of a Purkinje fiber with a maximum diastolic potential of −85 mV. Part (b) shows the abnormal automaticity that can occur when membrane potential is decreased: in *1*, the fiber is depolarized (at the arrow) to a membrane potential of −45 mV by injecting a long lasting current pulse through a microelectrode and three automatic action potentials occur, in *2*, a larger amplitude current pulse at the arrow reduces membrane potential to −40 mV, resulting in more sustained automatic activity; in *3*, a still larger current pulse at the arrow reduces membrane potential to −30 mV and automatic activity occurs at a still faster rate. Automaticity in atrial and ventricular muscle also occur when the membrane potential is decreased in a similar way (Reproduced with permission after Wit and Friedman (1975) © American Medical Association, Chicago, Illinois)

where R is the gas constant, F is the Faraday, T is the absolute temperature, $[K]_o$ and $[K]_i$ are the extracellular and intracellular K^+ concentrations, respectively; P_{Na}/P_k is the ratio of the permeability coefficients for Na^+ and K^+, and $[Na]_o$ and $[Na]_i$ are the extracellular and intracellular Na^+ concentrations, respectively.

The several ways in which the resting potential can be less negative according to this equation are that $[K]_o$ might be increased, $[K]_i$ might be decreased, or the ratio P_{Na}/P_K might be increased following either an increase in P_{Na} (sodium permeability of the sarcolemma) or a decrease in P_K (potassium permeability of the sarcolemma). Any one of these changes would by itself cause the resting potential to decline and more than one change might occur in diseased cell [58].

Although an increase in extracellular potassium concentration can reduce membrane potential, automatic firing in working atrial, ventricular, and Purkinje fibers usually does not occur when $[K]_o$ is elevated because of the increase in K^+ conductance (and, hence, net outward current) that results from an increase in $[K]_o{}^+$ [59]. However, atrial fibers in the mitral valve [60] and fibers in the AV node may have automatic activity even when $[K]_o$ is markedly elevated. A decrease in $[K]_i$ has been shown to occur in the Purkinje fibers which survive on the endocardial surface of infarcts and this decreases persists for at least 24 h after coronary occlusion [61]. The reduction in $[K]_i$ undoubtedly contributes to the low membrane potential in these cells, although changes in membrane conductance are also responsible [61]. These Purkinje fibers have abnormal automaticity [62, 63]. Preparations of diseased atrial and ventricular myocardium from human hearts show phase 4 depolarization and abnormal automaticity at membrane potentials in the range −50 to −60 mV [64–66]. It has been proposed that a decrease in membrane potassium conductance, P_K, is an important cause of the low membrane potentials in the atrial fibers [65].

Myocardial fibers with low resting potentials will not fire automatically if the sinus node drives them faster than their intrinsic abnormal, automatic rate. An abnormal automatic focus should manifest itself and cause an arrhythmia when the sinus rate decreases below the intrinsic rate of the focus or when the rate of the focus increases above that of the sinus node, as was discussed for latent pacemakers with normal automaticity. A similar interplay between maximum diastolic potential, threshold potential and rate of phase 4 depolarization determines the rate of impulse initiation by the abnormal pacemaker. However, there is an important distinction between the effects of the dominant sinus pacemaker on the two kinds of foci, that is abnormal automaticity is *not* overdrive-suppressed to the same extent as the normal automaticity that occurs at high levels of membrane potential [67–69]. Moreover, the extent of suppression of spontaneous diastolic depolarization by overdrive is directly related to the level of membrane potential at which the automatic rhythms occur [68, 69] (❷ Fig. 1.6). For example, Purkinje fibers showing automaticity at membrane potentials of −60 to −70 mV still manifest some overdrive suppression, although less than those fibers with automaticity at −90 mV. Automaticity in Purkinje fibers with membrane potentials less than −60 mV is only slightly suppressed by short periods of overdrive. These differences in the effects of overdrive may be related to the reduction in the amount of sodium entering the cell membrane as potential decreases, and therefore, the degree to which the sodium- potassium pump is stimulated. (As the

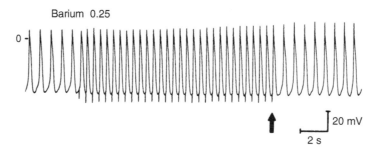

Barium 0.25

20 mV

2 s

■ Fig. 1.6

Effects of overdrive stimulation on abnormal automaticity occurring at a membrane potential of −52 mV. Abnormal automaticity was caused by adding 0.25 mmol BaCl$_2$ to the Tyrode's superfusate. The control cycle length is 810 ms. Stimulation cycle is 500 ms and the period of stimulation is denoted by the stimulus artifacts. The stimulation was stopped at the *arrow*. Note the absence of overdrive suppression (Reproduced with permission after Dangman and Hoffman (1982) © Futura, Mount Kisco, New York)

membrane potential is reduced and the Na^+ channels inactivated there is a decrease in the fast inward sodium current and hence a decrease in activation of the pump [70].) For markedly depolarized tissue showing no suppression after brief periods of overdrive, long periods of rapid overdrive can suppress automaticity either because Na^+ can enter the cell through the slow channel to stimulate the pump [70] or because calcium entering during the upstroke of slow response action potentials is exchanged for sodium, thereby elevating $[Na]_i$ [71].

At normal sinus rates there may be little overdrive suppression of pacemakers with abnormal automaticity. As a result of the lack of overdrive suppression, even transient sinus pauses or occasional long sinus cycle lengths may permit the ectopic focus to capture the heart for one or more beats. On the other hand, an ectopic pacemaker with normal automaticity would probably be quiescent during relatively short, transient sinus pauses because they are overdrive- suppressed. It is possible that the depolarized level of membrane potential at which abnormal automaticity occurs might cause entrance block into focus and prevent it form being overdriven by the sinus node [72]. This would lead to parasystole, an example of an arrhythmia caused by a combination of an abnormality of impulse conduction and initiation (discussed in more detail later in this chapter).

The firing rate of an abnormally automatic focus might also be enhanced above that of the sinus node, leading to arrhythmias in the absence of sinus node suppression or conduction block between the focus and surrounding myocardium. The automatic rate is a direct function of the level of membrane potential– the greater the depolarization, the faster the rate [51–55]. Experimental studies have shown firing rates in muscle and Purkinje fibers of 150–200 min^{-1} at membrane potentials less that -50 mV and these rates appear to be sufficiently rapid to enable these pacemakers to control the heart. Catecholamines also increase abnormal automaticity [73].

1.2.1.3   Some Clinical Characteristics of Arrhythmias Caused by Automaticity

Thus far, we have considered the influences of the sinus node pacemaker on subsidiary pacemakers with different automatic mechanisms. The sinus node probably exerts an inhibitory effect on the normal automatic mechanism by overdrive but has lesser inhibitory effects on the abnormal one. These known effects of overdrive on pacemaker mechanisms might sometimes be of use in distinguishing automatic arrhythmias caused by triggered activity or reentry (see ❷ Sect. 1.2.2) in the in situ heart, or in distinguishing arrhythmias caused by normal automaticity from those caused by abnormal automaticity [68]. If a tachycardia is caused by normal automaticity it could be predicted that the rate of tachycardia should be suppressed immediately after it is overdriven by electrical stimulation, even when the overdrive period is relatively short (❷ Fig. 1.7). The transient pause after overdrive should be followed by a gradual speeding up of the ectopic rhythm until the original rate is resumed. The duration of the transient pause and the time required for resumption of the original rate is directly related to the rate and duration of overdrive. It is important to stress, however, that the tachycardia is not terminated but only suppressed transiently. This behavior is a result of the increased activity of the sodium-potassium pump discussed previously. During overdrive of atrial or sinus tachycardias, acetylcholine may be released from electrically stimulated nerve endings and contribute further to the overdrive suppression [74].

The characteristic behavior of normally automatic pacemakers has been demonstrated in some clinical and experimental electrophysiological studies on both atrial and ventricular tachycardias [75, 76]. On the other hand, tachycardias caused by abnormal automaticity should not be suppressed by overdrive, unless the overdrive period is long and the rate fast [68]. The difficulty in suppressing such tachycardias by overdrive stems from a lesser amount of Na^+ entering the cells, as previously mentioned. Short periods of overdrive can even result in a transient speeding of the tachycardia rate (overdrive acceleration) [68]. Accelerated idioventricular rhythms or tachycardia in canine myocardial infarction are not easily overdrive-suppressed and therefore may be caused by abnormal automaticity [76].

In addition to overdrive, the response of the rhythm to programmed premature stimuli applied to the heart is sometimes useful in determining the mechanism of clinical arrhythmias [77]. Of major importance is the fact that automatic rhythms caused by either normal or abnormal automaticity cannot be terminated by premature impulses (nor can they be started by premature impulses–in contrast, see effects of stimuli on triggered activity and on reentry discussed in ❷ Sect. 1.2.2). Other than that, premature impulses induced at different times during diastole may transiently perturb the rhythm during the subsequent few cycles. Detailed descriptions of the effects of premature impulses in automatic impulse initiation have been published [78–80].

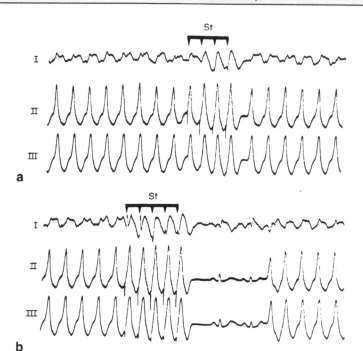

⬛ Fig. 1.7

Effects of overdrive on ventricular tachycardia that may be caused by automaticity. Leads I, II, and III of the ECG are shown. In (**a**), a burst of rapid stimuli St is followed by a short pause and then recurrence of tachycardia, In (**b**), a burst of five stimuli is followed by a greater suppression of tachycardia, allowing the occurrence of two sinus beats. Tachycardia then reappears (Reproduced with permission after Fontaine et al. (1984) © Futura, Mount Kisco, New York)

1.2.2   Afterdepolarizations and Triggered Activity

Afterdepolarizations are oscillations in membrane potential that are induced by, and follow, an action potential. These oscillations are divided into two categories: early afterdepolarizations, which precede full repolarization of the membrane; and delayed afterdepolarizations, which follow full repolarization. Both of these types of afterdepolarizations are, in turn, capable of initiating arrhythmias referred to as "triggered" [81]. Triggered arrhythmias must be initiated by a conducted or stimulated action potential (the trigger) and cannot arise during a period of quiescence such as that caused by sinus node inhibition [82]. This contrasts with normal or abnormal automaticity which have just been described.

1.2.2.1   Early Afterdepolarizations

Early afterdepolarizations most frequently occur during repolarization of an action potential which has been initiated from a high level of membrane potential (usually −75 to −90 mV). They may appear as an oscillation at the plateau level of membrane potential or later during phase 3 of repolarization. Under certain conditions these oscillations can lead to a second upstroke or action potential (see ❷ Fig. 1.8). When the oscillation is large enough, the decrease in membrane potential leads to an increase in inward (depolarizing) current and a second action potential occurs prior to complete repolarization of the first.

This second action potential occurring during repolarization is triggered in the sense that is evoked by an early after-depolarization which, in turn is induced by the preceding action potential. Without the preceding action potential there would be no second upstroke. The second action potential may also be followed by other action potentials, all occurring at the low level of membrane potential characteristic of the plateau of phase 3 (❷ Fig. 1.8). The sustained rhythmic activity

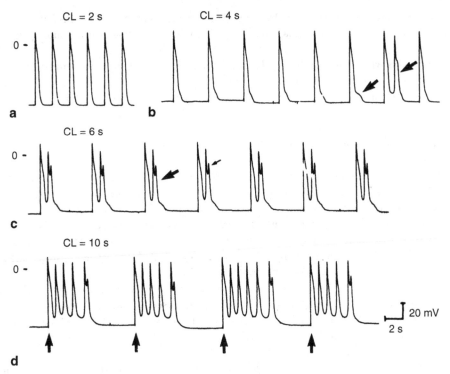

⬤ Fig. 1.8
Early afterdepolarizations in Purkinje fibers. Part (**a**) shows the transmembrane potential recorded from a Purkinje fiber stimulated at a cycle length (CL) of 2 s. Repolarization appears to be normal. In (**b**), when CL is increased to 4 s, an early after-depolarization appears during phase 3 of repolarization (*arrow*). At the right a second upstroke or triggered action potential arises from the early afterdepolarization (*arrow*). In (**c**), at a CL of 6 s, a single triggered action potential (arrow) occurs during phase 3 of each stimulated action potential. An early afterdepolarization also occurs during the plateau of the triggered action potential (*small arrow*). In (**d**), at a CL of 10 s, a burst of triggered action potentials occurs during phase 3 of each stimulated action potential (arrows point to stimulated action potentials) (Reproduced with permission after Damiano and Rosen (1984) © American Heart Association, Dallas, Texas)

that ensues may continue for a variable number of impulses and may terminate when the increase in membrane potential associated with repolarization of the initiating action potential returns membrane potential to a high level. Triggered activity may occur again when the next action potential is initiated from the high level membrane potential. Sometimes repolarization to this high level may not occur, and membrane potential may remain at the plateau level or at a level inter-mediate between the plateau and the resting potential. The sustained rhythmic activity may then continue at the reduced level of membrane potential.

There are some conceptual difficulties associated with triggered activity caused by early afterdepolarizations [81]. According to the definition of triggered activity, there is no problem in characterizing the second action potential that is induced by an early afterdepolarization and occurs during repolarization as being triggered. However, if a series of action potentials arises following this premature upstroke and before the cell repolarizes to a high resting potential, it might be wondered whether these action potentials are triggered or whether they occur only because the membrane potential has been shifted into a region where abnormal automatic activity occurs. The previous section pointed out how abnormal automaticity occurs at reduced membrane potentials. Certainly, based on the response of the sustained rhythm to pacing (see below), it is not readily differentiated from abnormal automaticity occurring at low membrane potentials. It is for this reason the authors think it appropriate to suggest that only the first action potential is triggered and the remaining are automatic. As a result, the major differentiation between triggered and abnormally automatic rhythms may be that the former result from interruption of repolarization by an oscillation (which is triggered) and the latter from depolarization of the membrane to the same range of potentials. Hence, the inciting events differ but the subsequent rhythm may be the same.

The ionic mechanisms which cause early afterdepolarizations likely result from abnormalities in the repolarizing membrane currents. During the plateau phase of the action potential, the rate of membrane repolarization is very slow and the net repolarizing membrane current is very small. This net current is outward throughout the range of membrane potentials between zero and the resting potential [59]. The net repolarizing current results from an imbalance between inward and outward currents. The inward current component includes a background Na^+ current, Na^+ current flowing through incompletely inactivated sodium channels [83] and the slow inward Ca^{2+} current [84]. The major outward currents are carried by potassium via rapidly activating (I_{Kr}) and slowly activating (I_{Ks}) delayed rectifier currents, which are voltage gated [85]. Also contributing to outward membrane current in the plateau range is the electrogenic sodium-potassium pump [86]. Normally the net outward membrane current shifts membrane potential progressively in a negative direction and the final rapid phase of action-potential repolarization takes place. An early afterdepolarization might occur if there is a shift in the current-voltage relationship resulting in a region of net inward current during the plateau range of membrane potentials. This would retard or prevent repolarization [59] and might lead to a secondary depolarization during the plateau phase or phase 3 if regenerative inward current is activated. The second upstroke and any subsequent action potentials that arise from the low levels of membrane potential during the plateau are Ca^{2+}-dependant; that is, the inward current responsible for the upstroke flows through the Ca^{2+} channel because that fast channel is inactivated [55]. Action potentials which arise during phase 3 might have upstrokes caused by current flowing through partially reactivated fast sodium channels or a combination of slow and fast channels. More recent research has suggested that either a Ca window current [87] alterations in Ca loading and Na/Ca exchange current [88] and/or calmodulin kinase activity [89] also may contribute to early afterdepolarizations.

Conditions that increase the inward current components or decrease the outward current components during repolarization are expected to induce the shift in the current- voltage relationship which causes early afterdepolarizations. Experimental drugs such as aconitine [90] and veratridine [91] cause early afterdepolarizations probably by increasing Na^+ conductance during the plateau phase. Although these drugs are not clinically important, their effects demonstrate that if similar increases in conductance were caused by cardiac pathology, triggered activity would occur. Early afterdepolarizations can also occasionally be seen in Purkinje fibers superfused with normal Tyrode's solution soon after they have been excised from the heart. These early afterdepolarizations might be caused by relatively nonspecific inward current flowing via incompletely healed cuts made at the ends of fibers, or through other regions injured by stretching or crushing during the dissection [82]. This suggests the interesting possibility that mechanical injury or stretch of Purkinje fibers in situ might cause triggering. Stretch of the cardiac fibers in the ventricles might occur in heart failure or in ventricular aneurysms. Mechanical injury might also occur in the area of an infarct or aneurysm.

Early afterdepolarizations leading to triggered activity in isolated cardiac preparations may also be caused by factors which are present in the heart in situ under some pathological conditions. Among these factors are hypoxia [92], high pCO_2 [93] and high concentrations of catecholamines [94]. Data are not yet available which elucidate how they exert their effects. Since catecholamines, hypoxia, and elevated pCO_2 may be present in an ischemic or infarct regions of the ventricles, it is possible that early afterdepolarization may cause some of the arrhythmias which occur soon after myocardial ischemia.

Some drugs that have been used clinically and that markedly prolong the time course for repolarization, such as the β-receptor blocking drug sotalol [95] and the antiarrhythmic N-acetyl procainamide [96], also cause early afterdepolarizations and triggered activity. These drugs have been shown to cause cardiac arrhythmias that may be triggered in experimental animals and in patients [97] (see ❷ Fig. 1.9). Single triggered impulses occurring as a result of early afterdepolarizations should induce premature depolarizations having fixed coupling intervals to the preceding beat (since they occur during repolarization of an action potential accompanying the preceding beat). Hence, a bigeminal rhythm would occur if each action potential caused by propagation of the normal sinus impulse were followed by a second upstroke caused by an early afterdepolarization. If a train of triggered action potentials occurs during repolarization, it would be expected to cause a paroxysm of tachycardia with the first impulse of tachycardia having a fixed coupling interval to the preceding eat. Tachycardias would terminate when repolarization of the triggering action potential occurs. Usually, the rate of activity during the repolarization of the triggering action potentials slows gradually before termination. Thus termination of the triggered tachycardias might be expected to be preceded by gradual slowing of the tachycardias.

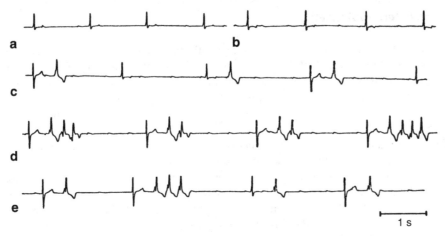

⬤ Fig. 1.9

Ventricular arrhythmias that might be caused by early afterdepolarizations in the dog (a), the control electrocardiogram of a dog with experimentally induced heart block; (b) and (c), traces after 50 mg kg^{-1} N-acetyl procainamide (NAPA) was injected intravenously; (d) and (e), traces taken after 100 mg kg^{-1} NAPA was administered. NAPA prolongs Purkinje fiber action potential duration, causing early afterdepolarization and triggered activity. In (c) coupled ventricular premature depolarizations caused by the NAPA are evident. In (d) and (e), short runs of ventricular tachycardia can be seen. The first impulse of tachycardia has a relatively fixed coupling to the QRS (Reproduced with permission after Dangman and Hoffman (1981) © Williams and Wilkins, Baltimore, Maryland)

Since the occurrence of early afterdepolarizations is facilitated by a decrease in the net repolarizing current, a slowing of the rate at which the triggering action potentials are elicited might also favor the occurrence of the afterdepolarizations (⬤ Fig. 1.8). As the drive rate slows, action potential duration is prolonged, reflecting a decrease in net outward current. It, therefore, seems likely that some tachycardias which occur after a period of bradycardia might be caused by early afterdepolarizations [98]. It is likely that tachycardias in patients with the congenital and acquired long QT interval syndromes (in which there is prolonged repolarization) are triggered [91]. Certainly, experimental animal studies [99, 100] as well as the clinical literature [101] point to early afterdepolarizations and triggered activity as a cause of torsades de pointes, the characteristic and often lethal arrhythmia of congenital and acquired LQTS. The clinical applicability of this mechanism was most dramatically brought home by the SWORD trial [102], in which d- Sotalol, a drug that blocks the HERG channel that carries I_{Kr} was found to cause excess deaths in a population of post-myocardial infarction patients.

It is instructive to attempt to predict the effects of stimulation of the heart on triggered arrhythmias caused by early afterdepolarizations, since various stimulation protocols are used in attempts to determine the mechanisms causing clinical arrhythmias. Overdrive stimulation during sinus rhythm should prevent occurrence of paroxysmal triggered tachycardias since rapid stimulation usually decreases the duration of the action potential; that is, an action potential of short duration does not favor the occurrence of early afterdepolarizations. However, once overdrive pacing is stopped, the paroxysms of tachycardias might spontaneously reappear as action potential duration again lengthens. The response of the triggered tachycardias to overdrive (during tachycardia) is similar to the response of abnormal automaticity to overdrive [103]; these rhythms are not easily terminated or suppressed by brief periods of overdrive but are suppressed transiently by periods of pacing in the range of 2–3 min. The tachyarrhythmias induced by early afterdepolarizations are not terminated readily by single interpolated stimulated impulses, but can be reset in much the same way as automatic rhythms. The similar response to overdrive pacing of the tachyarrhythmias induced by early afterdepolarizations and of abnormal automaticity is further evidence that the two phenomena are caused by a similar mechanism as mentioned above.

1.2.2.2 Delayed Afterdepolarizations

Delayed afterdepolarizations are oscillations in membrane potential that occur after repolarization of an action potential and are induced by that action potential (● Fig. 1.10). One or more oscillations may occur after each action potential. Delayed afterepolarizations may be subthreshold, but when they are large enough to bring the membrane potential to the threshold of a regenerative inward current, a nondriven (triggered) impulse arises which may also be followed by an afterdepolarization. The impulse is said to be triggered since it would not have occurred without the preceding action potential [55, 81, 82].

Delayed afterdepolarizations occur under a number of conditions in which there is either a large increase in the intracellular calcium, or an abnormality in the sequestration or release of calcium by the sarcoplasmic reticulum, or a combination of the two. One of the most widely recognized causes is toxic concentrations of cardiac glycosides [104–107]. Cardiac glycosides inhibit the Na^+-K^+ pump thereby leading to an increase in $[Na]_i$. This in turn increases the intracellular Ca^{2+} through a Na^+-Ca^{2+} exchange mechanism [108]. Delayed afterdepolarizations caused by digitalis can occur in Purkinje fibers and in working atrial and ventricular muscle fibers although Purkinje fibers seem to develop them at lower drug concentrations [107]. Other experimental maneuvers which inhibit the Na^+-K^+ pump also increase the intracellular calcium and cause delayed afterdepolarizations similar to those induced by digitalis. A prime example is exposure of cardiac fibers to a K^+-free extracellular environment [109].

Catecholamines can cause delayed afterdepolarizations [10, 110, 111], and delayed afterdepolarizations and triggered activity induced by catecholamine have been described in atrial fibers of the mitral valve [111] and coronary sinus [10], as well as other regions of the atria [82]. Ventricular muscle fibers and Purkinje fibers also can develop delayed afterdepolarizations in the presence of high concentrations of catecholamines [110, 111].

Delayed afterdepolarizations may also occur in the absence of drugs or catecholamines. They have been identified in fibers in the upper pectinate muscles bordering the crista terminalis in the rabbit heart [112], in hypertrophied ventricular myocardium [113], in human atrial myocardium [45], in Purkinje fibers surviving on the subendocardial surface of canine infarcts [114], and in atrial fibers in sleeves of myocardium extending into the pulmonary veins (in which early afterdepolarizations also have described) [115]. Triggered activity in the pulmonary veins has been hypothesized as a likely cause of paroxysmal atrial fibrillation [115, 116]. The exact relationship of hypertrophy or ischemia to the occurrence of delayed afterdepolarizations in not known yet in any detail, but in the former uptake and release of calcium by sarcoplasmic reticulum may be abnormal [117] and in the latter there may be an increase in $[Ca]_i$ secondary to an increase in $[Na]_i$ [118].

The mechanisms by which elevated intracellular Ca^{2+} causes delayed afterdepolarizations have been explored in studies utilizing voltage-clamp techniques to control the depolarization of the membrane and to measure ionic currents [109, 119–123]. Delayed afterdepolarizations result from a transient inward current which is activated by repolarization after a depolarizing voltage-clamp pulse (● Fig. 1.11). The voltage clamp pulse is somewhat comparable to an action potential. Increasing the magnitude of the depolarization in the plateau voltage range increases the magnitude of the current and causes the peak to be reached more rapidly. The transient inward current also increases in amplitude with increasing duration of the voltage clamp pulse or increasing pulse frequency (see below). All these changes in the characteristics of the clamp pulse may lead to an increase in $[Ca^{2+}]_i$, at least partly from an increase in the slow inward current [124]. The

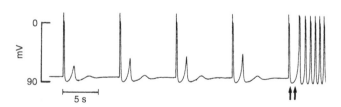

□ Fig. 1.10

Delayed afterdepolarizations caused by catecholamines recorded from an atrial fiber in an isolated, superfused preparation of canine coronary sinus tissue. The afterdepolarization amplitude is increasing with each stimulated impulse until it reaches threshold and causes triggered activity, as indicated by the *black arrows* at the *right*

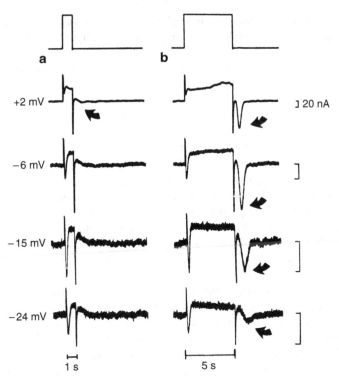

◘ Fig. 1.11

Some characteristics of the transient inward current in calf Purkinje fibers. The preparation was exposed to 1 μm strophanthidin, Traces a and b show the protocol. The membrane potential was clamped at a holding potential of −41 mV and depolarizing voltage-clamp pulses were imposed for either 1 s (a) or 5 s (b). The depolarization ranged from −24 to +2 mV as indicated on the *left side* of the figure. The membrane currents recorded during this clamp protocol are shown in each column. The transient inward (TI) current responsible for delayed afterdepolarizations is indicated by the arrows. The TI current is larger after longer duration voltage clamp pulses and after pulses to around −6 mV (Reproduced with permission after Lederer and Tsien (1976) © Cambridge University Press, London)

amplitude of the transient inward current is maximal at membrane potentials of −50 to −70 mV and decreases at both lower and higher membrane potentials, Thus, the transient inward current is significantly different from the pacemaker currents which cause automatic rhythms.

From these characteristics of the transient inward current, it can be predicted that the following will lead to an increase in delayed afterdepolarization amplitude and cause triggered activity:

(a) An increase in the amplitude and/or duration of the action-potential plateau [114];
(b) An increase in the frequency at which action potentials are induced;
(c) A decrease in the resting membrane potential in muscle or Purkinje fibers from normal levels around −80 mV to −90 mV to less than −70 mV [125].

The link between the depolarization pulse (whether caused by voltage clamp or by an action potential) and the subsequent transient inward current may involve release and reuptake of calcium from the sarcoplasmic reticulum. Normally, release is initiated by the depolarization phase of the action potential and reuptake is complete by the end of the action potential. However, if the sarcoplasmic reticulum is overloaded with calcium, it may not be able to take up all the calcium and/or there may be secondary release of calcium after repolarization [126]. Certainly, spontaneous Ca^{2+} release from the sarcoplasmic reticulum has been demonstrated both in single cardiac myocytes and in isolated cardiac trabeculae. Moreover, the occurrence of propagating Ca^{2+} waves in myocytes that induce delayed afterdepolarizations has been reported and validated [127].

The increased level of cytoplasmic calcium has been proposed to alter sarcolemmal permeability, causing activation of a nonspecific membrane channel that allow an inward rush of positive charge carried mainly by sodium, such that the delayed afterdepolarization occurs [128]. However, there are some dissenting opinions concerning the mechanism for the inward current during the afterdepolarization. It has also been proposed that this current results from electrogenic exchange of intracellular calcium for extracellular sodium that results in the net transfer into the cell of positive charge in the form of sodium ions, to generate an inward current [122, 129].

Delayed afterdepolarizations may not be large enough to reach threshold, in which case triggered activity does not occur. As indicated previously, triggering may result in fibers showing subthreshold afterdepolarization if the rate at which the fiber is driven is increased (❷ Fig. 1.12a). In cardiac fibers with a single afterdepolarization following each action potential, the amplitude of the afterdepolarization increases as the drive rate increases (unlike early afterdepolarizations which have the opposite relationship). At a sufficiently rapid drive rate the afterdepolarization attains a sufficient amplitude to reach threshold and triggering occurs (❷ Fig. 1.12a). A decrease in the length of even a single drive cycle, that is, a premature impulse, may increase the amplitude of the afterdepolarization of the action potential that follows the short cycle. As the premature impulse occurs earlier and earlier after the previous impulse, the amplitudes of the afterdepolarizations which follow the premature impulses increase and may reach threshold, initiating triggered activity (❷ Fig. 1.12b). The likelihood of a premature impulse initiating triggered activity increases at more rapid basic drive rates. In cardiac Purkinje fibers made digitalis toxic, at least two afterdepolarizations are usually present at relatively slow rates of drive. The first afterdepolarization is larger than the second. As the drive cycle length is decreased to around 500 ms, the amplitude of the first oscillation increases to its maximum and triggered activity may occur. If it does not occur and the drive cycle length is decreased further, the amplitude of the second afterdepolarization increases while the first declines, and triggered action potentials may arise from the second oscillation [130].

The increase in amplitude of delayed afterdepolarizations with increasing drive rate is also probably responsible for perpetuation of triggered activity once the nondriven action potential has occurred. Since the first nondriven action potential arises from the peak of a delayed afterdepolarization, the coupling interval between the upstroke of this triggered action potential and the upstroke of the triggering action potential is usually shorter than the drive cycle length which caused the first triggered impulse; that is, the first triggered action potential is, itself, premature. Hence, the afterdepolarization following the first nondriven action potential will be larger and a second triggered action potential will, therefore, occur at a short coupling interval. The process thus perpetuates itself.

There may be some differences in the characteristics of triggered activity caused by delayed afterdepolarizations, depending upon the cause. The initial period of triggered activity caused by catecholamines in atrial fibers is often characterized by a gradual decrease in the cycle length after which a relatively constant cycle length occurs [10, 131]. This decrease in cycle length may be accompanied by a decrease in maximum diastolic potential, (at least partly caused by accumulation of K^+ outside the cell during rapid activity owing to restricted diffusion in the extracellular space [132, 133]). The decrease in maximum diastolic potential contributes to the gradual acceleration in the rate of triggered activity since the rate increases as membrane potential decreases in the same way as we described for normal automaticity. Similar characteristics for triggered activity caused by factors other than catecholamines have also been described in atrial, ventricular, and Purkinje fibers. On the other hand, during triggered activity in Purkinje fibers exposed to toxic amounts of digitalis, there is not usually a gradual increase in rate, but rather, the maximum triggered rate is attained after a few impulses [134].

Triggered activity often terminates spontaneously. When catecholamine-induced triggered activity in atrial fibers of the coronary sinus terminates, the rate usually slows gradually before termination. This gradual slowing is accompanied by a progressive increase in the maximum diastolic potential. A delayed afterdepolarization usually follows the last triggered impulse [10, 131]. The spontaneous termination of triggered activity in canine coronary sinus fibers (and probably also in other types of cardiac fibers) is caused, at least in part, by an increase in the rate of electrogenic sodium extrusion [131]. Sodium pump activity is enhanced by the increase in intracellular Na^+ concentration which results from the increase in Na^+ influx during the rapid period of triggered activity. The increase in outward sodium pump current increases the maximum diastolic potential and reduces the rate of triggered activity; a sufficient increase in sodium pump current terminates the triggered activity [131]. Triggered activity caused by digitalis toxicity probably stops by another mechanism. Termination of a triggered burst is usually not associated with gradual slowing and hyperpolarization but often

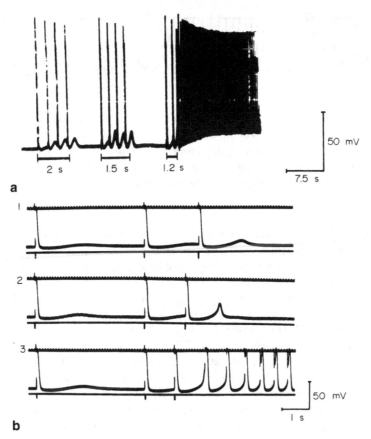

◘ Fig. 1.12
Part (a) shows the effects of stimulus rate on afterdepolarization amplitude. Part (b) shows the effects of premature stimulation on afterdepolarization amplitude and triggering. The transmembrane potentials shown were recorded from an atrial fiber in the canine coronary sinus superfused with Tyrode's solution containing norepinephrine. In (a), the cycle length is indicated beneath each group of impulses. The afterdepolarization following the last driven impulse has an amplitude of 10 m in the first case and 17 mV in the second. In the third case, sustained rhythmic activity is triggered. The rate is too rapid for the individual upstrokes to be apparent. Maximum diastolic potential decreases during the initial period of triggered activity. In (b), the bottom trace in each panel shows the stimulus pulses. Each panel shows the last two impulses of a series of ten impulses, driven at a cycle length of 4 s, that did not cause triggering. A premature impulse is then induced at progressively shorter coupling intervals. The amplitude of the afterdepolarizations during the basic drive varied from 2 to 6 mV. In *1*, the afterdepolarization following premature action potential induced 2 s after the last basic action potential has an amplitude of 11 mV. In *2*, at a shorter premature coupling interval of 1.4 s, the amplitude of the afterdepolarization following premature action potential is 31 mV. In *3*, at a shorter premature coupling of 1 s triggered activity occurs following the premature action potential (Reproduced with permission after Wit and Cranefield (1977) © American Heart Association, Dallas, Texas)

by speeding of the rate, a decrease in action potential amplitude and membrane depolarization. Termination is probably not related to activity of the Na^+ pump since the pump is inhibited by the digitalis, but may be caused by Na^+ or Ca^+ accumulation in the cell secondary to the rapid rate. A decreased transmembrane concentration gradient to either Na^+ or Ca^+ might diminish the afterdepolarization and finally lead to cessation of activity.

Since, as mentioned before, electrical stimulation of the heart is one way in which mechanisms of clinical arrhythmias have been studied, it is worth reviewing the effects of stimulation on triggered activity caused by delayed afterdepolarizations. Triggered tachycardias may be initiated by either an increase in heart rate or by premature impulses as described

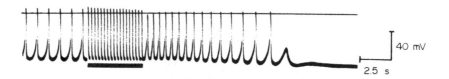

□ Fig. 1.13

Termination of triggered activity by overdrive stimulation. At the left the transmembrane potential from an atrial fiber in the canine coronary sinus is shown during a period of triggered activity. Rapid overdrive stimulation was accomplished during the period that is underlined. Immediately following this overdrive, the rate of triggered activity is accelerated. Later there is a gradual slowing of the rate and a simultaneous increase in maximum diastolic potential until triggered activity stops (Reproduced with permission after Wit et al. (1981) © American Heart Association, Dallas, Texas)

above, and therefore triggered arrhythmias might be started by stimulating the heart. Triggered activity can also be terminated by either premature or overdrive stimulation. It is sometimes possible to terminate triggered activity with a single premature stimulus [60]. Such a premature impulse is followed by an increased afterhyperpolarization which, in turn, is followed by an afterdepolarization that does not reach threshold because it arises from the more negative membrane potential of the preceding afterhyperpolarization. More frequently, premature impulses will simply reset the triggered rhythm in much the same way as they reset automatic rhythms. The ability of premature impulses to terminate triggered activity is increased if they are preceded by a period of rapid drive [135].

Triggered activity can also be terminated by overdrive (❷ Fig. 1.13). The effects of overdrive are dependant both on its rate and duration. During a short period of overdrive at a rate only moderately faster than the triggered rate there is often a decrease in the maximum diastolic potential; following the period of overdrive the rate of the triggered activity may be faster than it was before overdrive, perhaps because of the decrease in maximum diastolic potential. This postoverdrive acceleration is similar to the acceleration which can occur during abnormal automaticity. The accelerated rate then slows, and maximum diastolic potential increases until preoverdrive values are attained. If either the rate or duration of overdrive is increased to a critical degree, the decline in maximum diastolic potential during overdrive is greater as is the postoverdrive acceleration. In cardiac fibers in which triggered activity is caused by factors other than digitalis, such as catecholamines, the maximum diastolic potential then increases and the rate gradually slows until activity stops (❷ Fig. 1.13). The increase in maximum diastolic potential and the slowing and termination of triggered activity following a period of overdrive are caused by enhanced activity of the electrogenic sodium pump. This enhanced activity results from a transient increase in intracellular Na^+ caused by the increased number of action potentials during overdrive. The increased outward pump current following overdrive increases maximum diastolic potential and slows the rate as discussed above for spontaneous termination of triggered activity [131].

Although overdrive stimulation also terminates triggered activity caused by digitalis, the mechanism for the termination may not involve enhanced electrogenic Na^+ pump activity, since the pump is inhibited by the presence of digitalis. Termination caused by overdrive usually is associated with depolarization rather than hyperpolarization and generally occurs within several beats after the overdrive [135]. Termination may be caused by an increase in intracellular Na^+ or Ca^+ resulting from the increased number of action potentials during the overdrive.

1.3   Abnormalities of Repolarization and Their Genetic Determinants

As was demonstrated in ❷ Chap. 3, the past decade has seen a vast increment in our understanding of the molecular determinants of ion channels. ❷ Figure 1.14 demonstrates how either a decrease in outward current or an increase in inward current may result in prolongation of repolarization and an arrhythmia. Note that the prolonged repolarization in itself is not arrhythmogenic unless it initiates dispersion of repolarization sufficient to facilitate reentry and/or is associated with an early afterdepolarization that, in turn, initiates triggered activity.

We now appreciate that ion channelopathies associated with genetic or acquired alterations in channel structure can alter repolarization importantly and give rise to arrhythmias. A major impetus to this understanding came from the

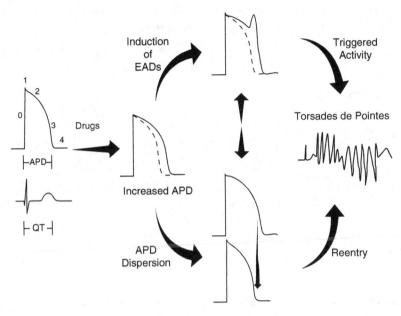

◘ Fig. 1.14
Potential mechanisms underlying the induction of torsades de pointes by drugs that prolong repolarization. Depicted here is an increase in action potential duration (APD) induced by drugs. As a result there can be the generation of early afterdepolarizations (EAD) and/or increased dispersion of APD. EAD can induce triggered activity and excess APD dispersion can induce reentry. Both mechanisms can result in torsades de pointes (Reproduced with permission from Ebert et al. (1998))

pioneering work of Schwartz and colleagues on the congenital long QT syndrome (LQTS) [136, 137]. Their work demonstrated that syndromes resulting from autosomal dominant inheritance resulted in long QT intervals on ECG, syncope, and death from an arrhythmia having the characteristic torsades de pointes morphology [136, 137]. We now understand that rather than a single disease entity characterized by a long QT interval on the electrocardiogram, lesions occur that are literally family-specific in potassium and sodium channels [138–141]. With regard to the potassium channels, two potassium channel pore-forming or α-subunits, (KvLQT1 and HERG) have been implicated in the LQT$_1$ and LQT$_2$ syndromes, respectively, while two beta subunits, minK and MiRP1 are involved in LQT$_5$ and LQT$_6$ respectively. In addition, the sodium channel, SCN5A has been found associated with the LQT3 syndrome. All these subunits contribute to the genesis of the arrhythmias in LQTS, although via different mechanisms. The K channels involved normally carry repolarizing currents, but lose function in LQTS such that there is a decrease in outward current through the ion channel in question, thereby prolonging the duration of repolarization. In contrast, the Na channel manifests an increase in inward current during the plateau of the action potential, giving rise to prolongation of repolarization.

The initial gene identified as associated with LQTS was the KvLQT1 gene [138] in which intragenic deletions, missense mutations, deletion mutations and insertion mutations all have been described (see [139] for summary). This family of abnormalities was incorporated in the LQT1 family of channelopathies. Based on the association of the beta-subunit, minK to impart normal function to KvLQT1, it was also hypothesized and later demonstrated [140] that mutations in minK can also contribute to LQTS (LQT5).

The second major potassium channel involved in LQTS was the HERG channel (LQT2). Intragenic deletions, missense mutations and duplications [139] all have been implicated here. The potassium channel subunit MiRP1 – largely associated with HERG – also has been shown to express missense mutations contributing to LQTS [141] (LQT6).

The remaining channelopathy noted has not been in a potassium channel, but in the sodium channel, SCN5A (LQT3). Missense mutations and intragenic deletions [139] have been shown to contribute to the persistence of inward current during the plateau of the action potential here.

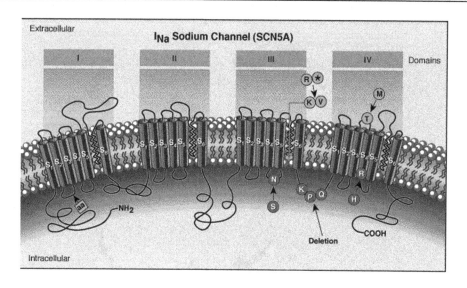

◘ Fig. 1.15

The predicted secondary structure of the cardiac sodium channel and locations of mutations causing idiopathic ventricular fibrillation (IVF) and chromsosome-3-linked long –QT syndrome (LQT). The channels consist of four putative transmembrane domains (DI-DIV), with each domain containing six transmembrane segments (S1-S-6). IVF mutations are shown in green and LQT- associated mutations in red (Reproduced with permission from Chen et al. (1998))

It is interesting to note that lesions close in locus to those in the SCN5A channel are not uniquely associated with LQTS (❯ Fig. 1.15). Rather, it has been demonstrated that in the Brugada syndrome, in which there is also familial inheritance, mutations in SCN5A are associated with a loss of function or rapid recovery from inactivation of the sodium channels. The arrhythmia is expressed far more in young adult males than in females and has shown a particular predilection for Asian populations [141, 142]. Hence subtle differences among loci in the SCN5A channel in Brugada's syndrome and LQTS result in major differences in terms of age, gender, and phenotypic expression of the arrhythmia seen.

A final arrhythmia to be mentioned is familial atrial fibrillation. The familial inheritance is well-established here, linkages to chromosomes 6 and 10 have been identified and abnormalities in at least one ion channel (I_{ks}) and the $KvLQT_1$ and mink subunits have been noted [143]. It is probable however that this information represents only a subset of patients with familial atrial fibrillation.

1.4   Alterations in Refractory Period

After the upstroke of the action potential, the sodium channels are inactivated, and the fast sodium current ceases to flow. Inactivation of the inward Ca^{2+} current and activation of outwardly directed potassium currents bring about repolarization. The sodium channels remain inactivated throughout the action potential plateau until repolarization increases membrane potential levels negative to about −60 mV. Inactivation is then gradually removed as repolarization continues. Complete removal of inactivation occurs when membrane potential returns to around −90 mV. During the plateau, when Na^+ channels are inactivated, the cell cannot be excited. The period during which the cell cannot respond to an impulse by initiating a propagated action potential is referred to as the "effective refractory period." During the latter phase of repolarization, progressive removal of inactivation allows increasingly large sodium currents to flow through the still partially inactivated sodium channels when the cells are excited. This is the "relative refractory period." The rate of rise of action potentials initiated during the relative refractory period is reduced because the Na^+ channels are only partially reactivated. Hence, the conduction velocity of these "premature" action potentials is low. In cells with slow response action potentials (sinus and AV nodes or depolarized myocardial fibers), the effective refractory period and recovery of excitability persists until after complete repolarization. Removal of inactivation of slow channels is time dependent as well as voltage-dependent, and as result the relative refractory period extends well into diastole.

Alterations of both the effective and relative refractory periods may contribute to the occurrence of reentry in several different ways. First, as indicated previously, a decrease in the effective refractory period can decrease the size of reentrant circuits enabling them to exist in many localized areas of the heart. In fact, if the effective refractory period is decreased sufficiently, more than one reentrant circuit can exist at a time in some regions [144, 145]. The effective refractory period of atrial muscle, for example, is decreased by the acetylcholine released during vagal stimulation. As a result, reentry in atrial muscle causing atrial fibrillation is more easily induced during vagal stimulation [146]. Many reentrant circuits probably exist simultaneously during this arrhythmia [144]. Action potential duration and effective refractory are decreased in the ventricle during the early minutes of acute ischemia [147], or in some of the ventricular muscle cells in chronically ischemic areas, probably contributing to the occurrence of reentry [148]. Action potential duration and the effective refractory period of Purkinje fibers just distal to a site of conduction block may be decreased by the effects of electrotonic interactions with muscle proximal to the site of block, enabling reentrant impulses to reexcite the Purkinje regions [149].

Marked differences in refractory periods of closely adjacent regions may contribute to the initiation of reentry by causing localized block of premature impulses – a mechanism for the transient or unidirectional block discussed earlier. Inhomogeneities in the effective refractory periods in adjacent regions occur in the atria during vagal stimulation because of the irregular distribution of nerve endings [150], and in the ventricle and Purkinje system during acute or chronic ischemia [62, 148]. Moreover, recent data suggest that with healing of myocardial infarct there is a sprouting of sympathetic nerves growing in areas that had been totally or partially demonstrated as a result of ischemia [151]. Depending in the distribution of this neural growth, increased heterogeneity of sympathetic input may occur.

When the effective refractory period of adjacent regions are sufficiently different, conduction of an early premature impulse may block in the region with the longest refractory periods but may proceed slowly through the relatively refractory myocardium in the region with the shorter refractory period (❷ Fig. 1.22). The slowly conducting impulse may return to excite tissue just distal to the region of block and then reexcite tissue proximal to the site of block. Sufficient time must elapse during propagation to permit this region proximal to the site of block to recover excitability. Inhomogeneities in refractory periods are also a probable cause of reentry initiated by early premature impulses in the sinus and AV nodes [152, 153].

1.5 Abnormal Impulse Conduction and Reentry

The second major cause of arrhythmias is abnormal impulse conduction. One means whereby conduction abnormalities can cause arrhythmias has already been discussed, namely, the escape of subsidiary pacemakers that occur when there is sinoatrial, or atrioventricular block. Abnormal impulse conduction can also cause reentrant excitation, a mechanism for arrhythmias that does not depend on pacemaker activity.

Before discussing abnormalities of impulse propagation it is important to review the normal propagation of the cardiac impulse. As a general rule it is understood that propagation is more rapid in fibers and through fiber bundles of large diameter than of small diameter [7]. However, given that the cell membrane is a good insulator, it is imperative that for propagation to proceed intercellular sites be present that have low resistances, permitting the flow of electrical current and of signaling molecules from cell to cell. These sites are the so-called gap junctions, regions at which the membranes of adjacent cells are closely apposed [154]. Examination of such sites reveals the presence of intercellular channels, whose anatomy is contributed to by one hemichannel provided by each cell (❷ Fig. 1.16). Each hemichannel is referred to as a connexon, each of which is formed by a rosette-like pattern of 6 transmembrane spanning proteins called connexins. A number of connexins occur in the cells of the body: those most numerous in heart are connexins 43 (most prominent in atrial and ventricular myocardium), 45 (most prominent in the sinoatrial node and the ventricular conducting system), and 40 (most prominent in sinoatrial node and atrial myocardium and ventricular conducting system)[155]. Gap junctional density is greatest at the longitudinal ends of myocytes, thereby facilitating propagation along the long axes of cardiac fibers. Gap junctions are also seen at the lateral margins of myocytes, but given their lower density, current flow transversely is a fraction of that longitudinally [154].

It is the combination of low resistance junctions and the upstroke velocity of an arriving action potential that contributes most immediately to the propagation of the cardiac impulse. However, the relationship between number of

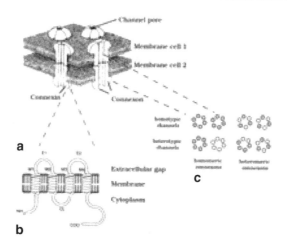

■ Fig. 1.16

Schematic illustration of gap junction structure. (a) Part of a gap junction plaque showing several channels interconnecting two cells and the composition of an individual channel from two half-channels (connexons) which are composed of connexin proteins. (b) Secondary structure of a single connexin protein. (c) Scheme explaining the composition of homotypic and heterotypic channels from homomeric and heteromeric connexons (Reproduced with permission from van Veen et al. (2001))

connexins present in any region of the heart and conduction velocity is complex, because there is a large margin of safety within the system. Specifically in myocardium it appears that the preponderance of connexins must be lost before conduction begins to slow [156]. Hence, extensive pathology must be present before a change is seen in the propagation of the cardiac impulse.

During sinus rhythm, the cardiac impulse usually dies out after the sequential activation of the atria and ventricles, because it is surrounded by tissue that it recently excited and which is therefore, refractory. A new impulse must arise in the sinus node for subsequent activation. Under special conditions the propagating impulse may not die out after complete activation of the heart but it may persist to reexcite (reenter) the atria or ventricles after the end of the refractory period [157]. The underlying principles that enable this reentrant excitation to occur can be illustrated with a simple experimental model consisting of a ring of excitable tissue. This model was first studied by physiologists during the early twentieth century and the results of these studies provided much of the basic information which has led to an understanding of reentrant mechanisms [158, 159]. In fact, more is being learned even today from studies on simple rings [160]. As shown in ❷ Fig. 1.17, if a ring of excitable tissue is stimulated at one point, two waves of excitation progress in opposite directions around the ring, but only one excitation of the ring occurs since the waves collide and die out. By temporarily applying pressure near the site of stimulation, however, an excitation can be induced to progress in only one direction. If the compression then is removed restoring conduction in this region, the impulse can then propagate around the ring, reenter tissue it previously excited and continue to circulate. Circular conduction of this kind has also been called circus movement.

Reentry does not occur normally in the heart. The pattern of conduction and the dying out of each impulse of sinus origin might be represented by the diagram in ❷ Fig. 1.17a. It is apparent that for reentry to occur a region of block must be present, at least, transiently. The block is necessary to provide the return pathway for the impulse to reenter the region it is to reexcite. Transient block, causing reentry, can occur in the heart after premature excitation (see below). Reentry also may occur when there is permanent block, but the block then must be unidirectional. In the ring experiment shown in ❷ Fig. 1.17, identical circus movement would occur if, instead of transient compression, permanent unidirectional conduction block were present. This means that conduction is blocked in one direction (from right to left in the diagram) but can proceed in the other (from left to right). It is obvious that if permanent block occurred in both directions reentry could not occur. Unidirectional block often occurs in cardiac fibers in which excitability and conduction are depressed. The electrophysiological mechanisms are discussed later in this chapter.

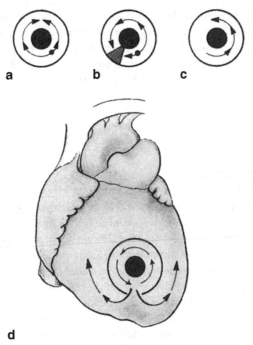

◘ Fig. 1.17

Schematic representation of reentry in a ring of cardiac tissue. The pattern of impulse propagation is indicated by the arrows and the small dot indicates the area in which the ring is stimulated. In (a), impulses propagate away from the point of stimulation in both directions and collide; no reentry occurs. In (b), in which the *shaded area* was compressed, the impulse propagates around in the ring in any one direction. Immediately, after stimulation the compression was relieved. Part (c) shows the circulating impulse returning to its point of origin and then continuing around the loop. Identical reentry would occur if the cross-hatched area were a region of permanent unidirectional conduction block, with the conduction block in the right-to-left direction. Part (d) shows how reentry in a loop of the kind described in (a)–(c) can cause arrhythmias if located in the heart. In this example, the loop is composed of ventricular muscle which is functionally separated from the rest of the ventricles along most of its border (*bold line*), perhaps as a result of fibrosis, but in functional continuity with the ventricles at its lower end. The *arrows* in (d) show how excitation waves propagate into the ventricles from continuously circulating impulses to cause ventricles tachycardia (Reproduced with permission after Wit (1979) © Excerpta Medica, Amsterdam)

In addition, for reentry to occur, the impulse must always find excitable tissue in the direction in which it is propagating. This requires the conduction time around the loop to be longer than the effective refractory period of the cardiac fibers that compromise the loop. If it is not, conduction of the reentering impulse would block. Normal heart muscle (excluding nodal fibers) has a refractory period which ranges from about 150–500 ms and a conduction velocity of at least $0.5–2.0 \text{ ms}^{-1}$. Therefore, the impulse conducting at a normal velocity of at least 0.5 ms^{-1} in reentrant pathway must conduct for at least 150 ms before it can return and reexcite a region it previously excited. This means the conduction pathway must be at least 7.5 cm long for reentry to occur in cardiac fibers with normal conduction and refractory properties. Such long reentrant pathways, functionally isolated from the rest of the heart, rarely exist. Clearly, the length of the pathway necessary for reentry can be shortened if the conduction velocity is slowed and/or the refractory period is reduced. For example, if conduction velocity is slowed to 0.05 ms^{-1} (as can occur in diseased cardiac fibers or in the normal sinus or AV node) the reentrant circuit need be no more than 7.5 mm in length. Circuits of this size can readily exist in the heart. Therefore, slowed conduction in combination with unidirectional block is a prerequisite which permits reentry to occur.

The "loop" of tissue which enables reentry to occur is called the reentrant circuit. It can be located almost anywhere in the heart and can assume a variety of sizes and shapes. The circuit may be an anatomical structure such as a ring of cardiac fibers in the peripheral Purkinje system. The circuit may also be functional and its existence, size, and shape be determined by electrophysiological properties of cardiac cells rather than anatomy. The size and location of an anatomical by defined reentrant circuit obviously remains fixed and results in what may be called "ordered reentry." The size and reentrant circuits dependent on functional properties rather than anatomy may also be fixed but they also may change with time leading to random reentry. Random reentry is probably most often associated with atrial or ventricular fibrillation, whereas ordered reentry can cause most other types of arrhythmias [3].

1.5.1　Mechanisms for Slow Conduction

There can be a number of causes for the slow conduction and block which predispose to the occurrence of reentry. The speed at which impulses propagate in cardiac fibers is dependent on certain features of their transmembrane action potentials and passive electrical properties [161]. Alterations in either (by cardiac pathology) can result in reentrant arrhythmias. An important feature of the transmembrane potential of working (atrial and ventricular) myocardial and Purkinje fibers which governs speed of propagation is the magnitude of the inward sodium current flowing through the fast sodium channels in the sarcolemma during the active potential upstroke and the rapidity with which this current reaches maximum intensity. The magnitude of this current flow determines the amplitude of phase 0 of the action potential; the speed of development of current flow is reflected in the rate at which the cell depolarizes (V_{max} of phase 0) [162]. The depolarization phase or upstroke of the action potential may be considered as resulting from the opening of specialized membrane channels (fast sodium channels) through which sodium ions rapidly pass form the extracellular fluid into the cell (❷ Fig. 1.18). The process of channel opening and closing has been described in a model devised by Hodgkin and Huxley for the nerve action potential [163]. According to this model, two "gates" control the passage of sodium ions through the channel. One gate m moves rapidly to open the channel; the other gate h moves slowly to close the channel. For an action potential to be initiated, a large enough area of membrane must be depolarized rapidly to threshold potential so that enough sodium channels are opened to give rise to the regenerative inward sodium current (m gates opened). After the upstroke of the action potential the sodium channels inactivate and the fast sodium current ceases to flow (h gates closed)(❷ Fig. 1.18).

　　The inward sodium current causes conduction of the cardiac impulse as follows: Impulse conduction occurs from one cell exciting the next by means of local currents which flow ahead of the action potential. These local currents depolarize the membrane potential to threshold potential to elicit the action potential. This process is illustrated in ❷ Fig. 1.19. An action potential is elicited at site A and is accompanied by a rapid inward sodium current I_{Na}. Part of this inward current flows along the fiber towards site B, which has not yet been excited. This intracellular flow is called the axial current I_a. Site A is the current source and site B, the current sink. The current at site B exits through the membrane either as capacitive current I_c which depolarizes the membrane potential or as membrane current flowing through ionic channels I_i. If the depolarization caused by the capacitive current is large enough to bring the membrane to its threshold potential an action potential will occur at site B. When the resting membrane resistance r_m (determined by channels that conduct ionic current near the resting potential) is high, a larger portion of the current passes out as capacitive current and is, therefore, more effective in eliciting an action potential. Also, when the resting membrane resistance is high, more axial current spreads for a longer distance along the fiber and excites more distant areas. There is also intracellular resistance to the axial current flow r_a which determines how far axial current spreads and its effectiveness in depolarizing the membrane at a distance. The cytoplasm offers minimal resistance to the spread of axial current. A larger portion of the resistance is located at the intercellular connections between myocardial fibers-gap junctions of the intercalated disks. Although extracellular resistance to current flow has an influence, it is normally significantly less than intracellular resistance.

　　The conduction velocity depends both on how much capacitive current flows out at unexcited sites ahead of the propagating wavefront and the distance at which the capacitive current can bring membrane potential to threshold. One important factor which influences the amount of axial and, therefore, capacitive current is the amount of fast inward current generated by the propagating action potential. A reduction of this inward current, leading to a reduction in the rate or amplitude of depolarization, may decrease axial current flow, slow conduction and lead to conduction block. Such a reduction may result from inactivation of sodium channels (❷ Fig. 1.18). The intensity of the inward Na^+ current depends on the fraction of Na^+ channels which are open when the cell is excited and the size of the Na^+ electrochemical potential

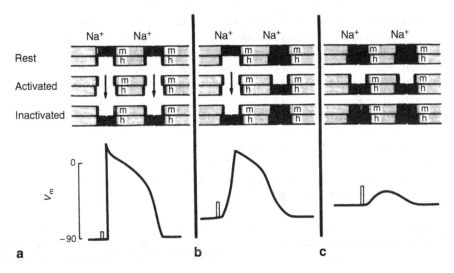

☐ Fig. 1.18

Schematic depiction of the Na$^+$ channels in the sarcolemma at rest, in the activated state and in the inactivated state. The "gates", m and h control channels opening and closing, respectively. At the bottom of the figure are representative action potentials. In (a) at a resting potential of −90 mV, most of the Na$^+$ channels can be activated causing an action potential with rapid upstroke. Activation is represented by open channels and the arrow depicting inward Na$^+$ current. When the membrane depolarizes during the upstroke of the action potential, the channels inactivate; the diagram shows that they are closed. In (b), resting potential is reduced to −70 mV and about 50% of the Na$^+$ channels cannot be activated. A depressed fast-response action potential with a slow upstroke occurs when the cell is excited because the inward Na$^+$ current is decreased. In (c), at a resting potential less than −60 mV; Na$^+$ channels cannot be activated and an action potential might not be elicited (Reproduced with permission after Wit and Rosen (1981) © American Heart Association, Dallas, Texas)

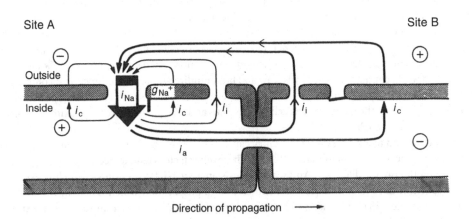

Direction of propagation ⟶

☐ Fig. 1.19

Schematic diagram of the propagation of an action potential along a cardiac muscle fiber: i_{Na}, sodium current; I_a, axial current i_c, capacitive current: I_i, ionic current: g_{Na+}, conductivity of the membrane to Na ions. The *larger arrow* indicates the large inrush of Na ions (I_{Na}) through membrane channels during the upstroke (Reproduced with permission after Frame and Hoffman (1984) © Nijhoff, The Hague)

gradient (relative concentration of Na^+ outside the cell, in the extracellular space, compared to Na^+ concentration inside the cell) [84, 164]. The fraction of Na^+ channels available for opening is determined largely by the level of membrane potential at which an action potential is initiated. Na^+ channels are inactivated either after the upstroke of an action potential or if the steady-state resting membrane potential is reduced. Immediately after the upstroke cardiac fibers are inexcitable because of Na^+ channel inactivation at the positive level of membrane potential. During repolarization progressive removal of inactivation allows increasingly large Na^+ currents to flow through the still partially inactivated Na^+ channels when the cells are excited. The inward Na^+ current and rate of rise of action potentials initiated during this relative refractory period are reduced because the Na^+ channels are only partly reactivated [164]. Hence the conduction velocity of these premature action potentials is low. Premature activation of the heart can therefore induce reentry because premature impulses conduct slowly in regions of the heart where the cardiac fibers are not completely repolarized (where Na^+ channels are to some extent inactivated) and their conduction may block in regions where cells have not repolarized to about −60 mV. Hence the prerequisites for reentry – slow conduction and block – can be brought about by premature activation.

Reentry might also occur in cardiac cells with persistently low levels of resting potential (which may be between −60 and −70 mV) caused by disease. At these resting potentials, a significant fraction of the Na^+ channels is inactivated, and therefore unavailable for activation by a depolarizing stimulus. The magnitude of the net inward current during phase 0 of the action potential is reduced and consequently both the speed and amplitude of the upstroke is diminished, decreasing axial current flow and slowing conduction significantly. Such action potentials with upstrokes dependent on inward current flowing via partially inactivated Na^+ channels are sometimes referred to as "depressed fast responses" (❷ Fig. 1.18). Further depolarization and inactivated of the Na^+ channel may decrease the excitability of cardiac fibers to such an extent that they may become a site of unidirectional conduction block [1]. Thus in a diseased region there may be some area of slow conduction and some area of conduction block, possibly depending on the level of resting potential. The combination may cause reentry.

After the upstroke of the action potential, membrane potential begins to return to the resting level during phase 1 repolarization because the sodium channels are inactivated and the fast (depolarizing) sodium current ceases to flow. However, this return is slowed by a second inward current which is smaller and slower than the fast sodium current and probably is carried by both sodium and calcium ions [165] (❷ Fig. 1.20). This secondary inward current flows through so-called slow channels that are distinct from the fast sodium channels. The threshold for activation of the slow inward current is in the range of −30 to −40 mV compared with −60 to −70 mV for the fast sodium current. This current inactivates much more slowly than the fast sodium current and gradually diminishes as the cell repolarizes. Under special conditions, it may also underlie the occurrence of the slow conduction that causes reentrant arrhythmias [49]. Although, the fast sodium current may be largely inactivated at membrane potentials near −50 mV, the slow inward current is not activated and is still available for activation [43, 84, 165]. Under certain conditions in cells with resting potentials less than −60 mV (such as when membrane conductance is very low or when catecholamines are present), this normally weak slow inward current may give rise the regenerative depolarization characteristic of a propagated action potential. This propagated action potential, dependent on slow inward current alone, is "the slow response" (❷ Fig. 1.20) [55]. Since this inward current is weak, conduction velocity is slow and both unidirectional and bidirectional conduction block may occur [163]. Slow response action potentials can occur in diseased cardiac fibers with low resting potentials but they also occur in some normal tissue of the heart, such as cells of the sinus and AV nodes where the maximum diastolic potential is normally less than about −70 mV [55, 166].

The slow conduction and block necessary for reentry can also be caused by factors other than the decrease in inward current accompanying a decrease in membrane potential. These other factors tend to decrease the magnitude and spread of axial current along the myocardial fiber. An increased resistance to axial current flow, which is expressed as "effective axial resistance" (resistance to current flow in the direction of propagation which is dependent on the intracellular and extracellular resistivities) may decrease conduction velocity [167, 168]. Whether an increase in extracellular resistance to current flow sufficient to impair conduction and cause arrhythmias occurs during pathological states is not yet known. It is likely, however, that sufficient increases in intracellular resistance can occur. Although the intracellular resistance depends on both the resistance of the cytoplasm and the resistance at the gap junctions which couple cells together, the change in intracellular resistance causing arrhythmias probably results mainly from changes in junctional resistance.

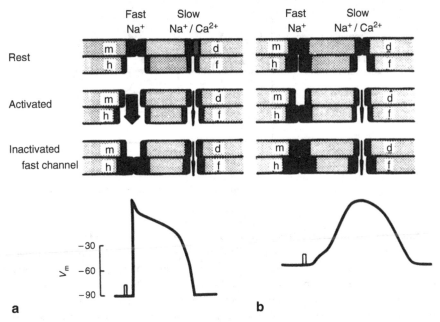

⬛ **Fig. 1.20**
Schematic depiction of the sarcolemma containing the fast Na' channels and the slow Na$^+$/Ca^{2+} channels. The "gates" m and h control Na$^+$ channel opening and closing, respectively. The "gates" d and f control Ca^{2+} channel opening and closing, respectively. Representative action potentials are shown at the bottom of the figure. In (a), the normal action potential, elicited from a resting potential of –90 mV is shown. At rest, both fast and slow channels are inactivated (represented by closed channels). After the fiber is stimulated the channels are activated (represented by open channels) and fast inward Na$^+$ current (*large arrows*) and slow inward Na$^+$/Ca^{2+} current (*small arrows*) cause the action potential upstroke and plateau. The fast channel inactivates before the slow channel. In (b), in a cell with a resting potential of –50 mV, the fast Na$^+$ channels are not activated when the fiber is stimulated. The slow channels can still be activated and current can pass through them to cause slow response action potentials (Reproduced with permission after Wit and Rosen (1981) © American Heart Association, Dallas, Texas)

During conduction of the impulse, axial current flows from one myocardial cell to the adjacent cell through the gap junctions at the intercalated disks (which normally have a relatively low resistance) [161] and, therefore, the resistance, extent and distribution of these junctions have a profound influence on conduction. This influence can be seen even in normal atrial or ventricular myocardium. In regions where cardiac muscle fibers are closely packed together and arranged parallel to each other in a uniform manner, conduction in the direction parallel to the myocardial fiber orientation (along the long axis of the myocardial fibers) is much more rapid than in the direction perpendicular to the long axis (❯ Fig. 1.21) [167–169]. This property is known as anisotropy. Conduction perpendicular to the long axis of the fibers can be slow as 0.1 ms^{-1} even though resting and action potentials of the muscles fibers are normal. The slow conduction is caused by an effective axial resistivity which is higher in the direction perpendicular to fiber orientation than parallel to fiber orientation. This higher axial resistivity results in part from fewer and shorter intercalculated disks connecting myocardial fibers in a side-to-side direction than in the end-to-end direction. Conduction in normal ventricular myocardium can, therefore, be slow enough to cause reentry as will be discussed in more detail later.

Pathological alterations in anatomy may also cause slow conduction by increasing axial resistance through effects on coupling between cells. Fibrosis in the heart separates myocardial fibers, reducing the number of disk connections and decreasing the extent or area of connections that remain (see ❯ Fig. 1.22a). An example is the effect of fibrosis, resulting from infarction, on the myocardial fibers in the infracted region. The broad, wide disks which occur at the longitudinal ends of normal cells no longer are present because of the deformation of the cells by the connective tissue. Only short

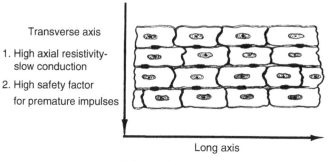

○ Fig. 1.21

Influence of anisotropic structure of cardiac muscle on conduction velocity. In the uniformly anisotropic cardiac muscle [137, 138] shown, the myocardial fibers are arranged parallel to each other and are packed closely together. Intercalated disks join cardiac cells both at their ends and in a side-to-side direction. The disks joining the fibers in the end-to-end direction are usually broad and numerous resulting in a low axial resistivity in this direction, whereas the disks connecting cells in a side-to-side direction are short and sometimes sparse, resulting in a higher axial resistivity in this direction. The high safety factor for premature impulses in the transverse axis means that, in this direction, premature impulses are not easily blocked (Reproduced with permission after Gardner et al. (1984) © Lea & Febiger, Philadelphia, Pennsylvania)

segments of intercalculated disks remain in some regions. Conduction is very slow despite the presence of normal resting potentials, probably because there is a high resistance to current flow through the shortened disks [170].

A combination of reduction in gap junctions plus microfibrosis occurring between myocytes is responsible for the slow conduction and reentry seen in, for example, healing myocardial infarction [171, 172]. In addition, the formation of gap junctions along the lateral margins of cells that had been uncoupled during the acute phase of ischemia can favor current flow from cell to cell along the lateral margins [173, 174]. Resultant very slow transverse conduction to the point of discontinuous propagation is a mechanism whereby reentry has been shown to occur (summarized in [175]). In addition to structural changes, a rise in intracellular calcium can slow conduction by increasing resistance to current flow through gap junctions in the disks, since calcium levels profoundly affect the resistance of the gap junction [176]. This may occur during prolonged periods of ischemia [177]. Cardiac glycosides also increase resistance at the disk by increasing intracellular calcium [33].

The effective axial resistivity is also dependent on the size and shape of the myocardial cells (○ Fig. 1.23). Resistance to current flow may increase markedly and conduction may be slowed in regions where cells branch or where there are abrupt increases in cell size or number. A detailed description of the mechanisms is given by Spach et al. [167, 168], and Joyner et al. [178, 179]. Some discussion of these factors can also be found in ○ Sect. 1.5.2.

1.5.2   Unidirectional Block of Impulse Conduction

According to the model illustrated in ○ Fig. 1.17, unidirectional conduction block (block of conduction in one direction along a bundle of cardiac fibers, while conduction in the other direction is maintained) is necessary for the occurrence of many kinds of reentry. Unidirectional block in part of the circuit leaves a return pathway through which impulse conducts to reenter previously excited areas. There are a number of mechanisms that might cause unidirectional block, some of which have been demonstrated directly and others of which are the products of theoretical considerations. The mechanisms involve changes in both active and passive properties of the cardiac cells.

The unidirectional block needed for the initiation of the reentrant tachycardia may be transient, as exemplified by block of a premature impulse that initiates a reentrant tachycardia. The conduction of an impulse, which is sufficiently

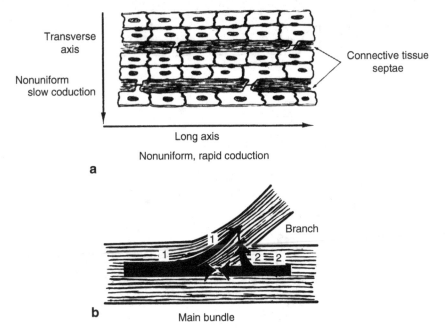

Fig. 1.22
Influences of myocardial structure on impulse conduction. Part (**a**) shows the separation of myocardial fiber bundles that can result from fibrosis. This may reduce the number of disk connections, thereby slowing impulse conduction. Part (**b**) shows how branching of a fiber bundle can influence propagation. The lines within the main bundle and the branch indicate the orientation of the myocardial fibers. Conduction occurs in the direction of the long axis of the fibers when the impulse conducts along the main bundle into the branch as indicated by *arrow 1*. Conduction in this direction is not influenced by the presence of the branch. When an impulse conducts from the main bundle into the branch as indicated by *arrow 2*, there is a sudden change in fiber orientation in the direction of propagation so that the impulse must conduct transversely to the long axis of the fibers as it enters the branch. The sudden increase in axial resistivity caused by the change might cause block, particularly when there is some depression of the action-potential upstroke (Reproduced with permission from Gardner et al. (1984) © Lea & Febiger, Philadelphia, Pennsylvania)

premature, is blocked where it encounters cells that are not excitable because of incomplete repolarization but may continue to propagate in other regions of the reentrant pathway if the fibers are more fully repolarized and, therefore, excitable (see ❷ Sect. 1.5.3). Functionally, the region where the premature impulse blocks is a region of unidirectional block if it can be excited later, after it has recovered excitability, by an impulse propagated from another direction as shown in ❷ Fig. 1.24.

Unidirectional conduction block in a reentrant circuit can also be persistent and independent of premature activation. In a bundle of atrial, ventricular or Purkinje fibers with normal electrophysiological properties, an impulse can conduct rapidly in either direction. However, there is usually some asymmetry in the conduction velocity and as a consequence, conduction in one direction may take slightly longer than in the other direction [1, 55, 161]. This is of no physiological significance. The asymmetry of conduction can be the result of several factors. Bundles of cardiac muscle are composed of interconnecting myocardial fibers (cells), packed in a connective tissue matrix. These calls have differing diameters and branch frequently. An impulse conducting in one direction encounters a different sequence of changes in cell diameter, branching and frequency and distribution of gap junctions than it does when traveling in the opposite direction. The "configuration of the pathways" in each direction is not the same [55]. As mentioned above, these structural features influence conduction by affecting the axial current. Theoretical analyses indicate that the conduction velocity of an impulse passing abruptly from a fiber of small diameter to one of large diameter transiently slows at the junction because the larger cable results in a larger sink in longitudinal axial current (there is more membrane for this current to depolarize to threshold if

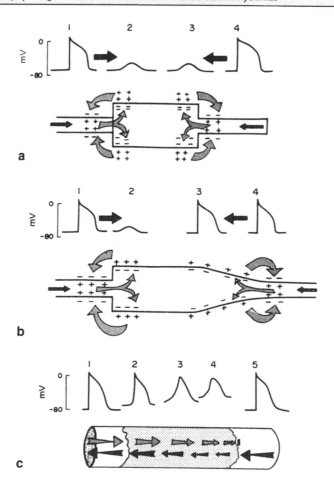

⬛ Fig. 1.23

Mechanisms for unidirectional conduction block. Part (a) shows the effects on conduction of a small diameter fiber coupled to a large diameter fiber. When the impulse is conducting (*solid arrows*) from left to right there is a sudden increase in membrane area which the current flow (*shaded arrows*) must depolarize to threshold for conduction to continue. If the membrane is not depolarized to threshold, conduction blocks as indicated by action potential 2 (above). The change in membrane area in (a) is symmetrical, that is, the large diameter cable is connected at its other end to another small diameter cable. Therefore, an impulse conducting from right to left in the diagram would also block. Part (b) shows an asymmetrical nonuniformity that might cause unidirectional block. Conduction from left to right blocks at the region where there is an abrupt increase in the cable diameter as in (a) (see the action potentials). However the transition from large to small cable at the opposite end is gradual. An impulse conducting from right to left can still depolarize the membrane to threshold despite a gradual increase in membrane area (see text). Part (c) shows unidirectional block caused by asymmetrical depression of the action-potential upstroke. The stippled region represents a poorly perfused part of the cable between two normal regions. During conduction from left to right, the action potentials are progressively more depressed. Normal action potential 1 can excite 2, 2 excites 3 and 3 excites 4, but the slowly rising low-amplitude upstroke of 4 does not generate sufficient axial current to bring membrane potential of 5 to threshold and conduction blocks. In the opposite direction, the large amplitude action potential at 5 generates sufficient current to excite 4. Impulse conduction continues through the depressed region to the opposite end where the upstroke of action potential 2 is large enough to excite the normal adjacent area 1

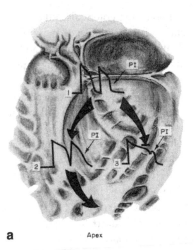
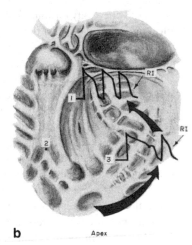

a   Apex   b   Apex

⬛ Fig. 1.24

Mechanism for functional unidirectional conduction block and initiation of reentry in the subendocardial Purkinje network surviving over an area of extensive myocardial infarction [154]. Both **(a)** and **(b)** show the endocardial surface of the left anterior papillary muscle (to the *left*) and the anterior interventricular septum (to the *right*). Subendocardial Purkinje fibers in different regions have action potentials with different durations and refractory periods. Action potentials recorded at sites 1 and 2 have shorter durations and refractory periods than at site 3. In **(a)**, an early premature impulse PI arising at 1 conducts into regions where action potentials have a longer duration (conduction pathways indicated by *large arrows*). The action potential at 3 is longer than at 2. Consequently the premature impulse can excite cells at 2 but conduction blocks at 3. This area becomes a site of unidirectional block because as shown in **(b)**, the premature impulse, after conducting through 2 arrives at 3 when these cells are excitable. It excites the cells at 3 in the retrograde direction and then returns to its site of origin (1) as a reentrant impulse RI (Reproduced with permission after Wit et al. (1974) © Mosby, St Louis, Missouri)

conduction of the impulse is to continue) [161, 178–181]. A similar slowing occurs when an impulse conducts into a region where there is an abrupt increase in branching of the myocardial syncytium; conduction transiently slows because of the larger current sink provided by the increased membrane area that must be depolarized. In the opposite direction, it can be predicted that conduction will speed transiently at the junction between larger and smaller cable because the smaller sink for axial current results in more rapid depolarization of the membrane to threshold [161, 178–180]. Theoretically, if there is a large enough difference in the diameter of the two cables, an impulse conducting in the small fiber will block at the junction with the larger fiber while in the opposite direction, excitation will proceed from the large diameter fiber to the small one [180]. For this model to explain unidirectional block, once the abrupt change in cell diameter or membrane area has occurred it does not return to its original one. In the heart, however, it is more likely that the properties are more or less the same on each side of the region through which the asymmetrical conduction has occurred [180]. If the abnormalities of that region are symmetrical around its midpoint (an abrupt increase in fiber diameter followed later by an abrupt decrease (❷ Fig. 1.23a), block would occur irrespective of direction. An asymmetrical uniformity is necessary for one-way conduction [181]. For example, there may be an abrupt increase in fiber diameter or effective axial resistance R_i followed by a gradual return to the original diameter (❷ Fig. 1.23b). In this model, block would occur in the direction in which there is an abrupt increase in the sink for the reasons described above. However, in the opposite direction the gradual increase in diameter would not cause block because the axial current would actually increase (there is a decrease in R_i as the cable diameter is increased as well as an increase in transmembrane current because of the larger membrane area) [180] (❷ Fig. 1.23).

It is doubtful, however, that abrupt changes of the magnitude required to cause block of the normal action potential exist because the safety factor for conduction is large; that is, there is a large excess of activating current over that required for propagation [161]. Dodge and Cranefield have pointed out that "only if an action potential is a relatively weak stimulus and the unexcited area is not easily excited will plausible changes in membrane resistance, cell diameter, or intercellular coupling block"[181]. There is the necessity for interaction of abnormal action potentials and decreased excitability with the preexisting anatomical impediments. When the resting potential of muscle fiber or Purkinje bundle is decreased, the reduced action potential upstroke results in a decreased axial current as described above and, therefore, the action potential is a weak stimulus. The normal directional differences in conduction are then exaggerated. At a critical degree of depression, conduction may fail in one direction while being maintained in the other (although it may be markedly slowed). At this critical degree of depression the reduced axial current is not sufficient to depolarize the membrane to threshold where the current sink is increased because of the structural changes described above, but the axial current is still more than adequate during conduction in the opposite direction (❷ Fig. 1.23c).

It also has been proposed that block may occur at branching points where there is an abrupt change in the orientation of the myocardial fibers if there is a sudden increase of axial resistivity [168]. For example, an impulse conducting along a muscle bundle in a direction parallel to the fiber orientation (low effective axial resistivity) may conduct into a branch of that bundle; at the branching point the orientation of the myocardial fiber may be perpendicular to the original direction of conduction and therefore, the effective axial resistivity suddenly becomes high (❷ Fig. 1.22b). Therefore, it seems that a sufficient decrease in axial current caused by depression of the action potential upstroke could result in conduction block of the impulse entering the branch from the direction in which there is the marked change in the fiber orientation, but no block from the opposite direction (❷ Fig. 1.22).

Although the possible mechanisms for unidirectional conduction block discussed so far all involved important influences on conduction of the structure of muscle bundles, unidirectional block is most likely to occur when action potential upstrokes are depressed. Asymmetrical depression of the upstroke may also be an important factor that causes unidirectional conduction block irrespective of anatomy [55]. Such asymmetrical depression of the action potential might occur because of asymmetrical distribution of a pathological event. As a simple example, the action-potential upstrokes in a bundle of fibers may be diminished as a result of a reduction of perfusion after coronary occlusion, but reduction may be more severe towards one end of the bundle than the other (❷ Fig. 1.23). A propagating impulse consisting of an action potential with the normal upstroke velocity enters the poorly perfused region and propagates through this region with decrement. That is, as it conducts from the less depressed to the more severely depressed end, the action-potential upstroke velocity and amplitude progressively decrease, as does the axial current caused by the upstroke [7]. When the impulse arrives at the opposite end of the depressed segment of the bundle with normal action potentials, the weak axial current may not be sufficient to depolarize the membrane to threshold. Conduction, therefore, blocks even though the normally perfused region is excitable. Conduction in the opposite direction, however, might still occur. The large axial current generated by the normal action potential flows for a considerable distance through the depressed region. These cells, in turn, may be able to excite adjacent fibers in the direction of propagation (❷ Fig. 1.23c).

1.5.3   Reentrant Arrhythmias

It has been indicated above that reentry can occur in different regions of the heart, utilizing either anatomical or functional pathways. It has also been shown that slow conduction and block may have a number of different cellular mechanisms. Conceivably, any of these mechanisms may occur in either an anatomical or functional reentrant pathway. Several examples of reentry caused by the different mechanisms will now be provided.

1.5.3.1   Anatomical Pathways

Reentrant excitation caused by the slow conduction and block which accompany depression of the action potential upstroke (either because of premature excitation or because of a persistent reduction in the resting membrane potential) may occur in gross anatomically distinct circuits (around an anatomical obstacle). Reentrant excitation involving an anatomically distinct circuit and obstacle is exemplified by reentry in a loop of cardiac fiber bundles such as the loop of Purkinje fiber bundles in the distal conduction system illustrated in ❷ Fig. 1.25a. In this model of an anatomic circuit, slow conduction and unidirectional block are caused by reducing the steady-state level of the resting potential [182]. The unidirectional block (shaded area) is located near the origin of branch B in the loop of Purkinje fiber bundles; an impulse cannot conduct through this area in the anterograde direction but it can in the retrograde direction. Slow conduction

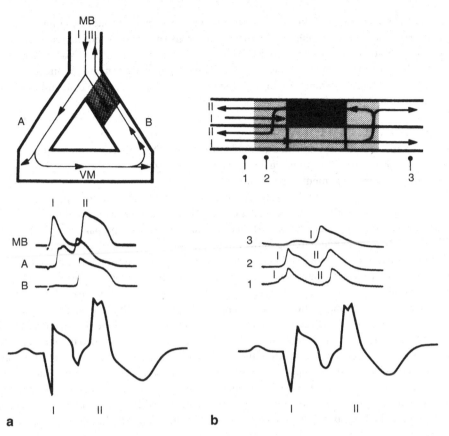

☐ Fig. 1.25

A possible mechanism for reentry in an anatomical pathway comprised of Purkinje fiber bundles and ventricular muscle. Part (a) shows a main bundle of Purkinje fibers (*MB*) which divides into two branches A and B before terminating on ventricular muscle (*VM*). A severely depressed area in which unidirectional conductional block occurs in the anterograde direction is located in branch B (*shaded area*). Conduction is slow throughout the rest of the loop because the Purkinje fibers have low resting potentials, and consequently, their action potentials have slow upstrokes. The arrows indicate the sequence of activation of the loop by the conducting impulse: *arrow I* represents an impulse of sinus origin entering the loop; *arrow II* is the reentering impulse leaving the loop (details of the mechanism by which reentry occurs are given in the text). Action potentials recorded from MB and branches A and B are shown below, together with an example of how the ECG might appear. Action potential I was recorded from the main bundle (MB) as impulse I entered the loop; the action potentials in A and B were recorded from Purkinje bundles A and B as the impulse conducted around the loop; and the action potential II in the MB trace was recorded from the main bundle when the impulse reexcited it. Impulse I would cause ventricular depolarization I on the ECG and impulse II would cause a ventricular extrasystole (ventricular depolarization II). Part (b) shows, at the *top*, how reentry can occur even in a single bundle of muscle or Purkinje fibers by the mechanism of reflection. The diagram depicts two adjacent fibers in a bundle. The entire *shaded area* is depressed and depression in the *darker area* of the upper fiber is so severe that unidirectional conduction block occurs there. The *arrows* indicate the sequence of activation in the bundle. *Arrows* labeled I show the impulse entering the bundle. Conduction of the impulse blocks in the fiber at the top in the severely depressed region but continues in the fiber at the bottom which is not as depressed. The impulse conducts transversely from the *bottom* fiber to the *top* fiber, once past the region *of* severe depression. It then conducts retrogradely through this severely depressed region in the top bundle. *Arrows* labeled II show the reentrant impulse returning to reexcite the left end *of* the bundle (see text). Action potentials recorded from sites 1, 2 and 3 in the lower fiber are shown below: action potentials labeled I were recorded as the impulse conducted from *left* to *right*; action potentials labeled II were recorded as the impulse returned to its origin. The bottom trace shows how such events might appear on the ECG (Reproduced with permission after Wit and Bigger (1975) © American Heart Association, Dallas, Texas)

occurs in the rest of the loop because of the low resting potentials. An impulse conducting into the loop via the main Purkinje fiber bundle (arrow showing impulse I) blocks near the origin of branch B and can enter only branch A through which it conducts slowly into the ventricular muscle (VM). The impulse then can invade branch B at its myocardial end. This branch had not been excited initially because of the unidirectional block at its origin and so the impulse can still conduct in a retrograde direction in branch B, through the region of unidirectional block, and then reexcite the main bundle from which it entered the loop (arrows showing impulse II).

The reentering impulse (II) will, of course, block if it returns to the main bundle while the fibers in that region are still effectively refractory. Hence, there is the necessity for slow conduction around the loop (slow conduction in only part of the loop, such as in the area of unidirectional block, would also suffice). The region of unidirectional block is necessary to prevent one part of the loop (branch B) from being invaded by the anterograde impulse and so provides a return excitable pathway for the reentering impulse as mentioned before.

When the reentrant impulse returns to the main bundle it may travel throughout the conduction system to reactivate the ventricles, causing a premature ventricular depolarization. It also may reinvade the bundle of Purkinje fibers through which it originally excited the ventricular muscle (branch A) and once again propagate back through the reentrant pathway. This may result in a continuous circling of the impulse around the loop and a tachycardia.

If conduction in this pathway – the loop of Purkinje fibers and ventricular muscle – is not sufficiently slow to permit reentry or if there is no strategically located site of unidirectional block, reentry might still be induced by premature activation. If the cardiac fibers are activated prematurely, before they have completely recovered excitability, the premature impulse will conduct slowly and unidirectional block may result because of the low safety margin for conduction in partially refractory tissue. Premature activation may, therefore, lead to reentry of kind illustrated in ❷ Fig. 1.25.

Anatomic circuits also might be formed by bundles of surviving muscle fibers in healed infarcts or in fibrotic regions of the atria or ventricles. The critical slow conduction and block may be caused by depressed transmembrane potentials such as in the atria of hearts with cardiomyopathy [183] or in increased effective axial resistivity such as in healed infarcts [170]. Gross anatomical circuits are also involved in reentry utilizing the bundle branch which may cause ventricular tachycardia [184], reentry utilizing an accessory AV connecting pathway which may cause supraventricular tachycardia [185], and reentry around the tricuspid ring which may cause atrial flutter [186]. The specific mechanisms involved are discussed in the publications referenced.

1.5.3.2 Functional Pathways

Gross anatomical loops and anatomical obstacles are not a prerequisite for the occurrence of reentry. Reentry caused by slow conduction and unidirectional block can also occur in unbranched bundles or "sheets" of muscle fibers. A kind of reentry called reflection occurs in unbranched bundles of Purkinje fibers in which conduction is slow because the resting and action potentials are depressed (❷ Fig. 1.25b) [1, 55]. During reflection, excitation occurring slowly in one direction along a bundle of fibers and is followed by excitation occurring in the opposite direction. The returning (reflected) impulse may be caused by reentry owing to functional longitudinal dissociation of the bundles [135].

Antzelevitch, Jalife and Moe described another mechanism which may cause reflection [187, 188]. Slow conduction does not occur along the entire bundle because of depressed transmembrane potentials, but rather there is a delayed activation of part of the bundle, resulting from electronic excitation of a region distal to an inexcitable segment (❷ Fig. 1.26). The segment, may be rendered inexcitable by a depressed resting potential and subsequent inactivation of the sodium current channels. If a segment of a bundle of Purkinje fibers is inexcitable and will not generate action potentials, impulses conducting along the bundle will block at that segment (❷ Fig. 1.26a, A). The blocked action potential, however, can generate axial current flow through the inexcitable segment of the fiber bundle which can act as a passive cable. The electronic manifestation of the blocked impulse decays along the cable in the inexcitable segment according to the length constant which is dependant to a large extent on the intracellular and extracellular resistances to current flow. If the inexcitable segment is sufficiently short relative to the length constant (less than 2 mm in the experiments of Antzelevitch et al. [187] and Jalife and Moe [188]), the current flow across the gap can depolarize the excitable fibers distal to the inexcitable region and can excite an action potential (❷ Fig. 1.26a). The magnitude of delay of the action potential is dependant to a large extent on the time-course and amplitude of the electrotonic current flow. The action potential initiated distal to the point of block not only will conduct distally along the fiber but can also itself cause retrograde axial current flow through

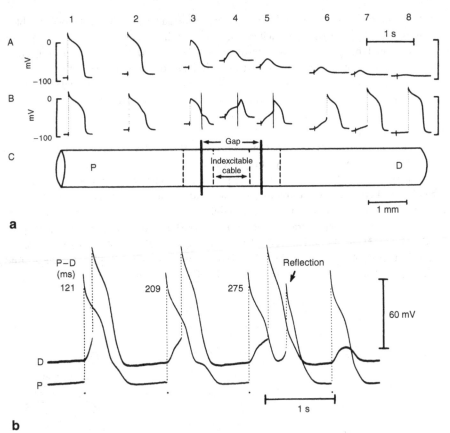

Fig. 1.26
Part (a) is a schematic representation of block and conduction across an inexcitable segment of a Purkinje fiber bundle. The bundle is represented in C. The inexcitable segment of the cable with a low membrane potential shown here was produced experimentally by exposing this central segment to a superfusion solution that mimicked an ischemic environment. An impulse initiated in the proximal segment P propagates to the border of the inexcitable region and conduction blocks there (action potentials *1, 2* and *3* in *A* and *B*). Axial current flows through the inexcitable cable, depolarizing electrotonically the membrane fibers distal (D) to the inexcitable region (action potentials *4, 5, 6, 7* in *A*). Depolarization may be large enough to bring the distal membrane to threshold, causing an action potential distal to the inexcitable region (potential *5, 6, 7* in *B*). When conduction across the inexcitable region is successful, axial current generated from the distal action potential may also flow back towards the proximal region through the gap. This current flow has a depolarizing effect as evidenced in action potential *3* in *B*; note the alteration in repolarization of this action potential that resembles an early afterdepolarization (Reproduced with permission after Antzelevitch and Mae (1981) © American Heart Association. Dallas, Texas). Part (**b**) shows the case when this reaches threshold, the axial current being sufficiently large, and causes an action potential during repolarization. Two action potentials are shown, one recorded from the proximal (P) and the other from the distal (D) side of the inexcitable region. Conduction delay between P and D increases with each stimulated impulse, from 121 to 275 ms. Note the delay in repolarization in the P trace after the second action potential. This reaches threshold after the third action potential (with 275 ms delay) resulting in an action potential arising during phase 3 of repolarization (labeled "reflection") (Reproduced with permission from Antzelevitch (1983) © Saunders, Philadelphia, Pennsylvania)

the inexcitable gap to depolarize the part of the fiber proximal to the gap at the site of the original block. If the sum of excitation timed in both directions across the inexcitable gap exceeds the refractory period of the proximal segment, an action potential will be elicited that propagates retrogradely along the fiber (❷ Fig. 1.26b). This reflected action potential reenters the part of the bundle that already was excited. Thus impulse transmission in both directions occurs over the same pathway unlike the types of reentry discussed previously. Reflection resulting from delays in activation caused by electrotonic transmission might be limited to areas where damage to the myocardial fiber is focal, as if the damage is too extensive electrotonic transmission across the inexcitable area would fail.

Another mechanism that can cause reentry in functional pathways is the "leading circle" mechanism originally described by Allessie et al. in experiments on atrial muscle [189–191]. Reentry is initiated by precisely timed premature impulses in regions which are activated normally at regular rates of stimulation. Initiation of reentry is made possible by the different refractory periods of atrial fibers in close proximity to one another [189]. The premature impulse that initiates reentry blocks in fibers with long refractory periods and conducts in fibers with shorter refractory periods, eventually returning to the initial region of block after excitability recovers there. The impulse may then continue to circulate around a central area which is kept refractory because it is constantly bombarded by impulses propagating toward it from all sides of the circuit (❷ Fig. 1.27). This central area provides a functional obstacle that prevents excitation from propagating across the fulcrum of the circuit. The circumference of the smallest (leading) circle around the functional obstacle may be as little as 6–8 mm and is a pathway in which the efficacy of stimulation of the circulating wavefront is just

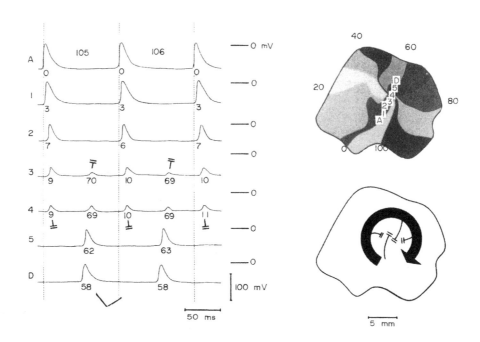

❏ Fig. 1.27

Reentry in isolated left atrial myocardium by the leading circle mechanism. At the *right*, above, is the map of the activation pattern of the atrium during circus movement. The impulse rotates continuously in a clockwise direction; each number and different *shading* indicates the time in milliseconds during which a given region is activated. Activation proceeds from 0 to 100 ms and one complete revolution takes 100 ms. At the *left*, the membrane potentials of seven fibers (marked A, D and 1–5) located on a straight line through the center of the circus movement are shown (the locations from which these action potentials were recorded are indicated on the map at the *upper right*). These records show that the fibers in the, central point of the circuit (3 and 4) show double responses of subnormal amplitude during circus movement. These responses result from conduction of the impulse from the circulating wave toward the center. At the *lower right* the activation pattern during circus movement is given schematically. It shows the circuit with the converging wavelets in the center (Reproduced with permission after Allessie et al. (1976) © American Heart Association, Dallas, Texas) sufficient to excite the tissue ahead. This tissue is still in its relative refractory phase. Conduction through the functional reentrant circuit is slowed, therefore, because impulses are propagating in partially refractory tissue. Single circuits of this kind might cause atrial tachycardia or flutter [192]. Functional reentrant circuits of the leading circle type may change their size and location and if they do, would fall under the general category of random reentry. Changes in size may result from changes in refractory period, as would be expected to occur if autonomic (particularly parasympathetic) activity increases. The existence of multiple circuits is made possible by conditions which shorten the refractory period and/or depress conduction velocity and thereby decrease the minimal dimensions of the leading circuit. Multiple circuits of the leading circle type may be the cause of atrial fibrillation during which "reentry occurs over numerous loops of various size and position wandering over the excitable surface" [144]. Functional reentrant circuits of the leading circle type might also occur in the ventricles as a result of similar mechanisms, and might even cause fibrillation.

The anisotropic properties of atrial and ventricular myocardium also may predispose to functional reentrant circuits [167, 171] as described previously how conduction velocity varies depending on the direction of impulse propagation relative to the long axis of the myocardial fibers; slow conduction occurs perpendicular to the long axis while more rapid conduction occurs parallel to this axis. In addition, although it may seem paradoxical, some experimental studies on isolated tissue have shown that despite more rapid conduction, early premature impulses block more readily in the direction of the long axis because the safety factor is lower in the direction of lower axial resistivity [167]. There is, however, some controversy concerning this point [193]. More detailed discussion on this subject has been published [167, 168, 193]. As a result of this heterogeneity of conduction, early premature impulses may block in some regions but conduct slowly through others. Conduction may be slow enough to allow the impulse eventually to excite areas of initial block and a functional reentrant circuit is established (❯ Fig. 1.28).

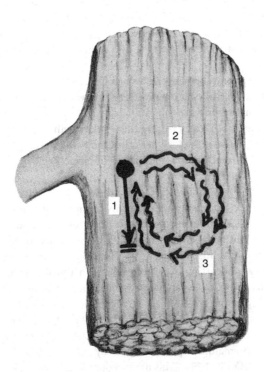

❑ Fig. 1.28
Diagram of reentry caused by anisotropic properties of cardiac muscle. An atrial trabeculum is shown. The direction of the long axis of the myocardial fibers is indicated by the *lines*. Conduction of an early stimulated premature impulse at the site where the *dot* is located blocks in the direction of the long axis of the myocardial fibers. Block is indicated by *arrow 1* and *horizontal lines*. Conduction of the premature impulse in the direction perpendicular to the long axis does not block but proceeds slowly (*arrow 2*), returning to the site of block after this region has recovered excitability (*arrow 3*)

An additional factor to be considered here is spiral wave reentry. Initially described as a physical-chemical phenomenon the principle behind spiral wave reentry is that for any rotating wave, the lip of the wave creates a spiral in moving through a surrounding medium [194]. The importance of this phenomenon may be appreciated by referring to leading circle reentry (❷ Fig. 1.27) where the core around which reentry occurs is rendered permanently inexcitable by centripetally conducting wavelets. In the leading circle setting, excitability is an essential determinant of reentry. However, wavefront curvature is also a critical factor in maintaining functional reentry [195] as even in the presence of excitable tissue, once a critical curvature is reached a wavefront may cease to propagate. In spiral wave reentry, the core is excitable (as opposed to the leading circle) but it is not excited: hence the fundamental difference between the two forms of reentry. Contributing to the occurrence of spiral wave reentry are such factors as tissue anisotropy, fibrosis and blood vessels [196].

1.5.3.3   Clinical Characteristics of Reentrant Excitation

Although it once was thought that arrhythmias caused by reentrant excitation could be distinguished readily from arrhythmias caused by other mechanisms either by their electrocardiographic characteristics or by the effects of clinical interventions, it now appears that this is not the case. For example, spontaneously occurring premature depolarizations occurring with fixed coupling to a preceding beat were thought to result mainly from reentrant excitation [197]. The coupling interval represented the time elapsed while the impulse was conducted through the reentrant circuit before reemerging to excite the heart. The coupling interval was fixed because the conduction pathway and conduction velocity did not change. However, it is now understood that conduction velocity through reentrant circuits can vary from beat to beat [1] and that the circuits sometimes may change in size, resulting in reentrant premature depolarizations with variable degrees of coupling. Furthermore, premature depolarizations with fixed coupling also to result from mechanisms other than reentry. One such example is triggered activity, described previously. Moreover, electrotonic interactions between conducted impulses and parasystolic foci also can cause fixed coupling [198, 199]. This mechanism will be explained in more detail in ❷ Sect. 1.6 dealing with arrhythmias caused by a combination of abnormalities of impulse initiation and impulse conduction.

Another distinguishing feature of reentrant tachycardias was believed to be their initiation by spontaneous or stimulated premature impulses occurring at critical cycle lengths. Yet it is now recognized that triggered activity can be induced in the same way. Properly timed premature impulses may initiate reentry by causing the necessary slow conduction and/or transient conduction block, if they are not present during the regular rhythm. Either or both may occur when the premature impulse encroaches on the relative refractory period of the tissue in the potential reentrant circuit. Overdrive stimulation also may cause reentry by inducing slow conduction or block. Reentry may be induced in either anatomical or functional circuits.

The influence of stimulated impulses on established tachycardias has also been considered to be a way in which reentrant excitation might be differentiated from other mechanisms causing arrhythmias. In general, it had been thought that termination of tachycardias by single stimulated premature impulses or by a period of overdrive stimulation (again, occurring at critical cycle lengths) identified reentry. However, it has been discussed how stimulation of the heart may not always affect reentrant tachycardias in this predicted way. The influence of stimulated impulses on reentry depends to a large extent on whether reentry is occurring in anatomical or functional circuits and whether or not an "excitable gap" is present in the circuit. The term "excitable gap" is used to describe a region in the reentrant circuit which has had the chance to recover full excitability before arrival of the reentering impulse [200]. During reentry caused by the leading circle mechanism in tissue with relatively uniform properties of conduction and refractoriness, no fully excitable gap exists because the crest of the reentrant impulse is conducting in the relatively refractory tissue it previously excited [189–191]. It is, therefore, very difficult for premature impulses induced by stimuli outside the reentrant circuit to penetrate the circuit and influence the tachycardia (❷ Fig. 1.29a). This may account for the failure of stimulated premature impulses to terminate rapid atrial flutter [201], or some sustained ventricular tachycardias which nevertheless for other reasons are believed to be caused by reentry [202].

On the other hand, there may often be an excitable gap in a circuit defined by anatomy in which the conduction time around the circuit takes longer than the full recovery time of cardiac fibers comprising the circuit. A properly timed premature impulse can then enter the circuit. The stimulated impulse might conduct around the circuit in the same way as the reentering impulse, thereby resetting the tachycardia, or it may block conduction of the reentering impulse and

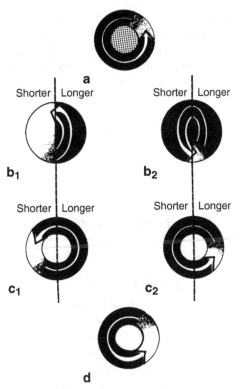

□ Fig. 1.29
Schematic representation of the effects of stimulated impulses on reentry in circuits with different properties. *Black* areas represent refractory tissue, *dotted* areas partially refractory tissue and white areas an excitable gap. Part **(a)** shows leading circle reentry over a functional pathway in which refractoriness is sufficiently uniform that there is no fully excitable gap. Parts **(b₁)** and **(b₂)** show functional pathway with an area of long refractoriness and an area of short refractoriness. In **(b₁)**, an excitable gap is present in the area with the short refractory period at the time the reentering impulse shown by the *arrow* is conducting in the region with the longer refractory period. The excitable gap is absent in **(b₂)** when the reentrant impulse is conducting through the region with the shorter refractory period. Parts **(c₁)** and **(c₂)** show an anatomic pathway with a region of long refractoriness and a region of short refractoriness. In **(c₁)**, an excitable gap exists in the region with the short refractory period while the reentering impulse, shown by the *arrow*, is conducting in the region with the longer refractory period. In **(c₂)**, an excitable gap is absent when the reentering impulse conducts through the region with the shorter refractory period **(c₂)**. Part **(d)** shows an anatomically defined pathway that is long enough in relation to the duration of refractoriness so that all parts of the pathway have a fully excitable gap (Reproduced with permission after Frame and Hoffman (1984) © Nijhoff, The Hague)

terminate the tachycardia. Termination of the tachycardia would be expected to occur when conduction of the stimulated impulse blocks in the circuit in the anterograde direction and collides with the reentering impulse in the retrograde direction (❷ Fig. 1.29d). These two examples of the possible lack of effect of stimulated impulses on leading circle reentry and termination of reentry in an anatomical pathway represents opposite extremes. Excitable gaps also may exist in functional circuits if there are large differences in the refractory periods or conduction velocities in different parts of the circuit [200]. A premature impulse then might be able to enter the circuit during the excitable gap in the region with the shorter refractory period while the reentrant impulse is conducting in the region with the longer refractory period or slower conduction velocity (❷ Fig. 1.29b). Conversely, no excitable gap exists in the circuit while the reentering impulse is conducting through the region with the shorter refractory period or more rapid conduction velocity. Some forms of atrial flutter, supraventricular tachycardias and ventricular tachycardias which can be terminated by premature impulses may be caused by reentry in functional circuits with an excitable gap. Excitable gaps might also be absent in some anatomic circuits if the impulse is conducting in relatively refractory tissue throughout the circuit because of a long refractory period or a short path length ($\bullet$ Fig. 1.29c$_2$) [200]. A means for considering the mechanism of an arrhythmia via its response to specific form of programmed electrical stimulation has been described by Waldo and associates [201, 202] as transient entrainment. By pacing at cycle lengths that permit capture of an arrhythmia and observing the characteristics of the paced beats as well as the pattern of interruption and reinitiation of the arrhythmias, reentry can be diagnosed with a high degree of certainty.

Overdrive stimulation can also terminate reentry when the stimulated impulses penetrate the reentrant circuit and block conduction [203]. The presence or absence of a fully excitable gap may also influence the effects of overdrive for the same reason discussed for single stimulated impulses.

1.6   Simultaneous Abnormalities of Impulse Initiation and Conduction

Abnormalities of impulse initiation and conduction are expected to coexist under certain conditions. Action potentials initiated by spontaneous diastolic depolarization or delayed afterdepolarizations may conduct very slowly or block if they arise at sufficiently low membrane potentials caused by diastolic depolarization [204, 205] Threshold potential also shifts to more positive values when the rate of diastolic depolarization is slow, ensuring that the action potentials arise from low membrane potentials. These action potentials have slow upstrokes and reduced amplitudes resulting from partial inactivation of the sodium channel. Slow conduction of the impulse arising from the abnormality in initiation may cause reentry [204]. Impulses propagating into regions with spontaneous diastolic depolarization or delayed afterdepolarization may also conduct slowly (and reenter) if they enter these regions late in the diastolic cycle, at a time when membrane potential has markedly deceased. If they invade these regions early in the cycle, prior to phase 4 depolarization, they will conduct more normally. The interrelationship between diastolic depolarization and conduction could be a cause of rate-dependent changes in conduction such as the appearance of right bundle branch block at long cycle lengths [206]. Impulses arising during phase 4 depolarization might also conduct more rapidly than normal, even when there is partial inactivation of the inward current if threshold potential is not shifted, since the amount of depolarizing current necessary to initiate an action potential would be reduced. This enhancement of conduction might occur when diastolic depolarization is relatively small.

The second major example of coexisting abnormalities of conduction and automaticity is the parasystolic focus. The existence of such a focus depends on the presence of entry block. The likelihood that the spontaneous impulses generated by the parasystolic focus will excite the heart depends on the ability of these impulses to propagate from the focus to surrounding fibers. If, because of marked phase 4 depolarization, the focus generates small, slowly rising action potentials, these may not be able to propagate or may propagate quite slowly. The degree of exit block thus might depend on the magnitude of phase 4 depolarization in the focus [3].

If a parasystolic focus with normal automaticity is coupled in an appropriate manner to the surrounding cardiac fiber, propagating activity of those fibers may influence the firing of the focus even though there is entry block [198, 199]. This may occur if there are electrotonic effects of the propagating impulses on phase 4 depolarization of the focus. Electrotonic current spread from action potentials arriving in the vicinity of the focus tends to depolarize the fibers in the focus during diastole (axial current flows toward the focus). The resulting subthreshold depolarization early in diastole inhibits subsequent phase 4 depolarization (possibly by inactivating the voltage dependent I_f), while late in diastole it shifts the membrane potential enough to cause activation of the fast inward current and thus accelerates firing ($\bullet$ Fig. 1.30). During phase 4 depolarization membrane resistance increases [43]. For this reason, as the action potential arrives at the site of entry block later and later during phase 4 depolarization of fibers in the parasystolic focus, it will cause a progressively larger change in their membrane potential. As the synchrony between the focus and the dominant rhythm changes and the propagating impulse arrives progressively later during phase 4, the cycle of the parasystolic focus will increase to a maximum, abruptly decrease to a minimum and then progressively increase to the control value [199]. This type of interaction between the dominant rhythm and the rhythm of the parasystolic focus means the parasystolic rhythms may show fixed or variable coupling or other complex interactions with the sinus rhythm. These are discussed in greater detail elsewhere [199]. Although electrotronic interactions are also expected to occur between the dominant rhythm and parasystolic

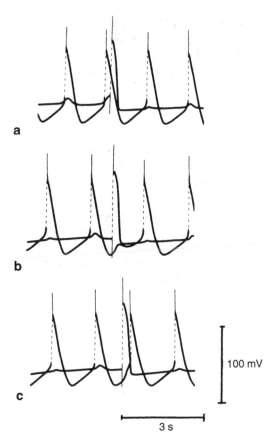

100 mV

3 s

☐ Fig. 1.30

Electrotonic interaction between propagated impulses and a parasystolic focus. In each part, transmembrane potentials recorded at two different sites are shown. The *top* traces in each show stimulated action potentials that cannot propagate into and excite a parasystolic focus; automatic firing in this focus is shown in the *bottom* traces. The focus also has a high grade of exit block as indicated by the failure of an action potential to occur in the top trace following a spontaneous impulse in the focus. The only action potentials seen in the top trace result from propagation from another site. In (**a**), the propagating impulse (*top trace*) occurs shortly after the impulse in the parasystolic focus and does not influence it. In (**b**), the propagating impulse occurs early during phase 4 depolarization in the focus. Electrotonic current spread from this impulse causes a sub-threshold depolarization early in diastole and this slows the rate of subsequent phase 4 depolarization. In (**c**), the propagating impulse occurs late in diastole of the parasystolic focus. Electrotonic current spread from the impulse accelerates the terminal portion of phase 4 depolarization and accelerates firing (Reproduced with permission after Jalife and Moe (1976) © American Research Association, Dallas, Texas)

focus with abnormal automaticity, the effects of the interactions cannot be predicted without an understanding of the voltage-dependence of the conductance causing the abnormal phase 4 depolarization.

1.7 Conclusion

The information we have discussed here on arrhythmogenic mechanisms has been derived mainly from experimental laboratory studies on isolated cardiac tissues and to a lesser extent from studies of intact animals, of ion channels and of the genetic determinants of specific arrhythmias. Approximately 20 years ago, in the first edition of this text, we wrote "there is a good possibility that pharmacological agents can be developed to modify the operation of these channels and suppress or abolish the arrhythmogenic mechanism"[207]. We stated this because we believed that "since the different mechanisms [for arrhythmias] utilize different channels with different properties, drugs which act specifically on one another of the mechanisms can be developed. Hence, rational therapy of arrhythmias in the future will consist in identifying the mechanism for a clinical arrhythmia by a specific clinical test and then selecting an appropriate drug to suppress that mechanism"[207].

Simply stated, we were naïve. As the CAST [208] and SWORD [102] trials have effectively demonstrated, attempts to use basic and clinical information available at the time to devise rational approaches to pharmacologic therapy resulted in excess mortality. This is not to say that newer and more selective and safer molecules will not be developed: but it is to admit that the goal is far more daunting than we had expected. In the meantime, the use of interventional techniques such as ablation [209] has had a high degree of success in selected arrhythmias and the advent of cardioverter-defibrillators has clearly improved the duration of life [210]. In other words, the device industry has provided interventions and expectations that pharmacology has not yet been able to deliver.

The final ingredient in our therapeutic mix is provided by the nascent field of gene and cell therapy. Although approaches here are very much in their infancy, early results hold out some promise that repair and replacement of, and therapy for, arrhythmogenic tissues may be within reach [211–216]. And having stated this, we very much still believe in our concluding statement of 20 years ago: "rational therapy of arrhythmias in the future will consist in identifying the mechanism for a clinical arrhythmia by a specific clinical test and then selecting an appropriate [intervention] to suppress that mechanism"[207].

Acknowledgements

The authors would like to thank Ms. Laureen Pagan for her careful attention to the preparation of this manuscript and Mr. Richard Haynes for illustration assistance.

References

1. Cranefield, P.F., A.L. Wit, and B.F. Hoffman, Genesis of cardiac arrhythmias. *Circulation*, 1973;**47**: 190–204.

2. Hoffman, B.F. and P.F. Cranefield, The physiological basis of cardiac arrhythmias. *Am. J. Med.*, 1964;**37**: 670–684.

3. Hoffman, B.F. and M.R. Rosen, Cellular mechanisms for cardiac arrhythmias. *Circ. Res.*, 1981;**49**: 1–15.

4. DiFrancesco, D. and C. Ojeda, Properties of the current i_f in the sino-atrial node of the rabbit compared with those of the current i_k in Purkinje fibers. *J. Physiol. London*, 1980;**308**: 35–37.

5. Biel, M., A. Schneider, and C. Wahl, Cardiac HCN channels: structure, function, and modulation. *Trends Cardiovas. Med.*, 2002;**12**: 206–212.

6. Yanagihara, K. and H. Irisawa, Potassium current during the pacemaker depolarization in rabbit sinoatrial node cell. *Pflügers Arch.*, 1980;**388**: 255–260.

7. Hoffman, B.F. and P.F. Cranefield, *Electrophysiology of the Heart*. New York: McGraw-Hill, 1960.

8. Hogan, P.M. and L.D. Davis, Evidence for specialized fibers in the canine atrium. *Circ. Res.*, 1968;**23**: 387–396.

9. Kokubun, S., M. Nishimura, A. Noma, and A. Irisawa, The spontaneous action potential of rabbit atrioventricular node cells. *Jpn. J. Physiol.*, 1980;**30**: 529–540.

10. Wit, A.L. and P.F. Cranefield, Triggered and automatic activity in the canine coronary sinus. *Circ. Res.*, 1977;**41**: 435–445.

11. Wit, A.L., J.J. Fenoglio Jr., B.M. Wagner, and A.L. Bassett, Electrophysiological properties of cardiac muscle in the anterior mitral valve leaflet and the adjacent atrium in the dog: possible implications for the genesis of atrial dysrhythmias. *Circ. Res.*, 1973;**32**: 731–745.

12. Vassalle, M., The relationship among cardiac pacemakers: overdrive suppression. *Circ. Res.*, 1977;**41**: 269–277.

13. Erlanger, J. and J.R. Blackman, A study of relative rhythmicity and conductivity in various regions of the auricles of the mammalian heart. *Am. J. Physiol.*, 1907;**19**: 125–174.

14. Hope, R.R., B.J. Scherlag, N. EI-Sherif, and R. Lazzara, Hierarchy of ventricular pacemakers. *Circ. Res.*, 1976;**39**: 883–888.

15. DiFrancesco, D., A new interpretation of the pace-maker current in calf Purkinje fibers. *J. Physiol. London*, 1981;**314**: 359–376.

16. DiFrancesco, D., A study of the ionic nature of the pace-maker current in calf Purkinje fibers. *J. Physiol. London*, 1981;**314**: 377–393.

17. Qu, J., A. Barbuti, L. Protas, B. Santoro, I.S. Cohen, and R.B. Robinson, HCN2 overexpression in newborn and adult ventricular myocytes: distinct effects on gating and excitability. *Circ. Res.*, 2001;**89**: E8–E14.

18. Vassalle, M., Electrogenic suppression of automaticity in sheep and dog Purkinje fibers. *Circ. Res.*, 1970;**27**: 361–377.

19. Vassalle, M., D.L. Caress, A.J. Slovin, and J.H. Stuckey, On the cause of ventricular asystole during vagal stimulation. *Circ. Res.*, 1967;**10**: 228–241.

20. Glitsch, H.G., Characteristics of active Na transport in intact cardiac cells. *Am. J. Physiol.*, 1979;**236**: H189–H199.

21. Gadsby, D.C. and P.F. Cranefield, Direct measurement of changes in sodium pump current in canine cardiac Purkinje fibers. *Proc. Natl. Acad. Sci. USA* 1979;**76**: 1783–1787.

22. January, C.T. and H.A. Fozzard, The effects of membrane potential, extracellular potassium and tetrodotoxin on the intracellular sodium ion activity of sheep cardiac muscle. *Circ. Res.*, 1984;**54**: 652–665.

23. Jordan, J.L., I. Yamaguchi, W.J. Mandel, and A.E. McCullen, Comparative effects of overdrive on sinus and subsidiary pacemaker function. *Am. Heart J.*, 1977;**93**: 367–374.

24. Kodama, I., J. Goto, S. Ando, J. Toyama, and K. Yamada, Effects of rapid stimulation on the transmembrane action potentials of rabbit Sinus node pacemaker cells. *Circ. Res.*, 1980;**46**: 90–99.

25. Gang, E.S., J.A. Reiffel, F.D. Livelli Jr., J.T. Bigger Jr., Sinus node recovery times following the spontaneous termination of supraventricular tachycardia and following atrial overdrive pacing: a comparison. *Am. Heart J.* 1983;**105**: 210–215.

26. Breithardt, G., L. Seipel, and F. Loogen, Sinus node recovery time and calculated sinoatrial conduction time in normal subjects and patients with sinus node dysfunction. *Circulation*, 1977;**56**: 43–50.

27. Van Capelle, F.J.L. and D. Durrer, Computer simulation of arrhythmias in a network of coupled excitable elements. *Circ. Res.*, 1980;**47**: 454–466.

28. Wit, A.L. and P.F. Cranefield, Mechanisms of impulse initiation in the atrioventricular junction and the effects of acetylstrophanthidin. *Am. J. Cardiol.*, 1982;**49**: 921.

29. Toda, N. and T.C. West, Changes in sino-atrial node transmembrane potentials on vagal stimulation of the isolated rabbit atrium. *Nature*, 1965;**205**: 808–809.

30. Erlanger, J. and A.D. Hirschfelder, Further studies on the physiology of heart block in mammals. *Am. J. Physiol.*, 1906;**15**: 153–206.

31. Ferrer, M.I., *The Sick Sinus Syndrome.* Mount Kisco, NY: Futura, 1974.

32. Dahl, G. and G. Isenberg, Decoupling of heart muscle cells: correlation with increased cytoplasmic calcium activity and with changes of nexus ultrastructure. *J. Membr. Biol.*, 1980;**53**: 63–75.

33. Weingart, R., The actions of ouabain on intercellular coupling and conduction velocity in mammalian ventricular muscle. *J. Physiol. London*, 1977;**264**: 341–365.

34. Ellis, D., The etTects of external cations and ouabain on the intracellular sodium activity of sheep heart Purkinje fibers. *J. Physiol. London*, 1977;**273**: 211–240.

35. Tsien, R.W., ETTect of epinephrine on the pacemaker potassium current of cardiac Purkinje fibers. *J. Gen. Physiol.*, 1974;**64**: 293–319.

36. Pliam, M.B., D.J. Krellenstein, M. Vassalle, and C.M. Brooks, The influence of norepinephrine, reserpine and propranolol on overdrive suppression. *J. Electrocardiol.*, 1975;**8**: 17–24.

37. Armour, J.A., G.R. Hageman, and W.C. Randall, Arrhythmias induced by local cardiac nerve stimulation. *Am. J. Physiol.*, 1972;**223**: 1068–1075.

38. Randall, W.C., Sympathetic control of the heart, in, ed. *Neural Regulation of the Heart*, WC Randall, Editor. New York: Oxford University Press, 1977, pp. 45–94.

39. Vassalle, M., M.J. Levine, and J.H. Stuckey, On the sympathetic control of ventricular automaticity; the effects of stellate ganglion stimulation. *Circ. Res.*, 1968;**23**: 249–258.

40. Katzung, B.G., L.M. Hondeghem, and A.O. Grant, Cardiac ventricular automaticity induced by current of injury. *Pflügers Arch.*, 1975;**360**: 193–197.

41. Janse, M.J. and F.J.L. van Capelle, Electrotonic interactions across an inexcitable region as a cause of ectopic activity in acute regional myocardial ischemia. A study in intact porcine and canine hearts and computer models. *Circ. Res.*, 1982;**50**: 527–537.

42. Rosen, M.R., H. Gelband, C. Merker, and B.F. Hoffman, Mechanisms of digitalis toxicity: effects of ouabain on phase four of canine Purkinje fiber transmembrane potentials. *Circulation*, 1973;**47**: 681–689.

43. Vassalle, M., Cardiac pacemaker potentials at different extra- and intracellular K concentrations. *Am. J. Physiol.*, 1965;**208**: 770–775.

44. Deck, K.A., Anderungen des Ruhepotentials und der Kabeleigenschaften von Purkinje 'Faden bei der Dehnung. *Pflügers Arch.*, 1964;**280**: 131–140.

45. Mary-Rabine, L., A.J. Hordof, P. Danilo Jr., J.R. Maim, and M.R. Rosen, Mechanisms for impulse initiation in isolated human atrial fibers. *Circ. Res.*, 1980;**47**: 267–277.

46. Hoppe, U.C. and D.J. Beuckelmann, Characterization of the hyperpolarization-activated inward current in isolated human atrial myocytes. *Cardiovasc. Res.*, 1998;**38**: 788–801.

47. Yu, H., F. Chang, and I.S. Cohen, Pacemaker current I_f in adult canine cardiac ventricular myocytes. *J. Physiol.*, 1995;**485**: 469–483.

48. Cerbai, E., M. Barbieri, and A. Mugelli, Occurrence and properties of the hyperpolarization-activated current I_f in ventricular myocytes from normotensive and hypertensive rats during aging. *Circulation*, 1996;**94**: 1674–1481.

49. Cerbai, E., R. Pino, F. Porciatti, G. Sani, M. Toscano, M. Maccherini, G. Giunti, and A. Mugelli, Characterization of the hyperpolarization-activated current, I_f, in ventricular myocytes from human failing heart. *Circulation*, 1997;**95**: 568–571.

50. Cerbai, E., L. Sartiani, P. DePaoli, R. Pino, M. Maccherini, F. Bizzarri, F. DiCiolla, G. Davoli, G. Sani, and A. Mugelli, The properties of the pacemaker current I_f in human ventricular myocytes are modulated by cardiac disease. *J. Mol. Cell Cardiol.*, 2001;**33**: 441–448.

51. Katzung, B.G. and J.A. Morgenstern, Effects of extracellular potassium on ventricular automaticity and evidence for a pacemaker current in mammalian ventricular myocardium. *Circ. Res.*, 1977;**40**: 105–111.

52. Imanishi, S. and B. Surawicz, Automatic activity in depolarized guinea pig ventricular myocardium: characteristics and mechanisms. *Circ. Res.*, 1976;**39**: 751–759.

53. Brown, H.F. and S.J. Noble, Membrane currents underlying delayed rectification and pace-maker activity in frog atrial muscle. *J. Physiol. London*, 1969;**204**: 717–736.

54. Imanishi, S., Calcium-sensitive discharges in canine Purkinje fibers. *Jpn. J. Physiol.*, 1971;**21**: 443–463.

55. Cranefield, P.F., *The Conduction of the Cardiac Impulse: The Slow Response and Cardiac Arrhythmias.* Mount Kisco, NY: Futura, 1975.

56. Noble, D. and R.W. Tsien, The kinetics and rectifier properties of the slow potassium current in cardiac Purkinje fibers. *J. Physiol. London*, 1968;**195**: 185–214.

57. Hodgkin, A.L. and B. Katz, The effect of sodium ions on the electrical activity of the giant axon of the squid. *J. Physiol. London*, 1949;**108**: 37–77.

58. Gadsby, D.C. and A.L. Wit, Electrophysiologic characteristics of cardiac cells and the genesis of cardiac arrhythmias, in *Cardiac Pharmacology*, RD Wilkersen, Editor. New York: Academic Press, 1981, pp. 229–274.

59. Gadsby, D.C. and P.F. Cranefield, Two levels of resting potential in cardiac Purkinje fibers. *J. Gen. Physiol.*, 1977; **70**:725–746.

60. Wit, A.L. and P.F. Cranefield, Triggered activity in cardiac muscle fibers of the simian mitral valve. *Circ. Res.*, 1976;**38**: 85–98.

61. Dresdner, K.P., R.P. Kline, and A.L. Wit, Cytoplasmic K^+ and Na^+ activity in subendocardial canine Purkinje fibers from one day old infarcts using double-barrel ion selective electrodes: comparison with maximum diastolic potential. *Biophys. J.*, 1985;**47**: 463a.

62. Friedman, P.L., J.R. Stewart, and A.L. Wit, Spontaneous and induced cardiac arrhythmias in subendocardial Purkinje fibers surviving extensive myocardial infarction in dogs. *Circ. Res.*, 1973;**33**: 612–626.

63. Lazzara, R., N. EI-Sherif, and B.J. Scherlag, Electrophysiological properties of canine Purkinje cells in one-day-old myocardial infarction. *Circ. Res.*, 1973;**33**: 722–734.

64. Hordof, A.J., R. Edie, J.R. Maim, B.F. Hoffman, and M.R. Rosen, Electrophysiological properties and response to pharmacologic agents of fibers from diseased human atria. *Circulation*, 1976;**54**: 774–779.

65. Ten Eick, R.E. and D.H. Singer, Electrophysiological properties of diseased human atrium. I. Low diastolic potential and altered cellular response to potassium. *Circ. Res.*, 1979;**44**: 545–557.

66. Singer, D.H., C.M. Baumgarten, and R.E. Ten Eick, Cellular electrophysiology of ventricular and other dysrhythmias: studies on diseased and ischemic heart. *Prog. Cardiovasc. Dis.*, 1981;**24**: 97–156.

67. Carmeliet, E., The slow inward current: non-voltage-clamp studies, in *The Slow Inward Current and Cardiac Arrhythmias*, D.P. Zipes, J.C. Bailey, and V. Elharrar, Editors. The Hague: Nijhoff, 1980, pp. 97–110.

68. Hoffman, B.F. and K.H. Dangman, Are arrhythmias caused by automatic impulse generation? in *Normal and Abnormal Conduction In the Heart*, A. Paes de Carvalho, B.F. Hoffman, M. Lieberman, Editors. Mount Kisco, NY: Futura, 1982, pp. 429–448.

69. Dangman, K.H. and B.F. Hoffman, Studies on overdrive stimulation of canine cardiac Purkinje fibers: maximal diastolic potential as a determinant of the response. *J. Am. Coll. Cardiol.*, 1983;**2**: 1183–1190.

70. Falk, R.T. and I.S. Cohen, Membrane current following activity in canine cardiac Purkinje fibers. *J. Gen. Physiol.*, 1984;**83**: 771–799.

71. Mullins, L.J., *Ton Transport in Heart*. New York: Raven, 1981.

72. Ferrier, G.R. and J.E. Rosenthal, Automaticity and entrance block induced by focal depolarization of mammalian ventricular tissues. *Circ. Res.*, 1980;**47**: 238–248.

73. Hume, J. and B.G. Katzung, Physiological role of endogenous amines in the modulation of ventricular automaticity in the guinea-pig. *J. Physiol. London*, 1980;**309**: 275–286.

74. Lange, G., Action of driving stimuli from intrinsic and extrinsic sources on in situ cardiac pacemaker tissues. *Circ. Res.*, 1965;**17**: 449–459.

75. Goldreyer, B.N., J.J. Gallagher, and A.N. Damato, The electrophysiologic demonstration of atrial ectopic tachycardia in man. *Am. Heart J.*, 1973;**85**: 205–215.

76. Le Marec, H., K.H. Dangman, P. Danilo Jr., and M.R. Rosen, An evaluation of automaticity and triggered activity in the canine heart one to four days after myocardial infarction. *Circulation*, 1985;**71**: 1224–1236.

77. Wellens, H.J.J., Value and limitations of programmed electrical stimulation of the heart in the study and treatment of tachycardias. *Circulation*, 1978;**57**: 845–853.

78. Bonke, F.I.M., L.N. Bouman, H.E. vap Rijn, Change of cardiac rhythm in the rabbit after an atrial premature beat. *Circ. Res.*, 1969;**24**: 533–544.

79. Klein, H.O., D.H. Singer, B.F. Hoffman, Effects of atrial premature systoles on sinus rhythm in the rabbit. *Circ. Res.*, 1973;**32**: 480–491.

80. Klein, H.O., P.F. Cranefield, and B.F. Hoffman, Effect of extrasystoles on idoventricular rhythm. *Circ. Res.*, 1972;**30**: 651–615.

81. Cranefield, P.F., Action potentials, afterpotentials, and arrhythmias. *Circ. Res.*, 1977;**41**: 415–423.

82. Wit, A.L., P.F. Cranefield, and D.C. Gadsby, Triggered activity, in *The Slow Inward Current and Cardiac Arrhythmias*, D.P. Zipes, J.C. Bailey, and V. Elharrar, Editors. The Hague: Nijhoff, 1980, pp. 437–454.

83. Attwell, D., I. Cohen, D. Eisner, M. Ohba, and C. Ojeda, The steady state lTX-sensitive ("window") sodium current in cardiac Purkinje fibers. *Pftügers Arch.*, 1979;**379**: 137–142.

84. Reuter, H., Properties of two inward membrane currents in the heart. *Annu. Rev. Physiol.*, 1979;**41**: 413–424.

85. Jurkiewicz, N.K. and M.C. Sanguinetti, Rate-dependent prolongation of cardiac action potentials by a methanesulfonanilide class III antiarrhythmic agent. Specific block of rapidly activating delayed rectifier K+ current by dofetilide. *Circ. Res.*, 1993;**72**: 75–83.

86. Gadsby, D.C. and P.F. Cranefield, Electrogenic sodium extrusion in cardiac Purkinje fibers. *J. Gen. Physiol.*, 1979;**73**: 819–837.

87. January, C. and J.M. Riddle, Early afterdepolarizations: mechanisms of induction and block. A role for the L type Ca current. *Circ. Res.*, 1989;**64**: 977–990.

88. Volders, P.G., A. Kulcsar, M.A. Vos, K.R. Sipido, H.J. Wellens, R. Lazzara, and B. Szabo, Similarities between early and delayed after depolarizations induced by isoproterenol in canine ventricular myocytes. *Cardiovasc. Res.*, 1997;**34**: 348–359.

89. Wu, Y., D.M. Roden, and M.E. Anderson, CaM kinase inhibition prevents development of the arrhythmogenic transient inward current. *Circ. Res.*, 1999;**84**: 906–912.

90. Schmidt, R.F., Versuche mit Aconitin zum Problem der spontanen Erregungsbildung im Herzen. *Pftügers Arch.*, 1960;**271**: 526–536.

91. Matsuda, K., B.F. Hoffman, C.N. Ellner, M. Katz, C.Mc. Brooks, Veratrine induced prolongation of repolarisation in the mammalian heart, in *Proceeding of the 19th International Physiological Congress*, Montreal, 1953, pp. 596–597.

92. Trautwein, W., U. Gottstein, and J. Dudel, Der Aktionsstrom der Myokardfaser im Sauerstoffmangel. *Pflügers Arch.*, 1954;**260**: 40–60.

93. Coraboeuf, E. and J. Boistel, L'action des taux eleves de gaz carbonique sur Ie tissu cardiaque, etudiee a l'aide de microelectrodes intracellulaires. *C. R. Soc. Bioi. Paris*, 1953;**147**: 654–665.

94. Brooks, C.Mc., B.F. Hoffman, E.E. Suckling, and O. Orias, *Excitability of the Heart*. New York: Grune and Stratton, 1955.

95. Strauss, H.C., J.T. Bigger Jr., and B.F. Hoffman, Electrophysiological and beta-receptor blocking effects of MJ 1999 on dog and rabbit cardiac tissue. *Circ. Res.*, 1970;**26**: 661–678.

96. Dangman, K.H. and B.F. Hoffman, *In vivo* and *in vitro* antiarrhythmic and arrhythmogenic effects of *N*-acetyl procainamide. *J. Pharmacol. Exp. Ther.*, 1981;**217**: 851–862.

97. Elonen, E., P.J. Neuvonan, L. Tarssanen, and R. Kala, Sotalol intoxication with prolonged Q-T interval and severe tachyarrhythmias. *BMJ*, 1979;**1**: 1184.

98. Krikler, D.M. and P.V.L. Curry, *Torsatk de pointes*: an atypical ventricular tachycardia. *Br. Heart J.*, 1976;**38**: 117–120.

99. Brachmann, J., B.J. Scherlag, L.Y. Rosenshtraukh, R. Lazzara, Bradycardia-dependent triggered activity: relevance to drug-induced multiform ventricular tachycardia. *Circulation*, 1983;**68**: 846–856.

100. Volders, P.G., K.R. Sipido, M.A. Vos, R.L. Spatjens, J.D. Leunissen, E. Carmeliet, H.J. Wellens, Downregulation of delayed rectifier K(+) currents in dogs with chronic complete atrioventricular block and acquired torsades de pointes. *Circulation*, 1999;**100**: 2455–2461.

101. Belardinelli, L., C. Antzelevitch, M.A. Vos, Assessing predictors of drug-induced torsade de pointes. *Trends Pharmacol. Sci.*, 2003;**24**: 619–625.

102. Pratt, C.M., A.J. Camm, W. Cooper, P.L. Friedman, D.J. MacNeil, K.M. Moulton, B. Pitt, P.J. Schwartz, E.P. Veltri, and A.L. Waldo, Mortality in the survival with oral D-sotalol (SWORD) trial: why did patients die? *Am. J. Cardiol.*, 1998;**81**: 869–876.

103. Damiano, B.P. and M.R. Rosen, Effects of pacing on triggered activity induced by early afterdepolarizations. *Circulation*, 1984;**69**: 1013–1025.

104. Rosen, M.R., H. Gelband, and B.F. Hoffman, Correlation between effects of ouabain on the canine electrocardiogram and transmembrane potentials of isolated Purkinje fibers. *Circulation*, 1973;**47**: 65–72.

105. Ferrier, G.R., J.H. Saunders, and C. Mendez, A cellular mechanism for the generation of ventricular arrhythmias by acetylstrophanthidin. *Circ. Res.*, 1973;**32**: 600–609.

106. Davis, L.D., Effect of changes in cycle length on diastolic depolarization produced by ouabain in canine Purkinje fibers. *Circ. Res.*, 1973;**32**: 206–214.

107. Ferrier, G.R., Digitalis arrhythmias: role of oscillatory afterpotentials. *Prog. Cardiovasc. Dis.*, 1977;**19**: 459–474.

108. Akera, T. and T.M. Brody, The role of Na$^+$, K$^+$ ATPase in the inotropic action of digitalis. *Pharmacol. Rev.*, 1977;**29**: 187–220.

109. Eisner, D.A. and W.J. Lederer, Inotropic and arrhythmogenic effects of potassium-depleted solutions on mammalian cardiac muscle. *J. Physiol. London*, 1979;**294**: 255–277.

110. Nathan, D. and G.W. Beeler Jr., Electrophysiologic correlates of the inotropic effect of isoproterenal in canine myocardium. *J. Mol. Cell. Cardiol.*, 1975;**7**: 1–15.

111. Dangman, K.H., P. Danilo Jr., A.J. Hordof, L. Mary-Rabine, R.F. Reder, and M.R. Rosen, Electrophysiologic characteristics of human ventricular and Purkinje fibers. *Circulation*, 1982;**65**: 362–368.

112. Saito, T., M. Otoguro, and T. Matsubara, Electrophysiological studies on the mechanism of electrically induced sustained rhythmic activity in the rabbit right atrium. *Circ. Res.*, 1978;**42**: 199–206.

113. Aronson, R.S., Afterpotentials and triggered activity in hypertrophied myocardium from rats with renal hypertension. *Circ. Res.*, 1981;**48**: 120–127.

114. EI-Sherif, N., W.B. Gough, R.H. Zeiler, and R. Mehra, Triggered ventricular rhythm in I-day-old myocardial infarction in the dog. *Circ. Res.*, 1983;**52**: 566–579.

115. Chen, Y.J., S.A. Chen, M.S. Chang, and C.I. Lin, Arrhythmogenic activity of cardiac muscle in pulmonary veins of the dog: implication for the genesis of atrial fibrillation. *Cardiovas. Res.* 2000;**48**: 265–273.

116. Haissaguerre, M., P. Jais, D.C. Shah, A. Takahashi, M. Hocini, G. Quiniou, S. Garrigue, A. Le Mouroux, P. Le Metayer, and J. Clementy, Spontaneous initiation of atrial fibrillation by ectopic beats originating in the pulmonary veins. *N. Engl. J. Med.*, 1998;**339**: 659–666.

117. Braunwald, E., J. Ross Jr., and E.H. Sonnenblick, *Mechanisms of Contraction of the Normal and Failing Heart*. Boston, MA: Little, Brown, 1976.

118. Clusin, W.T., M. Buchbinder, A.K. Ellis, R.S. Kemoff, J.C. Giacomini, and D.C. Harrison, Reduction of ischemic depolarization by the calcium blocker diltiazem. Correlation with improvement of ventricular conduction and early arrhythmias in the dog. *Circ. Res.*, 1984;**54**: 10–20.

119. Kass, R.S., R.W. Tsien, and R. Weingart, Ionic basis of transient inward current induced by strophanthidin in cardiac Purkinje fibres. *J. Physiol. London*, 1978;**281**: 209–226.

120. Kass, R.S., W.J. Lederer, R.W. Tsien, and R. Weingart, Role of calcium ions in transient inward currents and after contractions induced by strophanthidin in cardiac Purkinje fibres. *J. Physiol. London*, 1978;**281**: 187–208.

121. Vassalle, M. and A. Mugelli, An oscillatory current in sheep cardiac Purkinje fibers. *Circ. Res.*, 1981;**48**: 618–631.

122. Karagueuzian, H.S. and B.G. Katzung, Voltage-damp studies of transient inward current and mechanical oscillations induced by ouabain in ferret papillary muscle. *J. Physiol. London*, 1982;**327**: 255–271.

123. Tseng, G.N. A.L. Wit, Characteristics of a transient inward current causing catecholamine induced triggered atrial tachycardia. *Circulation*, 1984;**70**(Suppl. II): 221.

124. Reuter, H., The dependence of slow inward current in Purkinje fibres on the extracellular calcium-concentration. *J. Physiol. London*, 1967;**192**: 479–492.

125. Ferrier, G.R., Effects of transmembrane potential on oscillatory afterpotentials induced by acetylstrophanthidin in canine ventricular tissues. *J. Pharmacol. Exp. Ther.*, 1980;**215**: 332–341.

126. Tsien, R.W., R.S. Kass, and R. Weingart, Cellular and subcellular mechanisms of cardiac pacemaker oscillations. *J. Exp. Biol.*, 1979;**81**: 205–215.

127. Ter Keurs, H.E.D.J. and P.A. Boyden, Ca^{2+} and arrhythmias, in *Foundations of Cardiac Arrhythmias*, P.M. Spooner and M.R. Rosen, Editors. New York: Marcel Dekker Inc, 2000, pp. 287–317.

128. Colquhoun, D., E. Neher, H. Reuter, and C.F. Stevens, Inward current channels activated by intracellular Ca in cultured cardiac cells. *Nature*, 1981;**294**: 752–754.

129. Arlock, P. and B.G. Katzung, Effects of sodium substitutes on transient inward current and tension in guinea-pig and ferret papillary muscle. *J. Physiol. London*, 1985;**360**: 105–120.

130. Rosen, M.R. and P. Danilo Jr., Digitalis-induced delayed afterdepolarizations, in *The Slow Inward Current and Cardiac Arrhythmias*, D.P. Zipes, J.C. Bailey, and V. Elharrar Editors. The Hague: Nijhoff, 1980, pp. 417–435.

131. Wit, A.L., P.F. Cranefield, and D.C. Gadsby, Electrogenic sodium extrusion can stop triggered activity in the canine coronary sinus. *Circ. Res.*, 1981;**49**: 1029–1042.

132. Kline, R.P., M.S. Siegal, J. Kupersmith, and A.L. Wit, Effects of strophanthidin on changes in extracellular potassium during triggered activity in the arrhythmic canine coronary sinus. *Circulation*, 1982;**66**(Suppl. 2): 356.

133. Kline, R.P. and M. Morad, Potassium efflux in heart muscle during activity: extracellular accumulation and its implications. *J. Physiol.*, 1978;**280**: 537–558.

134. Rosen, M.R. and R.F. Reder, Does triggered activity have a role in the genesis of cardiac arrhythmias? *Ann. Intern. Med.*, 1981;**94**: 794–801.

135. Moak, J.P. and M.R. Rosen, Induction and termination of triggered activity by pacing in isolated canine Purkinje fibers. *Circulation*, 1984;**69**: 149–162.

136. Schwartz, P.J., The idiopathic long, Q.T., syndrome: progress and questions. *Am. Heart J.*, 1985;**109**: 399–411.

137. Schwartz, P.J., Prevention of the arrhythmias in the long QT syndrome. in *Medical Management of Cardiac Arrhythmias*, H.E. Kulbertus, Editor. Edinburgh: Churchill Livingston, 1986, pp. 153–156.

138. Keating, M.T., D. Atkinson, C. Dunn, K. Timothy, G.M. Vincent, and M. Leppert, Linkage of a cardiac arrhythmia, the long QT, and the Harvey ras-1 gene. *Science*, 1991;**252**: 704–706.

139. Towbin, J.A. and K. Schwartz, Genetic approaches and familial arrhythmias, in *Foundations of Cardiac Arrhythmias*, P.M. Spooner and M.R. Rosen, Editors. New York: Marcel Dekker Inc, 2000, pp. 665–699.

140. Splawski, I., M. Tristani-Firouzi, M.H. Lehmann, M.C. Sanguinetti, and M.T. Keating, Mutations in the hminK gene cause long QT syndrome and suppress I_{Ks} function. *Nat. Genet.*, 1997;**17**: 338–340.

141. Abbott, G.W., F. Sesti, I. Splawski, M.E. Buck, M.H. Lehmann, K.W. Timothy, M.T. Keating, and S.A. Goldstein, MiRP1 forms I_{Kr} potassium channels with HERG and is associated with cardiac arrhythmia. *Cell*, 1999;**97**: 175–187.

142. Chen, Q., G.E. Kirsch, D. Zhang, R. Brugada, J. Brugada, P. Brugada, D. Potenza, A. Moya, M. Borggrefe, G. Breithardt, R. Ortiz-Lopez, Z. Wang, C. Antzelevitch, R.E. O'Brien, E. Schulze-Bahr, M.T. Keating, J.A. Towbin, and Q. Wang, Genetic basis and molecular mechanism for idiopathic ventricular fibrillation. *Nature* 1998;**392**: 293–296.

143. Ellinor, P.T. and C.A. Macrae, The genetics of atrial fibrillation. *J. Cardiovasc. Electrophysiol.*, 2003;**14**: 1007–1009.

144. Moe, G.K., On the multiple wavelet hypothesis of atrial fibrillation. *Arch. Int. Pharmacodyn.*, 1962;**140**: 183–188.

145. Moe, G.K., W.C. Rheinboldt, and J.A. Abildskov, A computer model of atrial fibrillation. *Am. Heart J.*, 1964; **67**: 200–220.

146. Coumel, P., P. Attuel, J. Lavallee, D. Flammang, J.F. Leclercq, and R. Slama, Syndrome d'arythmie auriculaire d'origine vagale. *Arch. Mal. Coeur Vaiss.*, 1978;**71**: 645–656.

147. Janse, M.J. and A.G. Kleber, Electrophysiological changes and ventricular arrhythmias in the early phase of regional myocardial ischemia. *Circ. Res.*, 1981;**49**: 1069–1081.

148. Myerburg, R.J., H. Gelband, K. Nilsson, et al., Long term electrophysiological abnormalities resulting from experimental myocardial infarction in cats. *Circ. Res.*, 1977;**41**: 73–84.

149. Sasyniuk, B.I. and C. Mendez, A mechanism for reentry in canine ventricular tissue. *Circ. Res.*, 1971;**28**: 3–15.

150. Alessi, R., M. Nusynowitz, J.A. Abildskov, G.K. Moe, Nonuniform distribution of vagal effects on the atrial refractory period. *Am. J. Physiol.*, 1958;**194**: 406–410.

151. Zhou, S., L.S. Chen, Y. Miyauchi, M. Miyauchi, S. Kar, S. Kangavari, M.C. Fishbein, B. Sharifi, and P.S. Chen, Mechanisms of cardiac nerve sprouting after myocardial infarction in dogs. *Circ. Res.*, 2004;**95**: 76–83.

152. Mendez, C. and G.K. Moe, Demonstration of a dual A-V nodal conduction system in the isolated rabbit heart. *Circ. Res.*, 1966;**19**: 378–393.

153. Allessie, M.A. and F.I.M. Bonke, Direct demonstration of sinus node reentry in the rabbit heart. *Circ. Res.*, 1979;**44**: 557–568.

154. Severs, N.J., S.R. Coppen, E. Dupont, H.I. Yeh, Y.S. Ko, T. Matsushita, Gap junction alterations in human cardiac disease. *Cardiovasc. Res.*, 2004;**62**: 368–377.

155. van Veen, A.A., H.V. van Rijen, and T. Opthof, Cardiac gap junction channels: modulation of expression and channel properties. *Cardiovasc. Res.*, 2001;**51**: 217–229.

156. Thomas, S.P., J.P. Kucera, L. Bircher-Lehmann, Y. Rudy, J.E. Saffitz, A.G. Kleber, Impulse propagation in synthetic strands of neonatal cardiac myocytes with genetically reduced levels of connexin43. *Circ. Res.*, 2003;**92**: 1209–1216.

157. Wit, A.L. and P.F. Cranefield, Reentrant excitation as a cause of cardiac arrhythmias. *Am. J. Physiol.*, 1978;**235**: H1–H17.

158. Mines, G.R., On circulating excitations in heart muscles and their possible relation to tachycardia and fibrillation. *Trans. R. Soc. Can.*, 1914; Ser. 3, 8: Sect. IV, 43–52.

159. Mayer, A.G., Rhythmical pulsation in Scyphomedusae-II. *Carnegie Inst. Washington. Papers Tortugas Lab.*, 1908;**I**: 113–131.

160. Page, R.L., L.H. Frame, and B.F. Hoffman, Circus movement in the tricuspid ring: an in vitro model. *J. Am. Coll. Cardiol.*, 1984;**3**: 478.

161. Fozzard, H.A., Conduction of the action potential, in *Handbook of Physiology. Section 2: The Cardiovascular System*, vol. I, *The Heart*, R.M. Berne and N. Sperelakis, Editors. Bethesda, MD: American Physiological Society, 1979, pp. 335–356.

162. Carmeliet, E. and J. Vereecke, Electrogenesis of the action potential and automaticity, in *Handbook of Physiology. Section 2: The Cardiovascular System*, vol. I, *The Heart*, R.M. Berne and N. Sperelakis, Editors. Bethesda, MD: American Physiological Society, 1979, pp. 269–334.

163. Hodgkin, A.L., *The Conduction of the Nervous Impulse*. Springfield, IL: Thomas, 1964.

164. Weidmann, S., The effect of the cardiac membrane potential on the rapid availability of the sodium-carrying system. *J. Physiol. London*, 1955;**127**: 213–224.

165. Tsien, R.W., Calcium channels in excitable cell membranes. *Annu. Rev. Physiol.* 1983;**45**: 341–358.

166. Zipes, D.P. and C. Mendez, Action of manganese ions and tetrodotoxin on atrioventricular nodal transmembrane potentials in isolated rabbit hearts. *Circ. Res.*, 1973;**32**: 447–454.

167. Spach, M.S., W.T. Miller 3rd, D.B. Geselowitz, R.C. Barr, J.M. Kootsey, and E.A. Johnson, The discontinuous nature of propagation in normal canine cardiac muscle: evidence for recurrent discontinuities of intracellular resistance that effect the membrane currents. *Circ. Res.*, 1981;**48**: 39–54.

168. Spach, M.S., W.T. Muller 3rd, P.C. Dolber, J.M. Kootsey, J.R. Sommer, C.E. Mosher Jr., The functional role of structural complexities in the propagation of depolarization in the atrium of the dog: cardiac conduction disturbances due to discontinuities of effective axial resistivity. *Circ. Res.*, 1982;**50**: 175–191.

169. Clerc, L., Directional differences of impulse spread in trabecular muscle from mammalian heart. *J. Physiol. London*, 1976;**2S5**: 335–346.

170. Ursell, P.C., P.I. Gardner, A. Albala, J.J. Fenoglio Jr., A.L. Wit, Structural and electrophysiological changes in the epicardial border zone of canine myocardial infarcts during infarct healing. *Circ. Res.*, 1985;**56**: 436–451.

171. Spach, M.S. and P.C. Dolber, Relating extracellular potentials and their derivatives to anisotropic propagation at a microscopic level in human cardiac muscle. Evidence for electrical uncoupling of side-to-side fiber connections with increasing age. *Circ. Res.*, 1986;**58**: 356–371.

172. Spach, M.S., P.C. Dolber, and J.F. Heidlage, Influence of the passive anisotropic properties on directional differences in propagation following modification of the sodium conductance in human atrial muscle. A model of reentry base on anisotropic discontinuous propagation. *Circ. Res.*, 1988;**62**: 811–832.

173. Spach, M.S. and M.E. Josephson, Initiating reentry: the role of nonuniform anisotropy in small circuits. *J. Cardiovasc. Electrophysiol.*, 1994;**5**: 182–209.

174. Lake, F.R., K.J. Cullen, N.H. de Klerk, M.G. McCall, D.L. Rosman, Atrial fibrillation and mortality in an elderly population. *Aust. NZ J. Med.*, 1989;**19**: 321–326.

175. Antzelevitch, C. and M.S. Spach, Impulse conduction: continuous and discontinuous, in *Foundations of Cardiac Arrhythmias*, P.M. Spooner and M.R. Rosen, Editors. New York: Marcel Dekker Inc, 2000, pp. 205–241.

176. Page, E. and Y. Shibata, Permeable junctions between cardiac cells. *Annu. Rev. Physiol.*, 1981;**43**: 431–441.

177. Wojtczak, J., Contractures and increase in internal longitudinal resistance of cow ventricular muscle induced by hypoxia. *Circ. Res.*, 1979;**44**: 88–95.

178. Joyner, R.W., Effects of the discrete pattern of electrical coupling on propagation through an electrical syncytium. *Circ. Res.*, 1982;**50**: 192–200.

179. Joyner, R.W., R. Veenstra, D. Rawling, and A. Chorro, Propagation through electrically coupled cells. Effects of a resistive barrier. *Biophys. J.*, 1984;**45**: 1017–1025.

180. Goldstein, S.S. and W. Rail, Changes of action potential shape and velocity for changing core conductor geometry. *Biophys. J.*, 1974;**14**: 731–757.

181. Dodge, F.A. and P.F. Cranefield, Nonuniform conduction in cardiac Purkinje fibers, in *Normal and Abnormal Conduction in the Heart*, A. Paes de Carvalho, B.F. Hoffman, and M. Lieberman, Editors. Mount Kisco, NY: Futura, 1982, pp. 379–395.

182. Wit, A.L., P.F. Cranefield, and B.F. Hoffman, Slow conduction and reentry in the ventricular conducting system II. Singly and sustained circus movement in networks of canine and bovine Purkinje fibers. *Circ. Res.*, 1972;**30**: 11–22.

183. Boyden, P.A., L.P. Tilley, A. Albala, S.K. Liu, J.J. Fenoglio Jr., and A. Wit, Mechanisms for atrial arrhythmias associated with cardiomyopathy: a study of feline hearts with primary myocardial disease. *Circulation*, 1984;**69**: 1036–1047.

184. Moe, G.K., C. Mendez, J. Han, and A.V. Aberrant, Impulse propagation in the dog heart: a study of functional bundle branch block. *Circ. Res.*, 1965;**16**: 261–286.

185. Gallagher, J.J., M. Gilbert, R.H. Svenson, W.C. Sealy, J. Kasell, A.G. Wallace, Wolff-Parkinson-White syndrome: the problem, evaluation, and surgical correction. *Circulation*, 1975;**51**: 767–785.

186. Frame, L.H., R.L. Page, P.A. Boyden, and B.F. Hoffman, A right atrial incision that stabilizes reentry around the tricuspid ring in dogs. *Circulation*, 1983;**68**(Suppl. 3): 361.

187. Antzelevitch, C., J. Jalife, G.K. Moe, Characteristics of reflection as a mechanism of reentrant arrhythmias and its relationship to parasystole. *Circulation*, 1980;**61**: 182–191.

188. Jalife, J. and G.K. Moe, Excitation, conduction, and reflection of impulses in isolated bovine and canine cardiac Purkinje fibers. *Circ. Res.*, 1981;**49**: 233–247.

189. Allessie, M.A., F.I.M. Bonke, and F.J.G. Schopman, Circus movement in rabbit atrial muscle as a mechanism of tachycardia II. The role of nonuniform recovery of excitability in the occurrence of unidirectional block, as studied with multiple microelectrodes. *Circ. Res.*, 1976;**39**: 168–177.

190. Allessie, M.A., F.I.M. Bonke, and F.J.G. Schopman, Circus movement in rabbit atrial muscle as a mechanism of tachycardia. *Circ. Res.*, 1973;**33**: 54–62.

191. Allessie, M.A., F.I.M. Bonke, and F.J.G. Schopman, Circus movement in rabbit atrial muscle as a mechanism of tachycardia. III. The "Leading Circle" concept: a new model of circus movement in cardiac tissue without the involvement of an anatomical obstacle. *Circ. Res.*, 1977;**41**: 9–18.

192. Allessie, M.A., W.J.E.P. Lammers, F.I.M. Bonke, and J. Hollen, Intra-atrial reentry as a mechanism for atrial flutter induced by acetylcholine and rapid pacing in the dog. *Circulation*, 1984;**70**: 123–135.

193. Van Capelle, F.J.L., *Slow conduction and cardiac arrhythmias*, thesis. Amsterdam: University of Amsterdam, 1983.

194. Davidenko, J.M., A.V. Pertsov, R. Salomonsz, W. Baxter, and J. Jalife, Stationary and drifting spiral waves of excitation in isolated cardiac muscle. *Nature*, 1992;**355**: 349–351.

195. Winfree, A.T., *When Time Breaks Down.* Princeton, NJ: Princeton University Press, 1987.

196. Janse, M.J. and E. Downer, Reentry, in *Foundations of Cardiac Arrhythmias*, P.M. Spooner and M.R. Rosen, Editors. New York: Marcel Dekker Inc, 2000, pp. 449–477.

197. Katz, L.N. and A. Pick, *Clinical Electrocardiography. I. The Arrhythmias* Philadelphia, PA: Lea & Febiger, 1956.

198. Jalife, J. and G.K. Moe, A biologic model of parasystole. *Am. J. Cardiol.*, 1979;**43**: 761–772.

199. Jalife, J. and G.K. Moe, Effect of electrotonic potentials on pacemaker activity of canine Purkinje fibers in relation to parasystole. *Circ. Res.*, 1976;**39**: 801–808.

200. Frame, L.H. and B.F. Hoffman, Mechanisms of tachycardia, in *Tachycardias*, B. Surawicz, C. Pratrap Reddy, and E.N. Prystowsky, Editors. Boston, MA: Nijhoff, 1984, pp. 7–36.

201. Waldo, A.L., W.A.H. Maclean, R.B. Karp, N.T. Kouchoukos, and T.N. James, Entrainment and interruption of atrial flutter with atrial pacing: studies in man following open heart surgery. *Circulation*, 1977;**56**: 737–745.

202. Waldo, A.L., Atrial flutter: entrainment characteristics. *J. Cardiovasc. Electrophysiol.*, 1997;**8**: 337–352.

203. Josephson, M.E., L.N. Horowitz, A. Farshidi, S.R. Spielman, E.L. Michelson, A.M. Greenspan, Sustained ventricular tachycardia: evidence for protected localized reentry. *Am. J. Cardiol.*, 1978;**42**: 416–424.

204. Singer, D.H., R. Lazzara, and B.F. Hoffman, Interrelationships between automaticity and conduction in Purkinje fibers. *Circ. Res.*, 1967;**21**: 537–558.

205. Saunders, J.H., G.R. Ferrier, G.K. Moe, Conduction block associated with transient depolarizations induced by acetylstrophanthidin in isolated canine Purkinje fibers. *Circ. Res.*, 1973;**32**: 610–617.

206. Rosenbaum, M.B., J.O., Lazzari, and M.V. Elizara, The role of phase 3 and phase 4 block in clinical electrocardiography, in *The Conduction System of the Heart: Structure, Function and Clinical Implications*, H.J.J. Wellens, K.I. Lie, M.J. Janse, Editors. Leyden: Stenfert Kroese, 1976, pp. 126–142.

207. Wit, A.L. and M.R. Rosen, Cellular electrophysiological mechanisms of cardiac arrhythmias, in *Comprehensive Electrocardiology, Theory and Practice in Health and Disease*, vol. 2, P.W. MacFarlane and T.D. Veitch Lawrie, Editors. Elmsford, NY: Pergamon Press, 1989, Chapter 20, pp. 801–841.

208. Akhtar, M., G. Breithardt, A.J. Camm, P. Coumel, M.J. Janse, R. Lazzara, R.J. Myerburg, P.J. Schwartz, A.L. Waldo, H.J. Wellens, et al., CAST and beyond implications of the cardiac arrhythmia suppression trial. Task force of the working group on arrhythmias of the European society of cardiology. *Circulation*, 1990;**81**: 1123–1127.

209. Manolis, A.S., P.J. Wang, and N.A. Estes 3rd, Radiofrequency catheter ablation for cardiac tachyarrhythmias. *Ann. Intern. Med.*, 1994;**121**: 452–461.

210. Moss, A.J., A. Vyas, H. Greenberg, R.B. Case, W. Zareba, W.J. Hall, M.W. Brown, S.A. McNitt, and M.L. Andrews, MADIT-II Research Group. Temporal aspects of improved survival with the implanted defibrillator (MADIT-II). *Am. J. Cardiol.*, 2004;**94**: 312–315.

211. Plotnikov, A.N., E.A. Sosunov, J. Qu, I.N. Shlapakova, E.P. Anyukhovsky, L. Liu, M.J. Janse, P.R. Brink, I.S. Cohen, R.B. Robinson, P. Danilo Jr., and M.R. Rosen, Biological pacemaker implanted in canine left bundle branch provides ventricular escape rhythms that have physiologically acceptable rates. *Circulation*, 2004;**109**: 506–512.

212. Potapova, I., A. Plotnikov, Z. Lu, P. Danilo Jr., V. Valiunas, J. Qu, S. Doronin, J. Zuckerman, I.N. Shlapakova, J. Gao, Z. Pan, A.J. Herron, R.B. Robinson, P.R. Brink, M.R. Rosen, and I.S. Cohen, Human mesenchymal stem cells as a gene delivery system to create cardiac pacemakers. *Circ. Res.*, 2004;**94**: 952–959.

213. Murata, M., E. Cingolani, A.D. McDonald, J.K. Donahue, E. Marbán, Creation of a genetic calcium channel blocker by targeted gem gene transfer in the heart. *Circ. Res.*, 2004;**95**: 398–405.

214. Kehat, I., L. Khimovich, O. Caspi, A. Gepstein, R. Shofti, G. Arbel, I. Huber, J. Satin, J. Itskovitz-Eldor, and L. Gepstein, Electromechanical integration of cardiomyocytes derived from human embryonic stem cells. *Nat. Biotechnol.*, 2004;**22**: 1282–1289.

215. Dobert, N., M. Britten, B. Assmus, U. Berner, C. Menzel, R. Lehmann, N. Hamscho, V. Schachinger, S. Dimmeler, A.M. Zeiher, F. Grunwald, Transplantation of progenitor cells after reperfused acute myocardial infarction: evaluation of perfusion and myocardial viability with FDG-PET and thallium SPECT. *Eur. J. Nucl. Med. Mol. Imaging*, 2004;**31**: 1146–1151.

216. Wollert, K.C., G.P. Meyer, J. Lotz, S. Ringes-Lichtenberg, P. Lippolt, C. Breidenbach, S. Fichtner, T. Korte, B. Hornig, D. Messinger, L. Arseniev, B. Hertenstein, A. Ganser, and H. Drexler, Intracoronary autologous bone-marrow cell transfer after myocardial infarction: the BOOST randomised controlled clinical trial. *Lancet*, 2004;**364**: 141–148.

2 Clinical Cardiac Electrophysiology

Andrew C. Rankin · F. Russell Quinn · Alan P. Rae

P. W. Macfarlane et al. (eds.), *Cardiac Arrhythmias and Mapping Techniques*, DOI 10.1007/978-0-85729-877-5_2,
© Springer-Verlag London Limited 2012

2.1 Introduction

Clinical cardiac electrophysiology (EP) techniques, involving intracardiac recording and electrical stimulation, have been of major importance in elucidating the mechanisms of cardiac arrhythmias. They not only have led to improved interpretation of the surface electrocardiogram (ECG) but have evolved to play a major role in the therapy of tachycardias. This role has changed in recent years, with a decline in EP-guided therapy for ventricular tachyarrhythmias but an increase in diagnostic use prior to curative catheter ablation.

2.2 History of Clinical Electrophysiology

Direct recording of intracavitary electrograms was first reported in 1945 by Lenègre and Maurice [1]. Developments in recording techniques subsequently permitted the registration of these potentials from all the cardiac chambers [2–5]. Although the integration of the atrioventricular (AV) conducting system had been described in 1906 by Tawara [6], the His-bundle electrogram was not recorded until 1958 by Alanis, Gonzalez, and Lopez in the isolated canine heart [7]. His-bundle recordings in man were obtained using an electrode catheter in 1960 [8], but the standard endocardial catheter technique for recording a His-bundle potential was first described by Scherlag and coworkers in 1969 [9]. Subsequently, electrode catheter recordings of electrograms from the sinus node [10] and from accessory AV pathways [11] have been obtained.

Initially, the major clinical application of "His-bundle electrocardiography" was as a descriptive method for the diagnosis of AV conduction disturbances [12, 13]. Subsequently electrophysiological techniques were used to assess sinoatrial disease [14], and the development of programmed electrical stimulation to initiate tachycardia allowed the study of the mechanisms of arrhythmias.

The induction of ventricular fibrillation by electrical currents was demonstrated as early as 1899 by Prevost and Battelli [15], but the electrical induction and termination of arrhythmias essentially started in the early 1950s. Reentry as a mechanism for tachyarrhythmias was proposed initially by Mines [16] and the presence of potential substrate for reentry was identified by Moe and coworkers [17] in 1956. Subsequently, in 1963, the initiation and termination of supraventricular tachycardia was demonstrated in a canine model [18]. A seminal study by Durrer et al. [19] in 1967 demonstrated that supraventricular tachycardia could be initiated and terminated by the introduction of premature beats in patients with the Wolff-Parkinson-White syndrome. Evidence for the reentrant basis for the majority of paroxysmal supraventricular tachycardias was provided by Bigger and Goldreyer using a systematic approach with programmed stimulation and His-bundle recording [20]. These techniques were translated to patients with ventricular tachycardia in 1972 by Wellens et al. [21] who suggested that the mechanism underlying this arrhythmia was also reentry [22]. A macroreentrant mechanism was described by Akhtar and colleagues in 1976 with the demonstration of the "V_3 phenomenon" or bundle branch reentrant beat [23], although clinically occurring tachycardias of this type are uncommon [24]. The microreentrant basis for the majority of ventricular tachycardias in patients with underlying coronary artery disease was demonstrated in a series of studies from Josephson and Horowitz and coworkers [25–28].

The ability to reproducibly initiate ventricular arrhythmias by programmed electrical stimulation, using repetitive extrastimuli with varying coupling intervals, led to EP-guided drug therapy. The arrhythmia would be induced in the drug-free state, and then the effect of drug therapy on subsequent inducibility was used to select long-term treatment. Non-randomized studies appeared to support this practice [29, 30] but more recent randomized studies have not confirmed benefit from this approach [31–34], leading to the virtual demise of the electrophysiology study as the determinant of therapy for life-threatening arrhythmias. At the same time, the development of catheter ablation techniques has increased the use of clinical electrophysiology testing to identify the targets for this curative therapy [35].

2.3 Methodology

2.3.1 Electrophysiological Equipment

At its most basic, a clinical EP study requires equipment to allow recording of cardiac activity and delivery of electrical stimulation to the heart. A standard ECG recorder, a temporary external pacing unit, and a transvenous pacing catheter would suffice for a simple EP study, such as the measurement of the sinus node recovery time in the evaluation of the sick sinus syndrome. However, such simple procedures are now rarely performed, and modern clinical electrophysiology equipment is designed to undertake more complex studies, with recordings from multiple intracardiac electrode catheters, and programmed electrical stimulation for the induction and investigation of tachyarrhythmias.

In a modern EP system, dedicated computer systems have replaced multi-channel analogue chart- and tape-recorders. Surface electrodes and intracardiac catheters are connected to the computer system via an electrically isolated patient-interface unit. Multiple ECG leads and intracardiac electrograms can be displayed on-screen, stored to hard disk, or printed out. The simultaneous display of the signals with several surface ECGs permits the evaluation of the timing and morphology of the surface signals relative to the intracardiac electrograms. Usually, at least three approximately orthogonal surface leads are displayed, with additional limb and precordial ECG leads if required for tachycardia morphology analysis. For routine studies, bipolar intracardiac signals are amplified and band-pass filtered in the frequency range 30–500 Hz, which allows optimum definition of the intracardiac electrograms. Additional information can be obtained from unipolar electrograms, using either Wilson's central terminal or an electrode catheter placed distant from the heart, e.g., in the inferior vena cava, as the reference potential. By using different filtering of the unipolar potential, essentially the same as a standard ECG (0.5–25 Hz), valuable information can be obtained from the electrogram morphology, not only the timing [36].

For studies involving the assessment of refractory periods and tachycardia induction, simple temporary pacing units are not sufficient, and a more sophisticated programmable stimulator is required. This should provide isolated outputs to prevent leakage currents that might cause arrhythmias, with the capability of delivering at least three extrastimuli at independently variable intervals during spontaneous or paced rhythms, and with provision for a wide range of paced cycle lengths.

The studies should be performed in a dedicated EP laboratory, cardiac catheterization laboratory, or procedure room with fluoroscopy. In addition, it should be emphasized that the personnel should have the necessary specialist training and that full resuscitative equipment should be available. Recommendations have been published for training and clinical competence in invasive electrophysiology studies [37, 38].

2.3.2 The Electrophysiology Study

Patients are studied in the post-absorptive state with no, or only mild, sedation (e.g., with benzodiazepines). If patients have been on antiarrhythmic drugs, these should be withdrawn prior to study for a period of at least five half-lives, if arrhythmia induction is planned. Other cardioactive drugs that are not used as antiarrhythmics may be continued.

Electrode catheters are inserted percutaneously using standard catheterization techniques under local anesthesia, and are positioned in selected areas of the heart under fluoroscopic guidance (❷ Fig. 2.1). Depending on the type of study and the intracardiac recordings required, two to five catheters are usually inserted. The conventional EP catheter is quadripolar, which allows the distal pair of electrodes to deliver the stimuli for pacing and the proximal pair of electrodes to obtain bipolar electrogram recordings. Pre-shaped curves aid the placement of catheters in different positions in the heart. There are large varieties of specialized electrode catheters in routine use. For example, a multipolar tricuspid annulus catheter may aid ablation of atrial flutter (❷ Fig. 2.1c), and a circular multipolar catheter may be used to guide pulmonary vein isolation (❷ Fig. 2.1d). Ablation catheters are deflectable to aid their placement, and have a larger electrode at their tip, usually 4 mm. Larger 8 mm tip, or irrigated tip, catheters are also used, to create larger and deeper lesions.

The number of catheters, and the site of placement, varies depending on the clinical requirements. If the only clinical question is whether or not a ventricular arrhythmia is inducible then a single quadripolar catheter to the right ventricular

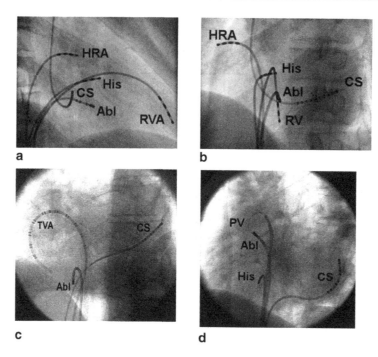

Fig. 2.1

Radiographs of EP catheters. (a) Right Anterior Oblique (*RAO*) and (b) Left Anterior Oblique (*LAO*) views of catheters placed for a diagnostic and RF ablation procedure. Catheters have been positioned to high right atrium (*HRA*), tricuspid annulus to record a His-bundle potential (*His*), coronary sinus (*CS*), right ventricular apex (RVA), and for ablation of AV nodal slow pathway (*Abl*). (c) Multipolar catheters placed at tricuspid valve annulus (*TVA*), coronary sinus (CS), and an ablation catheter (Abl) placed across the cavo-tricuspid isthmus for ablation of atrial flutter (LAO view). (d) Pulmonary vein (PV) catheter placed via a transseptal sheath at the right upper pulmonary vein to guide the ablation catheter (Abl) during a pulmonary vein isolation procedure. Catheters also positioned at coronary sinus (CS) and His bundle (His), seen in LAO view

(RV) apex may suffice, but if further assessment of cardiac electrophysiology or diagnosis is required then more catheters are used. Many EP laboratories have routinely placed three catheters (high right atrial, His bundle, and RV apex) for an initial study, with a fourth catheter placed in the coronary sinus to provide recordings from left atrium and ventricle when investigating supraventricular tachycardia (❯ Fig. 2.1a, b). With the expanding indications for electrophysiological procedures, catheter choice and placement have become more specific, to maximize the diagnostic information required to proceed to ablation and to avoid unnecessary catheter use, in order to reduce complications and cost [39]. Much time was previously spent on assessments of the electrophysiological properties of the heart, which now may be omitted to concentrate on the identification and ablation of the arrhythmia substrate. For example, a single catheter approach has been described for left-sided accessory pathway ablation, omitting all EP assessment prior to ablation [40].

2.3.2.1 His-Bundle Recording

The cornerstone of EP testing has been a stable, accurate His-bundle recording. To achieve this, a multipolar catheter is inserted via the femoral vein and is manipulated across the tricuspid valve into the right ventricle. While maintaining clockwise torque to hold the catheter against the tricuspid ring, the catheter is slowly withdrawn until the His-bundle signal between the atrial and ventricular electrograms is recorded (❯ Fig. 2.2). With a proximal His-bundle recording, the atrial and ventricular components of the electrogram should be of nearly equal amplitude. The normal His-bundle deflection is 10–25 ms in duration and, in the absence of a bypass pathway, the HV interval should be at least 35 ms.

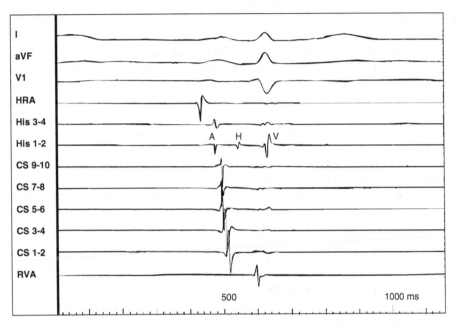

☐ Fig. 2.2
Recordings in sinus rhythm. Three ECG leads (I, aVF, and V1) and intracardiac bipolar electrograms from high right atrium (HRA), proximal and distal electrodes of the His-bundle catheter (His 3-4, 1-2), pairs of electrodes of a decapolar catheter in the coronary sinus (CS 1-10), and right ventricular apex (RVA) are shown. Atrial activation begins in the high right atrium, followed by septal activation at the His and then spreading across the left atrium

If this interval is less than 35 ms, the deflection may be a right bundle branch potential. Validation may be obtained by selective His-bundle pacing – the interval between stimulus and ventricular component should be identical to the basal HV interval [41].

2.3.2.2 Intracardiac Chamber Recording

A right atrial catheter may be positioned at the superior posterolateral region near the sinus node (❷ Fig. 2.1a, b). The left atrium can be entered directly from the right atrium through a patent foramen ovale or by means of a trans-septal procedure, but in most cases left atrial stimulation and recording are obtained from a catheter positioned in the coronary sinus (❷ Figs. 2.1 and ❷ 2.2). This is of particular value with supraventricular tachycardia, when an accessory pathway is suspected, and a catheter with multiple electrodes, e.g., octapolar or decapolar, is placed in the coronary sinus to facilitate mapping. The coronary sinus catheter was previously most commonly inserted from above (❷ Fig. 2.1a, b), via the left antecubital, subclavian, or right internal jugular veins, but increasingly the femoral vein approach is used, deploying a deflectable multipolar catheter (❷ Fig. 2.1c, d). Some laboratories use the coronary sinus catheter to pace the atria, and hence dispense with the right atrial catheter, in order to simplify procedures [39]. The standard catheter position in the right ventricle is with the tip in the RV apex, because it provides a stable, easily reproducible site. The RV outflow tract is also utilized, particularly for arrhythmia induction. For certain studies, such as ventricular stimulation or tachycardia mapping, a left ventricular (LV) electrode catheter is required [42]. It is inserted by the standard retrograde arterial approach usually from the femoral artery but occasionally by means of a brachial arteriotomy. Access to the LV can also be achieved by crossing the mitral valve after a trans-septal puncture, and in some cases epicardial pacing of the LV can be obtained via a branch of the CS. LV catheterization during routine EP studies is not standard.

2.3.2.3   Stimulation

Pacing and programmed stimulation is normally performed with rectangular stimuli having a 1–2 ms pulse width and an amplitude of twice the late diastolic threshold. The electrode catheters are positioned in appropriate regions of low threshold for stimulation. In general, these thresholds should be less than 2, 1, and 4 mA for catheters positioned in the right atrium, right ventricle, and coronary sinus, respectively. Repositioning of catheters, and interventions such as antiarrhythmic therapy, may alter stimulation thresholds and these should be rechecked after such maneuvers. Changing thresholds may influence certain electrophysiological parameters such as refractory periods. Although the use of pulse amplitude of twice the diastolic threshold is a routine practice in many laboratories, some investigators have advocated using higher pulse amplitudes, since an increase in current strength may facilitate the induction of ventricular tachyarrhythmias by permitting the introduction of extrastimuli at shorter coupling intervals [43]. However, in some patients, ventricular arrhythmias were not inducible at the higher strength although an arrhythmia was induced at twice the diastolic threshold [44]. A major concern with the use of high pulse amplitudes is the possibility of an increased induction of nonclinical arrhythmias [45].

2.3.3   Electrophysiology Study Protocols

An EP study protocol must be flexible and should be selected in accordance with the particular problem to be evaluated. Unfortunately, there has been little standardization in study protocols between laboratories, particularly in relation to ventricular stimulation, and this has contributed to the concerns about the evidence base for its clinical utility. However, while EP-guided therapy for ventricular arrhythmias has declined, the role of the electrophysiology study in the diagnosis of tachycardia and the identification of a substrate for ablation has increased. The baseline diagnostic information obtained will depend on the number of catheters placed, and the stimulation protocols utilized, but may include an assessment of the AV conduction system, evaluation of the refractory periods of its components and induction, definition of mechanism, and termination of tachyarrhythmia.

2.3.3.1   Baseline AV Conduction Intervals

(a) *PA interval and intra-atrial conduction times*

The depolarization of the atrium usually occurs earliest in the region of the sinus node either at the high right atrium, the node itself or the mid-lateral aspect of the right atrium [46]. The PA interval, measured from the onset of the P wave in the surface ECG to the atrial electrogram recorded from the His-bundle electrode (AV junction) catheter is a measure of the intra-atrial conduction time [47]. It is not sensitive to changes in autonomic tone. The sequence of atrial activation times at various right and left atrial sites may be more useful than the PA interval. An example of a normal atrial activation pattern is shown in ❷ Fig. 2.2 and an example of an abnormal pattern during atrioventricular re-entrant tachycardia (AVRT) is shown in ❷ Fig. 2.3.

(b) *AH interval*

Since the depolarization of the AV node cannot be demonstrated using standard electrophysiological techniques, the AH interval is employed for the functional evaluation of AV nodal conduction. The AH interval is measured from the first high-frequency deflection in the atrial electrogram recorded from the His-bundle catheter to the first deflection of the His-bundle electrogram (❷ Fig. 2.2). The normal range of the AH interval is 60–125 ms. The AH interval is markedly influenced by changes in autonomic tone. The AH interval shortens with sympathetic stimulation and lengthens with parasympathetic (vagal) stimulation. Therefore, it may vary profoundly during an EP study depending on the balance of autonomic tone in relation to the patient's level of sedation, anxiety, and other factors.

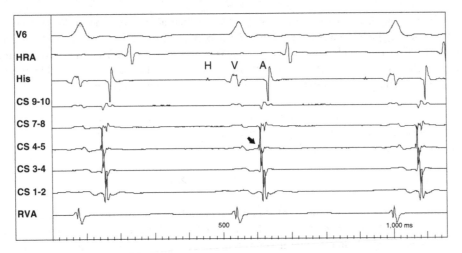

Fig. 2.3
Atrioventricular (AV) tachycardia, with a left-sided accessory pathway. Electrograms from high right atrium (HRA), His-bundle catheter (His), a decapolar coronary sinus catheter (CS 1-10), and RV apex. Earliest atrial activation (arrowed) is recorded from the middle pair of electrodes of the coronary sinus catheter (CS 4-5), indicating a left-sided pathway

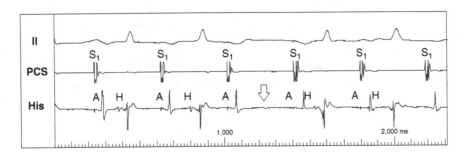

Fig. 2.4
Wenckebach-type AV block with atrial pacing. The drive cycle length (S_1-S_1) is 390 ms, pacing from proximal coronary sinus electrodes (PCS). The AH interval increases until block occurs (arrow) of AV nodal conduction

During atrial pacing at increasing rates (incremental pacing), the normal physiological response is a progressive lengthening in the AH interval at successive rates until AV nodal block occurs. This block occurs usually at rates of 130–170 beats per minute (bpm) and has Wenckebach periodicity, with beat-to-beat AH prolongation prior to block (❯ Fig. 2.4). With alterations in autonomic tone, however, physiological AV nodal block can occur in normal individuals outside this range. At more rapid atrial pacing rates 2:1 or higher degrees of AV nodal block can occur (❯ Fig. 2.4b). The development of AV nodal Wenckebach periods at cycle lengths of 600 ms or longer raises the possibility of a conduction disturbance, especially if they persist after the administration of atropine. AV nodal block at cycle lengths of 300 ms or shorter is suggestive of enhanced AV nodal conduction, sometimes called Lown-Ganong-Levine syndrome [48]. Whether this syndrome merely constitutes one end of the spectrum of AV nodal conduction or is caused by the presence of an atrio-His accessory pathway bypassing part or all of the AV node remains speculative [49].

(c) HV interval

The HV interval, a measure of infranodal conduction, assesses conduction through the His bundle, the bundle branches, and the terminal Purkinje system. The normal His-bundle width is 10–25 ms. The total HV interval is measured from the first deflection of the His bundle to the earliest indication of ventricular activation either in the surface or intracardiac leads (❷ Fig. 2.2). For adults, the HV interval ranges from 35 to 55 ms. An interval less than 35 ms suggests that either the electrogram is obtained from the right bundle branch, or there is an accessory AV connection bypassing at least part of the His-Purkinje system. The HV interval is not influenced by autonomic tone and should not vary within or between studies. With atrial pacing, the HV interval normally remains constant, although at high-paced rates HV interval lengthening with infra-His block may occur in normal individuals. The development of functional bundle branch or complete infra-His block can also occur because of abrupt shortening of the paced cycle length. The facilitation of AV nodal conduction, for instance by catecholamine stimulation, permitting the penetration of impulses into the His-Purkinje system can also increase the likelihood of functional His-Purkinje block.

(d) *Intraventricular conduction*

To measure intraventricular conduction, endocardial mapping of both ventricles is required, which is not usually part of a routine study. The Q-RVA conduction time may be measured, from the onset of ventricular activation to the RV apical electrogram, but is of limited clinical value, in contrast to the QRS duration from the surface ECG, which may have prognostic value [50].

(e) *Ventriculoatrial conduction*

In the absence of an accessory pathway, ventriculoatrial (VA) conduction utilizes the normal AV conduction system retrogradely. VA conduction may be absent in normal individuals with intact anterograde conduction and conversely may be present in patients with anterograde AV block [51]. In general, AV conduction is better than VA conduction.

During incremental ventricular pacing, in the majority of patients, VA conduction time progressively lengthens until the development of VA block, although the degree of prolongation of VA conduction is relatively less than that seen with AV conduction. The site of retrograde VA block may be located in either the His-Purkinje system or the AV node, but since retrograde His-bundle electrograms are only infrequently recorded during ventricular pacing, this localization can only be inferred indirectly. As with AV conduction, the retrograde His-Purkinje system is sensitive to abrupt changes in cycle length.

2.3.3.2   Refractory Period Assessment

The refractory periods of the cardiac chambers and the components of the AV conduction system are evaluated by the technique of premature stimulation. Refractoriness is influenced by several factors including the intensity of the extrastimuli and the cycle length of the spontaneous or paced rate at which the refractory period is measured. There is a basic difference in the responses of myocardium and nodal tissue to increasing rate or increasing prematurity: in atrial or ventricular muscle there is a decrease in the refractory periods, in contrast to the AV node where there is an increase in refractory intervals and conduction time (decremental conduction).

By convention, the notation used is as follows: S_1 is the basic stimulus and S_2 is the first premature stimulus; S_1-S_1 is the paced cycle length; S_1-S_2 is the coupling interval between the last complex of the paced cycle and the premature stimulus S_2. The corresponding notations for the atrial, His-bundle, and ventricular electrograms are A_1-A_1 and A_1-A_2, H_1-H_1 and H_1-H_2, and V_1-V_1 and V_1-V_2, respectively (e.g., ❷ Fig. 2.5).

(a) *Effective refractory period*

The effective refractory period (ERP) is defined as the longest premature coupling interval, S_1-S_2, which fails to produce a propagated response. For the atrium, therefore, the ERP is the longest S_1-S_2, which fails to produce an A_2 (❷ Fig. 2.5c); the AV nodal ERP is the longest A_1-A_2, which fails to produce an H_2 (❷ Fig. 2.5b); and the ERP of the His-Purkinje system is the longest H_1-H_2, which fails to elicit a ventricular response. The ERP of the components of the AV conduction system, except for the AV node, shorten with decreasing drive cycle lengths.

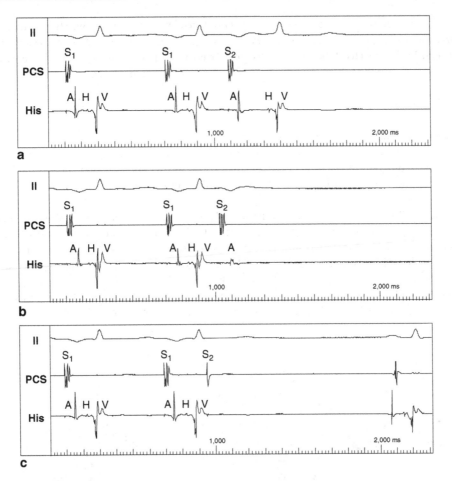

◻ Fig. 2.5
Responses to atrial premature beats. Following an 8-beat drive train, S_1-S_1, cycle length 600 ms, from proximal coronary sinus electrodes (PCS), a premature stimulus is delivered (S_1-S_2). With a coupling interval of 380 ms (a) there is prolongation of the AH interval, compared to during the drive train. With a shorter coupling interval of 320 ms (b) the AV nodal effective refractory period (ERP) is reached and there is block of conduction, with only atrial capture - note the absence of a His potential, demonstrating that the block is at the level of the AV node. When the coupling interval is shortened further to 260 ms (c) the atrium is also refractory, with no atrial capture

(b) *Relative refractory period*

The relative refractory period (RRP) is the longest premature coupling interval at which delay in conduction (prolongation of conduction time) of the extrastimulus occurs. The RRP of the atrium is, therefore, the longest S_1-S_2 at which S_2-A_2 is greater than S_1-A_1. For the AV node, the RRP is the longest A_1-A_2 at which A_2-H_2 is greater than A_1-H_2 and the RRP of the His-Purkinje system is the longest H_1-H_2 at which H_2-V_2 is greater than H_1-V_2.

(c) *Functional refractory period*

In contrast to the ERP and the RRP, the functional refractory period (FRP) is an indication of the conduction within tissue, not the refractoriness of the tissue. Although a misnomer, the term refractory period has remained in conventional usage.

The FRP is defined as the shortest output-coupling interval produced by a tissue in response to programmed extrastim-ulation. The atrial FRP is the shortest A_1-A_2 produced by any S_1-S_2. The AV nodal FRP is the shortest H_1-H_2 in response to any A_1-A_2 and the FRP of the His-Purkinje system is the shortest V_1-V_2 in response to any H_1-H_2. Frequently, the FRP of the AV node is longer than the ERP of the His-Purkinje system preventing measurement of the His-Purkinje ERP.

(d) Programmed atrial premature stimulation

Programmed atrial stimulation is performed by scanning diastole with a premature stimulus introduced initially late in diastole after 6–10 beats of either spontaneous rhythm or an atrial drive cycle. The coupling interval of the premature stimulus is progressively shortened by 10–20 ms. The introduction of premature stimuli in the atrium in the region of the sinus node during sinus rhythm permits the evaluation of the sinoatrial conduction time (see ❷ Chap. 4).

Decreasing the coupling interval of atrial premature stimuli produces progressive delay in AV nodal conduction man-ifested by lengthening of the A_2-H_2 interval (❷ Fig. 2.6). The H_1-H_2 interval initially shows progressive shortening in response to shortening of the A_1-A_2 interval until a nadir is reached, when the increase in AH interval is greater than the decrease in A_1-A_2, followed by a slow increase in the H_1-H_2 intervals. By definition, this nadir corresponds to the FRP of the AV node. Further shortening of A_1-A_2 may produce block in the AV node (ERP of the AV node).

Changes in the cycle length of the drive train tend to have a variable effect on the FRP, but with shortening of the drive train cycle length, there is invariably a lengthening of the ERP of the AV node [52]. The probability, therefore, of

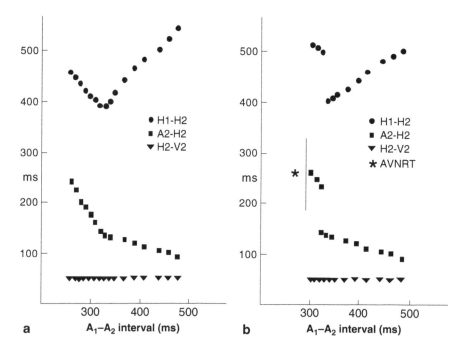

❑ Fig. 2.6
Responses of the AV conduction system to atrial extrastimuli in a normal individual (a) and a patient with dual AV nodal physiology (b). With progressive shortening of the coupling interval (A_1-A_2) there is initial associated shortening of the H_1-H_2 interval, but as the A_1-A_2 shortens further there is relatively greater increase in the AH interval, which results in prolongation of the H_1-H_2 interval. In the normal individual (a) a minimum value of the H_1-H_2 interval is reached (380 ms), which is the functional refractory period (FRP) of the AV node. The presence of dual AV nodal pathways (b) is shown by a sudden increase in the AH (and correspondingly the HV) intervals. At a critical delay, this is associated with the initiation of AV nodal reentrant tachycardia (AVNRT) (asterisk)

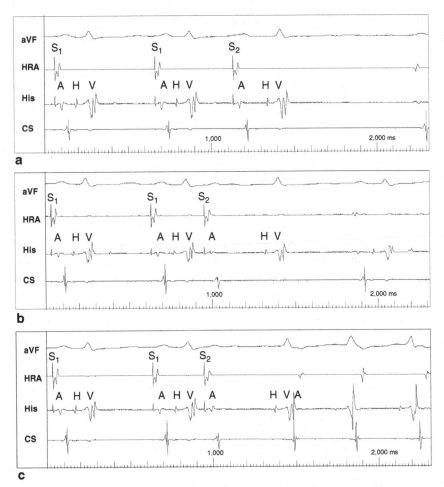

◘ Fig. 2.7

Responses to atrial premature beat demonstrating dual AV nodal pathways and initiation of AVNRT. With a relatively long coupling interval of 470 ms (a) there is conduction down the fast pathway, with a normal AH interval. With a short coupling interval of 320 ms (b) there is marked prolongation of the AH interval, indicating conduction down the slow pathway. With further shortening of the coupling interval to 310 ms (c) there is initiation of AVNRT. Surface lead aVF and electrograms from high right atrium (HRA), His bundle, and coronary sinus (CS) are shown

encountering the ERP of the AV node is increased by employing faster drive trains. In a proportion of patients, especially those with AV nodal reentrant tachycardia (AVNRT), the response to atrial premature stimulation demonstrates a discontinuous curve suggesting two electrophysiologically distinct AV nodal pathways [53, 54]. In patients with dual pathways, the AH interval progressively grows longer until there is a sudden "jump" in the AH interval in response to a small decrement in the premature coupling interval (◗ Figs. 2.6 and ◗ 2.7). This sudden increase in AH interval reflects block in the "fast" AV nodal pathway, which has a longer refractory period than the "slow" pathway. The presence of dual AV nodal pathways in itself does not imply the presence of AVNRT but only the potential substrate. In some patients, dual AV nodal pathways may not be manifest in the baseline state but can be exposed by alterations in autonomic tone or with drug therapy [55]. Despite the presence of discontinuity in AV conduction, retrograde VA conduction commonly is continuous [53]. However, the finding of discontinuous retrograde conduction curves in a minority of patients identified differences in the site of atrial insertion, with the slow pathway retrograde activation via the area of the coronary sinus os and the fast pathway in the region of the His-bundle recording [56]. This anatomical differentiation between the pathways provides the basis of selective slow pathway ablation in the treatment of AVNRT [57]. Further experience has revealed the potential complexities of arrhythmia substrate with a diversity of AV nodal pathways described [58, 59].

In contrast to the AV node, there is usually no change in conduction in the His-Purkinje system to atrial premature stimulation (❯ Fig. 2.6). Uncommon patterns of response include progressive delay in conduction with lengthening of the HV interval, an abrupt change in the HV interval, and complete block of infranodal conduction. The development of aberrant conduction or block within the His-Purkinje system is more likely during sinus rhythm or longer drive train cycle lengths because the refractoriness of the tissue is directly related to the preceding cycle length. At slower rates, the relative or ERPs may then be longer than the FRP of the AV node. Conduction delay or block within the His-Purkinje system therefore is not necessarily an abnormal response. Functional delay or block in the right bundle tends to occur more frequently than in the left bundle.

(e) *Programmed ventricular premature stimulation*

Programmed ventricular stimulation is performed in a similar manner to atrial stimulation. Ventricular stimuli are introduced after 6–10 beats of spontaneous rhythm or a ventricular drive train at progressively shorter coupling intervals until ventricular refractoriness occurs. For routine studies, ventricular stimulation is performed at the RV apex. The ventricular ERP at the apex is usually less than 300 ms and, in an otherwise normal ventricle, refractoriness varies little at other sites.

Retrograde refractory periods may be difficult to determine because the His-bundle electrogram is frequently obscured by the ventricular electrogram. With progressive shortening of the V_1-V_2 (S_1-S_2) interval, the retrograde His-bundle electrogram H_2 may emerge from the ventricular electrogram, and with further shortening the V_2-H_2 interval will progressively lengthen until either ventricular refractoriness or retrograde His-Purkinje block occurs. Not infrequently, in the latter circumstances, with further shortening of V_1-V_2, the H_2 will reappear because of proximal conduction delay (gap phenomenon: see ❯ Sect. 2.3.3.2.f). Retrograde AV nodal conduction (H_2-A_2) may show either progressive slowing of conduction with an increasing H_2-A_2 interval, or an almost constant relatively short H_2-A_2 interval, or discontinuous curves analogous to the anterograde dual AV nodal pathways. Retrograde atrial activation in the absence of an accessory pathway is usually first observed in the His-bundle electrogram (❯ Fig. 2.8).

Ventricular premature stimulation can induce a variety of repetitive responses. AV nodal echo beats in relation to retrograde dual pathways may be initiated, although a sustained tachycardia rarely occurs. Frequently, in patients with normal conduction, the "V_3 phenomenon," or bundle branch reentrant beat, (❯ Fig. 2.9) may be observed [23]. This repetitive ventricular response is caused by the development of a macro-reentrant circuit involving the His bundle and bundle branches. Block in the right bundle branch is followed by retrograde conduction of the impulse by the left bundle with retrograde conduction to the His bundle and subsequent completion of the reentrant circuit by

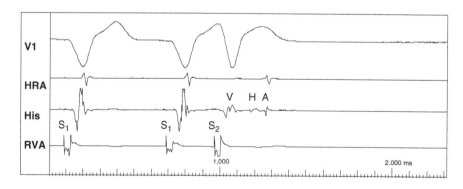

❏ Fig. 2.8

Retrograde conduction in response to a ventricular premature beat. Following the ventricular extrastimulus, coupling interval 280 ms, retrograde His bundle and atrial activation are seen

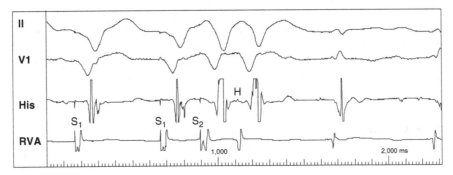

◻ Fig. 2.9
Bundle branch reentrant beat in response to a single ventricular extrastimulus. Following the extrastimulus (S2), coupling interval 230 ms, there is retrograde His-bundle activation (H) preceding the reentrant beat, which has a left bundle branch block morphology

anterograde conduction down the now-recovered right bundle branch. Therefore, the repetitive response has a left bundle branch block morphology with an HV interval the same or longer than the HV interval observed during sinus rhythm.

(f) *Gap phenomenon*

During programmed extrastimulation, block of the impulse may occur but then be followed by the resumption of conduction with shorter coupling intervals of the premature stimuli. This is known as the gap phenomenon. It is caused by the development of conduction delay proximal to the site of block, allowing the distal tissue to recover and conduct [60]. For example, as A_1-A_2 is shortened, block may occur at the level of the His bundle. With further shortening of A_1-A_2, the resulting increase in the A_2-H_2 interval produces lengthening of the H_1-H_2 such that it exceeds the refractory period of the distal tissue with the resumption of conduction. Several gaps have been identified in relation to the components of the AV conduction system, both in the anterograde [60, 61] and retrograde directions [62]. The gap phenomenon is a physiological response and is not of pathological significance.

2.3.3.3 Induction, Definition of Mechanism, and Termination of Tachyarrhythmias

The stimulation protocol used to induce tachycardia will depend on the specific arrhythmia. Programmed stimulation of the ventricle can induce ventricular tachycardia or fibrillation, and this has been used to guide therapy and assess risk (❷ Figs. 2.10 and ❷ 2.11). A common protocol would use up to three extrastimuli (S_2, S_3, S_4), at two drive cycle-lengths (S_1-S_1, e.g., 600 and 450 ms) at two ventricular sites, such as RV apex and outflow tract. However, a variety of other protocols have been used, with different drive cycle lengths and number of extrastimuli [63]. More aggressive protocols, with faster drive rates and increased number of extrastimuli, particularly if tightly coupled, may induce nonspecific arrhythmia, such as ventricular fibrillation [64]. The diversity of protocols, and the concerns about the specificity of induced arrhythmia, have contributed to the decline in the clinical use of ventricular stimulation. Induced tachycardia may be terminated by further ventricular stimulation, either extrastimuli or overdrive pacing (❷ Fig. 2.10b) [63]. There is the risk of causing acceleration of the arrhythmia, particularly if the tachycardia is fast (❷ Fig. 2.11b). With respect to other tachycardias, supraventricular tachycardias may be induced by atrial or ventricular extrastimuli, and atrial arrhythmias can be induced by atrial extrastimuli or rapid atrial pacing. Catecholamine stimulation, using isoproterenol infusion, may be necessary for arrhythmia induction. Tachycardia induction, diagnosis, and termination, and techniques of mapping to identify targets for ablation, are discussed further below, and in ❷ Chaps. 1 and ❷ 3.

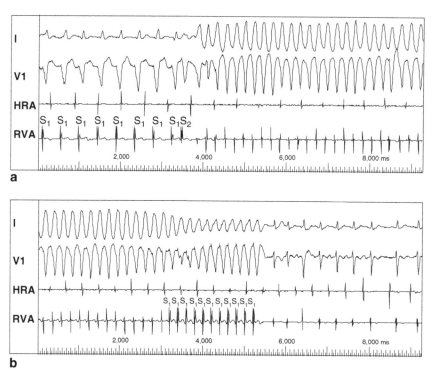

◘ Fig. 2.10

Initiation and termination of sustained ventricular tachycardia. Following an 8-beat drive train, cycle length 450 ms, a single premature ventricular beat, coupling interval 250 ms, initiates VT (**a**). There is ventricular-atrial dissociation, as seen in the recording from high right atrium (HRA). A burst of rapid ventricular pacing (**b**) terminates the VT and restores normal sinus rhythm

2.3.4   Safety of Electrophysiological Testing

Clinical cardiac electrophysiological testing involves invasive techniques and therefore has a potential for complication, which is inherent in any cardiac catheterization procedure. Venous thrombosis is the most common complication, with an incidence ranging between 0.5 and 2.5% [65, 66]. Factors which may influence the development of thrombosis include not only the patient population being studied but also specific aspects of the procedure, such as the use of systemic anticoagulation and the duration the electrode catheters are in situ [65, 66]. Arterial injury occurs in 0.1–0.4% of patients either because of local trauma during attempts at arterial cannulation or inadvertently during femoral venous catheterization [66]. Cardiac perforation has been observed in 0.2% of patients, although tamponade was less common and emergency pericardiocentesis was required only rarely [67]. The risk of complications has increased with the addition of ablation procedures to the diagnostic EP study, which may include complications specific to the procedure, such as inadvertent AV block with ablation of AV nodal pathways, or thromboembolic complications with left-sided ablations, or pericardial tamponade with transseptal puncture [68, 69]. In a prospective study of nearly 4,000 procedures, the risk of complications increased from 1.1% for diagnostic EP procedures to 3.1% with radiofrequency ablation [70]. Risk was increased with older age patients and with the presence of systemic disease. The target of ablation also increases the risk, with higher complications for AVNRT compared to AVRT, and for scar-related VT compared to idiopathic VT [68]. Pulmonary vein isolation and left atrial ablation for atrial fibrillation may also expose the patient to increased risk of up to 6%, including specific risks like pulmonary vein stenosis and atrio-esophageal fistula [71, 72].

Complications specifically related to ventricular stimulation studies, such as the induction of heart block or nonclinical arrhythmias, are usually transient and not of clinical importance, despite the need for cardioversion in

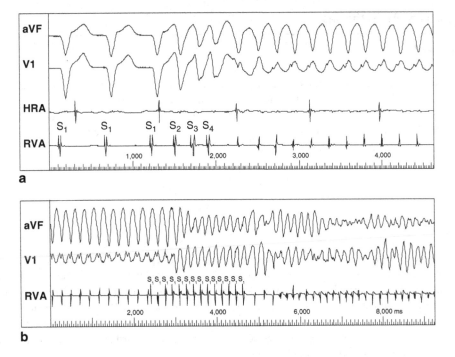

◘ Fig. 2.11
Initiation of VT with triple extrastimuli (**a**), and acceleration to ventricular fibrillation with burst pacing (**b**)

over 50% of these patients [66]. The risk of death during EP testing is low (0.1–0.2%), despite the induction of malignant ventricular arrhythmias.

2.5 Indications for Electrophysiology Studies

The indications for EP studies can be considered in three categories:

1. Diagnostic – to determine the mechanism of an arrhythmia, either tachycardia or bradycardia
2. Therapeutic – to identify the substrate of the arrhythmia prior to ablation, or to guide therapy selection
3. Risk stratification – to determine the risk of life-threatening arrhythmia

The role of EP testing in each of these categories has changed, due to progress in diagnostic methodologies, the results of clinical studies and the advances in treatment options. For example, implantable event-recorders now have an important role in the diagnosis of unexplained syncope [73], and often replace the relatively nonspecific invasive EP study [74]. The exception may be patients with syncope and prior myocardial infarction (MI), where induction of monomorphic VT can indicate an arrhythmic etiology. However, there is evidence of benefit from the implantable defibrillator in many such patients without the need for an EP study [75], further reducing the role of invasive testing. There is clearly overlap between the diagnostic and the therapeutic indications in that establishing the diagnosis may lead to curative catheter ablation. With respect to risk stratification, the value of the EP study in predicting adverse outcome has been questioned, because of the recognition of persisting risk of sudden death despite a negative EP study in a variety of conditions, including ventricular arrhythmias occurring post-infarction [31], or associated with dilated cardiomyopathy [76] or Brugada syndrome [77]. When considering specific arrhythmias, each of these categories (diagnosis, therapy, and risk assessment) may have a role.

2.5.1   Diagnosis of Arrhythmias

2.5.1.1   Bradycardia

The role of invasive EP studies in the diagnosis of bradycardias has declined in recent years. The ACC/AHA/HRS 2008 pacing guidelines include the measurement of HV interval ($\geq$ 100 ms), the diagnosis of infranodal conduction block post-MI and the presence of major abnormalities of sinus node function as factors in the decision as to whether to implant a permanent pacemaker in selected situations [78]. Assessment of sinoatrial dysfunction and AV conduction disease is described in ❯ Chaps. 4 and ❯ 6 respectively.

2.5.1.2   Tachycardia

The specific diagnostic electrophysiological procedures undertaken will depend on the clinical question and therapeutic aim, usually determined by the previously documented arrhythmia. Tachycardias with narrow QRS complexes are described as supraventricular tachycardias, and include atrial and junctional tachycardias. The latter include AVRT, utilizing an accessory pathway, and AVNRT, whose substrate is dual AV nodal pathways. Wide-complex tachycardias may also be supraventricular, with aberrant AV conduction such as bundle branch block or pre-excitation, but may be ventricular in origin. The surface ECG has limitations in diagnosing such broad complex tachycardias, and invasive electrophysiological studies may be of particular value in this context.

(a) *Identification of substrate*

In a patient with supraventricular tachycardia, the presence of a substrate for reentry, such as an accessory pathway, may be manifest by an abnormal intracardiac activation sequence of either atrial or ventricular electrograms. For example, in the presence of pre-excitation, the earliest ventricular activation during sinus rhythm will be at the site of the ventricular insertion of the pathway (❯ Fig. 2.12), or with a concealed pathway the earliest atrial activation during ventricular pacing may be used to identify the site of the pathway. The most common pathway location is left-sided, in which case the

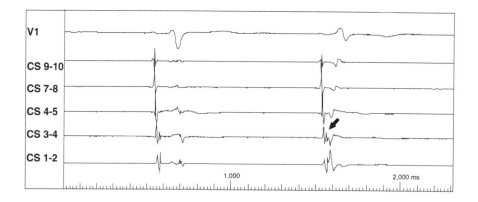

◻ Fig. 2.12

Intermittent pre-excitation with a left-sided accessory pathway. The first beat is not pre-excited and left ventricular (LV) activation in the coronary sinus (CS) electrograms is late. The second beat is pre-excited, with a delta wave on the surface ECG (V1), and earliest ventricular activation is recorded from the distal coronary sinus electrodes (arrowed) indicating a left-lateral accessory pathway

earliest activation will be identified from the coronary sinus catheter electrograms. If the activation sequences are normal during sinus rhythm and ventricular pacing, with earliest retrograde atrial activation recorded at the His-bundle catheter, then atrial programmed stimulation may identify the presence of dual AV nodal physiology, as the substrate for AVNRT (❯ Fig. 2.7). The identification of the tachycardia substrate may allow curative catheter ablation. If there is neither an accessory pathway nor AVNRT, then an atrial arrhythmia is likely, and it may be necessary to induce the tachycardia to allow mapping and ablation. However, if typical atrial flutter has been documented, it is not necessary to induce the arrhythmia, since it is recognized that the cavo-tricuspid isthmus is an essential component of the reentry circuit and the target for ablation.

(b) *Mechanisms of tachycardia*

Reentry is the most common mechanism underlying clinical sustained tachyarrhythmias. It is a characteristic of reentrant arrhythmias that they can be initiated by premature beats. Atrial reentrant and junctional tachycardias, AVNRT or AVRT, can commonly be initiated by atrial premature beats. The latter tachycardias are dependent on critical delay in the AV conduction induced by the premature beat, which allows subsequent retrograde conduction up the accessory pathway or the fast retrograde AV nodal pathway. Ventricular premature beats may also induce AVRT, and infrequently AVNRT, or may initiate reentrant ventricular tachycardia (❯ Fig. 2.10), particularly in the presence of a ventricular substrate such as scarring from an old MI. Less commonly, arrhythmias are due to focal increased automaticity, or to triggered activity. Tachycardias that originate from an automatic focus may be less likely to be inducible by programmed stimulation but may be initiated by catecholamine stimulation, using an infusion of isoproterenol, a β-adrenoceptor agonist. Triggered arrhythmias, which may depend on oscillations of intracellular calcium induced by preceding beats, may also be initiated by pacing protocols.

(c) *Atrial activation during tachycardia*

Once a sustained tachycardia has been induced, the mechanism may be clear from the atrial activation timing and sequence. With typical ("slow–fast") AVNRT, atrial activation may be coincident with or precede ventricular activation, and the earliest atrial activation is commonly seen from the His-bundle catheter (❯ Fig. 2.7). With AVRT, the atrial activation sequence is determined by the site of the accessory pathway, and is commonly eccentric (❯ Fig. 2.3), although a paraseptal pathway may have a retrograde activation sequence similar to that via the normal conducting system. Atrial tachycardia may remain a differential diagnosis of such tachycardias, and electrophysiological maneuvers have been described, which may aid the diagnosis. A ventricular premature beat timed to coincide with the His-bundle electrogram can alter the timing of the atrial activation only in the presence of an accessory pathway, since retrograde conduction via the normal conducting system will be refractory (❯ Fig. 2.13). Differentiating between an atrial tachycardia and AVNRT or AVRT can be achieved by observing the responses following cessation of a short burst of ventricular pacing, faster than the tachycardia rate and with 1:1 VA conduction [79]. With atrial tachycardia, on termination of ventricular pacing the retrograde atrial signal is followed by an atrial tachycardia beat, which conducts to the ventricle – an A-A-V response – whereas AVNRT and AVRT show an A-V response (❯ Fig. 2.14). There are limitations to this technique, including a "pseudo A-A-V" response in patients with AVNRT and long HV intervals, when identification of A-H or A-A-H responses is more accurate [80]. Differentiation between atypical AVNRT from AVRT utilizing a posterior paraseptal accessory pathway may be aided by the appearance of V-H-A with ventricular premature beats in the former [81]. The presence of a concealed paraseptal pathway can be assessed in sinus rhythm by pacing via the His-bundle catheter and comparing the retrograde atrial activation timing with His-bundle capture and local ventricular capture [82]. Atrial flutter has a faster atrial rate and is characterized by intermittent AV conduction, commonly 2:1. The atrial activation sequence is typically counterclockwise around the tricuspid annulus. Ventricular tachycardia may have retrograde conduction to the atria, with earliest activation at the His-bundle catheter, or there may be VA dissociation.

(d) *Entrainment*

The evidence of the reentrant basis of the majority of clinical atrial and ventricular tachycardias came from studies of the phenomenon of entrainment [83]. Waldo et al, in a series of studies initially of post-operative atrial flutter [84] and

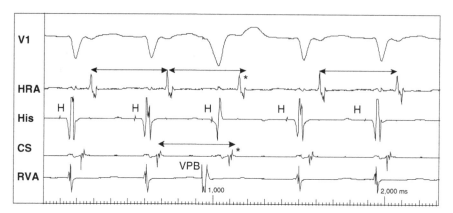

Fig. 2.13

His-coincident ventricular premature beat (VPB) during atrio-ventricular reentrant tachycardia (AVRT). A premature stimulus in the right ventricle pulls ventricular activation earlier, timing with the anterograde activation of the His bundle. The following atrial activation (*asterisks*) occurs at an interval shorter than the tachycardia cycle length (*arrows*). This confirms the presence of an accessory pathway, since the normal conducting system would be refractory and unable to conduct retrogradely

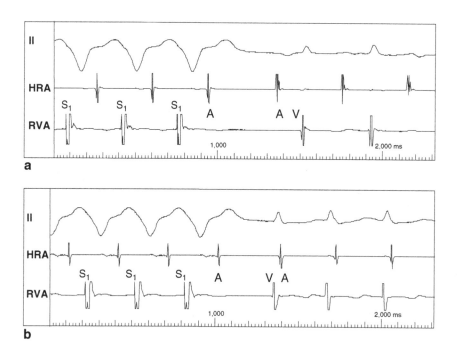

Fig. 2.14

A technique for the diagnosis of atrial tachycardia. During atrial tachycardia (**a**), following termination of ventricular pacing with retrograde atrial activation, there is a A-A-V response. During AVNRT (**b**) there is a A-V-A response

subsequently of supraventricular [85] and ventricular tachycardia [86], described three criteria for entrainment: (1) constant fusion during the transient entrainment of a tachycardia except for the last captured beat (which was entrained but not fused), (2) progressive fusion at different entrainment rates, and (3) interruption of the tachycardia associated with local conduction block followed by activation from a different direction [85]. A fourth criterion was added based on the electrogram equivalent of progressive fusion [87]. Demonstration that any of these criteria were met by pacing during a sustained tachycardia was evidence of a reentrant mechanism.

The demonstration of entrainment required that the reentry circuit had an excitable gap, allowing capture from pacing outside of the circuit. Local activation sequences within the tachycardia circuit were unchanged, with the rate increased to that of the pacing, but the surface electrogram was a fusion of the morphologies determined by the local pacing site and the tachycardia. Since the last paced beat entered the circuit but the output did not fuse with a subsequent paced beat, the beat following pacing had the morphology of the tachycardia but was at the pacing cycle length (❷ Fig. 2.15). The degree of fusion varied depending on the pacing rate, with the morphology more closely resembling that of the paced beats with increased rate (progressive fusion). At a critical rate, the paced impulse may collide with the tachycardia wavefront producing block and termination of the tachycardia. Subsequent activation was from the direction of pacing, and had a shorter coupling interval.

With the development of mapping techniques it became apparent that if the pacing site was within the reentry circuit then none of the criteria could be met, so-called "concealed entrainment" [88] or "entrainment with concealed fusion". In this case the morphology and activation sequences of the entrained rhythm would be identical to the tachycardia, but at the pacing rate. The local return cycle would be at the tachycardia cycle length, and not the pacing rate (❷ Fig. 2.16). A prolonged return cycle indicates that the pacing site was not within the reentry circuit [89]. The demonstration of concealed entrainment may be of value in confirming a site for successful catheter ablation [90, 91].

(e) *Syncope of undetermined etiology*

The role of EP studies in the diagnosis of syncope has diminished, but may still be of value in selected patients [74, 92, 93]. Tilt testing to diagnose neurocardiogenic syncope and implanted loop recorders to allow correlation between symptoms and cardiac rhythm have contributed to the decline in the use of invasive studies. The expanding indications for implantable devices to treat ventricular arrhythmias have reduced the need to demonstrate inducible ventricular arrhythmias in patients in whom they are suspected. The clinical significance of an induced arrhythmia or an identified conduction abnormality may be uncertain, reflecting the low sensitivity and specificity of EP testing. The diagnostic yield is particularly low in the absence of structural heart disease [94, 95].

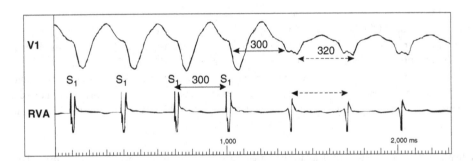

◻ Fig. 2.15
Entrainment of ventricular tachycardia. During pacing at cycle length 300 ms the ECG has a different morphology compared to during tachycardia. The beat following the last stimulus is at the pacing cycle length, but has the morphology of the tachycardia. Pacing cycle length indicated by *filled arrow,* **and tachycardia cycle length by** *interrupted arrows*

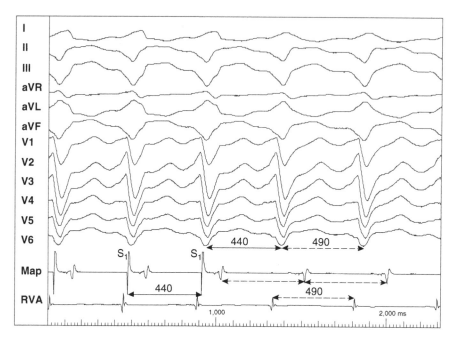

Fig. 2.16
Concealed entrainment. Pacing using the mapping catheter (Map) at cycle length 440 ms produces an ECG morphology nearly identical to that during tachycardia. The return cycle of the local electrogram recorded from the mapping catheter is at almost the tachycardia cycle length (*interrupted arrows*). This is consistent with pacing within the reentry circuit, and the delay between the stimulus and the ventricular activation, as indicated by the surface ECG, suggests the site is at the entrance to an area of slow conduction

2.5.2   Therapeutic Role of Electrophysiology Studies

2.5.2.1   Catheter Ablation

A major change in the role of EP studies has followed the development of catheter ablation for the curative treatment of cardiac arrhythmias [35, 96, 97]. Techniques and principles developed for the diagnosis of arrhythmias now are applied in a more specific manner to identify the substrate for ablation. A more anatomical, rather than electrophysiological, approach may be applied to the ablation of some arrhythmias, including AVNRT [98], atrial flutter [99] or fibrillation [100], and ventricular tachycardia [101]. Technologies have been developed to aid the mapping of complex arrhythmia substrates, and are described in ❷ Chap. 3. However, many arrhythmias can be successfully treated by catheter ablation using conventional electrophysiological techniques to aid the mapping and identification of the ablation target, using the following methods.

(a) *Earliest activation.* The site of successful ablation of an accessory pathway or a focal atrial or ventricular tachycardia is usually determined by the identification of the site of earliest activation (❷ Figs. 2.3 and ❷ 2.17). The use of unipolar signals from the distal ablation catheter (filtered like a standard ECG) is of value, as the presence of an R wave identifies a site unlikely to be successful, whereas successful sites have a QS pattern (❷ Fig. 2.18) [102].

(b) *Pace mapping.* This is based on the principle that pacing at the site of origin of the tachycardia should produce the identical ECG morphology to the clinical arrhythmia. It is of value in the ablation of focal ventricular tachycardia, such as RV outflow tachycardia (❷ Fig. 2.17). One advantage is the option to continue mapping in the absence of the arrhythmia, particularly if the tachycardia is poorly tolerated by the patient.

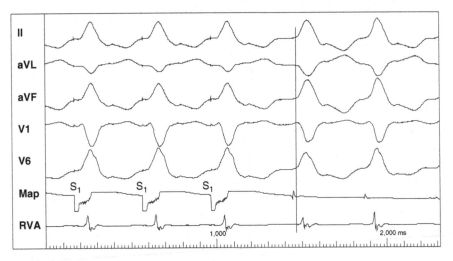

Fig. 2.17

Pace mapping at a site of early activation during RV outflow tachycardia. Pacing through the mapping catheter (*Map*) produces a morphology nearly identical to that during tachycardia. The local activation at this site is early, preceding the onset of the QRS complexes (*vertical line*)

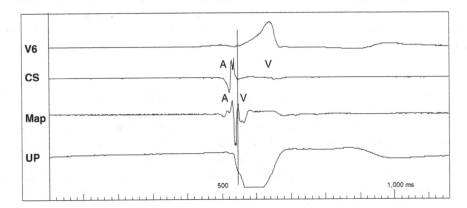

Fig. 2.18

Site of ablation of an accessory pathway. The ventricular activation recorded from the coronary sinus (*CS*) catheter indicates that LV activation is late. Mapping catheter (*Map*) is at a site on the RV annulus where ventricular activation is earlier, preceding the onset of the delta wave (vertical line). The unipolar signal has a PQS morphology, consistent with the site of the pathway, indicating a likely successful site for ablation

(c) *Electrogram-guided ablation.* For a number of tachycardias, the above methods may be of limited value, particularly if the substrate is a macro-reentrant circuit, and specific characteristics of potentially successful ablation sites have been described. Examples include (1) AVNRT, where a characteristic complex signal with a slow pathway potential has been described [57], (2) Mahaim tachycardia, which uses an atrio-fascicular bypass tract, and can be ablated on the tricuspid annulus guided by a Mahaim potential [103, 104], and (3) Idiopathic LV (fascicular) tachycardia, where ablation is guided by Purkinje and pre-Purkinje potentials [105, 106].

(d) *Entrainment mapping.* With reentrant arrhythmias, activation mapping may be of limited value, and the aim is to identify a component of the circuit, which may be the site of successful ablation. The demonstration of "entrainment with concealed fusion" as described above, may identify an area within the circuit, or a prolonged post-pacing interval may provide evidence that the site is outside the circuit and therefore unlikely to be a successful ablation

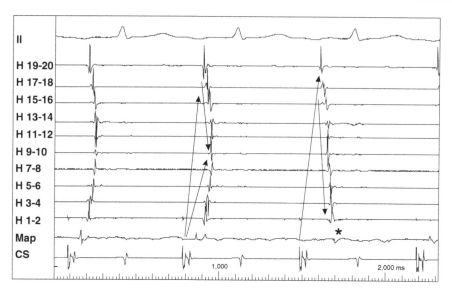

■ Fig. 2.19

Cavo-tricuspid isthmus block during radiofrequency ablation for atrial flutter. A double-decapolar "Halo" catheter (H 1-20) is recording activation from around the tricuspid annulus, during pacing from the coronary sinus (CS) catheter. In the first two beats, there is activation around the annulus in both clockwise and counterclockwise directions, indicated by the *arrows*. During the third beat, there is only counterclockwise activation, indicating isthmus block. This is confirmed by the local electrogram from the mapping catheter (*Map*) at the site of the ablation, which becomes widely split (*asterisk*)

site. Such "entrainment mapping" may be of particular value in identifying sites for ablation in atrial and ventricular reentrant tachycardias, [89, 90, 107].

(e) *Assessment of ablation success.* EP techniques can be used to assess whether a catheter ablation has been successful in a number of ways. In the case of an accessory pathway, the absence of abnormal ventricular or atrial activation indicates successful pathway block. Non-inducibility of tachycardia is the end-point for ablation of AVNRT, or reentrant VT. With AVNRT, it is not necessary to abolish slow pathway conduction since persisting dual AV nodal physiology but non-inducibility of AVNRT is an acceptable end-point, correlating with long-term benefit [57]. Abolition of spontaneous or isoproterenol-induced arrhythmia, such as automatic tachycardias like RVOT tachycardia, may indicate success. In atrial flutter, in which the cavo-tricuspid isthmus is part of the reentrant circuit, termination of the arrhythmia during ablation by itself did not correlate with good long-term outcome [108], whereas demonstration of bi-directional isthmus block post-ablation indicated long-term benefit [109]. Thus, in this case, successful ablation can be performed in the absence of the arrhythmia, using the change in atrial activation recorded from a multipolar tricuspid annulus catheter (❷ Fig. 2.1c) during coronary sinus pacing as the indication of isthmus block (❷ Fig. 2.19).

2.5.2.2 Guidance of Therapy

The practice of EP-guided drug therapy for ventricular arrhythmias has now largely been abandoned. The ability to induce life-threatening arrhythmias by ventricular stimulation [21], led to the premise that the EP study could be used to assess the efficacy of drug therapy [30, 110]. During the 1980s, much time was spent in EP labs performing multiple ventricular stimulation studies in patients with prior ventricular arrhythmias. When sustained arrhythmia was induced at baseline in a drug-free state, re-induction was attempted following intravenous drug administration, commonly procainamide [111]. Oral drug treatment was then initiated and EP studies were repeated at intervals, depending on the response [112]. Such serial drug testing took many days, or weeks if amiodarone was also tested. Observational data indicated that patients whose arrhythmias were non-inducible on drug therapy [29], or whose tachycardia rate was slowed to improve hemo-dynamic tolerability [113–115], had a better outcome compared to those who continued to have inducible life-threatening arrhythmia. However, randomized studies have failed to confirm the prognostic benefit from EP-guided drug therapy [34, 116, 117]. In addition, there was evidence that patients whose arrhythmias were non-inducible may remain at risk of life-threatening arrhythmia recurrence [31, 118]. In addition, data from the AVID registry indicated that stable VT may not be a benign arrhythmia, with a mortality of over 30% at 3 years [119]. There are also concerns regarding the specificity of induced arrhythmias in relation to the stimulation protocols [64] and the day-to-day reproducibility of the technique [120, 121]. The development of the implantable cardioverter defibrillator (ICD) provided a superior therapy to dug treatment for high-risk patients [116].

It has been suggested that an EP study may be of value in identifying those patients with VT who may respond to anti-tachycardia pacing (ATP) [63]. However, reproducibility of response to ATP is variable, and may not be predictive [122]. In particular, induced fast VT had a lower success rate of ATP, but studies have shown a high percentage success (73%) with spontaneous fast VT [123, 124]. In addition, survivors of cardiac arrest from VF, without prior documented clinical VT, may have recurrent monomorphic VT, which is poorly predicted by EP studies [125], and which may be successfully terminated by ATP [123].

2.5.3 Risk Stratification

The role of EP testing in risk stratification remains controversial. The ability of the EP study to induce life-threatening arrhythmia may offer a method to identify patients at high risk of sudden death, of particular value in those patients who have not yet had an arrhythmia but have been identified as being at risk.

2.5.3.1 Wolff-Parkinson-White Syndrome

In patients with the Wolff-Parkinson-White syndrome there is a recognized risk of sudden death. A minority of patients have an accessory pathway with a short refractory period allowing a rapid ventricular response to atrial flutter or fibrilla-tion [126], which may degenerate from pre-excited atrial fibrillation to ventricular fibrillation [127]. Noninvasive testing, including ambulatory monitoring and exercise testing [128], may reveal intermittent pre-excitation, indicating a relatively long accessory pathway refractory period, in up to 20%, but in the majority of patients the properties of their pathway cannot be determined without invasive EP assessment. A pathway ERP of less than 270 ms, or the shortest RR interval less than 250 ms during induced atrial fibrillation, identified increased risk [129]. In symptomatic patients, this is less of an issue, since catheter ablation can be curative and removes the risk from the pathway. The asymptomatic patient presents more of a dilemma. Conventional wisdom has been that the risk to an asymptomatic patient is low and does not merit even the low risk associated with catheter ablation. However, recent reports have challenged this view, providing evidence to support a more aggressive approach to ablation in the asymptomatic patient [130, 131].

2.5.3.2 Ventricular Arrhythmias

(a) *Post-myocardial infarction*

Sudden death due to lethal ventricular arrhythmia continues to be a major cause of mortality following MI. The peri-infarct area of myocardium provides a substrate for reentrant arrhythmias. Although ventricular fibrillation (VF) is commonly the identified fatal arrhythmia, there is evidence that the initial arrhythmia is often fast monomorphic ventric-ular tachycardia (VT), which then degenerates into VF. Thus, ventricular stimulation may induce VT or VF in survivors of cardiac arrest post-MI. Such potentially lethal arrhythmias may also be inducible in patients who have not yet had a cardiac arrest, and therefore may identify those at risk. The initiation of VT or VF has been shown to identify a popu-lation of post-infarction patients at risk of sudden death by spontaneous development of ventricular tachyarrhythmias

[132, 133]. With the availability of the ICD, there is a need to identify high-risk patients likely to benefit from expensive device therapy post-MI, so-called primary prevention. Studies utilizing combinations of risk factors, including LV dysfunction, non-sustained VT, and inducibility, have shown that it is possible to identify a high-risk population which can benefit from the ICD [134]. The Multicenter Automatic Defibrillator Implantation Trial (MADIT) [135] and the Multicenter Unsustained Tachycardia Trial (MUSTT) [116] required an EP study with inducible VT and showed mortality benefit with the ICD. However, MADIT II required only LV dysfunction post-MI as an entry criterion, without the need to demonstrate inducibility of arrhythmia, and showed a 31% reduction in the risk of death post-MI with the ICD [75]. In this study, 82% of patients who received an ICD had an EP study, and unexpectedly, ICD therapy for VF was less common in inducible than in noninducible patients [32]. Furthermore, the induction of VF was less predictive of subsequent arrhythmia than the induction of monomorphic VT, confirming the relatively nonspecific nature of induced VF. Finally, observational data from the MUSTT registry showed that patients post-MI who did not have inducible arrhythmia at EP study had a similar mortality to those who had inducible VT/VF [31], providing further evidence against the role of invasive EP testing following MI.

(b) *Cardiomyopathy*

Sudden death from ventricular arrhythmia is a cause of mortality in both dilated and hypertrophic cardiomyopathy. While EP studies to induce ventricular arrhythmia have been advocated for both these conditions, there is now recognition that ventricular stimulation is of limited value, due to its unacceptably low sensitivity and specificity [136, 137]. However, the finding of paced electrogram fractionation may be of prognostic value [138, 139]. Non-inducibility at EP study in patients with dilated cardiomyopathy may be even less predictive of freedom from sudden death than in the post-MI patients [136]. Mortality benefit from the ICD has been shown in patients with heart failure, including dilated cardiomyopathy, without the requirement of an EP study [140]. In hypertrophic cardiomyopathy, indications for the ICD are based on clinical risk factors, including family history, syncope, septal thickness, non-sustained VT, or hemodynamical instability at exercise testing [141].

Arrhythmogenic right ventricular dysplasia or cardiomyopathy (ARVC) is a genetically linked abnormality affecting the RV predominantly and is characterized by monomorphic ventricular tachycardia and a risk of sudden death [142]. EP-guided therapy has been shown to be of clinical value, but suffers from the same limitations as in the post-MI situation, and there is increasing use of the ICD, without a prior EP study [143, 144].

(c) *Arrhythmogenic channelopathies*

A major advance in recent years has been the increased understanding of genetic disorders, which may cause life-threatening arrhythmia due to electrophysiological changes at the level of ion channels and receptors, in the absence of structural heart disease. These include the long QT syndrome, Brugada syndrome, and catecholaminergic polymorphic ventricular tachycardia. Ventricular stimulation has little role in the management of these conditions [145, 146], except in the Brugada syndrome, where it remains controversial. This is a condition characterized by baseline ECG abnormalities (RBBB with ST elevation) and can cause lethal ventricular arrhythmias [147, 148]. The only treatment is an ICD. Inducible arrhythmia has been shown to be of value in the identification of risk by some [149], but not confirmed by others [77, 150].

References

1. Lenègre, J. and P. Maurice, De quelques resultats obtenus par la dérivation directe intracavitaire des courants électriques de l'oreillette et du ventricle droits. *Arch. Mal. Coeur Vaiss.*, 1945;**38**: 298–302.

2. Battro, A. and H. Bidoggia, Endocardiac electrocardiogram obtained by heart catheterization in man. *Am. Heart J.*, 1947;**33**: 604–632.

3. Hecht, H.H., Potential variations of the right auricular and ventricular cavities in man. *Am. Heart J.*, 1946;**32**: 39–51.

4. Zimmerman, H.A. and H.K., Hellerstien, Cavity potentials of the human ventricles. *Circulation*, 1951;**3**: 95–104.

5. LeVine, H.D. and W.T. Goodale, Studies in intracardiac electrography in man; IV. The potential variations in the coronary venous. *Circulation*, 1950;**2**: 48–59.

6. Tawara, S., *Das Reizleitungssystem des Säugetierherzens. Ein Anatomisch-Histologische Studie über das Atrioventrikularbundel und die Purkinjeschen Fäden*. Jena, Germany: Verslag Gustav Fischer, 1906.

7. Alanis, J., H. Gonzalez, and E. Lopez, The electrical activity of the bundle of His. *J. Physiol.*, 1958;**142**: 127–140.

8. Giraud, G., P. Puech, H. Latour, and J. Hertault, Variations de potentiel liées à l'activité du système de conduction auriculo-ventriculaire chez l'homme. *Arch. Mal. Coeur Vaiss.*, 1960;**53**: 757–776.

9. Scherlag, B.J., S.H. Lau, R.H. Helfant, et al., Catheter technique for recording His bundle activity in man. *Circulation*, 1969;**39**: 13–18.

10. Reiffel, J.A., E. Gang, J. Gliklich, et al., The human sinus node electrogram: A transvenous catheter technique and a comparison of directly measured and indirectly estimated sinoatrial conduction time in adults. *Circulation*, 1980;**62**: 1324–1334.

11. Prystowsky, E.N., K.F. Browne, and D.P. Zipes, Intracardiac recording by catheter electrode of accessory pathway depolarization. *J. Am. Coll. Cardiol.*, 1983;**1**: 468–470.

12. Damato, A.N., S.H. Lau, R. Helfant, et al., A study of heart block in man using His bundle recordings. *Circulation*, 1969;**39**: 297–305.

13. Narula, O.S., B.J. Scherlag, P. Samet, and R.P. Javier, Atrioventricular block. Localization and classification by His bundle recordings. *Am. J. Med.*, 1971;**50**: 146–165.

14. Mandel, W., H. Hayakawa, R. Danzig, and H.S. Marcus, Evaluation of sino-atrial node function in man by overdrive suppression. *Circulation*, 1971;**44**: 59–66.

15. Prevost, J.-L. and F. Battelli, La mort par les courants electriques: Courants alternatifs à haute tension. *J. Physiol. Pathol. Gen.*, 1899;**1**: 427.

16. Mines, G.R., On dynamic equilibrium in the heart. *J. Physiol. (London)*, 1913;**46**: 349–383.

17. Moe, G.K., J.B. Preston, and H. Burlington, Physiologic evidence for a dual A-V transmission system. *Circ. Res.*, 1956;**4**: 357–375.

18. Moe, G.K., W. Cohen, and R.L. Vick, Experimentally induced paroxysmal A-V nodal tachycardia in the dog. *Am. Heart J.*, 1963;**65**: 87–92.

19. Durrer, D., L. Schoo, R.M. Schuilenburg, and H.J. Wellens, The role of premature beats in the initiation and the termination of supraventricular tachycardia in the Wolff-Parkinson-White syndrome. *Circulation*, 1967;**36**: 644–662.

20. Bigger, J.T., Jr. and B.N. Goldreyer, The mechanism of supraventricular tachycardia. *Circulation*, 1970;**42**: 673–688.

21. Wellens, H.J., R.M. Schuilenburg, and D. Durrer, Electrical stimulation of the heart in patients with ventricular tachycardia. *Circulation*, 1972;**46**: 216–226.

22. Wellens, H.J., D.R. Duren, and K.I. Lie, Observations on mechanisms of ventricular tachycardia in man. *Circulation*, 1976;**54**: 237–244.

23. Akhtar, M., A.N. Damato, W.P. Batsford, et al., Demonstration of re-entry within the His-Purkinje system in man. *Circulation*, 1974;**50**: 1150–1162.

24. Lloyd, E.A., D.P. Zipes, J.J. Heger, and E.N. Prystowsky, Sustained ventricular tachycardia due to bundle branch reentry. *Am. Heart J.*, 1982;**104**: 1095–1097.

25. Josephson, M.E., L.N. Horowitz, A., Farshidi, and J.A. Kastor, Recurrent sustained ventricular tachycardia. 1. Mechanisms. *Circulation*, 1978;**57**: 431–440.

26. Josephson, M.E., L.N. Horowitz, and A. Farshidi, Continuous local electrical activity. A mechanism of recurrent ventricular tachycardia. *Circulation*, 1978;**57**: 659–665.

27. Horowitz, L.N., M.E. Josephson, and A.H. Harken, Epicardial and endocardial activation during sustained ventricular tachycardia in man. *Circulation* 1980;**61**: 1227–1238.

28. Josephson, M.E., L.N. Horowitz, A. Farshidi, et al., Sustained ventricular tachycardia: Evidence for protected localized reentry. *Am. J. Cardiol.*, 1978;**42**: 416–424.

29. Wilber, D.J., H. Garan, D. Finkelstein, et al., Out-of-hospital cardiac arrest. Use of electrophysiologic testing in the prediction of long-term outcome. *N. Engl. J. Med.*, 1988;**318**: 19–24.

30. Horowitz, L.N., M.E. Josephson, A. Farshidi, et al., Recurrent sustained ventricular tachycardia 3. Role of the electrophysiologic study in selection of antiarrhythmic regimens. *Circulation*, 1978;**58**: 986–997.

31. Buxton, A.E., K.L. Lee, L. DiCarlo, et al., Electrophysiologic testing to identify patients with coronary artery disease who are at risk for sudden death. Multicenter Unsustained Tachycardia Trial Investigators. *N. Engl. J. Med.*, 2000;**342**: 1937–1945.

32. Daubert, J.P., W. Zareba, W.J. Hall, et al., Predictive value of ventricular arrhythmia inducibility for subsequent ventricular tachycardia or ventricular fibrillation in Multicenter Automatic Defibrillator Implantation Trial (MADIT) II patients. *J. Am. Coll. Cardiol.*, 2006;**47**: 98–107.

33. Brodsky, M.A., L.B. Mitchell, B.D. Halperin, M.H. Raitt, and A.P. Hallstrom Prognostic value of baseline electrophysiology studies in patients with sustained ventricular tachyarrhythmia: The Antiarrhythmics Versus Implantable Defibrillators (AVID) trial. *Am. Heart J.*, 2002;**144**: 478–484.

34. Mason, J.W., A comparison of electrophysiologic testing with Holter monitoring to predict antiarrhythmic-drug efficacy for ventricular tachyarrhythmias. Electrophysiologic Study versus Electrocardiographic Monitoring Investigators. *N. Engl. J. Med.*, 1993;**329**: 445–451.

35. Morady, F., Radio-frequency ablation as treatment for cardiac arrhythmias. *N. Engl. J. Med.*, 1999;**340**: 534–544.

36. Stevenson, W.G. and K. Soejima, Recording techniques for clinical electrophysiology. *J. Cardiovasc. Electrophysiol.*, 2005;**16**: 1017–1022.

37. Campbell, R.W., R. Charles, J.C. Cowan, et al., Clinical competence in electrophysiological techniques. *Heart*, 1997;**78**: 403–412.

38. Tracy, C.M., M. Akhtar, J.P. DiMarco, et al., American College of Cardiology/American Heart Association 2006 Update of the Clinical Competence Statement on invasive electrophysiology studies, catheter ablation, and cardioversion: A report of the American College of Cardiology/American Heart Association/American College of Physicians Task Force on Clinical Competence and Training. *Circulation*, 2006;**114**:1654–1668.

39. Ng, G.A., E.W. Lau, and M.J. Griffith, A streamlined "3-catheter" approach in the electrophysiological study and radiofrequency ablation of narrow complex tachycardia. *J. Intervent. Card. Electrophysiol.*, 2002;**7**: 209–214.

40. Kuck, K.H. and M. Schluter, Single-catheter approach to radiofrequency current ablation ofleft-sided accessory pathways

in patients with Wolff-Parkinson-White syndrome. *Circulation*, 1991;**84**: 2366–2375.

41. Narula, O.S., B.J. Scherlag, and P. Samet, Pervenous pacing of the specialized conducting system in man. His bundle and A-V nodal stimulation. *Circulation*, 1970;**41**: 77–87.

42. Michelson, E.L., S.R. Spielman, A.M. Greenspan, et al., Electrophysiologic study of the left ventricle: Indications and safety. *Chest*, 1979;**75**: 592–596.

43. Herre, J.M., D.E. Mann, J.C. Luck, et al., Effect of increased current, multiple pacing sites and number of extrastimuli on induction of ventricular tachycardia. *Am. J. Cardiol.*, 1986;**57**: 102–107.

44. Morady, F., L.A. Dicarlo, Jr., L.B. Liem, R.B. Krol, and J.M. Baerman, Effects of high stimulation current on the induction of ventricular tachycardia. *Am. J. Cardiol.*, 1985;**56**: 73–78.

45. Kennedy, E.E., L.E. Rosenfeld, C.A. McPherson, S.I. Stark, and W.P. Batsford, Mechanisms and relevance of arrhythmias induced by high-current programmed ventricular stimulation. *Am. J. Cardiol.*, 1986;**57**: 598–603.

46. Josephson, M.E., D.L. Scharf, J.A. Kastor, and J.G. Kitchen, Atrial endocardial activation in man. Electrode catheter technique of endocardial mapping. *Am. J. Cardiol.*, 1977;**39**: 972–981.

47. Bekheit, S., J.G. Murtagh, P. Morton, and E. Fletcher, Measurements of sinus impulse conduction from electrogram of bundle of His. *Br. Heart J.*, 1971;**33**: 719–724.

48. Benditt, D.G., L.C. Pritchett, W.M. Smith, A.G. Wallace, and J.J. Gallagher, Characteristics of atrioventricular conduction and the spectrum of arrhythmias in Lown-Ganong-Levine syndrome. *Circulation*, 1978;**57**: 454–465.

49. Wiener, I., Syndromes of Lown-Ganong-Levine and enhanced atrioventricular nodal conduction. *Am. J. Cardiol.*, 1983;**52**: 637–639.

50. Kashani, A., and S.S. Barold, Significance of QRS complex duration in patients with heart failure. *J. Am. Coll. Cardiol.*, 2005;**46**: 2183–2192.

51. Gupta, P.K., and J.I. Haft, Retrograde ventriculoatrial conduction in complete heart block: Studies with His bundle electrography. *Am. J. Cardiol.*, 1972;**30**: 408–411.

52. Denes, P., D. Wu, R. Dhingra, R.J. Pietras, and K.M. Rosen, The effects of cycle length on cardiac refractory periods in man. *Circulation*, 1974;**49**: 32–41.

53. Denes, P., D. Wu, R.C. Dhingra, R. Chuquimia, and K.M. Rosen, Demonstration of dual A-V nodal pathways in patients with paroxysmal supraventricular tachycardia. *Circulation*, 1973;**48**: 549–555.

54. Scheinman, M.M. and Y. Yang, The history of AV nodal reentry. *Pacing Clin. Electrophysiol.*, 2005;**28**: 1232–1237.

55. Wu, D., P. Denes, R. Bauernfeind, et al., Effects of atropine on induction and maintenance of atrioventricular nodal reentrant tachycardia. *Circulation*, 1979;**59**: 779–788.

56. Sung, R.J., H.L. Waxman, S. Saksena, and Z. Juma, Sequence of retrograde atrial activation in patients with dual atrioventricular nodal pathways. *Circulation*, 1981;**64**: 1059–1067.

57. Jackman, W.M., K.J. Beckman, J.H. McClelland, et al., Treatment of supraventricular tachycardia due to atrioventricular nodal reentry, by radiofrequency catheter ablation of slow-pathway conduction. *N. Engl. J. Med.*, 1992;**327**: 313–318.

58. Heidbuchel, H. and W.M. Jackman, Characterization of subforms of AV nodal reentrant tachycardia. *Europace*, 2004;**6**: 316–329.

59. Nawata, H., N. Yamamoto, K. Hirao, et al., Heterogeneity of anterograde fast-pathway and retrograde slow-pathway conduction patterns in patients with the fast-slow form of atrioventricular nodal reentrant tachycardia: Electrophysiologic and electrocardiographic considerations. *J. Am. Coll. Cardiol.*, 1998;**32**: 1731–1740.

60. Wu, D., P. Denes, R. Dhingra, and K.M. Rosen, Nature of the gap phenomenon in man. *Circ. Res.*, 1974;**34**: 682–692.

61. Akhtar, M., A.N. Damato, W.P. Batsford, et al., Unmasking and conversion of gap phenomenon in the human heart. *Circulation*, 1974;**49**: 624–630.

62. Akhtar, M., A.N. Damato, A.R. Caracta, W.P. Batsford, and S.H. Lau, The gap phenomena during retrograde conduction in man. *Circulation*, 1974;**49**: 811–817.

63. Josephson, M.E., *Clinical Cardiac Electrophysiology. Techniques and Interpretations*, 4th Edition, Philadelphia, PA: Lippincott Williams & Williams, 2008.

64. Brugada, P., M. Green, H. Abdollah, and H.J. Wellens, Significance of ventricular arrhythmias initiated by programmed ventricular stimulation: The importance of the type of ventricular arrhythmia induced and the number of premature stimuli required. *Circulation*, 1984;**69**: 87–92.

65. DiMarco, J.P., H. Garan, and J.N. Ruskin, Complications in patients undergoing cardiac electrophysiologic procedures. *Ann. Intern. Med.*, 1982;**97**: 490–493.

66. Horowitz, L.N., H.R. Kay, S.P. Kutalek, et al., Risks and complications of clinical cardiac electrophysiologic studies: A prospective analysis of 1,000 consecutive patients. *J. Am. Coll. Cardiol.*, 1987;**9**: 1261–1268.

67. Horowitz, L.N., Safety of electrophysiologic studies. *Circulation*, 1986;**73**: II28–II31.

68. Hindricks, G., The Multicentre European Radiofrequency Survey (MERFS): Complications of radiofrequency catheter ablation of arrhythmias. The Multicentre European Radiofrequency Survey (MERFS) investigators of the Working Group on Arrhythmias of the European Society of Cardiology. *Eur. Heart J.*, 1993;**14**: 1644–1653.

69. Scheinman, M.M. and S. Huang, The 1998 NASPE prospective catheter ablation registry. *Pacing Clin. Electrophysiol.*, 2000;**23**: 1020–1028.

70. Chen, S.A., C.E. Chiang, C.T. Tai, et al., Complications of diagnostic electrophysiologic studies and radiofrequency catheter ablation in patients with tachyarrhythmias: An eight-year survey of 3,966 consecutive procedures in a tertiary referral center. *Am. J. Cardiol.*, 1996;**77**: 41–46.

71. Cappato, R., H. Calkins, S.A. Chen, et al., Worldwide survey on the methods, efficacy, and safety of catheter ablation for human atrial fibrillation. *Circulation*, 2005;**111**: 1100–1105.

72. Quinn, F.R. and A.C. Rankin, Atrial fibrillation ablation in the real world. *Heart*, 2005;**91**: 1507–1508.

73. Boersma, L., L. Mont, A. Sionis, E. Garcia, and J. Brugada, Value of the implantable loop recorder for the management of patients with unexplained syncope. *Europace*, 2004;**6**: 70–76.

74. Strickberger, S.A., D.W. Benson, I. Biaggioni, et al., AHA/ACCF Scientific Statement on the evaluation of syncope. *Circulation*, 2006;**113**: 316–327.

75. Moss, A.J., W. Zareba, W.J. Hall, et al., Prophylactic implantation of a defibrillator in patients with myocardial infarction and reduced ejection fraction. *N. Engl. J. Med.*, 2002;**346**: 877–883.

76. Grimm, W., J. Hoffmann, V. Menz, K. Luck, and B. Maisch, Programmed ventricular stimulation for arrhythmia risk prediction in patients with idiopathic dilated cardiomyopathy and non-sustained ventricular tachycardia. *J. Am. Coll. Cardiol.*, 1998;**32**: 739–745.

77. Kanda, M., W. Shimizu, K. Matsuo, et al., Electrophysiologic characteristics and implications of induced ventricular fibrillation in symptomatic patients with Brugada syndrome. *J. Am. Coll. Cardiol.*, 2002;**39**: 1799–1805.

78. Epstein, A.E., J.P. DiMarco, K.A. Ellenbogen, et al., ACC/AHA/HRS 2008 Guidelines for Device-Based Therapy of Cardiac Rhythm Abnormalities: a report of the American College of Cardiology/American Heart Association Task Force on Practice Guidelines (Writing Committee to Revise the ACC/AHA/NASPE 2002 Guideline Update for Implantation of Cardiac Pacemakers and Antiarrhythmia Devices): developed in collaboration with the American Association for Thoracic Surgery and Society of Thoracic Surgeons. Circulation 2008;117: e350–408.

79. Knight, B.P., A. Zivin, J. Souza, et al., A technique for the rapid diagnosis of atrial tachycardia in the electrophysiology laboratory. *J. Am. Coll. Cardiol.*, 1999;**33**: 775–781.

80. Vijayaraman, P., B.P. Lee, G. Kalahasty, M.A. Wood, and K.A. Ellenbogen, Reanalysis of the "pseudo A-A-V" response to ventricular entrainment of supraventricular tachycardia: Importance of his-bundle timing. *J. Cardiovasc. Electrophysiol.*, 2006;**17**: 25–28.

81. Owada, S., A. Iwasa, S. Sasaki, et al., "V-H-A Pattern" as a criterion for the differential diagnosis of atypical AV nodal reentrant tachycardia from AV reciprocating tachycardia. *Pacing Clin. Electrophysiol.*, 2005;**28**: 667–674.

82. Hirao, K., K. Otomo, X. Wang, et al., Para-Hisian pacing. A new method for differentiating retrograde conduction over an accessory AV pathway from conduction over the AV node. *Circulation*, 1996;**94**: 1027–1035.

83. Waldo, A.L., From bedside to bench: Entrainment and other stories. *Heart Rhythm*, 2004;**1**: 94–106.

84. Waldo, A.L., W.A. MacLean, R.B. Karp, N.T. Kouchoukos, and T.N. James, Entrainment and interruption of atrial flutter with atrial pacing: Studies in man following open heart surgery. *Circulation*, 1977;**56**: 737–745.

85. Waldo, A.L., V.J. Plumb, J.G. Arciniegas, et al., Transient entrainment and interruption of the atrioventricular bypass pathway type of paroxysmal atrial tachycardia. A model for understanding and identifying reentrant arrhythmias. *Circulation*, 1983;**67**: 73–83.

86. Waldo, A.L., R.W. Henthorn, V.J. Plumb, and W.A. MacLean, Demonstration of the mechanism of transient entrainment and interruption of ventricular tachycardia with rapid atrial pacing. *J. Am. Coll. Cardiol.*, 1984;**3**: 422–430.

87. Henthorn, R.W., K. Okumura, B. Olshansky, et al., A fourth criterion for transient entrainment: The electrogram equivalent of progressive fusion. *Circulation*, 1988;**77**: 1003–1012.

88. Okumura, K., R.W. Henthorn, A.E. Epstein, V.J. Plumb, and A.L. Waldo, Further observations on transient entrainment: Importance of pacing site and properties of the components of the reentry circuit. *Circulation*, 1985;**72**: 1293–1307.

89. Stevenson, W.G., H. Khan, P. Sager, et al., Identification of reentry circuit sites during catheter mapping and radiofrequency ablation of ventricular tachycardia late after myocardial infarction. *Circulation*, 1993;**88**: 1647–1670.

90. Waldo, A.L. and R.W. Henthorn, Use of transient entrainment during ventricular tachycardia to localize a critical area in the reentry circuit for ablation. *Pacing Clin. Electrophysiol.*, 1989;**12**: 231–244.

91. Morady, F., A. Kadish, S. Rosenheck, et al., Concealed entrainment as a guide for catheter ablation of ventricular tachycardia in patients with prior myocardial infarction. *J. Am. Coll. Cardiol.*, 1991;**17**: 678–689.

92. Brignole, M., P. Alboni, D. Benditt, et al., Guidelines on management (diagnosis and treatment) of syncope. *Eur. Heart J.*, 2001;**22**: 1256–1306.

93. Brignole, M., P. Alboni, D.G. Benditt, et al., Guidelines on management (diagnosis and treatment) of syncope—update 2004. *Europace*, 2004;**6**: 467–537.

94. Gulamhusein, S., G.V. Naccarelli, P.T. Ko, et al., Value and limitations of clinical electrophysiologic study in assessment of patients with unexplained syncope. *Am. J. Med.*, 1982;**73**: 700–705.

95. Linzer, M., E.H. Yang, N.A. Estes, III, et al., Diagnosing syncope. Part 2: Unexplained syncope. Clinical Efficacy Assessment Project of the American College of Physicians. *Ann. Intern. Med.*, 1997;**127**: 76–86.

96. Jackman, W.M., X.Z. Wang, K.J. Friday, et al., Catheter ablation of accessory atrioventricular pathways (Wolff-Parkinson-White syndrome) by radiofrequency current. *N. Engl. J. Med.*, 1991;**324**: 1605–1611.

97. Calkins, H., J. Sousa, R. el Atassi, et al., Diagnosis and cure of the Wolff-Parkinson-White syndrome or paroxysmal supraventricular tachycardias during a single electrophysiologic test. *N. Engl. J. Med.*, 1991;**324**: 1612–1618.

98. Epstein, L.M., M.D. Lesh, J.C. Griffin, R.J. Lee, and M.M. Scheinman, A direct midseptal approach to slow atrioventricular nodal pathway ablation. *Pacing Clin. Electrophysiol.*, 1995;**18**: 57–64.

99. Kirkorian, G., E. Moncada, P. Chevalier, et al., Radiofrequency ablation of atrial flutter. Efficacy of an anatomically guided approach. *Circulation*, 1994;**90**: 2804–2814.

100. Pappone, C., S. Rosanio, G. Oreto, et al., Circumferential radiofrequency ablation of pulmonary vein ostia: A new anatomic approach for curing atrial fibrillation. *Circulation*, 2000;**102**: 2619–2628.

101. Soejima, K., M. Suzuki, W.H. Maisel, et al., Catheter ablation in patients with multiple and unstable ventricular tachycardias after myocardial infarction: Short ablation lines guided by reentry circuit isthmuses and sinus rhythm mapping. *Circulation*, 2001;**104**: 664–669.

102. Haissaguerre, M., J.F. Dartigues, J.F. Warin, et al., Electrogram patterns predictive of successful catheter ablation of accessory pathways. Value of unipolar recording mode. *Circulation*, 1991;**84**: 188–202.

103. McClelland, J.H., X. Wang, K.J. Beckman, et al., Radiofrequency catheter ablation of right atriofascicular (Mahaim) accessory pathways guided by accessory pathway activation potentials. *Circulation*, 1994;**89**: 2655–2666.

104. Heald, S.C., D.W. Davies, D.E. Ward, C.J. Garratt, and E. Rowland, Radiofrequency catheter ablation of Mahaim tachycardia by targeting Mahaim potentials at the tricuspid annulus. *Br. Heart J.*, 1995;**73**: 250–257.

105. Nakagawa, H., K.J. Beckman, J.H. McClelland, et al., Radiofrequency catheter ablation of idiopathic left ventricular

tachycardia guided by a Purkinje potential. *Circulation*, 1993;**88**: 2607–2617.

106. Nogami, A., S. Naito, H. Tada, et al., Demonstration of diastolic and presystolic Purkinje potentials as critical potentials in a macroreentry circuit of verapamil-sensitive idiopathic left ventricular tachycardia. *J. Am. Coll. Cardiol.*, 2000;**36**: 811–823.

107. Stevenson, W.G., P.T. Sager, and P.L. Friedman, Entrainment techniques for mapping atrial and ventricular tachycardias. *J. Cardiovasc. Electrophysiol.*, 1995;**6**: 201–216.

108. Calkins, H., A.R. Leon, A.G. Deam, et al., Catheter ablation of atrial flutter using radiofrequency energy. *Am. J. Cardiol.*, 1994;**73**: 353–356.

109. Poty, H., N., Saoudi, M. Nair, F. Anselme, and B. Letac, Radiofrequency catheter ablation of atrial flutter. Further insights into the various types of isthmus block: Application to ablation during sinus rhythm. *Circulation*, 1996;**94**: 3204–3213.

110. Fisher, J.D., H.L. Cohen, R. Mehra, et al., Cardiac pacing and pacemakers II. Serial electrophysiologic-pharmacologic testing for control of recurrent tachyarrhythmias. *Am. Heart J.*, 1977;**93**: 658–668.

111. Waxman, H.L., A.E. Buxton, L.M. Sadowski, and M.E. Josephson, The response to procainamide during electrophysiologic study for sustained ventricular tachyarrhythmias predicts the response to other medications. *Circulation*, 1983;**67**: 30–37.

112. Breithardt, G., L. Seipel, R.R. Abendroth, and F. Loogen, Serial electrophysiological testing of antiarrhythmic drug efficacy in patients with recurrent ventricular tachycardia. *Eur. Heart J.*, 1980;**1**: 11–24.

113. Waller, T.J., H.R. Kay, S.R. Spielman, et al., Reduction in sudden death and total mortality by antiarrhythmic therapy evaluated by electrophysiologic drug testing: criteria of efficacy in patients with sustained ventricular tachyarrhythmia. *J. Am. Coll. Cardiol.*, 1987;**10**: 83–89.

114. Borggrefe, M., H.J. Trampisch, and G. Breithardt, Reappraisal of criteria for assessing drug efficacy in patients with ventricular tachyarrhythmias: Complete versus partial suppression of inducible arrhythmias. *J. Am. Coll. Cardiol.*, 1988;**12**: 140–149.

115. Handlin, L.R., W.N. Brodine, H. Gibbs, and J.L. Vacek, Slowing of ventricular tachycardia as a possible endpoint for serial drug testing at electrophysiological study. *Pacing Clin. Electrophysiol.*, 1992;**15**: 864–869.

116. Buxton, A.E., K.L. Lee, J.D. Fisher, et al., A randomized study of the prevention of sudden death in patients with coronary artery disease. Multicenter Unsustained Tachycardia Trial Investigators. *N. Engl. J. Med.*, 1999;**341**: 1882–1890.

117. Lee, K.L., G. Hafley, J.D. Fisher, et al., Effect of implantable defibrillators on arrhythmic events and mortality in the multicenter unsustained tachycardia trial. *Circulation*, 2002;**106**: 233–238.

118. Morady, F., L. DiCarlo, S. Winston, J.C. Davis, and M.M. Scheinman, Clinical features and prognosis of patients with out of hospital cardiac arrest and a normal electrophysiologic study. *J. Am. Coll. Cardiol.*, 1984;**4**: 39–44.

119. Raitt, M.H., E.G. Renfroe, A.E. Epstein, et al., "Stable" ventricular tachycardia is not a benign rhythm: Insights from the antiarrhythmics versus implantable defibrillators (AVID) registry. *Circulation*, 2001;**103**: 244–252.

120. McPherson, C.A., L.E. Rosenfeld, and W.P. Batsford, Day-to-day reproducibility of responses to right ventricular programmed electrical stimulation: Implications for serial drug testing. *Am. J. Cardiol.*, 1985;**55**: 689–695.

121. Mann, D.E., V. Hartz, E.A. Hahn, and M.J. Reiter, Effect of reproducibility of baseline arrhythmia induction on drug efficacy predictions and outcome in the Electrophysiologic Study Versus Electrocardiographic Monitoring (ESVEM) trial. *Am. J. Cardiol.*, 1997;**80**: 1448–1452.

122. Schaumann, A., M.F. von zur, B. Herse, B.D. Gonska, and H. Kreuzer, Empirical versus tested antitachycardia pacing in implantable cardioverter defibrillators: A prospective study including 200 patients. *Circulation*, 1998;**97**: 66–74.

123. Wathen, M.S., M.O. Sweeney, P.J. DeGroot, et al., Shock reduction using antitachycardia pacing for spontaneous rapid ventricular tachycardia in patients with coronary artery disease. *Circulation*, 2001;**104**: 796–801.

124. Wathen, M.S., P.J. DeGroot, M.O. Sweeney, et al., Prospective randomized multicenter trial of empirical antitachycardia pacing versus shocks for spontaneous rapid ventricular tachycardia in patients with implantable cardioverter-defibrillators: Pacing Fast Ventricular Tachycardia Reduces Shock Therapies (PainFREE Rx II) trial results. *Circulation*, 2004;**110**: 2591–2596.

125. Raitt, M.H., G.L. Dolack, P.J. Kudenchuk, J.E. Poole, and G.H. Bardy, Ventricular arrhythmias detected after transvenous defibrillator implantation in patients with a clinical history of only ventricular fibrillation. Implications for use of implantable defibrillator. *Circulation*, 1995;**91**: 1996–2001.

126. Wellens, H.J. and D. Durrer, Wolff-Parkinson-White syndrome and atrial fibrillation. Relation between refractory period of accessory pathway and ventricular rate during atrial fibrillation. *Am. J. Cardiol.*, 1974;**34**: 777–782.

127. Klein, G.J., T.M. Bashore, T.D. Sellers, et al., Ventricular fibrillation in the Wolff-Parkinson-White syndrome. *N. Engl. J. Med.*, 1979;**301**: 1080–1085.

128. Jezior, M.R., S.M. Kent, and J.E. Atwood, Exercise testing in Wolff-Parkinson-White syndrome: Case report with ECG and literature review. *Chest*, 2005;**127**: 1454–1457.

129. Blomstrom-Lundqvist, C., M.M. Scheinman, E.M. Aliot, et al., ACC/AHA/ESC guidelines for the management of patients with supraventricular arrhythmias-executive summary. *J. Am. Coll. Cardiol.*, 2003;**42**: 1493–1531.

130. Pappone, C., V. Santinelli, S. Rosanio, et al., Usefulness of invasive electrophysiologic testing to stratify the risk of arrhythmic events in asymptomatic patients with Wolff-Parkinson-White pattern: Results from a large prospective long-term follow-up study. *J. Am. Coll. Cardiol.*, 2003;**41**: 239–244.

131. Pappone, C., F. Manguso, R. Santinelli, et al., Radiofrequency ablation in children with asymptomatic Wolff-Parkinson-White syndrome. *N. Engl. J. Med.*, 2004;**351**: 1197–1205.

132. Richards, D.A., D.V. Cody, A.R. Denniss, et al., Ventricular electrical instability: A predictor of death after myocardial infarction. *Am. J. Cardiol.*, 1983;**51**: 75–80.

133. Richards, D.A., K. Byth, D.L. Ross, and J.B. Uther, What is the best predictor of spontaneous ventricular tachycardia and sudden death after myocardial infarction? *Circulation*, 1991;**83**: 756–763.

134. Bailey, J.J., A.S. Berson, H. Handelsman, and M. Hodges, Utility of current risk stratification tests for predicting major arrhythmic events after myocardial infarction. *J. Am. Coll. Cardiol.*, 2001;**38**: 1902–1911.

135. Moss, A.J., W.J. Hall, D.S. Cannom, et al., Improved survival with an implanted defibrillator in patients with coronary disease at high risk for ventricular arrhythmia. Multicenter Automatic

Defibrillator Implantation Trial Investigators. *N. Engl. J. Med.*, 1996;**335**: 1933–1940.

136. Chen, X., M. Shenasa, M. Borggrefe, et al., Role of programmed ventricular stimulation in patients with idiopathic dilated cardiomyopathy and documented sustained ventricular tachyarrhythmias: Inducibility and prognostic value in 102 patients. *Eur. Heart J.*, 1994;**15**: 76–82.

137. Behr, E.R., P. Elliott, and W.J. McKenna, Role of invasive EP testing in the evaluation and management of hypertrophic cardiomyopathy. *Card. Electrophysiol. Rev.*, 2002;**6**: 482–486.

138. Saumarez, R.C. and A.A. Grace, Paced ventricular electrogram fractionation and sudden death in hypertrophic cardiomyopathy and other non-coronary heart diseases. *Cardiovasc. Res.*, 2000;**47**: 11–22.

139. Saumarez, R.C., L. Chojnowska, R. Derksen, et al., Sudden death in noncoronary heart disease is associated with delayed paced ventricular activation. *Circulation*, 2003;**107**: 2595–2600.

140. Bardy, G.H., K.L. Lee, D.B. Mark, et al., Amiodarone or an implantable cardioverter-defibrillator for congestive heart failure. *N. Engl. J. Med.*, 2005;**352**: 225–237.

141. Elliott, P.M., J. Poloniecki, S. Dickie, et al., Sudden death in hypertrophic cardiomyopathy: Identification of high risk patients. *J. Am. Coll. Cardiol.*, 2000;**36**: 2212–2218.

142. Kies, P., M. Bootsma, J. Bax, M.J. Schalij, and E.E. van der Wall, Arrhythmogenic right ventricular dysplasia/cardiomyopathy: Screening, diagnosis, and treatment. *Heart Rhythm*, 2006;**3**: 225–234.

143. Corrado, D., L. Leoni, M.S. Link, et al., Implantable cardioverter-defibrillator therapy for prevention of sudden death in patients with arrhythmogenic right ventricular cardiomyopathy/dysplasia. *Circulation*, 2003;**108**: 3084–3091.

144. Wichter, T., M. Paul, C. Wollmann, et al., Implantable cardioverter/defibrillator therapy in arrhythmogenic right ventricular cardiomyopathy: Single-center experience of long-term follow-up and complications in 60 patients. *Circulation*, 2004;**109**: 1503–1508.

145. Bhandari, A.K., W.A. Shapiro, F. Morady, et al., Electrophysiologic testing in patients with the long QT syndrome. *Circulation*, 1985;**71**: 63–71.

146. Sumitomo, N., K. Harada, M. Nagashima, et al., Catecholaminergic polymorphic ventricular tachycardia: Electrocardiographic characteristics and optimal therapeutic strategies to prevent sudden death. *Heart*, 2003;**89**: 66–70.

147. Brugada, J., P. Brugada, and R. Brugada, The syndrome of right bundle branch block ST segment elevation in V1 to V3 and sudden death—the Brugada syndrome. *Europace*, 1999;**1**: 156–166.

148. Wilde, A.A., C. Antzelevitch, M. Borggrefe, et al., Proposed diagnostic criteria for the Brugada syndrome: Consensus report. *Circulation*, 2002;**106**: 2514–2519.

149. Brugada, P., R. Brugada, L. Mont, et al., Natural history of Brugada syndrome: The prognostic value of programmed electrical stimulation of the heart. *J. Cardiovasc. Electrophysiol.*, 2003;**14**: 455–457.

150. Priori, S.G., C. Napolitano, M. Gasparini, et al., Natural history of Brugada syndrome: Insights for risk stratification and management. *Circulation*, 2002;**105**: 1342–1347.

3 Intracardiac Mapping

Oliver R. Segal · Michael Koa-Wing · Julian Jarman · Nicholas Peters · Vias Markides ·
D. Wyn Davies

P. W. Macfarlane et al. (eds.), *Cardiac Arrhythmias and Mapping Techniques*, DOI 10.1007/978-0-85729-877-5_3,

3.1 Catheter-Based Mapping Techniques

3.1.1 The Development of Catheter-Based Mapping Techniques

Following the inception of cardiac catheterization in the 1940s, catheter-based techniques were developed to record electrical activity from the endocardial surface using electrode catheters. One of the first exponents of this technique was Scherlag, who used electrode catheters to record activity from the His bundle in man [1]. At the same time, programmed electrical stimulation was being developed by Wellens' group, to both induce and terminate supraventricular tachycardias (SVT) in patients with Wolff-Parkinson-White Syndrome [2], and then later in patients with ventricular tachycardia (VT) [3]. Catheter recordings were then used to determine the refractory periods of the atria, ventricles, and the His–Purkinje tissue, and the functional characteristics of the A-V conducting system. This led to the investigation of the effects of pharmacological agents on these functional parameters and their efficacy in terminating and preventing arrhythmias.

The use of multiple catheters inside the heart allowed investigators to compare activation timings at different sites and represented the first step in mapping arrhythmias. This simple technique allowed the approximate localization of accessory pathways in patients with Wolff-Parkinson-White Syndrome and, subsequently, led Josephson et al. to describe endocardial mapping techniques for VT arising from the left ventricle [4]. However, the use of single or multiple catheters for mapping arrhythmias has important limitations. It is usually only applicable to sustained, monomorphic arrhythmias that are hemodynamically stable where there is time for sequential mapping. Furthermore, the spatial resolution of individual catheters may not be sufficient to elucidate the mechanism or substrate and origin of complex arrhythmias, especially infarct-related VT. To overcome these limitations in VT, some investigators developed criteria for identifying sites critical for arrhythmogenesis during sinus rhythm, namely, the presence of abnormal fractionated electrograms [5–7].

3.1.2 Conventional Contact Catheter Mapping

Intracardiac mapping using conventional contact catheters remains the cornerstone of diagnostic electrophysiology and ablation. The placement of catheters in different cardiac chambers with simultaneous recording enables determination of the origin of many types of arrhythmia. However, considerable knowledge and experience is required to interpret this information, and many different techniques designed to tackle the same forms of tachycardia have evolved.

3.1.3 Vascular Access

The placement of catheters within the right heart and coronary sinus requires cannulation of a central vein. The right and left femoral veins are typically used for the placement of most catheters, although the subclavian veins may be particularly useful for the placement of electrodes within the coronary sinus.

Access to the left atrium and ventricle can be obtained either via the retrograde trans-aortic route (although mapping of the left atrium using this technique is usually difficult) or via the transseptal route, where puncture of the intra-atrial septum is usually required unless a patent foramen ovale or atrial septal defect is present, in which case access may be achieved directly. Importantly, once catheters are placed within the left-sided circulation, anticoagulation with heparin is required to prevent thrombotic and embolic complications.

3.1.4 Contact Catheters

A variety of diagnostic catheters are available from many different manufacturers. In their simplest form, they comprise a fixed-curve bipolar catheter, with which it is possible to both record electrical activity and pace the heart using a bipolar or unipolar configuration.

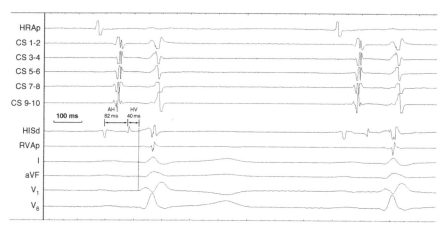

◘ Fig. 3.1

Typical electrograms recorded from a conventional diagnostic electrophysiology study. Abbreviations: *AH*, interval between septal atrial and His electrograms; *CS*, coronary sinus; *Hisd*, distal His bundle electrogram; *HRA*, high right atrium; *HV*, interval between the His electrogram and the earliest ventricular activity inscribed from any intracardiac or surface lead, in this case, V₁, which demonstrates right bundle branch block to be present; *RVAp*, proximal right ventricular apical electrogram. Four ECG leads are labeled conventionally

However, fixed curve quadripolar catheters are typically used for recording electrical activity from the high right atrium, the AV node/bundle of His, and the apex of the right ventricle (❷ Fig. 3.1). The addition of the two extra electrodes provides more electrical information from the chamber in which they have been placed, and this in turn provides greater information to gauge the direction of activation within a cardiac chamber. In addition, this offers the ability to pace and record simultaneously from closely adjacent electrodes. A quadripolar catheter placed at the bundle of His may also be able to record electrical potentials from the proximal right bundle branch, which is useful in some circumstances.

In contrast, a multipolar catheter, such as a decapolar catheter, is typically used for recording electrical activity within the coronary sinus, enabling the length of the vein to be spanned by the recording electrodes. The coronary sinus is the only place where left atrial and ventricular activity can be recorded from standard venous cannulation. It is therefore logical to obtain as much information as possible from a single catheter so that, for example, in patients with left-sided accessory pathways, a decapolar catheter within the coronary sinus lies close to the mitral annulus, facilitating pathway localization. Some centres now routinely use deflectable diagnostic decapolar catheters for use within the coronary sinus, which can make cannulation of the coronary sinus from the femoral route significantly easier.

Specialized multipolar mapping catheters are available that have been designed to guide specific types of catheter ablation. The "Halo" catheter is a 20-pole deflectable curvilinear mapping catheter, which is designed to sit around the tricuspid valve annulus and is used most frequently during typical atrial flutter ablation, although it can be useful in any procedure in which global right atrial recording is required or to guide the localization of right-sided accessory pathways [8]. The "Lasso" catheter is also a multipolar, curvilinear mapping catheter designed to sit at the os of the pulmonary veins to guide the ablation of atrial fibrillation (AF) by pulmonary venous isolation.

3.2   Recording Systems

A system that simultaneously records the standard 12 surface ECG waveforms in addition to a large number of channels for recording intracardiac signals is necessary for performing diagnostic and therapeutic electrophysiological procedures. A number of different recording systems are commercially available, and signals are amplified and filtered over a wide and variable frequency range (from under 1 Hz to 200 kHz), digitized, displayed, and stored.

3.3 Electrogram Recording and Morphology

Electrical activity within the heart can be recorded with unipolar or bipolar configurations. Unipolar electrograms are recorded between a single pole from within the heart and a distant pole typically located intravascularly but outside the heart to minimize surface electrical noise generated by skeletal muscle or an alternating current power supply.

The morphology of unipolar electrograms provides information about the direction of the wavefront of activation coming toward or away from the catheter by the same principle as seen on the standard surface ECG. A wavefront that comes toward the catheter will produce a positive deflection, while a negative deflection occurs when the wavefront travels away from it. Thus, when attempting to map a focal tachycardia, i.e., a tachycardia that originates from a specific focus and propagates centrifugally, a QS morphology indicates the location of the focus. Accordingly, an RS morphology is recorded from all other sites. There are important caveats to this rule that include the need for adequate tissue contact, minimal high-pass filtering, and the presence of "far-field" electrograms that can obscure small amplitude signals. Examples of the latter include ventricular far-field signals recorded from the overlying right atrial appendage or ventricular electrograms from healthy tissue obscuring small potentials from zones of slow conduction within reentrant VT circuits. Bipolar signals also provide information on wavefront propagation, but here, the orientation of the bipole relative to wavefront propagation is a major determinant of the signal shape.

The majority of intracardiac recordings are made with bipolar electrograms. Although their morphology provides limited information about wavefront direction, they indicate the time of local endocardial activation better than unipolar signals.

3.4 Catheter Mapping

Sites critical to the maintenance of a tachycardia can be elucidated by careful interpretation of surface ECG morphology and electrogram timing in combination with specialized pacing maneuvers. In addition, pacing is routinely used to initiate and terminate tachycardias, and the type of pacing maneuver that succeeds in doing so can give information about the likely substrate of the arrhythmia. For instance, arrhythmias that are readily and repeatedly induced using programmed stimulation are most frequently a result of reentry. Triggered rhythms may require appropriate drugs or sometimes physical maneuvers, such as straight leg raising, to aid inducibility.

The process of arrhythmia diagnosis depends significantly on the interpretation of electrogram timing. As bipolar recordings are used in the majority of cases, electrogram morphology is not usually considered in this diagnostic process, although sometimes the combination of unipolar and bipolar recordings are helpful, for example, in ablation of typical right atrial flutter (see below). Usually, complimentary methods of mapping are used to help in the diagnosis of arrhythmias. These are described below.

3.4.1 Activation Sequence Mapping

During focal tachycardias, the origin of the tachycardia is the site at which the earliest electrogram can be localized. This site is found using a roving mapping catheter, and the timing of successive electrograms recorded from this catheter are compared with a stable and relevant reference signal, be it another intracardiac electrogram or surface ECG feature. For instance, focal atrial tachycardias can be mapped by comparing the roving catheter electrogram to the earliest P wave onset on the surface ECG during tachycardia or perhaps to the electrogram recorded from a stable catheter placed within either atrium. If unipolar recording is utilized with minimal high-pass filtering, the presence of a QS morphology belies the source of the tachycardia. In another example, activation mapping can be used to locate the focus of idiopathic VT occurring in structurally normal hearts, especially when these tachycardias arise in the right or left ventricular outflow tracts. One approach to mapping these tachycardias is to progressively move two mapping and ablation catheters and compare electrogram timings between the two catheters that are gradually moved to the site with the earliest activation.

Arrhythmias that are caused by reentry do not have an "earliest" or "latest" signal as there is continuous electrical activity around a barrier to conduction, be it a fixed or functional barrier or a combination of the two. Nevertheless, activation mapping is still useful in locating sites critical to tachycardia maintenance in reentrant arrhythmias as long as the operator has knowledge of the substrate that supports these arrhythmias. In the case of infarct-related ventricular tachycardia, the circuit is composed of a "systolic" portion in essentially healthy myocardium and a "diastolic" portion in which activation proceeds along a corridor of diseased tissue, usually at the infarct scar border zone and protected by fixed or functional block (see below). Electrograms recorded from this area are found prior to the earliest onset of the QRS complex on the surface ECG. The "diastolic" pathway is the narrowest part of the VT reentrant circuit and the target for ablation. Electrograms occurring in diastole are searched for as they may indicate the location of the diastolic pathway (DP), which is critical to arrhythmia maintenance. However, electrograms in diastole may also represent recordings from blind-ending "bystander" pathways that are not required for tachycardia but usually lie close to the tachycardia's "diastolic" pathway. Specialized pacing maneuvers are required to make this differentiation, which are outlined in detail below.

3.4.2   Pacemapping

The principle of pacemapping is that stimulation at the site of origin of a tachycardia produces a 12-lead ECG that is identical to the tachycardia itself. Stimulation must be performed at a similar cycle length to tachycardia, otherwise localized conduction characteristics may alter ECG morphology. Although bipolar pacing is employed most often for this, it must be remembered that endocardial capture can be from either of the two poles.

Pacemapping is most helpful when used, in addition to activation mapping, in mapping focal tachycardias occurring in structurally normal hearts. As the rest of the myocardium has normal conduction characteristics, pacing at the focus of the arrhythmia should result in a surface ECG morphology identical to tachycardia, or, more commonly, to ectopy arising from the same site. It is important to examine all 12 leads of the surface ECG during tachycardia/ectopy and pacing, and even the smallest difference in P or QRS shape can imply that the catheter is not exactly on the focus. One disadvantage of this technique is that the artifact caused by the pacing stimulus can hamper this comparison.

It is important to also be aware that in the presence of structural heart disease, for instance in infarct-related ventricular tachycardia, areas of "functional block" exist during tachycardia but not during sinus rhythm [9, 123]. These areas act as barriers to conduction protecting an area of myocardium to allow reentry. This is important in post-myocardial infarction (MI) VT and in typical atrial flutter [10]. Therefore, pacemapping from sinus rhythm in these scenarios would produce very different ECG morphologies to those during tachycardia, indicative of different activation sequences.

3.4.3   Entrainment Mapping

This method of mapping is reserved for reentrant arrhythmias. Reentrant circuits typically have "fast" and "slow" components, the latter allowing time for tissue that would otherwise be refractory to recover, permitting the circuit to continue. As described, the different components of these circuits may be separated by fixed anatomical obstacles or zones of functional block. As the activation wavefront travels around the circuit, it encounters continuously excitable tissue ahead of it. This area of tissue that exists between the advancing head of the activation wavefront and the retreating, refractory tail is known as the "excitable gap." It is believed that all macro-reentrant circuits contain such an excitable gap, although the size and conduction characteristics within it may vary not only between different types of reentrant arrhythmia but even at different locations within an individual circuit [11, 124].

Pacing maneuvers may therefore interact with the excitable gap, and the resulting change to activation indicates whether stimulation occurred within the circuit or from outside. It can even discriminate between pacing from the true diastolic pathway and bystander areas (see below).

A single premature extrastimulus may "reset" a reentrant circuit. Resetting is the term used to describe the effect that a premature stimulus has when it reaches the circuit and encounters excitable tissue, the excitable gap. It will both collide with the previous tachycardia wavefront in a retrograde (antidromic) direction and advance the orthodromic activation of the tachycardia [12–14]. The circuit will be "reset" if the excitable gap is fully excitable. The return cycle is the interval between the extrastimulus and the onset of the next beat of tachycardia, and its properties define the characteristics of the excitable gap as this interval corresponds with the time required to reach the circuit, conduct through it, and exit it.

Entrainment, therefore, refers to the ability to continuously reset a tachycardia circuit with pacing at a cycle length just shorter than tachycardia (overdrive pacing). The presence of fusion between the native tachycardia and the paced complex defines entrainment and ensures that activation wavefronts from pacing are interacting with the tachycardia circuit, and is strongly supportive of a reentrant mechanism [15–17]. Focal arrhythmias cannot manifest fusion during overdrive pacing, and tachycardia is suppressed or accelerated by this maneuver.

Entrainment has been described in atrial flutter [18], reentrant atrial tachycardia [19], atrioventricular reentry [17], and reentrant ventricular tachycardia [20–24], and has also been demonstrated in patients with atrioventricular nodal reentrant tachycardia (AVNRT) [20, 25]. Observations during pacing proximal to the site of slow conduction in a reentrant circuit led Waldo's group to propose first a set of three criteria [26], and subsequently a fourth criterion for transient entrainment [21], as follows:

1. The presence of constant fusion beats on the ECG while pacing during tachycardia, at a constant rate that is faster than the tachycardia and that fails to interrupt it, except for the last paced beat that is entrained but not fused.
2. The demonstration of progressive fusion while pacing during tachycardia at two rates that are faster than the tachycardia but do not terminate it.
3. The interruption of a tachycardia during pacing at a rate faster than that of the tachycardia is associated with localized conduction block to a site for one beat, followed by activation of that site by the next pacing impulse from a different direction and with a shorter conduction time.
4. While pacing during tachycardia from a constant site at two rates, both of which are faster than the tachycardia and do not interrupt it, a change in electrogram morphology at, and conduction to, an electrogram recording site is observed.

However, successful entrainment in itself does not prove that the pacing site is located within the circuit, simply that reentry exists. In order to determine whether the pacing site is in such a location, further examination of the fused ECG complexes, the return cycle interval, and the relationship of the pacing stimulus to intracardiac electrograms are required and are outlined below.

Pacing from within a protected part (usually the "diastolic" portion) of the circuit entrains the circuit without change to the surface ECG morphology, as the stimulated orthodromic wavefronts follow exactly the same pathway as the tachycardia wavefronts. This is termed entrainment with concealed fusion or concealed entrainment [27]. The antidromic wavefront from the stimulus collides with the native tachycardia wavefront within the boundaries of the protected pathway and, therefore, does not interrupt the outer portion of activation responsible for the majority of ECG morphology. However, pacing at a connected bystander site will also entrain with concealed fusion.

When pacing within the tachycardia circuit, the return cycle approximates the tachycardia cycle length (TCL) (within 30 ms). Consequently, if pacing from a bystander position, the return cycle is longer than the tachycardia cycle length. However, the return cycle alone cannot discriminate between outer systolic portions of the circuit and the narrow diastolic isthmuses. It is therefore necessary to examine the interval between the pacing stimulus and a fixed reference point, for instance, the stimulus-QRS interval in the setting of reentrant VT (described later).

It should be noted that overdrive pacing must be performed at a cycle length close to that of tachycardia due to the possibility that a shorter pacing cycle length may provoke decremental conduction within the circuit, thereby altering the intervals described above.

3.5 Alternative Mapping Technologies

To overcome the limitations of conventional mapping techniques, principally the ability to record electrogram data from small parts of each cardiac chamber and the usual need for sustained tachycardia, alternative mapping approaches have been developed. They are based on two principles. Electroanatomic mapping systems collect sequential electrogram data from an entire cardiac chamber if necessary to define the underlying electrical substrate, while noncontact and basket catheter mapping systems are designed to collect global electrogram data from even a single cardiac cycle.

3.5.1   Defining the Electrical Substrate Using Electroanatomic Mapping

Electroanatomic systems (CARTO, LocaLisa, Realtime Position Management, and NavX System) [28–31] correlate activation with acquired chamber geometries. They are not suitable for activation mapping during unstable rhythms, but data acquired during sinus rhythm can be used to target ablation.

In creating a global activation map by sequentially collecting activation times on a three-dimensional geometry of a cardiac chamber or chambers, the entire circuit of macro-reentrant arrhythmia can be visualized. Using voltage data, these systems can delineate scar, thereby highlighting the important scar boundary regions where, for instance, VT diastolic pathway activity predominates. Focal or linear lines of ablation can then be created at these regions to abolish reentrant circuits, the latter typically extended to electrically silent areas, for example, the mitral valve annulus or dense scar. This method overcomes the need for mapping during tachycardia by defining potential arrhythmogenic substrates.

3.5.2   Electroanatomic Mapping

The CARTO™ system (Biosense Webster, Diamond Bar, California, USA) works on the principle that a metal coil placed in a magnetic field will generate an electrical current. The magnitude of this current depends on the coil's orientation within the magnetic field and the field's strength. In this system, the coil is located in a specialized catheter tip and three magnets of varying strength are arranged under the patient. The catheter acts as a locator as it is dragged along the endocardial surface, and electrogram data is acquired at each point to facilitate sequential creation of isochronal and voltage maps. Therefore, as with conventional contact catheter techniques, detailed activation mapping of hemodynamically unstable VT is not possible using this system. Instead, substrate mapping (voltage data) and pacemapping during sinus rhythm are employed to identify areas thought to be critical to tachycardia maintenance. These mapping systems also offer the benefit of catheter navigation, thereby limiting x-ray exposure to both patients and medical personnel.

Electroanatomical mapping has been used for mapping and ablation of a range of supraventricular arrhythmias including focal and reentrant atrial tachycardias [32, 33], atrial flutter [31, 34], and accessory pathway ablation [35]. In addition, it has also been extensively used in the treatment of unstable infarct-related ventricular tachycardia using voltage maps created during sinus rhythm [36–39], which hitherto had essentially been "unmappable" using conventional techniques.

3.5.3   LocaLisa

LocaLisa is a non-fluoroscopic catheter location system [29] that utilizes the principle that when an external current is applied across a medium with predictable impedance, a voltage drop occurs [29]. The electrical field strength at a particular point is proportional to the relative position within the medium.

Three orthogonal skin electrode pairs are attached to the patient to produce three-dimensional currents. A 1 mA current is passed between electrodes to create a high-frequency transthoracic electric field. When catheters are moved within the electrical field, sensors incorporated into the catheter tip detect changes in voltage. Each electrode pair emits slightly different signals between 30 and 32 kHz, which are detected by the sensor catheters. Signals are then processed, and the components of different frequencies can be differentiated. The amplitude of each electrical signal is then recorded digitally. The three-dimensional position of any intracardiac catheter can then be computed from the field strength along each orthogonal axis. Sites of interest and previous catheter positions, such as radiofrequency ablation sites, can be marked and used for reference. The system has been used in ablating atrial tachycardia and atrial flutter [40–42], and has also been used to guide pulmonary vein isolation for patients with atrial fibrillation [43].

3.5.4   Global Data Acquisition from a Single Cardiac Cycle

Global mapping systems (basket catheter mapping and noncontact mapping (NCM)) [44, 45] were developed to provide simultaneous data from an entire cardiac chamber from just a single beat of sinus rhythm or tachycardia.

This ability allowed rapid and detailed mapping of an entire VT circuit without the need for tachycardia to be sustained, and such systems are therefore ideally suited for mapping complex and poorly tolerated arrhythmias, such as infarct-related VT.

3.5.5   Basket Catheter Mapping

The basket or multielectrode mapping catheter consists of eight equidistant collapsible splines, or arms, each with four or eight electrode pairs creating a 32–64-bipolar-electrode catheter. A suitably sized basket is deployed via a guiding sheath into the relevant chamber, enabling endocardial mapping.

Studies in swine have shown that this technology is capable of rapidly generating isochronal endocardial maps [46, 47], and unipolar pacing can be performed from each of the electrodes for both pacemapping or entrainment. It has been used to map focal and macro-reentrant atrial tachycardias, atrial arrhythmias in congenital heart disease, and idiopathic outflow tract VT [48–51]. However, there have been relatively few studies using this form of mapping technology to guide VT ablation in man. This is because nonuniform, unpredictable, and relatively uncontrollable spline contact limits spatial resolution of complex activation in structural heart disease and limits the ability to perform pacemapping and entrainment in severely deformed ventricles [45].

3.6   Noncontact Mapping

Noncontact mapping (NCM) is dependent on three important mathematical principles: the Laplace equation, the boundary element method, and the classic solid angle theory [52–55].

Laplace calculated that the voltage measured at an outer boundary (e.g., the endocardium) can be applied to a formula that accurately calculates the voltage everywhere inside a chamber cavity – the Laplace equation [52]. Cavitary potentials are a summation of the electric potential from around the entire endocardial surface and dependent on the distance from each endocardial source point, a principle known as spatial averaging.

The boundary element method describes the process in which a simple formula applied to multiple elements within a boundary and then combined, can provide an accurate assessment of information along the whole boundary [52]. Thus, when calculating voltage from an endocardial surface, the endocardium is divided into multiple elements and a simple expression for voltage and current is applied to each element to estimate the electrical behavior within and between each element. These estimates are combined for an accurate depiction of endocardial potentials.

The classic solid angle theory [53, 54] describes the phenomenon that changes in cardiac potential are detected earliest by an electrode in closest proximity to the source of activation. This site has the greatest negative potential change that decreases with distance. If position and orientation of each electrode is known, the site of origin and sequential activation within a cardiac chamber can be determined [55]. The use of the boundary element method as an inverse solution to Laplace's equation has enabled the reconstruction of surface endocardial electrograms from intracavitary potentials and led to the development of multielectrode intracavitary probes.

Using a collapsible multielectrode array (MEA) with a braid of 64 wires woven around an 8 ml balloon (recreating 3,360 virtual endocardial electrograms), three-dimensional chamber geometries are constructed on a computer worksta-tion. Far-field electrogram data from the array are fed into the amplifier system, sampled at 1.2 kHz, and filtered. A ring electrode on the proximal shaft of the 9F array catheter in the inferior vena cava (IVC) is used as a reference for unipolar electrogram recordings. Because the far-field electrograms detected by the array are of low amplitude and frequency, the potentials are enhanced and resolved mathematically. This allows the construction of high-resolution endocardial isopo-tential and isochronal maps. Using a locator signal, the system can also guide a contact mapping and ablation catheter, with limited need for fluoroscopy, to points on the virtual endocardium that may be suitable sites for ablation.

The system has been used to map macro-reentrant VT complicating ischemic heart disease, where it has proved valuable in identifying the target diastolic pathway and guiding its ablation [44, 56], and has also mapped other VTs in normal hearts [57, 58]. With the array deployed in the atrium, the noncontact system can delineate the substrates

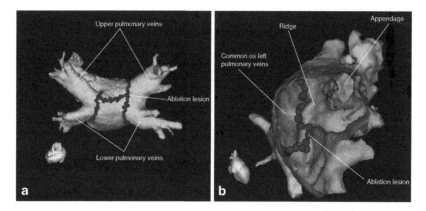

◘ Fig. 3.2

(a) External view of digitally derived anatomy of left atrium and pulmonary veins with linear ablation lesions depicted in red. (b) Internal view of digitally derived anatomy of left atrium showing the os of a common left pulmonary vein and the entrance into the left atrial appendage. Linear ablation lesions are depicted in *red*

of focal [59], macro-reentrant atrial tachycardia [60], focally initiated atrial fibrillation [61, 62], and atrial fibrillation and typical atrial flutter [63–65], and guide mapping and ablation of tachycardias due to intra-atrial reentry after Fontan surgery [66].

3.6.1   CARTO Merge™

The CARTO Merge™ system integrates computed tomography (CT) or magnetic resonance imaging (MRI) digital images of the heart structures into the mapping study so that a patient's actual anatomy and the conventional mapping geometry can be combined.

Once the images are imported into the CARTO system, each cardiovascular structure can be identified and segmented out until the structures of interest, for example, the left atrium and pulmonary veins, are selected and retained. Its three-dimensional hull is then integrated into the mapping study at the time of the procedure. Using fluoroscopy, fixed anatomical landmarks are identified and acquired as geometric location points. These points are then registered with their corresponding sites on the CT/MRI image, and the two then "merged" together so that the catheter tip can be navigated on-screen within the digital anatomical image (◘ Fig. 3.2).

Electroanatomical mapping with CT/MRI image integration is particularly useful in performing ablation procedures in which anatomical information is important, such as ablation of AF, and in patients with complex anatomy, such as those with congenital heart disease.

3.6.2   EnSite Verismo™ Segmentation Tool

This software works in a similar way to the CARTO Merge software, although direct integration of the mapping data with the CT/MR-derived images is just becoming available.

3.7   Conventional Mapping for Specific Arrhythmias

3.7.1   Mapping of Atrioventricular Nodal Reentrant Tachycardia (AVNRT)

In patients with AVNRT, during performance of an anterograde conduction curve, a jump in AH conduction (indicating anterograde block in the "fast" AV nodal pathway and conduction via a slow pathway) will initiate AVNRT in 70% of

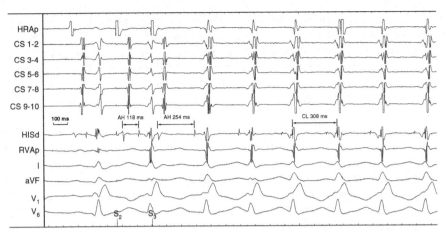

◑ Fig. 3.3

Abbreviations: *AVNRT*, atrioventricular nodal reentry tachycardia; *CL*, cycle length; otherwise as for ◗ Fig. 3.1. Initiation of typical slow-fast AVNRT by two premature atrial extrastimuli (S₁ & S₂) delivered during sinus rhythm. A jump in AH interval is seen after S₂, which is followed by typical slow-fast AVNRT (see text) at a cycle length of 308 ms

patients (◗ Fig. 3.3). A minimum 50 ms increase in the AH interval after a 10–20 ms shortening in the A1A2 interval is required for a "jump" to be diagnostic. However, single echo beats, i.e., a single cycle of anterograde conduction over the slow pathway followed by retrograde conduction over the fast pathway, are normal. The administration of isoprenaline or atropine may allow AVNRT to be sustained following further pacing. It should also be noted that variants of typical (slow-fast) AVNRT exist, in which the conduction properties and refractory periods overlap such that a jump may not be observed. It is standard practice to proceed to ablation only when tachycardia is readily and repeatedly inducible predominantly, so that a clear end point is provided, i.e., a lack of inducibility following ablation. If tachycardia cannot be induced despite the maneuvers described above, it is advisable not to proceed and to repeat the procedure at a later date.

Typical AVNRT consists of a long AH interval and synchronous, or nearly synchronous, atrial and ventricular conduction with a short VA interval. The latter reflects rapid retrograde fast pathway conduction coincident with rapid anterograde His–Purkinje activation. The presence of bundle branch block will cause HV prolongation and delay of ventricular electrograms depending on which bundle branch is affected but cycle length will not be affected. Retrograde atrial activation should occur in a concentric pattern during typical AVNRT.

Atypical AVNRT (fast-slow) in which anterograde conduction occurs over the fast pathway and retrograde via the slow pathway results in a "long RP" tachycardia on the ECG with corresponding change in intracardiac electrogram. The earliest atrial activation is typically more posteroinferior than in slow-fast AVNRT reflecting the relative location of the slow and fast pathways. The same surface appearance can be produced by orthodromic AVRT with a slowly conducting accessory pathway and low atrial tachycardia with 1:1 AV conduction.

Finally, if a narrow complex tachycardia is induced with an eccentric retrograde atrial activation pattern, either AVRT or AVNRT with a bystander accessory pathway is present. The latter, which is a rare entity, would be expected to demonstrate a degree of fusion between the retrograde activation via the accessory pathway and the fast AV nodal pathway. During any apparent junctional reentry tachycardia, it is important to examine for the presence of an accessory pathway. Sensed, single ventricular extrastimuli are introduced during tachycardia at shorter intervals until one produces ventricular depolarization that is synchronous with the His bundle electrogram. At this point, the ventricular stimulus cannot conduct retrogradely over the AV node as the His bundle is activating anterogradely. Therefore, if this maneuver alters the timing of the subsequent atrial electrogram from that anticipated, an accessory pathway should be suspected. However, this phenomenon is dependent on the size of the excitable gap present, intraventricular conduction properties, the site of pacing, and location of the accessory pathway. In typical AVNRT, the excitable gap is usually relatively small and the RV apical catheter, a considerable distance from the circuit. Therefore, the advancement of atrial activation can only occur with extremely premature extrastimuli. In contrast, an accessory-pathway-mediated tachycardia utilizes the His–Purkinje system, and therefore the circuit is much closer to the RV catheter. This phenomenon has been developed into a useful tool known as the preexcitation index (PI), to aid discrimination of different types of accessory-pathway-mediated AVRT and AVNRT [67]. The PI is defined as the tachycardia cycle length minus the longest coupled ventricular extrastimulus to result in advancement of atrial activation. A PI of >100 ms is typically seen with AVNRT, 75 ms or greater with left free wall accessory pathways, and <45 ms with septal APs [67]. Finally, failure to advance atrial activation with ventricular extrastimuli does not exclude AVRT, especially if the accessory pathway has decremental properties, or is located on the left free wall.

The response to entrainment is a further additional pacing maneuver that is useful to discriminate between different types of SVT. When AVNRT or AVRT is entrained from the ventricle, it will typically terminate with a V-A-V response, i.e., the last entrained atrial activation will return directly to the ventricle as there are two pathways connecting atrium to ventricle. However, when an atrial tachycardia, which by definition is not dependent on conduction via the AV node or ventricles for maintenance, is entrained, it will typically demonstrate a V-A-A-V response as the last entrained A will subsequently block anterogradely in the AV node. There are important distinctions to this rule, especially if atrial tachycardia occurs in the presence of dual AV node physiology.

The post-pacing interval (PPI) following entrainment (ventricular pacing) is also extremely useful to help differentiate AVNRT from AVRT. This interval represents the time taken to travel to the circuit from the pacing site, once around the circuit, and then the time back to the recording site. Thus, if the tachycardia cycle length (TCL) is subtracted from the PPI, this interval represents twice the time to conduct to and from the circuit, thereby giving a useful indication of how far away the circuit is. It is important to remember that the prematurity of the ventricular pacing results in decrementation elsewhere, especially in the AV node, so the previous definition of PPI-TCL is not entirely accurate. Nevertheless, this calculation has been shown to be extremely useful in differentiating atypical AVNRT from AVRT utilizing a septal accessory pathway, in which the former all had a PPI-TCL of >115 ms [68]. This technique has subsequently been refined to account for decrementation at the AV node [69, 125].

Once AVNRT has been confirmed and if appropriate given the patient's symptomatology, modification of the slow pathway can be performed to permanently interrupt the circuit. Different methods have been described to effect slow pathway modification based on analysis of electrograms [70, 71] or by anatomical guidance [72, 73]. Usually, a combination of these techniques is used. During sinus rhythm, a deflectable ablation catheter is advanced in the RAO (right anterior oblique) projection into the base of the right ventricle at the infero-posterior part of Koch's triangle and withdrawn slowly until small atrial electrograms are identified, typically later than those recorded at the His catheter [74]. The catheter is then moved progressively superiorly on the septal tricuspid annulus until a so-called "dome and spike" morphology is seen, thought to indicate an atrial electrogram closely followed by a slow pathway potential. It is not uncommon to find such potentials in alternative positions depending on the course of the right posterior extension of the AV node. Fairly frequently, this includes sites superior to the coronary sinus os. Successful slow pathway modification, usually associated with an irregular junctional rhythm during RF energy delivery, can be achieved at these sites. The presence of slow junctional activity during energy delivery tends to indicate a successful ablation site. The exact cause of this phenomenon is not clear, but is thought to be due to the effects of thermal injury on inputs to the AV node. It is almost always seen with energy delivery at successful sites at which its duration is longer, but is also seen in up to 65% of unsuccessful sites [75]. Thus, although lack of junctional activity during energy delivery almost invariably suggests an ineffective application, the converse is not necessarily true. Therefore, it is common practice not to continue energy delivery at sites in which junctional activity is not observed after approximately 15 s, and to proceed with caution if the rhythm is rapid, as this may indicate proximity to the compact AV node.

There is increasing risk of inadvertent heart block as the compact AV node is approached [76]. As such, it is absolutely critical that continuous radiographic screening and electrogram analysis is performed during energy delivery so that it can be immediately terminated should the catheter be displaced, AH prolongation is seen, there is absence of atrial depolarization during junctional rhythm, or AV block occurs. Occasionally, ablation within the coronary sinus ostium itself or even less commonly on the left side of the atrial septum is required to achieve successful ablation.

Mid-septal ablation sites appear to be associated with a higher and earlier occurrence of junctional rhythm and higher success rates than more posterior sites [77]. The cycle length of junctional activity during slow pathway ablation (around 500 ms) tends to be longer than that observed with fast pathway ablation (around 400 ms) [78], although there remains some debate about this [74]. Rates below 350 ms suggest proximity to the compact AV node and are associated with the development of conduction block [79].

3.7.2 Wolff-Parkinson-White Syndrome and Concealed Accessory Pathways

In patients with the Wolff-Parkinson-White Syndrome, the accessory pathway can be localized before the diagnostic electrophysiology study using surface electrocardiographic features. Analysis of the delta wave vector and QRS polarity has enabled the construction of various algorithms to help predict the ventricular insertion site of these pathways [80–86]. Morphological ECG analysis is however dependent on the degree of preexcitation, which is dependent on a combination of heart rate, pathway location, and AV nodal function. Atrial pacing during EP study can maximize preexcitation, thereby aiding analysis.

3.7.2.1 Mapping

A standard four-wire electrophysiology study is generally performed using catheters placed at the high right atrium, His bundle area, coronary sinus, and right ventricular apex (❷ Fig. 3.4).

If the ECG in sinus rhythm is normal, the presence of eccentric atrial activation during ventricular pacing should alert the operator to the possibility of a "concealed" accessory pathway, which is capable of only retrograde conduction and, therefore, does not cause ventricular preexcitation. If the earliest anterograde ventricular activation or retrograde atrial activation is recorded from the coronary sinus, the CS (coronary sinus) catheter should then be positioned such that the earliest atrial or ventricular electrograms can be recorded and are "bracketed" by later electrograms on either side of this site. The electrode site recording the earliest A or V electrogram then becomes a useful target for more detailed mapping and ablation. The same principle can be applied to the tricuspid valve annulus using Halo catheters for the localization of right-sided accessory pathways [8].

Atrial and ventricular pacing is performed to characterize the accessory pathway refractory period, induce tachycardia, and to exclude the presence of other arrhythmias. The operator should be alert to the possibility of alternative SVT, for example, atrial tachycardia and AVNRT being conducted with a bystander accessory pathway. It is therefore important that scanning ventricular extrastimuli and responses to entrainment, as described previously, are analyzed to confirm the properties of the circuit being examined.

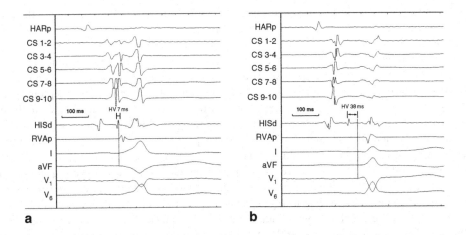

◘ Fig. 3.4
(a) Electrograms recorded from a patient with preexcitation by a right-sided pathway. Abbreviations as for ❷ Fig. 3.1. The earliest ventricular activation is seen at the right ventricular apex with a very short HV interval. Delta waves are seen at the QRS onset. **(b)** Electrograms from the patient recorded in ❷ Fig. 3.2a after successful ablation of the accessory pathway. The QRS and HV interval are now normal. The increased AV interval is most obviously seen in the CS electrograms

Once tachycardia has been induced, it is important to attempt to prove that it is accessory pathway mediated. Prolongation of the V-A interval that occurs with the development of bundle branch block ipsilateral to the site of the accessory pathway confirms this. This is also demonstrated by a His synchronous ventricular extrastimulus that terminates tachycardia without atrial capture, or delays the subsequent atrial electrogram.

More detailed mapping of the site of an accessory pathway is facilitated using a deflectable mapping and ablation catheter, usually with a 4 mm tip. Right-sided pathways are mapped along the tricuspid annulus typically from a femoral approach, although a subclavian approach may occasionally be required for greater catheter stability in some right free wall pathways. Left-sided pathways may be mapped from within the coronary sinus (especially postero-septal pathways), using a retrograde trans-aortic approach or via transseptal puncture, the latter being used most commonly for mapping and ablating left lateral pathways. Mapping itself can be performed during sinus rhythm, atrial or ventricular pacing, and orthodromic or antidromic AVRT depending on which of these provides the best identification of the earliest atrial or ventricular activation electrogram.

Bipolar recording is typically used, and the earliest atrial or ventricular electrogram recorded from the mapping catheter is continuously compared to a fixed reference point. In anterogradely conducting accessory pathways, this is often the earliest delta wave onset on the surface ECG. For concealed pathways, a fixed atrial electrogram is used, for example, the earliest atrial electrogram recorded on the CS catheter. In addition to this, morphological electrogram features are also analyzed including electrogram stability indicating tissue contact, the interval between atrial and ventricular components, and the presence of a high-frequency depolarization between these components. The latter may represent a "pathway potential," but it must be possible to dissociate this from both atrial and ventricular components of the electrogram to be sure of this. When mapping in an antero-septal or mid-septal location, the His depolarization must also be considered as a possible cause. A balanced signal, i.e., an electrogram in which the atrial and ventricular components have similar amplitude, suggests true apposition to the AV ring. However, accessory pathways can be successfully ablated from the atrial or ventricular sides of the annulus. Furthermore, pathways can lie obliquely across the AV ring such that the atrial and ventricular insertion sites are not obviously radiographically contiguous. Unipolar pacing can play an important role in the mapping of accessory pathways in which the presence of a QS morphology indicates the location of the pathway insertion site. The differentiation of atrial and ventricular components at sites close to the pathway is sometimes difficult and can be facilitated using atrial extrastimuli or burst pacing causing accessory pathway block.

Mapping of septal accessory pathways presents the additional hazard of the adjacent AV nodal structures, and even greater care must be taken during energy delivery. Postero-septal accessory pathways account for 25–30% of all accessory AV connections [87], and although equally successfully treated by catheter ablation, are often associated with long procedural times. This is related to the complexity of the anatomy of the postero-septal region in addition to the difficulty in delivering adequate energy deep in the postero-septal space. In the majority of cases and in spite of the morphology of the surface ECG, postero-septal accessory pathway electrograms can be reached from a right-sided approach, either at the right postero-septal right atrium or within the proximal coronary sinus. However, mapping of the left-sided postero-septal region is required in some cases. Some of these pathways lie epicardially, and catheters must be maneuvered into subbranches of the coronary venous system, especially if diverticulae are present, in which case retrograde coronary sinus angiography beforehand can be very useful. Accessory pathways arising in the anterior or mid-septum are less common (approximately 6–7%) and frequently conduct anterogradely. Due to the proximity of such pathways to the AV node and its connections, atrial and ventricular activation sequences (depending on which chamber is being paced) can closely mimic each other making differentiation difficult. The technique of para-Hisian pacing can be useful in this regard. Pacing at low outputs captures only adjacent ventricular muscle, which, in the absence of an accessory pathway, conducts relatively slowly to the His–Purkinje system before proceeding retrogradely to the atrium. Pacing at high outputs, however, captures the His bundle itself, leading to rapid retrograde conduction. If an adjacent septal accessory pathway is present, rapid conduction to the atrium will occur regardless of whether low or high outputs are used. This technique can be used both diagnostically prior to ablation as well as a confirmatory test following ablation. A similar technique can be performed with pacing from the base and apex of the right ventricle, the latter lying adjacent to the distal ramifications of the His–Purkinje system allowing rapid retrograde conduction.

Right free wall accessory pathways present their own special difficulties. Mapping of this portion of the tricuspid valve annulus is hampered by the difficulty in manipulating catheters such that they slide along the annulus smoothly and in achieving stability at sites of interest. The use of a multipolar circumferential catheter that sits around the annulus may sometimes be necessary to help localize and bracket the pathway region [8], and the use of catheter sheaths can greatly enhance stability. Furthermore, right free wall pathways may often be multiple, especially when Ebstein's anomaly is present in which identification of the true AV groove may prove extremely difficult. Occasionally, mapping from the ventricular side of the AV groove is necessary to ablate these pathways, which is achieved using the catheter inversion technique.

3.7.3 Atrial Flutter

Typical atrial flutter is a macro-reentrant circuit within the right atrium. Although very high success rates are now achieved routinely using ablation for this arrhythmia, the precise substrate that underlies it remains unclear. It is accepted that the tricuspid valve annulus forms the anterior boundary of the circuit and that a critical slowly conducting isthmus [88] exists between this and the inferior vena cava, the Eustachian ridge, and the ostium of the coronary sinus, and is targeted for ablation [89, 90]. The exact nature of the posterolateral barrier of the circuit remains less clear and relates to the crista terminalis and whether this represents a zone of fixed or functional block. Nevertheless, detailed mapping of the circuit is infrequently required if typical surface ECG features are present during tachycardia, including a regular "saw-tooth" pattern of atrial activity with negative polarity in the inferior limb leads and positive polarity in lead V1. If these features are present, many operators will not attempt the initiation of tachycardia or further mapping and proceed directly to ablation across the isthmus. However, if mapping is required, a circumferential multipolar catheter placed *en face* to the tricuspid valve annulus aids significantly. As the name suggests, counterclockwise atrial flutter (accounting for approximately 90% of typical atrial flutter [91]) demonstrates counterclockwise activation and importantly septal activation that proceeds in a caudo-cranial direction. Clockwise flutter demonstrates septal activation in the opposite direction. If required, entrainment using atrial pacing from the isthmus will confirm this if concealed fusion is manifest on the surface ECG. Demonstration of concealed entrainment from this region, in which there is a long stimulus to F wave interval [92], ensures that ablation that transects this region will prevent the arrhythmia recurring.

3.7.3.1 Mapping to Guide Radiofrequency Ablation

There are several different mapping strategies that can be adopted to aid typical atrial flutter ablation. One practice is to place a quadripolar catheter in the coronary sinus, a multipolar curvilinear "Halo" catheter around the tricuspid valve annulus, and a pentapolar 8 mm tip deflectable ablation catheter across the isthmus. The latter has four electrodes at the tip and a fifth along the shaft of the catheter to act as a reference electrode within the IVC to record unipolar signals from the isthmus (see below). An additional pole in the IVC acts as an indifferent electrode enabling unipolar mapping electrograms to be generated from the ablation catheter to more accurately guide ablation.

Ablation can be performed either during atrial flutter or, if in sinus rhythm, during pacing from the coronary sinus. The deflectable ablation catheter is passed into the base of the right ventricle such that it abuts the inferior aspect of the tricuspid valve annulus at a 5 to 6 o'clock position in an LAO (left anterior oblique) 30° projection. The desired electrogram recorded at the start of the procedure should demonstrate a large ventricular component and a small atrial signal. During continuous energy delivery, the ablation catheter is then withdrawn slowly into the right atrium across the isthmus ensuring good tissue contact and maintenance of the 5 or 6 o'clock position in the LAO projection. Electrograms recorded from the catheter tip are analyzed during ablation at each site to look for the development of split potentials indicating the creation of a line of block. As the catheter reaches the Eustachian ridge and the junction of the isthmus and the IVC, the catheter is de-flexed to maintain good apposition with the tissue surface. This may need confirmatory views in an RAO 30° projection. Care must be taken during ablation at this region, which is often painful for the patient. In addition, the catheter can suddenly fall back within the IVC, at which point energy delivery must be ceased immediately.

If performed during atrial flutter, it is expected that the arrhythmia will terminate during this procedure. However, this does not necessarily mark the end point of the procedure. Once sinus rhythm has occurred, continuous pacing from the coronary sinus is performed and electrograms from the Halo catheter are examined. Prior to the completion of a line of block across the isthmus, activation from the coronary sinus proceeds in two wavefronts across the superior and inferior aspects of the tricuspid valve annulus producing a fusion pattern with latest atrial activation at the lateral wall. This is demonstrated by a "chevron" pattern of atrial electrograms along the Halo catheter. The creation of a continuous line of block across the isthmus prevents activation proceeding along the inferior aspect of the right atrium with propagation

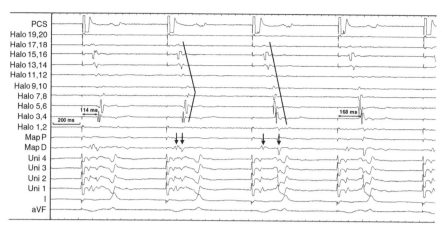

⬛ Fig. 3.5

Abbreviations: Halo, electrograms recorded from a 20-pole curvilinear catheter (the "Halo") placed around the tricuspid annulus; Map P & Map D, electrograms recorded from the proximal and distal map bipoles, respectively; PCS, proximal CS electrogram; Uni, unipolar electrograms recorded between each of the mapping/ablation catheter's four poles and an indifferent electrode in the inferior vena cava. The development of block to clockwise conduction during radiofrequency ablation seen by straightening of the chevron of the Halo electrograms (see text). Also note the separation of two components of the Map electrograms as block develops, most easily seen in Map P & Map D in this example

occurring exclusively in a counterclockwise direction. This is manifest by a straightening of the chevron into a line of atrial electrograms with the earliest at the septal side of the Halo catheter (its proximal poles) and the latest recorded from the Halo's distal poles just lateral to the line of block that has been created (❯ Fig. 3.5). This appearance indicates the presence of unidirectional block in the clockwise direction. However, unidirectional block alone as an end point is not sufficient to prevent long-term recurrence [89]. To explore for bidirectional block, pacing is then performed from different bi-poles (typically poles 1,2 and 5,6 or 7,8) on the Halo catheter. If counterclockwise block is also present, the Halo will activate in an exclusively clockwise direction and, when pacing from the distal poles 1,2, a longer interval will be measured between the pacing stimulus and the CS electrogram than when pacing from the more proximal poles.

Another indication of isthmus block is the finding of equally spaced split potentials from each of the mapping catheter's electrodes when it is placed along the line of block. When the line of block is incomplete, these split potentials can guide the operator to the point where conduction persists. This will be identified by a location where the electrogram is relatively normal and of greater amplitude than the neighboring treated tissue, and the two components of the split potential will be closer together (and even continuous) than the split potentials from the other poles betraying nearby conduction across the line of block.

Alternatively, this procedure can be performed using bipolar electrogram recording only from the ablation catheter looking for signal degradation during energy delivery and the creation of double potentials across the isthmus. If necessary, the expense of the procedure can be limited by performing the procedure without a catheter in the coronary sinus during tachycardia or sinus rhythm. Pacing from either side of the line is performed by advancing the Halo catheter across the isthmus, with the tip either within the coronary sinus itself or against the interatrial septum. This technique however requires repeated movement and repositioning of the Halo catheter, which adds to the complexity of the procedure and to the interpretation of the timing of the intracardiac signals. It is even possible to perform the entire procedure with just an ablation and coronary sinus catheter.

3.7.3.2 Atypical Atrial Flutter

This group of reentrant tachycardias can occur in the left or right atrium and are most commonly seen in the context of organic heart disease, previous cardiac surgical intervention, or previous linear atrial ablation, rather than in the structurally normal heart. The circuits that underlie such tachycardias are dependent on the presence of fixed anatomical barriers and lines of functional block. Gaps in the latter may lead to atypical circuits, and generally the use of advanced mapping systems (contact or noncontact) can significantly aid diagnosis and ablation. However, conventional mapping techniques can be utilized, especially activation mapping and entrainment. As with typical atrial flutter, a multipolar circumferential catheter can be extremely useful for mapping around the tricuspid valve annulus and right atrial free wall. Atypical reentrant left atrial flutters are fairly frequently encountered following linear ablation for atrial fibrillation. Due to the complexity of the underlying substrate, mapping these arrhythmias is often helped by an advanced mapping system.

3.7.4 Focal Atrial Tachycardias

Focal atrial tachycardias are most commonly present in the middle age, and although they can arise from any site within the left or right atrium, they are most commonly right sided [93], especially related to the crista terminalis (❯ Fig. 3.6). A small proportion of patients will have multiple foci. The majority are thought to be due to abnormal automaticity and, therefore, susceptible to the effects of the autonomic nervous system. As such, drugs such as isoproterenol may be necessary for induction, and programmed stimulation may not be useful although overdrive pacing can be used for tachycardia termination. Conversely, triggered or micro-reentrant focal atrial tachycardias are inducible with programmed stimulation, which, in the case of the former, may cause tachycardia acceleration.

Analysis of P wave morphology on the surface ECG, if available, is invaluable prior to intracardiac mapping to determine the general location of the focus. If tachycardia is sustained, activation mapping using a roving 4 mm tip deflectable mapping catheter is the preferred technique, utilizing the P wave onset as the fixed reference point and unipolar recording looking for a QS complex at the site of the focus. As with atrial flutter, multipolar catheters placed in relevant parts of the atrium can significantly aid this technique. Once the focus has thought to have been identified, entrainment mapping can be used for confirmation. In addition to these techniques and especially in the case of non-sustained tachycardia, pacemapping can be performed comparing paced P waves with those of tachycardia. For obvious reasons, it is necessary that sufficient AV block has occurred at some point during tachycardia such that an unperturbed P wave can be seen without interference from an adjacent QRS complex. It is also important that the lowest output to achieve local capture is used to prevent recruitment of larger areas of myocardium. This technique can feasibly be performed even if only a single culprit ectopic has previously been recorded, but in these cases, the use of noncontact mapping is extremely helpful. This

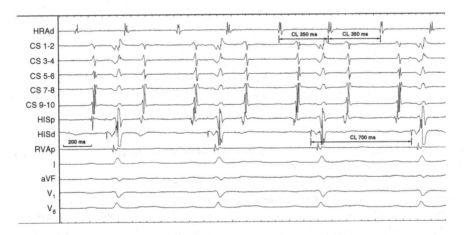

◻ Fig. 3.6

Abbreviations: HISp, proximal His electrogram; HRAd, distal HRA electrogram; otherwise as for ❯ Fig. 3.1. A right atrial tachycardia of CL 350 ms conducted with 2:1 AV block producing a ventricular CL of 700 ms. Note that right atrial activation (in HRA) is well in advance of left atrial activation (in CS channels) confirming a right atrial (or SVC) origin

mapping technique, described in detail below, simultaneously records activity from an entire cardiac chamber, enabling localization of a focus from a single ectopic beat. Electroanatomical mapping of stable sustained atrial tachycardias can aid the identification of the source.

3.7.5   Atrial Fibrillation

It is only relatively recently that ablative techniques have been developed to prevent the recurrence of atrial fibrillation (AF) [70]. Initial interest focused purely on the role of ectopy arising from the pulmonary veins and ablation to isolate them from the left atrium [94]. This strategy alone is not sufficient to effect a cure in many patients, especially those with persistent or permanent AF. For those, further techniques have been developed to compartmentalize the left atrium in an effort to prevent reentry [95], a strategy not dissimilar to the surgical Maze procedure [96].

Mapping of AF itself is not necessary for these ablation strategies to be performed. If pulmonary vein isolation is desired, circumferential mapping catheters can be placed at the ostia of the pulmonary veins to guide ostial or antral ablation and to establish the presence of entry and exit block facilitated by pacing outside and from within the vein, respectively. A purely anatomical approach relies on the creation of contiguous linear lesions, something that is really only possible using a three-dimensional mapping system (see below). Apart from testing the completeness of block across these lines, which is not necessarily recommended by all proponents, pacing and mapping is not required.

More recently, however, focus has shifted to modification of the underlying substrate that is thought to support AF. These techniques, including that recently proposed by Nademanee et al. [97], have sought to identify areas of complex fractionated electrograms during AF within regions of the left and right atria to be used as target sites for ablation. The underlying hypothesis is that these areas represent zones of slow conduction and turning points responsible for the reentrant wavelets of AF. Nademanee et al. reported that 95% of the patients had sinus rhythm restored without cardioversion during the procedure using this technique and 91% of patients were free from all arrhythmia at 1 year. It remains to be seen whether these results can be duplicated, or tested prospectively in a randomized controlled trial. However, the future of AF ablation may involve much more detailed intracardiac mapping than is necessary for those techniques most commonly practiced at present.

3.7.5.1   Focally Initiated Atrial Fibrillation

In most patients with AF, episodes are initiated by ectopic depolarization originating from within the muscular sleeves of a pulmonary vein (PV) or veins. In some patients, AF is also perpetuated by a rapidly firing focus within these muscular sleeves [94, 98]. Both these processes can be identified by mapping within the PVs. The "normal" PV activation sequence of atrial followed by PV electrograms is reversed during "culprit" PV activity. Ablation to disconnect such a PV should prevent the recurrence of AF, but the recognition that multiple PVs can generate AF at different times means that most ablation procedures will aim to disconnect all PVs. Occasionally, such foci may be identified in non-pulmonary veins sites, such as the superior vena cava or coronary sinus and vein/ligament of Marshall. Identification of the approximate location of these foci may be possible prior to the procedure using P wave vector analysis, including those arising from the pulmonary veins [99].

3.7.6   Conventional Diagnostic Electrophysiology Study for Ventricular Tachycardia and Ventricular Stimulation Studies

It is recommended that coronary angiography is performed prior to attempts to initiate VT in patients in whom coronary heart disease is either suspected or known because of increased risk of inducing unstable rhythms or VF in patients who might have critical coronary heart disease. When significant coronary artery disease is identified, revascularization should be undertaken before proceeding to further electrophysiological evaluation.

As for the investigation of SVT, quadripolar diagnostic catheters are placed at the right ventricular apex, His bundle area, and the high right atrium. Catheters at these three positions provide electrogram data that enables rapid discrimination between ventricular and supraventricular arrhythmias (especially preexcited tachycardias or those conducted

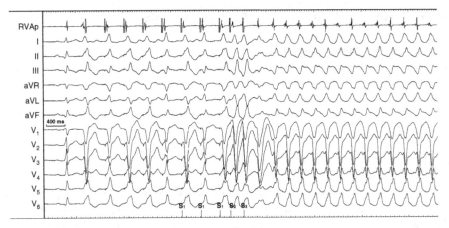

◘ Fig. 3.7

Abbreviations: as for other figures with conventional 12-lead ECG labeling. A drive train of eight paced beats is delivered to the right ventricular outflow tract (RVOT) at a CL of 400 ms. Two premature stimuli (S2 & S3) are then delivered, initiating VT. This has a similar but not identical morphology to the paced beats, suggesting that it originates somewhere from the RVOT

with aberrancy) or tachycardias arising from the AV junction. Due to the risk of inducing hemodynamically unstable arrhythmias, remote self-adherent defibrillation electrodes fitted to the patient and connected to an external defibrillator during the study are mandatory. In some centres, it is routine to also have invasive blood pressure monitoring during such a study to enable rapid assessment of an arrhythmia's hemodynamic status, especially when ablation is planned.

Baseline intervals are measured as before with special consideration paid to the presence of bundle branch block and HV prolongation during sinus rhythm, which will alter the appearance of induced supraventricular arrhythmias. Ventricular pacing should be performed using the extrastimulus technique to exclude the presence of a concealed accessory pathway, as described previously. Pacing is performed at twice diastolic threshold as higher current delivery may prevent VT induction [100]. VT initiation is performed using the Wellens protocol [3]. During this, sustained or non-sustained ventricular arrhythmias may be observed following the introduction of extrastimuli to the right ventricular apex and, if necessary, the right ventricular outflow tract (RVOT) (◘ Fig. 3.7), thereby increasing the sensitivity of the protocol [101]. Pacing is discontinued when a sustained ventricular arrhythmia is induced and blood pressure and the patient's conscious level recorded. External DC cardioversion should be immediately available if VF or hemodynamically unstable VT is induced. The addition of drugs such as isoproterenol may also be required.

It is important to be aware that the risk of inducing non-clinical VT or VF increases with the use of multiple extrastimuli so that, under those circumstances, the specificity of the test is reduced, although the sensitivity increases [102]. Knowledge of the pre-procedural clinical arrhythmia is thus important in the interpretation of such findings.

3.7.7 Mapping of Ventricular Tachycardia

The preferred method for mapping ventricular tachycardia depends on the underlying substrate and, therefore, the likely mechanism of the arrhythmia. VT occurring in the structurally normal heart, also known as idiopathic VT, can arise from several different sites. The commonest are from the right ventricular outflow tract and the left posterior fascicle, although left ventricular outflow tachycardias occur commonly. VT occurring in the context of structural heart disease also has a wide variety of subtypes and mechanisms including infarct-related/ischemic VT (reentry), bundle branch reentrant VT, VT associated with right ventricular dysplasia, Chagasic heart disease (reentrant or triggered), and is in association with dilated cardiomyopathy. In the following sections, we focus on the commonest VT subtypes, namely, idiopathic RVOT tachycardia, bundle branch reentry, and post-myocardial infarction VT.

3.7.7.1 Idiopathic Right Ventricular Outflow Tract Tachycardia

RVOT tachycardia accounts for approximately 10% of patients presenting with VT. They are focal in nature due to cyclic c-AMP-mediated triggered activity and typically present as a repetitive monomorphic tachycardia, i.e., characterized by frequent ventricular ectopy and salvoes of non-sustained VT interspersed with sinus rhythm [103, 104]. They most commonly originate from the septal portion of the RVOT below the pulmonary valve, but other locations have been identified including the anterior, posterior, and free walls of the RVOT, and from the epicardial surface. Although all forms typically manifest an LBBB (left bundle branch block) and inferior axis morphology on the surface ECG, there is a wide degree of subtle heterogeneity to other ECG features, such as the presence of notching, precordial R transition, and QRS frontal axis [51, 105, 106]. Although frequently incessant, induction may be facilitated by programmed stimulation or with the administration of isoproterenol.

Mapping may be performed conventionally, with a basket catheter or with complex mapping systems. Noncontact mapping can be particularly useful if RVOT ectopy is infrequent. Conventional mapping is performed using a standard quadripolar catheter at the RVA (right ventricular apex) for programmed stimulation and as a timing reference with one or two 4 mm tip deflectable mapping and ablation catheters in the RVOT. Following analysis of surface ECG morphology, the ablation catheter or catheters are navigated to the region of interest and a combination of activation mapping and pacemapping is used to locate the exact origin of tachycardia. Unipolar recording at the site of origin will display a QS morphology. Activation mapping is referenced to either the RVA catheter electrogram or preferably to the earliest ventricular onset on the surface ECG. However, due to the size of the catheter tip, activation mapping alone cannot be relied upon and a perfect pacematch should be sought before proceeding to ablation. Pacemapping should be performed at diastolic threshold, or just above, and at similar rates to tachycardia to enable direct comparison (❷ Fig. 3.8).

3.7.7.2 Bundle Branch Reentrant VT

This form of VT most commonly occurs in the setting of idiopathic dilated cardiomyopathy and is usually manifest with an LBBB morphology. Most patients have complete or a partial bundle branch block pattern on the surface

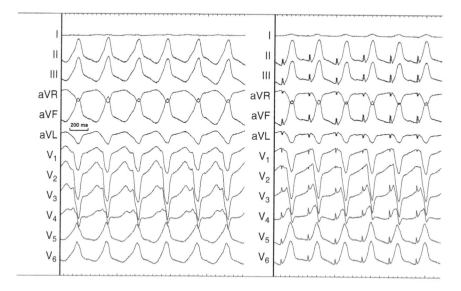

❑ Fig. 3.8
Pacemapping of RVOT tachycardia. The 12-lead ECG of tachycardia is in the left panel, and the attempt at pacemapping is in the right panel. The CL is the same in both. The QRS morphologies are similar but not identical. There are differences seen in leads V_4 and slightly in V_3, V_5, and V_6, suggesting that the catheter needs to be moved to a nearby location to produce a perfect pacematch in all 12 leads

ECG and a prolonged HV interval (75–80 ms) [107]. However, this probably reflects slow conduction rather than true block, which would preclude this arrhythmia. The macro-reentrant circuit that underlies this VT consists of retrograde conduction in the left bundle branch (LBB) followed by anterograde conduction via the right bundle branch (RBB). The circuit is completed via ventricular muscle between the distal ends of the bundle branches. In a minority of patients, an RBBB (right bundle branch block) form, which has an identical circuit but in the opposite direction is seen.

Induction is effected by programmed stimulation using extrastimuli and is dependent on achieving a critical conduction delay in the His–Purkinje network. Occasionally, atrial pacing or drugs that slow His–Purkinje conduction may be required (isoproterenol, Class IA agents). Mapping is performed with catheters at the RVA, His bundle, RBB, and preferably LBB. Activation should proceed from His bundle to RBB to RVA to LBB. Spontaneous changes in the V-V interval are preceded and predicted by change in the H-H interval. Ablation of the right bundle or sometimes left bundle branch terminates the tachycardia and prevents the arrhythmia recurring.

3.7.7.3 Infarct-Related Ventricular Tachycardia

Ventricular tachycardia is most commonly seen in the setting of underlying coronary artery disease with prior remote myocardial infarction (MI) and is due to macro-reentry within or at the border of the MI scar. Mapping of infarct-related VT using conventional methods continues to present significant challenges. This is related to several factors including hemodynamic intolerance, the size of the ventricles (and therefore the difficulty in navigating catheters to sites of interest), the complexity of the underlying circuit, and the difficulty in identifying its critical diastolic portion. Although once offered in an attempt to cure VT, it is now recognized that despite successful ablation, new VT occurs in a large proportion of patients during follow-up [56]. As such, ablation is now mostly performed in patients with existing implantable cardioverter defibrillators (ICDs) experiencing frequent ICD shocks, or using substrate ablation techniques during sinus rhythm (SR) (see below).

Determination of an endocardial exit site of a specific VT using morphological features of the surface ECG is less reliable than for VT in the structurally normal heart, largely due to the influence of scar and the frequent development of functional conduction block to complete the tachycardia circuit. However, three algorithms, which attempt this, enabling rapid localization of a VT to an approximate region of the left or right ventricle prior to insertion of catheters have been published [108–110].

Due to its reentrant mechanism, infarct-related VT is usually inducible by programmed stimulation. With conventional mapping, both activation and entrainment mapping techniques are needed to delineate the reentrant circuit. Pacemapping during sinus rhythm is unreliable in identifying either the diastolic pathway or exit site regions for the reasons outlined below.

Complex mapping systems can be particularly helpful in characterizing these complex substrates, especially when mapping hemodynamically unstable or non-sustained VT. In the former, electroanatomic substrate mapping during sinus rhythm may be deployed to identify regions of scar, the infarct border zone, and corridors of myocardium within dense scar that have persistent but impaired conduction. These regions are then targeted for ablation using linear lesions that are connected to electrically silent areas. In non-sustained VT, noncontact mapping offers the only realistic method of identifying key parts of the circuit, even from a single cardiac cycle.

3.7.8 Conventional Mapping of Infarct-Related VT

Continuous surface 12-lead ECG recording is mandatory in these studies both for approximate determination of VT exit site location as well for activation, pacemapping, and entrainment mapping. A quadripolar catheter is typically positioned at the RVA for programmed stimulation and termination and as a timing reference. Access to the left ventricle is achieved using either the retrograde trans-aortic or transseptal approaches. Each offers an advantage in reaching some parts of the LV more easily. It is advantageous to continuously monitor systemic and pulmonary arterial blood pressure throughout the procedure, as elevation of pulmonary artery pressure during VT is the first sign of hemodynamic deterioration and indicates the need to terminate VT and allow recovery during sinus rhythm before VT is re-induced and mapped again.

3.7.8.1 Activation Mapping

Once the clinical VT has been initiated, a mapping catheter is advanced to the approximate exit site region. From this reference point, the aim is to identify the critical diastolic pathway region of the circuit characterized by low-amplitude, high-frequency, fractionated electrograms that occur during diastole. Such electrograms are not specific for the critical diastolic pathway and may also be found at inner and outer loop sites as well as at bystander regions. These cannot be differentiated from the central common pathway using activation mapping alone; these require complimentary pacing techniques. To further complicate matters, a significant proportion of circuits have diastolic pathway regions located intramurally or subepicardially that are not identifiable using endocardial mapping techniques. Once identified, entrainment mapping is utilized to prove whether or not they are critical to circuit maintenance.

3.7.8.2 Pacemapping

In contrast to VT in the context of a structurally normal heart, pacemapping is not reliable in the setting of healed myocardial infarction. This is due to the necessity for functional lines of block to maintain the VT circuit. Functional block is not present during sinus rhythm [111, 112] so that paced activation wavefronts during sinus rhythm can propagate across these areas, resulting in a different surface QRS morphology [113].

3.7.8.3 Entrainment Mapping of VT

Pacing during VT, however, can be utilized to determine the portion of the circuit where the catheter is situated. During VT, pacing from a site remote to the circuit will collide with the reentrant wavefront, resulting in fusion with a resultant change in surface QRS morphology. The presence of constant QRS fusion during pacing defines entrainment and ensures that activation wavefronts from pacing are interacting with the tachycardia circuit. Criteria for recognition of entrainment during VT are summarized in ❱ Table 3.1.

The post-pacing interval (PPI) is the interval after the last paced extrastimulus that entrains VT and the next depolarization at the pacing site [27]. When pacing within the tachycardia circuit, the PPI approximates the tachycardia cycle length. Consequently, if pacing from a bystander position, the PPI is longer than VT cycle length. However, the PPI alone cannot discriminate between outer systolic portions of the circuit and the narrow diastolic isthmuses.

Pacing from within the diastolic portion of the circuit entrains the circuit without change to the surface QRS morphology, as the paced orthodromic wavefront activates the circuit in an identical sequence as the VT wavefronts. This is called concealed fusion or concealed entrainment [27]. The antidromic wavefront from the stimulus collides with the VT wavefront within the boundaries of the diastolic pathway and, therefore, does not interrupt the systolic portion of activation responsible for QRS morphology. Pacing at a bystander site within areas of scar adjacent to and connecting to the critical diastolic pathway will also entrain the tachycardia without change in the surface QRS morphology. These locations can be distinguished by analysis of the intervals between the diastolic electrograms, the pacing stimuli, and QRS onset. When pacing from the critical diastolic pathway, the interval between the diastolic electrogram and the QRS onset will be identical to the interval between the pacing stimulus and the QRS onset because the respective activation wavefronts travel over the same path. In the case of a bystander pathway, this is activated from the critical diastolic pathway while

◻ Table 3.1

Criteria for demonstrating entrainment of VT

1. Fixed fusion at a given paced cycle length
2. Progressive fusion at faster paced cycle lengths
3. Resumption of the VT on cessation of pacing with a non-fused QRS complex
4. For tachycardia in which fusion on the ECG is not observed: Fixed fusion demonstrated by analysis of the electrograms at the site of origin

⬛ Table 3.2

Characteristics of entrainment from the diastolic pathway of a VT circuit

1. Entrainment with concealed fusion
2. Post-pacing interval = VT cycle length ±30 ms
3. Stimulus-QRS = Electrogram-QRS
4. Stimulus-QRS/VT cycle length = 31–70%
5. Isolated potential during VT

activation continues along the critical diastolic pathway to the exit site to generate the QRS complex. When pacing from a bystander location, the activation wavefront has to travel back to reach the critical diastolic pathway before then proceeding to generate an identical QRS morphology. Therefore, the pacing-QRS interval is longer than the electrogram-QRS interval in a bystander pathway. However, such pathways do indicate that the mapping catheter is close to the ablation target of the critical diastolic pathway.

The stimulus-QRS interval is the conduction time from the pacing site to the VT exit site. It is therefore short when near the exit and longer at the entry site or from within the diastolic pathway. Therefore, the ratio of the stimulus-QRS interval as a proportion of the VT cycle length can help determine the location of the pacing site from sites within the inner loop. Characteristics of entrainment from the diastolic pathway are shown in ❷ Table 3.2.

The utility of these pacing maneuvers has been demonstrated in the work of El Shalakany et al. in which ablation sites were compared using the following criteria: an exact QRS match during entrainment, a return cycle within 10 ms of the VT cycle length, and the presence of presystolic potentials with the E-QRS interval less than or equal to 10 ms of the stimulus-to-QRS (S-QRS) interval. When all three criteria were met, VT could be terminated with a single radiofrequency lesion in all patients, whereas the lesion was almost invariably unsuccessful when all three criteria were not met [114].

3.7.9 VT Ablation Using Complex Mapping Systems

Initial data from series using noncontact mapping to guide VT ablation have been encouraging with high initial success rates. Schilling et al. [44] used noncontact mapping to target VT and achieved an initial success rate of 77% of all VT in which diastolic pathway activity was mapped. Strickberger's group [115] successfully ablated 15 of 19 targeted VT (78%). The remaining 4 VT could not be ablated due to inability to maneuver the catheter to the target site, proximity of the target site to the bundle of His, or due to a complication causing termination of the procedure. On follow-up, VT recurrence was significantly reduced, as was the requirement for defibrillator therapy. In the 12 patients with ICDs implanted prior to ablation, defibrillator therapy frequency was reduced from 19 ± 32 per month to 0.6 ± 1.4 per month in 1 month of follow-up.

The CARTO system was used by Soejima et al. [36] to generate voltage maps during sinus rhythm to target VT ablation. VT was induced and, if possible, a potential reentrant isthmus was identified. If unstable, pacemapping along the low voltage border of scar was performed looking for an identical pacematch to that of the induced VT in addition to a stimulus to QRS delay of greater than 40 ms. Standard RF, irrigated, or cooled-tip catheter energy was delivered to these sites during sinus rhythm; then short ablation lines were created extending from these sites parallel to the scar border zone over 1–2 cm until pacing at 10 mA at 2 ms stimulus strength failed to capture in that region. If the target site was within 2–3 cm of the mitral annulus, lesions were extended to the annulus to interrupt a potential submitral isthmus, as first demonstrated by Wilber et al. [116]. Programmed stimulation was repeated, and if VT was re-induced, further mapping and ablation was repeated with RF lines extended. Electrically unexcitable scar (EUS) was identified in all 14 patients, and all 20 VT circuit isthmuses were located adjacent to these regions. However, it was difficult to discriminate between low-amplitude, fractionated electrograms that represented scar and those that indicated the diastolic pathway. Nevertheless, RF ablation lines connecting selected EUS regions abolished all inducible VTs in 10 patients (71%) and spontaneous VT was markedly reduced during follow-up (142 ± 360 to 0.9 ± 2.0 episodes per month).

3.7.10   Mapping and Ablation of Hemodynamically Unstable VT

As described above, conventional mapping is not feasible for unstable ventricular arrhythmias. Several groups have published series on the use of substrate mapping during sinus rhythm and noncontact mapping of unstable VT followed by rapid termination.

3.7.10.1   Electroanatomic Mapping

Marchlinski et al. used the CARTO system to produce voltage maps of the LV with the creation of linear ablation lines from areas of dense scar (defined by a voltage amplitude of <0.5 mV) to areas of normal endocardium or anatomic boundaries [37]. In addition, ECG morphology during VT and pacemapping in SR guided sites of ablation. Nine of 16 patients had VT in the context of healed MI, and the remaining had dilated cardiomyopathy. Thirteen patients had poorly tolerated VT and of these, seven had VT-inducible post-ablation, five of which were fast VT only. All patients had ICDs, and during follow-up of median 8 months (range 3–36), only two patients with unstable VT had a recurrence, giving a success rate in this subset of 85%. Up to 87 RF lesions were required per patient, mean 54.6 ± 24.1 per patient.

Arenal et al. studied 18 patients considered to have unmappable VT, either because the target VT was not inducible or the target VT was not tolerated [38]. A further six patients with well-tolerated VT were studied to enable activation mapping and entrainment for comparison. The authors hypothesized that low-amplitude electrograms with an isolated, delayed component (E-IDC) along scar border were more specific for VT isthmus' slow conduction than low-amplitude electrograms alone (commonly found along scar border). Such electrograms were characterized by double or multiple components separated by very-low-amplitude signals and could be found in sinus rhythm. Again, the CARTO system was used to generate voltage maps (complete scar defined as voltage ≤0.1 mV, dense scar as voltage ≥0.1 mV and ≤0.5 mV), and E-IDC located during SR or RVA pacing were marked on the map for rapid location, with areas up to 1 cm around these sites then explored and labeled. When complete, pacemapping was performed starting at sites with the latest isolated, delayed component (E-LIDC) and moving to adjacent sites when pacemapping was not identical to clinical VT. Attempts at VT induction were performed at E-IDC sites with an identical pacematch, to look for presystolic or mid-diastolic electrograms during VT and to examine the stimulus-to-QRS interval. Concealed entrainment was attempted when the VT was sufficiently well tolerated. Ablation was then performed at all sites with E-IDC at which pacemapping reproduced the target VT and the stimulus-to-QRS interval was ≥50 ms, or at any E-IDC site that became mid-diastolic during VT. Between 1 and 35 RF lesions were applied per patient, and none of the six patients with hemodynamically unstable VT was inducible after ablation. Of the 18 patients with unmappable VT, two patients had a recurrence of their clinical VT during follow-up and a further five patients had a recurrence of a previously unrecorded VT.

Most recently, Brunckhorst et al. have used another marker of slow conduction to help identify targets for VT ablation during sinus rhythm [39]. Twelve patients were studied in whom 51 VT were inducible. All clinical VT were resistant to drug therapy causing ICD shocks in all. Stimulus-to-QRS interval (S-QRS) delays were analyzed during pacemapping at multiple areas in the left ventricle. Pacing was performed at 890 sites (74 ± 23 per patient) of which 93% of sites achieved capture. There was no S-QRS delay at 56% of pacing sites, a delay of ≥40 ms at 44%, and a delay of ≥80 ms at 15% of sites, the latter two groups usually being clustered together. The areas of conduction delay were compared to locations of target areas (areas within 2 cm of a reentrant isthmus, defined by entrainment and ablation) and overlapped in 13 of 14 cases. Sites with a delay ≥80 ms were more frequently in a target area, although a close pacematch was only seen in 41% of sites in these areas and an exact match in only 9%. Furthermore, 46% of sites with a close pacing match were outside the target area, emphasizing the limitations of pacemapping of VT in patients with structural heart disease. Ablation was performed at a mean of 10 ± 3 sites in the target area, rendering seven patients non-inducible at the end of the procedure and at least one VT was abolished in a further five patients. Over 6 months follow-up, three patients died and VT recurred at the time of death in two of these patients. The remaining nine patients remained free from VT despite a mean of 18 ± 16 VT episodes in the 6 months prior to ablation.

Although having limitations, these techniques have allowed the treatment of patients deemed unsuitable for conventional ablation. They have also improved our understanding of the subtleties of the underlying substrate that support scar-related VT.

3.7.10.2 Noncontact Mapping

Della Bella et al. have reported on the use of noncontact mapping to guide ablation of hemodynamically unstable VT in 17 patients, of whom 11 had infarct-related VT [117]. VT was induced and terminated after 15–20 s, and activation analyzed off-line. Ablation was performed in SR either by a line across the diastolic pathway (DP) (if identified) or around the exit point. If the patient was non-inducible at the end of the procedure, an ICD was not implanted. Separating out the different underlying etiologies, an exit point was defined in all 21 post-MI VT and DP activity identified in 17 (80%). Successful ablation was achieved in 67% of VT and in 53% of patients, with a partial success in one further patient. Ablation was not performed, or was unsuccessful in 42% of patients, and importantly, the success rate of ablation was higher with linear lesions across the DP (78%) compared with encircling lesions around the exit (16%).

During follow-up, seven out of nine successfully ablated patients remained free from arrhythmia recurrence, as did the patient with a partial success, and all remained free of the target VT. ICD shock frequency was significantly reduced. The results from this study demonstrate that noncontact-mapping-guided ablation of unstable VT is feasible with success highly dependent on the identification of DP activity, as with stable VT [44]. However, in patients with frequent ICD shocks from rapid, hemodynamically unstable VT, this technology does provide a therapeutic option if drug therapy is limited.

3.7.11 Epicardial Mapping of VT

Access to the epicardium can be obtained either from the coronary sinus and its tributaries, through the coronary arteries, or through direct pericardial puncture. The use of multipolar electrodes in the former can help facilitate positioning of endocardial catheters [118]. Intracoronary guide-wire mapping using standard angioplasty guidewires recording unipolar signals has also been reported to guide intracoronary ethanol ablation [126]. Pericardial puncture with direct epicardial mapping was originally described in the treatment of VT in the context of Chagasic heart disease [120]. However, it has now been used successfully in conjunction with substrate mapping of the endocardium in infarct-related VT [121, 122].

3.8 Conclusions

Intracardiac mapping has revolutionized our understanding of the mechanisms of abnormal arrhythmias and led directly to curative procedures in the majority through ablation. Intracardiac mapping techniques are based on analysis of electrogram timing (and, in some cases, morphology) during sinus rhythm, pacing, and during tachycardia in conjunction with morphological features and timing of surface ECG features. Conventional diagnostic electrophysiology is further based on three basic types of mapping: activation mapping, pacemapping, and entrainment. Complex mapping systems now exist that enable mapping of electrophysiological data from an entire cardiac chamber or from a single beat of tachycardia, so that previously "unmappable" rhythms may now be successfully treated.

References

1. Scherlag, B.J., S.H. Lau, R.H. Helfant, et al., Catheter technique for recording His bundle activity in man. *Circulation*, 1969;**39**: 13–18.

2. Durrer, D., L. Schoo, R.M. Schuilenburg, et al., The role of premature beats in the initiation and the termination of supraventricular tachycardia in the Wolff-Parkinson-White syndrome. *Circulation*, 1967;**36**: 644–662.

3. Wellens, H.J., R.M. Schuilenburg, and D. Durrer, Electrical stimulation of the heart in patients with ventricular tachycardia. *Circulation*, 1972;**46**: 216–226.

4. Josephson, M.E., L.N. Horowitz, and A. Farshidi, Continuous local electrical activity. A mechanism of recurrent ventricular tachycardia. *Circulation*, 1978;**57**: 659–665.

5. Cassidy, D.M., J.A. Vassallo, J.M. Miller, et al., Endocardial catheter mapping in patients in sinus rhythm: Relationship to underlying heart disease and ventricular arrhythmias. *Circulation*, 1986;**73**: 645–652.

6. Cassidy, D.M., J.A. Vassallo, A.E. Buxton et al., Catheter mapping during sinus rhythm: relation of local electrogram duration to ventricular tachycardia cycle length. *Am. J. Cardiol.*, 1985;**55**: 713–716.

7. Cassidy, D.M., J.A. Vassallo, A.E. Buxton, et al., The value of catheter mapping during sinus rhythm to localize site of origin of ventricular tachycardia. *Circulation*, 1984;**69**: 1103–1110.

8. Wong, T., W. Hussain, V. Markides, et al., Ablation of difficult right-sided accessory pathways aided by mapping of tricuspid annular activation using a Halo catheter: Halo-mapping of right sided accessory pathways. *J. Interv. Card. Electrophysiol.*, 2006;**16**: 175–182.

9. Stevenson, W.G., P.T. Sager, P.D. Natterson, et al., Relation of pace mapping QRS configuration and conduction delay to ventricular tachycardia reentry circuits in human infarct scars. *J. Am. Coll. Cardiol.*, 1995;**26**: 481–488.

10. Liu, T.Y., C.T. Tai, B.H. Huang, et al., Functional characterization of the crista terminalis in patients with atrial flutter: implications for radiofrequency ablation. *J. Am. Coll. Cardiol.*, 2004;**43**: 1639–1645.

11. Peters, N.S., J. Coromilas, M.S. Hanna, et al., Characteristics of the temporal and spatial excitable gap in anisotropic reentrant circuits causing sustained ventricular tachycardia. *Circ. Res.*, 1998;**82**: 279–293.

12. Almendral, J.M., N.J. Stamato, M.E. Rosenthal, et al., Resetting response patterns during sustained ventricular tachycardia: relationship to the excitable gap. *Circulation*, 1986;**74**: 722–730.

13. Almendral, J.M., M.E. Rosenthal, N.J. Stamato, et al., Analysis of the resetting phenomenon in sustained uniform ventricular tachycardia: incidence and relation to termination. *J. Am. Coll. Cardiol.*, 1986;**8**: 294–300.

14. Rosenthal, M.E., N.J. Stamato, J.M. Almendral, et al., Resetting of ventricular tachycardia with electrocardiographic fusion: incidence and significance. *Circulation*, 1988;**77**: 581–588.

15. Almendral, J.M., C.D. Gottlieb, M.E. Rosenthal, et al., Entrainment of ventricular tachycardia: explanation for surface electrocardiographic phenomena by analysis of electrograms recorded within the tachycardia circuit. *Circulation*, 1988;**77**: 569–580.

16. MacLean, W.A., V.J. Plumb, and A.L. Waldo, Transient entrainment and interruption of ventricular tachycardia. *Pacing Clin. Electrophysiol.*, 1981;**4**: 358–366.

17. Waldo, A.L., V.J. Plumb, J.G. Arciniegas, et al., Transient entrainment and interruption of the atrioventricular bypass pathway type of paroxysmal atrial tachycardia. A model for understanding and identifying reentrant arrhythmias. *Circulation*, 1983;**67**: 73–83.

18. Waldo, A.L., W.A. MacLean, R.B. Karp, et al., Entrainment and interruption of atrial flutter with atrial pacing: studies in man following open heart surgery. *Circulation*, 1977;**56**: 737–745.

19. Henthorn, R.W., V.J. Plumb, J.G. Arciniegas, et al., Entrainment of "ectopic atrial tachycardia": evidence for re-entry. *Am. J. Cardiol.*, 1982;**49**: 920.

20. Brugada, P., A.L. Waldo, and H.J. Wellens, Transient entrainment and interruption of atrioventricular node tachycardia. *J. Am. Coll. Cardiol.*, 1987;**9**: 769–775.

21. Henthorn, R.W., K. Okumura, B. Olshansky, et al., A fourth criterion for transient entrainment: the electrogram equivalent of progressive fusion. *Circulation*, 1988;**77**: 1003–1012.

22. Okumura, K., B. Olshansky, R.W. Henthorn, et al., Demonstration of the presence of slow conduction during sustained ventricular tachycardia in man: use of transient entrainment of the tachycardia. *Circulation*, 1987;**75**: 369–378.

23. Waldo, A.L., R.W. Henthorn, V.J. Plumb, et al., Demonstration of the mechanism of transient entrainment and interruption of ventricular tachycardia with rapid atrial pacing. *J. Am. Coll. Cardiol.*, 1984;**3**: 422–430.

24. Waldo, A.L. and R.W. Henthorn, Use of transient entrainment during ventricular tachycardia to localize a critical area in the reentry circuit for ablation. *Pacing Clin. Electrophysiol.*, 1989;**12**: 231–244.

25. Portillo, B., J. Mejias, N. Leon-Portillo, et al., Entrainment of atrioventricular nodal reentrant tachycardias during overdrive pacing from high right atrium and coronary sinus. With special reference to atrioventricular dissociation and 2:1 retrograde block during tachycardias. *Am. J. Cardiol.*, 1984;**53**: 1570–1576.

26. Okumura, K., R.W. Henthorn, A.E. Epstein, et al., Further observations on transient entrainment: importance of pacing site and properties of the components of the reentry circuit. *Circulation*, 1985;**72**: 1293–1307.

27. Stevenson, W.G., H. Khan, P. Sager, et al., Identification of reentry circuit sites during catheter mapping and radiofrequency ablation of ventricular tachycardia late after myocardial infarction. *Circulation*, 1993;**88**: 1647–1670.

28. Gepstein, L., G. Hayam, and S.A. Ben Haim, A novel method for nonfluoroscopic catheter-based electroanatomical mapping of the heart. In vitro and in vivo accuracy results. *Circulation*, 1997;**95**: 1611–1622.

29. Wittkampf, F.H., E.F. Wever, R. Derksen, et al., LocaLisa: new technique for real-time 3-dimensional localization of regular intracardiac electrodes. *Circulation*, 1999;**99**: 1312–1317.

30. de Groot, N., M. Bootsma, E.T. van der Velde, et al., Three-dimensional catheter positioning during radiofrequency ablation in patients: first application of a real-time position management system. *J. Cardiovasc. Electrophysiol.*, 2000;**11**: 1183–1192.

31. Ventura, R., T. Rostock, H.U. Klemm, et al., Catheter ablation of common-type atrial flutter guided by three-dimensional right atrial geometry reconstruction and catheter tracking using cutaneous patches: a randomized prospective study. *J. Cardiovasc. Electrophysiol.*, 2004;**15**: 1157–1161.

32. Kottkamp, H., G. Hindricks, G. Breithardt, et al., Three-dimensional electromagnetic catheter technology: electroanatomical mapping of the right atrium and ablation of ectopic atrial tachycardia. *J. Cardiovasc. Electrophysiol.*, 1997;**8**: 1332–1337.

33. Marchlinski, F., D. Callans, C. Gottlieb, et al., Magnetic electroanatomical mapping for ablation of focal atrial tachycardias. *Pacing Clin. Electrophysiol.*, 1998;**21**: 1621–1635.

34. Nakagawa, H. and W.M. Jackman, Use of a three-dimensional, nonfluoroscopic mapping system for catheter ablation of typical atrial flutter. *Pacing Clin. Electrophysiol.*, 1998;**21**: 1279–1286.

35. Worley, S.J., Use of a real-time three-dimensional magnetic navigation system for radiofrequency ablation of accessory pathways. *Pacing Clin. Electrophysiol.*, 1998;**21**: 1636–1645.

36. Soejima, K., M. Suzuki, W.H. Maisel, et al., Catheter ablation in patients with multiple and unstable ventricular tachycardias after myocardial infarction: short ablation lines guided by reentry circuit isthmuses and sinus rhythm mapping. *Circulation*, 2001;**104**: 664–669.

37. Marchlinski, F.E., D.J. Callans, C.D. Gottlieb, et al., Linear ablation lesions for control of unmappable ventricular tachycardia in patients with ischemic and nonischemic cardiomyopathy. *Circulation*, 2000;**101**: 1288–1296.

38. Arenal, A., E. Glez-Torrecilla, M. Ortiz, et al., Ablation of electrograms with an isolated, delayed component as treatment of unmappable monomorphic ventricular tachycardias in patients with structural heart disease. *J. Am. Coll. Cardiol.*, 2003;**41**: 81–92.

39. Brunckhorst, C.B., W.G. Stevenson, K. Soejima, et al., Relationship of slow conduction detected by pace-mapping to ventricular tachycardia re-entry circuit sites after infarction. *J. Am. Coll. Cardiol.*, 2003;**41**: 802–809.

40. Leonelli, F.M., G. Tomassoni, M. Richey, et al., Usefulness of three-dimensional non-fluoroscopic mapping in the ablation of typical atrial flutter. *Ital. Heart J.*, 2002;**3**: 360–365.

41. Leonelli, F.M., G. Tomassoni, M. Richey, et al., Ablation of incisional atrial tachycardias using a three-dimensional nonfluoroscopic mapping system. *Pacing Clin. Electrophysiol.*, 2001;**24**: 1653–1659.

42. Natale, A., L. Breeding, G. Tomassoni, et al., Ablation of right and left ectopic atrial tachycardias using a three-dimensional nonfluoroscopic mapping system. *Am. J. Cardiol.*, 1998;**82**: 989–992.

43. Macle, L., P. Jais, C. Scavee, et al., Pulmonary vein disconnection using the LocaLisa three-dimensional nonfluoroscopic catheter imaging system. *J. Cardiovasc. Electrophysiol.*, 2003;**14**: 693–697.

44. Schilling, R.J., N.S. Peters, and D.W. Davies, Feasibility of a noncontact catheter for endocardial mapping of human ventricular tachycardia. *Circulation*, 1999;**99**: 2543–2552.

45. Schalij, M.J., F.P. van Rugge, M. Siezenga, et al., Endocardial activation mapping of ventricular tachycardia in patients: first application of a 32-site bipolar mapping electrode catheter. *Circulation*, 1998;**98**: 2168–2179.

46. Aiba, T., W. Shimizu, A. Taguchi, et al., Clinical usefulness of a multielectrode basket catheter for idiopathic ventricular tachycardia originating from right ventricular outflow tract. *J. Cardiovasc. Electrophysiol.*, 2001;**12**: 511–517.

47. Eldar, M., D.G. Ohad, A.J. Greenspon, et al., Percutaneous multielectrode endocardial mapping and ablation of ventricular tachycardia in the swine model. *Adv. Exp. Med. Biol.*, 1997;**430**: 313–321.

48. Yamane, T., S. Miyanaga, K. Inada, et al., A focal source of atrial fibrillation in the superior vena cava: isolation and elimination by radiofrequency ablation with the guide of basket catheter mapping. *J. Interv. Card. Electrophysiol.*, 2004;**11**: 131–134.

49. Nishida, K., A. Fujiki, H. Nagasawa, et al., Complex atrial reentrant circuits evaluated by entrainment mapping using a multielectrode basket catheter. *Circ. J.*, 2004;**68**: 168–171.

50. Zrenner, B., G. Ndrepepa, M.A. Schneider, et al., Mapping and ablation of atrial arrhythmias after surgical correction of congenital heart disease guided by a 64-electrode basket catheter. *Am. J. Cardiol.*, 2001;**88**: 573–578.

51. Yoshida, Y., M. Hirai, Y. Murakami, et al., Localization of precise origin of idiopathic ventricular tachycardia from the right ventricular outflow tract by a 12-lead ECG: a study of pace mapping using a multielectrode "basket" catheter. *Pacing Clin. Electrophysiol.*, 1999;**22**: 1760–1768.

52. Sigl, R., *Introduction to Potential Theory: Fundamental Mathematical and Physical Topics for the Study of Physical Geodesy.* Tunbridge Wells: Abacus Press, 1973.

53. Plonsey, R., An extension of the solid angle potential formulation for an active cell. *Biophys. J.*, 1965;**5**: 663–667.

54. Scher, A. and M. Spach, Cardiac depolarization and repolarization and the electrogram, in *Handbook of Physiology*, R.M. Berne, Editor. Bethesda, MD: American Physiological Society, 1979, p. 37.

55. Colli-Franzone, P., L. Guerri, C. Viganotti, et al., Potential fields generated by oblique dipole layers modeling excitation wavefronts in the anisotropic myocardium. Comparison with potential fields elicited by paced dog hearts in a volume conductor. *Circ. Res.*, 1982;**51**: 330–346.

56. Segal, O.R., A.W. Chow, V. Markides, et al., Long-term results after ablation of infarct-related ventricular tachycardia. *Heart Rhythm*, 2005;**2**: 474–482.

57. Betts, T.R., P.R. Roberts, S.A. Allen, et al., Radiofrequency ablation of idiopathic left ventricular tachycardia at the site of earliest activation as determined by noncontact mapping. *J. Cardiovasc. Electrophysiol.*, 2000;**11**: 1094–1101.

58. Chen, M., B. Yang, J. Zou, et al., Non-contact mapping and linear ablation of the left posterior fascicle during sinus rhythm in the treatment of idiopathic left ventricular tachycardia. *Europace*, 2005;**7**: 138–144.

59. Segal, O.R., V. Markides, P. Kanagaratnam, et al., Multiple distinct right atrial endocardial origins in a patient with atrial tachycardia: mapping and ablation using noncontact mapping. *Pacing Clin. Electrophysiol.*, 2004;**27**: 541–544.

60. Tai, C.T., T.Y. Liu, P.C. Lee, et al., Non-contact mapping to guide radiofrequency ablation of atypical right atrial flutter. *J. Am. Coll. Cardiol.*, 2004;**44**: 1080–1086.

61. Schneider, M.A., G. Ndrepepa, B. Zrenner, et al., Noncontact mapping-guided catheter ablation of atrial fibrillation associated with left atrial ectopy. *J. Cardiovasc. Electrophysiol.*, 2000;**11**: 475–479.

62. Markides, V., R.J. Schilling, A.W.C. Chow, P. Kanagaratnam, D. Lamb, N.S. Peters, and D.W. Davies, Non-contact mapping of the human left atrium to guide ablation of focal atrial fibrillation. *Circulation*, 2000;**102**(18 Suppl. II): 575.

63. Schilling, R.J., A.H. Kadish, N.S. Peters, et al., Endocardial mapping of atrial fibrillation in the human right atrium using a non-contact catheter. *Eur. Heart J.*, 2000;**21**: 550–564.

64. Schilling, R.J., N.S. Peters, J. Goldberger, et al., Characterization of the anatomy and conduction velocities of the human right atrial flutter circuit determined by noncontact mapping. *J. Am. Coll. Cardiol.*, 2001;**38**: 385–393.

65. Schumacher, B., W. Jung, T. Lewalter, et al., Verification of linear lesions using a noncontact multielectrode array catheter versus conventional contact mapping techniques. *J. Cardiovasc. Electrophysiol.*, 1999;**10**: 791–798.

66. Betts, T.R., P.R. Roberts, S.A. Allen, et al., Electrophysiological mapping and ablation of intra-atrial reentry tachycardia after Fontan surgery with the use of a noncontact mapping system. *Circulation*, 2000;**102**: 419–425.

67. Miles, W.M., R. Yee, G.J. Klein, et al., The preexcitation index: an aid in determining the mechanism of supraventricular tachycardia and localizing accessory pathways. *Circulation*, 1986;**74**: 493–500.

68. Michaud, G.F., H. Tada, S. Chough et al., Differentiation of atypical atrioventricular node re-entrant tachycardia from orthodromic reciprocating tachycardia using a septal accessory pathway by the response to ventricular pacing. *J. Am. Coll. Cardiol.*, 2001;**38**: 1163–1167.

69. Gonzalez-Torrecilla, E., A. Arenal, F. Atienza, et al., First postpacing interval after tachycardia entrainment with correction for atrioventricular node delay: a simple maneuver for differential diagnosis of atrioventricular nodal reentrant tachycardias

versus orthodromic reciprocating tachycardias. *Heart Rhythm*, 2006;**3**: 674–679.

70. Haissaguerre, M., F. Gaita, B. Fischer, et al., Elimination of atrioventricular nodal reentrant tachycardia using discrete slow potentials to guide application of radiofrequency energy [see comments]. *Circulation*, 1992;**85**: 2162–2175.

71. Jackman, W.M., K.J. Beckman, J.H. McClelland, et al., Treatment of supraventricular tachycardia due to atrioventricular nodal reentry, by radiofrequency catheter ablation of slow-pathway conduction. *N. Engl. J. Med.*, 1992;**327**: 313–318.

72. Jazayeri, M.R., S.L. Hempe, J.S. Sra, et al., Selective transcatheter ablation of the fast and slow pathways using radiofrequency energy in patients with atrioventricular nodal reentrant tachycardia [see comments]. *Circulation*, 1992;**85**: 1318–1328.

73. Wathen, M., A. Natale, K. Wolfe, et al., An anatomically guided approach to atrioventricular node slow pathway ablation. *Am. J. Cardiol.*, 1992;**70**: 886–889.

74. Hintringer, F., J. Hartikainen, D.W. Davies, et al., Prediction of atrioventricular block during radiofrequency ablation of the slow pathway of the atrioventricular node. *Circulation*, 1995;**92**: 3490–3496.

75. Jentzer, J.H., R. Goyal, B.D. Williamson, et al., Analysis of junctional ectopy during radiofrequency ablation of the slow pathway in patients with atrioventricular nodal reentrant tachycardia. *Circulation*, 1994;**90**: 2820–2826.

76. Willems, S., H. Shenasa, H. Kottkamp, et al., Temperature-controlled slow pathway ablation for treatment of atrioventricular nodal reentrant tachycardia using a combined anatomical and electrogram guided strategy. *Eur. Heart J.*, 1996;**17**: 1092–1102.

77. Poret, P., C. Leclercq, D. Gras, et al., Junctional rhythm during slow pathway radiofrequency ablation in patients with atrioventricular nodal reentrant tachycardia: beat-to-beat analysis and its prognostic value in relation to electrophysiologic and anatomic parameters. *J. Cardiovasc. Electrophysiol.*, 2000;**11**: 405–412.

78. Schumacher, B., J. Tebbenjohanns, D. Pfeiffer, et al., Junctional arrhythmias in radiofrequency modification of the atrioventricular node. *Z. Kardiol.*, 1995;**84**: 977–985.

79. Lipscomb, K.J., A.M. Zaidi, A.P. Fitzpatrick, et al., Slow pathway modification for atrioventricular node re-entrant tachycardia: fast junctional tachycardia predicts adverse prognosis. *Heart*, 2001;**85**: 44–47.

80. Iturralde, P., V. Araya-Gomez, L. Colin, et al., A new ECG algorithm for the localization of accessory pathways using only the polarity of the QRS complex. *J. Electrocardiol.*, 1996;**29**: 289–299.

81. d'Avila, A., J. Brugada, V. Skeberis, et al., A fast and reliable algorithm to localize accessory pathways based on the polarity of the QRS complex on the surface ECG during sinus rhythm. *Pacing Clin. Electrophysiol.*, 1995;**18**: 1615–1627.

82. Xie, B., S.C. Heald, Y. Bashir, et al., Localization of accessory pathways from the 12-lead electrocardiogram using a new algorithm. *Am. J. Cardiol.*, 1994;**74**: 161–165.

83. Arruda, M.S., J.H. McClelland, X. Wang, et al., Development and validation of an ECG algorithm for identifying accessory pathway ablation site in Wolff-Parkinson-White syndrome. *J. Cardiovasc. Electrophysiol.*, 1998;**9**: 2–12.

84. Chiang, C.E., S.A. Chen, W.S. Teo, et al., An accurate stepwise electrocardiographic algorithm for localization of accessory pathways in patients with Wolff-Parkinson-White syndrome from a comprehensive analysis of delta waves and R/S ratio during sinus rhythm. *Am. J. Cardiol.*, 1995;**76**: 40–46.

85. Fitzpatrick, A.P., R.P. Gonzales, M.D. Lesh, et al., New algorithm for the localization of accessory atrioventricular connections using a baseline electrocardiogram [published erratum appears in *J. Am. Coll. Cardiol.* 1994 Apr;23(5):1272]. *J. Am. Coll. Cardiol.*, 1994;**23**: 107–116.

86. Diker, E., M. Ozdemir, U.K. Tezcan, et al., QRS polarity on 12-lead surface ECG. A criterion for the differentiation of right and left posteroseptal accessory atrioventricular pathways. *Cardiology*, 1997;**88**: 328–332.

87. Jackman, W.M., X.Z. Wang, K.J. Friday, et al., Catheter ablation of accessory atrioventricular pathways (Wolff-Parkinson-White syndrome) by radiofrequency current. *N. Engl. J. Med.*, 1991;**324**: 1605–1611.

88. Feld, G.K., M. Mollerus, U. Birgersdotter-Green, et al., Conduction velocity in the tricuspid valve-inferior vena cava isthmus is slower in patients with type I atrial flutter compared to those without a history of atrial flutter. *J. Cardiovasc. Electrophysiol.*, 1997;**8**: 1338–1348.

89. Nakagawa, H., R. Lazzara, T. Khastgir, et al., Role of the tricuspid annulus and the eustachian valve/ridge on atrial flutter. Relevance to catheter ablation of the septal isthmus and a new technique for rapid identification of ablation success [see comments]. *Circulation*, 1996;**94**: 407–424.

90. Olgin, J.E., J.M. Kalman, L.A. Saxon, et al., Mechanism of initiation of atrial flutter in humans: site of unidirectional block and direction of rotation. *J. Am. Coll. Cardiol.*, 1997;**29**: 376–384.

91. Saoudi, N., F. Cosio, A. Waldo, et al., A classification of atrial flutter and regular atrial tachycardia according to electrophysiological mechanisms and anatomical bases; a Statement from a Joint Expert Group from The Working Group of Arrhythmias of the European Society of Cardiology and the North American Society of Pacing and Electrophysiology. *Eur. Heart J.*, 2001;**22**: 1162–1182.

92. Feld, G.K., R.P. Fleck, P.S. Chen, et al., Radiofrequency catheter ablation for the treatment of human type 1 atrial flutter. Identification of a critical zone in the reentrant circuit by endocardial mapping techniques [see comments]. *Circulation*, 1992;**86**: 1233–1240.

93. Chen, S.A., C.T. Tai, C.E. Chiang, et al., Focal atrial tachycardia: reanalysis of the clinical and electrophysiologic characteristics and prediction of successful radiofrequency ablation. *J. Cardiovasc. Electrophysiol.*, 1998;**9**: 355–365.

94. Haissaguerre, M., P. Jais, D.C. Shah, et al., Spontaneous initiation of atrial fibrillation by ectopic beats originating in the pulmonary veins. *N. Engl. J. Med.*, 1998;**339**: 659–666.

95. Pappone, C., S. Rosanio, G. Oreto, et al., Circumferential radiofrequency ablation of pulmonary vein ostia: a new anatomic approach for curing atrial fibrillation. *Circulation*, 2000;**102**: 2619–2628.

96. Cox, J.L., R.B. Schuessler, D.G. Lappas, et al., An 8 1/2-year clinical experience with surgery for atrial fibrillation. *Ann. Surg.*, 1996;**224**: 267–273.

97. Nademanee, K., J. McKenzie, E. Kosar, et al., A new approach for catheter ablation of atrial fibrillation: mapping of the electrophysiologic substrate. *J. Am. Coll. Cardiol.*, 2004;**43**: 2044–2053.

98. Lau, C.P., H.F. Tse, and G.M. Ayers, Defibrillation-guided radiofrequency ablation of atrial fibrillation secondary to an atrial focus. *J. Am. Coll. Cardiol.*, 1999;**33**: 1217–1226.

99. Lee, S.H., C.T. Tai, W.S. Lin, et al., Predicting the arrhythmogenic foci of atrial fibrillation before atrial transseptal procedure: implication for catheter ablation [In Process Citation]. *J. Cardiovasc. Electrophysiol.*, 2000;**11**: 750–757.

100. Morady, F., L.A. Dicarlo Jr., L.B. Liem, et al., Effects of high stimulation current on the induction of ventricular tachycardia. *Am. J. Cardiol.*, 1985;**56**: 73–78.

101. Doherty, J.U., M.G. Kienzle, H.L. Waxman, et al., Programmed ventricular stimulation at a second right ventricular site: an analysis of 100 patients, with special reference to sensitivity, specificity and characteristics of patients with induced ventricular tachycardia. *Am. J. Cardiol.*, 1983;**52**: 1184–1189.

102. Herre, J.M., D.E. Mann, J.C. Luck, et al., Effect of increased current, multiple pacing sites and number of extrastimuli on induction of ventricular tachycardia. *Am. J. Cardiol.*, 1986;**57**: 102–107.

103. Lerman, B.B., K. Stein, E.D. Engelstein, et al., Mechanism of repetitive monomorphic ventricular tachycardia. *Circulation*, 1995;**92**: 421–429.

104. Lerman, B.B., L. Belardinelli, G.A. West, et al., Adenosine-sensitive ventricular tachycardia: evidence suggesting cyclic AMP-mediated triggered activity. *Circulation*, 1986;**74**: 270–280.

105. Jadonath, R.L., D.S. Schwartzman, M.W. Preminger, et al., Utility of the 12-lead electrocardiogram in localizing the origin of right ventricular outflow tract tachycardia. *Am. Heart J.*, 1995;**130**: 1107–1113.

106. Dixit, S., E.P. Gerstenfeld, D.J. Callans, et al., Electrocardiographic patterns of superior right ventricular outflow tract tachycardias: distinguishing septal and free-wall sites of origin. *J. Cardiovasc. Electrophysiol.*, 2003;**14**: 1–7.

107. Tchou, P., M. Jazayeri, S. Denker, et al., Transcatheter electrical ablation of right bundle branch. A method of treating macroreentrant ventricular tachycardia attributed to bundle branch reentry. *Circulation*, 1988;**78**: 246–257.

108. Kuchar, D.L., J.N. Ruskin, and H. Garan, Electrocardiographic localization of the site of origin of ventricular tachycardia in patients with prior myocardial infarction. *J. Am. Coll. Cardiol.*, 1989;**13**: 893–903.

109. Miller, J.M., F.E. Marchlinski, A.E. Buxton, et al., Relationship between the 12-lead electrocardiogram during ventricular tachycardia and endocardial site of origin in patients with coronary artery disease. *Circulation*, 1988;**77**: 759–766.

110. Segal, O.R., A.W. Chow, T. Wong, et al., A novel algorithm for determining endocardial VT exit site from 12 lead surface ECG characteristics in human, infarct-related ventricular tachycardia. *J. Cardiovasc. Electrophysiol.*, 2007;**18**: 161–168.

111. Callans, D.J., M. Zardini, C.D. Gottlieb, et al., The variable contribution of functional and anatomic barriers in human ventricular tachycardia: an analysis with resetting from two sites. *J. Am. Coll. Cardiol.*, 1996;**27**: 1106–1111.

112. Ciaccio, E.J., M.M. Scheinman, V. Fridman, et al., Dynamic changes in electrogram morphology at functional lines of block in reentrant circuits during ventricular tachycardia in the infarcted canine heart: a new method to localize reentrant circuits from electrogram features using adaptive template matching. *J. Cardiovasc. Electrophysiol.*, 1999;**10**: 194–213.

113. Morady, F., A. Kadish, S. Rosenheck, et al., Concealed entrainment as a guide for catheter ablation of ventricular tachycardia in patients with prior myocardial infarction. *J. Am. Coll. Cardiol.*, 1991;**17**: 678–689.

114. El Shalakany, A., T. Hadjis, P. Papageorgiou, et al., Entrainment/mapping criteria for the prediction of termination of ventricular tachycardia by single radiofrequency lesion in patients with coronary artery disease. *Circulation*, 1999;**99**: 2283– 2289.

115. Strickberger, S.A., B.P. Knight, G.F. Michaud, et al., Mapping and ablation of ventricular tachycardia guided by virtual electrograms using a noncontact, computerized mapping system. *J. Am. Coll. Cardiol.*, 2000;**35**: 414–421.

116. Wilber, D.J., D.E. Kopp, D.N. Glascock, et al., Catheter ablation of the mitral isthmus for ventricular tachycardia associated with inferior infarction. *Circulation*, 1995;**92**: 3481–3489.

117. Della, B.P., R. De Ponti, J.A. Uriarte, et al., Catheter ablation and antiarrhythmic drugs for haemodynamically tolerated post-infarction ventricular tachycardia; long-term outcome in relation to acute electrophysiological findings. *Eur. Heart J.*, 2002;**23**: 414–424.

118. de Paola, A.A., W.D. Melo, M.Z. Tavora, et al., Angiographic and electrophysiological substrates for ventricular tachycardia mapping through the coronary veins. *Heart*, 1998;**79**: 59–63.

119. Wong, T., A.W. Chow, V. Markides, R.J. Schilling, N.S. Peters, and D.W. Davies, Human ventricular tachycardia ablation guided by intracoronary artery guide-wire mapping. *Pacing Clin. Electrophysiol.*, 2002;**25**: 524.

120. Sosa, E., M. Scanavacca, A. d'Avila, et al., Endocardial and epicardial ablation guided by nonsurgical transthoracic epicardial mapping to treat recurrent ventricular tachycardia. *J. Cardiovasc. Electrophysiol.*, 1998;**9**: 229–239.

121. Cesario, D.A., M. Vaseghi, N.G. Boyle, et al., Value of high-density endocardial and epicardial mapping for catheter ablation of hemodynamically unstable ventricular tachycardia. *Heart Rhythm*, 2006;**3**: 1–10.

122. Schweikert, R.A., W.I. Saliba, G. Tomassoni, et al., Percutaneous pericardial instrumentation for endo-epicardial mapping of previously failed ablations. *Circulation*, 2003;**108**: 1329–1335.

123. Segal, O.R., A.W. Chow, N.S. Peters and D.W. Davies, Mechanisms that initiate ventricular tachycardia in the infarcted human heart. *Heart Rhythm*, 2010;**7**: 57–64.

124. Segal, O.R., A.W. Chow, V. Markides, D.W. Davies and N.S. Peters, Characterisation of the effects of single ventricular extrastimuli on endocardial activation in human, infarct-related ventricular tachycardia. *J. Am. Coll. Cardiol.*, 2007;**49**: 1315–1323.

125. Segal, O.R., L.J. Gula, A.C. Skanes, A.D. Krahn, R. Yee and G.J. Klein, Differential ventricular entrainment – a maneuver to differentiate AV node reentrant tachycardia from orthodromic reciprocating tachycardia. *Heart Rhythm*, 2009;**6**: 493–500.

126. Segal, O.R., T. Wong, A.W. Chow, J. Jarman, R.J. Schilling, V. Markides, N.S. Peters and D.W. Davies, Intra-coronary guidewire mapping – A novel technique to guide ablation of human ventricular tachycardia. *J. Interv. Card. Electrophysiol.*, 2007;**18**: 143–154.

4 Sinus and Atrial Arrhythmias

F. Russell Quinn · Andrew D. McGavigan · Andrew C. Rankin

P. W. Macfarlane et al. (eds.), *Cardiac Arrhythmias and Mapping Techniques*, DOI 10.1007/978-0-85729-877-5_4,
© Springer-Verlag London Limited 2012

4.1   Introduction

Although rarely fatal, disorders of sinus node function and atrial arrhythmias are causes of much morbidity. They are the most common causes of clinical bradyarrhythmias and tachyarrhythmias, respectively. Sinus node dysfunction accounts for over half of permanent pacemaker implants worldwide [1], while atrial fibrillation occurs secondary to the progression of most cardiac conditions [2]. The sinus node and the atrium are closely related, both anatomically and functionally, and disorders of one interfere with the functioning of the other. This fact is of particular relevance to the electrocardiographic study of sinus and atrial activity.

The electrocardiographic diagnosis both of sinus disorders and atrial arrhythmias depends on the P wave as evidence of atrial activation, since sinus node activity itself is not recorded on the surface ECG. The presence or absence of P waves, their morphology and timing, including their relation to ventricular activation as manifest by the PR interval, provide sufficient information for the diagnosis of most sinus and atrial disturbances. While the application of invasive electrophysiological techniques to the assessment of sinus node function [3, 4] and atrial arrhythmias [5] has provided a wealth of information about their origins and the mechanisms underlying arrhythmias in general, it is now recognized that non-invasive studies, including electrocardiography and ambulatory monitoring, are sufficient for the investigation of the majority [6, 7]. Invasive electrophysiological study may be useful for cases in which there are diagnostic or management problems [8], and as a prelude to curative catheter ablation. With catheter ablation techniques playing an increasing role in the management of certain atrial arrhythmias, there has been renewed interest in P wave morphology on the surface ECG as a guide to the origin and mechanism of focal and reentrant atrial rhythm disturbances.

4.2   Normal Sinus Rhythm and Sinus Arrhythmias

4.2.1   Electrophysiology of the Sinus Node

Activation of the normal cardiac cycle originates in the sinus node, a small discrete mass of specialized pacemaker (P) cells situated at the junction of the high right atrium (HRA) and superior vena cava [9, 10]. Sinus nodal cells are characterized by a membrane potential of around −60 mV at its most negative; that is, they are relatively depolarized compared to other non-nodal cardiac tissues which have a membrane potential of −80 to −100 mV [11]. At such a potential, fast sodium channels are largely inactivated and the action potential of the P cells is dependent on slower inward calcium currents [12, 13]. On repolarization after an action potential, slow spontaneous depolarization occurs during diastole until threshold is reached and another action potential occurs. This diastolic depolarization is often described as the pacemaker potential, or phase 4 of the action-potential cycle. Several ion currents have been implicated in the pacemaker potential, including potassium conductances, the hyperpolarization-activated cation current, I_f [14] and the sustained inward current, I_{st} [12, 15]. In addition, rhythmic release of calcium from intracellular stores, and its subsequent reuptake, may also play a role in generating the pacemaker potential [16]. Other cardiac tissues may also exhibit pacemaker potentials, notably atrioventricular (AV) nodal and Purkinje-fiber cells, but at a slower rate than in the sinus node. Thus, the rate of sinus firing determines the rate of the rest of the heart. In the absence of a sinus beat, however, these lower pacemakers may generate "escape" rhythms.

The activity originating in the sinus nodal cells is conducted out to the surrounding atrium through transitional (T) cells, which have electrophysiological properties intermediate between the pacemaker cells and the quiescent atrial tissue [17]. The site of the primary pacemaker may shift between groups of pacemaker cells within the sinus node, or into the T cells or even the atrium. Disorders of sinus function may result from a failure of impulse generation by the nodal (P) cells, or a failure of conduction of the impulse from sinus to atrial cells, via the T cells [4].

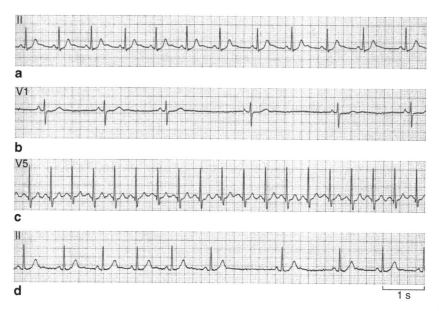

◘ Fig. 4.1

Sinus rhythm: (**a**) normal sinus rhythm, 72 bpm; (**b**) sinus bradycardia, 36 bpm; (**c**) sinus tachycardia, 114 bpm; (**d**) sinus arrhythmia, rate 66 bpm on inspiration, 38 bpm on expiration. ECG leads shown on each strip recording

4.2.2   Normal Sequence of Atrial Activation and P Wave Morphology

The cardiac impulse in normal sinus rhythm originates in the sinus node, spreads directly to the right atrium and thence to the left atrium, before being conducted through the AV node and His-Purkinje system to the ventricles. This activation sequence is clearly seen in electrophysiological studies using multiple sites for intracardiac recordings. Atrial activation occurs first in the high right atrium, followed by the low right atrium at the AV junction, before it is seen in the proximal and finally the distal coronary sinus electrograms, the latter representing left atrial activation. Activation of the His bundle is then detected, followed by spread of excitation to the ventricles (see ❷ Fig. 2.2). The origin of the atrial activation in the HRA determines the P wave axis, the normal axis being from 0 to +90°. Thus, the P wave is usually upright in leads I, II and aVF, and inverted in aVR. In the horizontal plane, the activation from right to left produces upright P waves in the left-sided chest leads V_3–V_6. The P wave may also be upright in V_1–V_2, but is more commonly inverted or biphasic. Normal sinus rhythm has regular P waves, preceding the QRS complexes by a constant PR interval of 120–200 ms (❷ Fig. 4.1a). The P wave configuration should be constant in any given lead, other than minor changes in axis with respiration.

4.2.3   Autonomic Control of Sinus Rate

The sinus node has both sympathetic and parasympathetic innervations which control the rate of sinus firing by altering the rate of depolarization of the pacemaker potential. The parasympathetic vagal influence is dominant at rest, slowing the intrinsic rate, as shown by the increase in heart rate with atropine [18]. Sympathetic innervation and circulating catecholamines increase heart rate during exercise and stress. Autonomic tone has a major influence on sinus node function and an awareness of this fact is important in the assessment of sinus node dysfunction.

Variations of autonomic tone may also cause the location of the pacemaker to shift within the sinus node, or to an ectopic atrial focus. As vagal discharge slows the pacemaker cells, another region under less vagal control may take over pacing. The P wave configuration may change only slightly with "wandering sinus pacemaker," but with "wandering atrial pacemaker" the P wave morphology and axis will change, as beats originate from ectopic atrial foci.

4.2.4 Normal Sinus Heart Rate

The normal heart rate in the adult is widely accepted as 60–100 beats per minute (bpm), lower than this being defined as bradycardia, and faster as tachycardia. However, not all physicians would agree with this stated range. A WHO/ISFC Task Force [19] thought that the inherent rate of the sinoatrial (SA) node had a "representative" range of 50–100 bpm. Spodick et al. measured the resting heart rate of 500 consecutive asymptomatic subjects, who were aged 50–80 years, and were free from cardiac medication. They found a range (2 standard deviations below and above the mean) of 46–93 bpm for men, and 51–95 bpm for women [20]. There was no association between age and the resting heart rate. Others have reported similar findings with ageing in healthy subjects, but in those with heart disease the resting heart rate falls with age (reviewed by Brignole [21]).

4.2.5 Sinus Bradycardia

A sinus rate of <60 bpm is defined as sinus bradycardia. Normal P waves precede each QRS complex with a constant PR interval (❷ Fig. 4.1b). Sinus bradycardia occurs in normal children [22] and adults [23, 24] during sleep, with heart rate commonly down to 30–40 bpm and also in athletes, owing to enhanced vagal tone [25]. Vagal overactivity may also be pathophysiological, producing profound sinus bradycardia during vasovagal episodes or acute inferior myocardial infarction [26]. Unexplained sinus bradycardia is the most common manifestation of sinus node dysfunction [21, 27, 28].

4.2.6 Sinus Tachycardia

The electrocardiographic features of sinus tachycardia are a heart rate of >100 bpm with a normal P wave morphology and axis and a normal PR interval (❷ Fig. 4.1c). Sinus tachycardia is normal in young children, while in adults it is seen in response to neural or hormonal influences. Physiological or pathological stresses, such as physical exercise, anxiety, fever, hypotension, heart failure or thyrotoxicosis all cause sinus tachycardia. The rate may be transiently slowed by carotid sinus massage. The rate of sinus tachycardia may be up to 200 bpm in young adults during maximal exercise. Maximal heart rate on exercise tends to decrease with age [29], an approximate guide being 208-(0.7 × age) bpm [30].

4.2.7 Sinus Arrhythmia

During normal sinus rhythm the P-P interval is relatively constant, but variations, termed sinus arrhythmia, may occur. This is a common arrhythmia, usually arising from physiological variations in autonomic tone [22, 23]. There is phasic variation in the P-P interval, the difference in sinus cycle length being ≥120 ms, with normal P waves and PR interval (❷ Fig. 4.1d). It is most commonly related to the respiratory cycle, with an increase in sinus rate during inspiration owing to reflex inhibition of vagal tone and a slowing of rate with expiration [31]. Non-respiratory sinus arrhythmia may also occur, secondary to heart disease, for example, acute myocardial infarction or digoxin toxicity.

A further form of variation in sinus rate, known as ventriculophasic sinus arrhythmia, is noted when there is prolongation of a sinus cycle which has no corresponding ventricular contraction. This is most commonly seen in complete AV block (❷ Fig. 4.2) [32]. The P-P interval of a cycle which includes a QRS complex is shorter than the following cycle which does not. A similar lengthening of P-P interval may be noted following a premature ventricular contraction with a compensatory pause. Proposed mechanisms for ventriculophasic sinus arrhythmia include mechanical and/or hemodynamic effects of ventricular systole on the sinus node and changes in baroreceptor-mediated vagal activity. In an interesting study, de Marchena et al. studied the phenomenon in patients who had received a cardiac transplant [33]. The P-P interval of the recipient's retained atrial tissue (which has preserved vagal innervation to its sinus node, but lacks flow in its sinus node artery) was found to be independent of the donor heart's ventricular activity. This lack of ventriculophasic effect suggests that hemodynamic rather than autonomic effects on the sinus node may be most important.

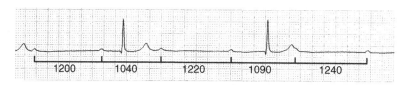

◨ Fig. 4.2

Ventriculophasic sinus arrhythmia. Cardiac monitor tracing in a patient with complete heart block and a narrow-complex escape rhythm, showing variations in the atrial rate in response to ventricular systole – the P-P intervals (indicated in ms) which contain a QRS complex are shorter than those which do not

4.2.8   Inappropriate Sinus Tachycardia and Postural Orthostatic Tachycardia Syndrome

Inappropriate sinus tachycardia, also referred to as chronic nonparoxysmal sinus tachycardia, occurs in otherwise healthy people and is apparently a result of increased automaticity of the sinus node, due to defective autonomic control [34, 35]. The clinical features are of resting sinus tachycardia, and an exaggerated response to minimal activity, in the absence of other causes, such as hyperthyroidism, heart failure, anaemia, cardioactive drugs, or infection. The electrocardiogram shows P waves with an axis and morphology corresponding to those during sinus rhythm. Ambulatory monitoring or exercise testing shows a gradual onset and termination of the tachycardia. A related, and often overlapping, condition is the postural orthostatic tachycardia syndrome (POTS) which is characterised by an increase in the sinus rate by 30 bpm, or to greater than 120 bpm, when the patient stands up from a supine position. This increase in heart rate occurs in the absence of significant orthostatic hypotension [35]. These conditions may persist for months or years, and can cause troublesome symptoms but have a good prognosis. Treatments often include volume expansion, beta-blockers and other peripherally- or centrally-active agents to modify vascular tone. Studies of catheter-based modification of the sinus node have generally yielded disappointing long-term results [35].

4.2.9   Sinus Node Reentrant Tachycardia

Sinus node reentrant tachycardia accounts for around 5–15% of supraventricular tachycardias and is characterized by a modest increase in heart rate to 100–150 bpm, P waves which are similar, though not necessarily identical, to those during sinus rhythm and a RP/PR ratio of >1 [36–38]. As with other reentrant tachycardias, it can be initiated and terminated during electrophysiological study by premature atrial stimuli [39]. The atrial activation sequence is identical to that during sinus rhythm, originating in the HRA. It is not usually associated with sinus node dysfunction and is seen more commonly during electrophysiological study than as a spontaneous arrhythmia [40]. If treatment is required, sinus node reentrant tachycardia can be managed with drugs or by ablative therapy [38].

4.3   Sinus Node Dysfunction

Disturbance of sinus node function is a common cause of symptomatic arrhythmias and may be a result of a failure of sinus automaticity, or of a failure of propagation of the impulse from the sinus node to the atrium (SA block), or a combination of both. There are many etiological or associated conditions and the cause of sinus node dysfunction may be classified as intrinsic, related to pathological changes in sinus and atrial tissue, or extrinsic, with disturbance of sinus function being attributable to the influence of other factors, commonly autonomic overactivity, or cardioactive drugs [41]. Both intrinsic and extrinsic forms may be chronic, with slow progression, or acute, with sudden onset usually related to predisposing factors such as ischemia, inflammation, surgical trauma or drugs.

    In view of the multifactorial etiology of sinus node dysfunction, it is not surprising that no single underlying histological abnormality has been identified, but rather a variety of findings have been reported. In most cases, the node is of normal size with marked loss of nodal cells and replacement by fibrosis. With normal ageing, the sinus node undergoes striking loss of myocardial cells, with an increase in fibrous tissue [42]. In patients with sinus node dysfunction, there may be virtual total fibrosis of the node, with the proportion of nodal cells being as low as 5%. By contrast to these fibrotic nodes of normal size, the sinus node may be hypoplastic, presumably as a congenital abnormality [43]. Rarely, the node appears to be morphologically normal, with fibrosis or fatty infiltration around the nodal tissue [44]. Fibrotic involvement of atrium itself and AV nodal regions is commonly found in patients with sinus nodal fibrosis [42, 43], consistent with the common coexistence of AV conduction abnormalities [45, 46], or atrial tachyarrhythmias [47]. Acute sinus node dysfunction may result from inflammatory involvement of the node in pericarditis [48] or myocardial infarction, but only rarely is it a result of atheroma or thrombosis of the sinus node coronary artery branch itself [42, 43]. The sinus node can also be affected by systemic infiltrative conditions, such as amyloidosis [49] and hemochromatosis [50], leading to sinus node dysfunction, and a variety of arrhythmias.

In addition to abnormal autonomic influences as extrinsic causes of sinus dysfunction, it has been hypothesized that an abnormal response to the regulatory influence of adenosine, locally released by active myocardium, may underlie intrinsic sinus node disease [51]. Evidence to support an increased sensitivity to adenosine comes from the demonstration of marked bradycardia and sinus pauses produced by intravenous adenyl compounds [52], and the therapeutic response to theophylline, an adenosine antagonist, in some patients [53, 54]. Finally, the possibility of an autoimmune mechanism has been raised by the finding of autoantibodies against sinus node in over 25% of patients with sinus dysfunction or bradycardia [55].

4.3.1 Sick Sinus Syndrome

The term "sick sinus syndrome" was first coined in the 1960s by Lown [56], to describe acute sinus disturbance after cardioversion, and was subsequently applied by Ferrer [57] to patients with chronic SA dysfunction. Although, strictly, it should be confined to patients with intrinsic sinus node dysfunction, the term has been commonly applied to any patient with symptoms attributable to disorders of sinus node function [58, 59]. The clinical picture of sick sinus syndrome includes a variety of arrhythmias [21, 27] with multifactorial etiologies [59]. The sick sinus syndrome may be diagnosed in symptomatic patients with any of the following electrocardiographic findings:

(a) Inappropriate sinus bradycardia,
(b) Sinus arrest with or without an ectopic atrial or junctional escape rhythm,
(c) Sinoatrial exit block,
(d) Alternating bradycardia and atrial tachyarrhythmia (the "bradycardia-tachycardia syndrome") [47, 60].

In addition, chronic atrial fibrillation with slow ventricular response in the absence of drug therapy usually indicates underlying sinoatrial dysfunction, and attempts at cardioversion typically produce a slow, unstable rhythm [56]. In patients with sinus node dysfunction there is commonly depression of the lower latent pacemakers and the failure of "escape" rhythms results in symptomatic bradycardia. Abnormalities of AV conduction are also found in over half of patients with sick sinus syndrome [45, 46], although more recent evidence suggests that in those with intact AV conduction, it remains stable with time, especially in those without concomitant bundle branch block [61]. Carotid sinus hypersensitivity may mimic, or unmask, sinus node dysfunction [62, 63].

The bradycardia-tachycardia syndrome comprises about half of the patients with sick sinus syndrome [59]. Symptoms may occur with the tachycardia, commonly atrial fibrillation or flutter, or especially with the bradycardia, as long pauses may result following spontaneous termination of the tachycardia (❯ Fig. 4.3). The tachycardia may simply be predisposed to by the bradycardia, occurring as an "escape" arrhythmia, and may be suppressed by atrial pacing [64]. In other cases, the finding of atrial histopathology [42] indicates that atrial arrhythmias may be the result of the general pathological process. It is probable that the development of atrial arrhythmias is the natural progression of the condition [65], but this progression occurs only very slowly [66].

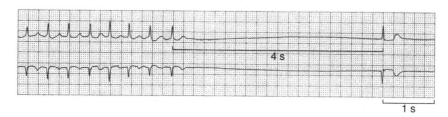

■ Fig. 4.3
Ambulatory monitor tracing, showing a pause of 4 s after spontaneous termination of atrial fibrillation in the bradycardia-tachycardia syndrome. The pause is followed by a junctional escape beat

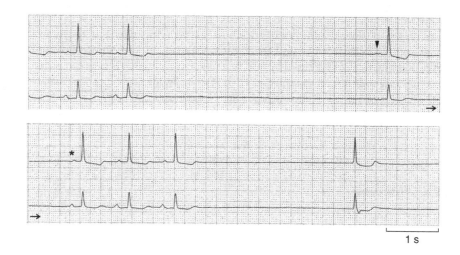

■ Fig. 4.4
Sinus arrest, as seen on ambulatory monitor tracing. The lower trace is continuous with the upper trace. After two sinus beats there is a pause of 4.9 s, followed by an ectopic atrial escape beat (*arrowhead*). The first spontaneous sinus beat (*) occurs after a total of 6.9 s. A further pause of 3.4 s occurs, followed by a junctional escape beat

4.3.2   Sinus Arrest

Failure of impulse formation by the sinus node results in the absence of atrial activation and a pause is seen on the ECG (❯ Fig. 4.4). Sinus arrest may produce periods of ventricular asystole of variable duration, depending on the time taken for recovery of sinus automaticity, or appearance of an escape rhythm from a lower pacemaker. Since the regular sinus discharge has been interrupted, the duration of the pause has no arithmetical relation to the basic sinus cycle length.

4.3.3   Sinoatrial Block

Block of SA conduction may result in the failure of atrial depolarization, despite continuing sinus automaticity. Sinoatrial block may be classified as first degree, second degree or third degree, with delayed conduction, intermittent or complete block, analogous to AV block. Only second-degree SA block can be diagnosed from the ECG, although first-degree conduction delay may be assessed by electrophysiological study. Second-degree SA block can be further subclassified as type I (Wenckebach) or type II, which is again analogous to second-degree AV block. Type II SA block is the most frequently

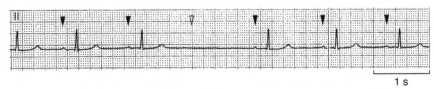

1 s

Fig. 4.5

Sinoatrial block (type II). The sinus pause is twice the preceding sinus cycle length (P waves are indicated by filled *arrowheads*), owing to exit block of sinus activity preventing the expected P wave (*open arrowhead*)

seen, with intermittent block occurring without preceding conduction delay. This is in contrast to AV block, where type I second-degree block is the more common. Sinoatrial block is diagnosed from the ECG by the intermittent absence of the P wave and subsequent QRS complex. The duration of the pause is an exact multiple of the preceding sinus cycle length, since sinus activity continues despite the failure of atrial activation (**○** Fig. 4.5). Type I (Wenckebach) SA block has increasing delay in SA conduction with successive beats until there is failure of atrial activation and an absent P wave. Since sinus activity is not apparent on the ECG, the diagnosis is established by a progressive decrease in P-P interval prior to the dropped beat, owing to the characteristic periodicity of the Wenckebach phenomenon, whereby, although conduction is progressively delayed, the beat-by-beat increment in delay decreases [67]. The pause with type I SA block will, therefore, be less than twice the preceding P-P interval.

4.3.4 Diagnosis of Sinus Node Dysfunction

The investigation of patients with suspected sick sinus syndrome must be directed to the demonstration of abnormalities of sinus function and the establishment of the correlation between the patient's symptoms and the arrhythmias. The rhythm abnormalities are often intermittent and the resting ECG may be normal. The likelihood of detecting arrhythmias is increased by longer periods of ECG recording, and ambulatory Holter monitoring reveals the diagnosis in many more patients [68, 69]. The development of implanted loop recorders has allowed more prolonged ECG monitoring (up to 3 years) and can increase the diagnostic yield in patients with normal baseline tests [70, 71]. The results of these tests, however, must be interpreted carefully since sinus bradycardia, sinus arrest and SA block may all be normal findings [24], particularly in young people [22, 23] or athletes [25]. Sinus pauses of >2 s are generally abnormal and indicate sinus node dysfunction [72, 73], but it is important to document the relationship of the patient's symptoms to an arrhythmia, as asymptomatic pauses do not require treatment [74].

Abnormal heart-rate responses to exercise [75], atropine [76, 77] or isoprenaline [77, 78] are common in the sick sinus syndrome, although these tests are of questionable clinical utility [21]. The combination of atropine (0.04 mg/kg) and propranolol (0.2 mg/kg) produces complete autonomic blockade and reveals the intrinsic heart rate (IHR), which has a well-defined normal range that decreases with age [79]. The IHR can be predicted from a linear regression equation:

$$IHR = 118.1 - (0.57 \times age)$$

Patients with intrinsic sinus node dysfunction have an abnormally slow IHR, whereas it is normal in those with extrinsic vagally-induced dysfunction [80, 81]. The effects of carotid sinus pressure should also be determined (**○** Fig. 4.6). Carotid sinus hypersensitivity is present in around 33% of patients with sick sinus syndrome, although the two conditions appear to be pathophysiologically distinct [21].

In the majority of patients, noninvasive investigation is sufficient to establish the diagnosis of sick sinus syndrome [6, 7, 81]. Invasive testing is now seldom employed in this context, however in some circumstances it may help clarify the clinical diagnosis. For example, in patients with syncope thought to be due to sick sinus syndrome in whom ambulatory ECG monitoring has failed to record an event, the demonstration of markedly abnormal sinus node function in an invasive electrophysiology study may support the diagnosis and strengthen the case for implantation of a permanent pacemaker [4, 7]. The most commonly used tests involve atrial pacing to measure sinus automaticity (the sinus node recovery

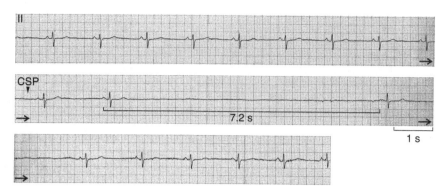

■ Fig. 4.6

Carotid sinus hypersensitivity. Traces are continuous. Carotid sinus pressure (CSP) results in sinus suppression, with a pause of 7.2 s

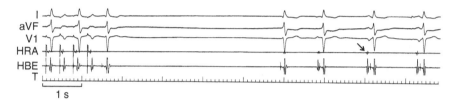

■ Fig. 4.7

Sinus node recovery time (SNRT). Following cessation of atrial pacing at a cycle length of 350 ms for 30 s, there is a pause of 6.9 s before the first spontaneous sinus beat (*arrowed*). The figure shows surface leads I, aVF and V1, and intracardiac recordings from the high right atrium (HRA) and His bundle electrogram (HBE). Time-bar (T) indicates seconds (large divisions)

time) and sinoatrial conduction (SA conduction time). Direct sinus node recordings [4, 82, 83] have added greatly to the understanding of the electrophysiological abnormalities in the sick sinus syndrome [84] but are not in routine clinical use [21]. The main invasive tests of sinus node function will be outlined below, but for more in depth reviews, the reader is directed elsewhere [4, 85–87].

4.3.5   Electrophysiological Assessment of Sinus Node Function

4.3.5.1   Sinus Node Recovery Time

Since the automaticity of cardiac pacemaker cells may be transiently suppressed by pacing at rates faster than their own firing rate [88], an assessment of sinus automaticity can be obtained by examining the time taken for recovery following a period of overdrive suppression by rapid atrial pacing [3]. The interval from the last paced P wave to the first spontaneous sinus P wave is the sinus node recovery time (SNRT). If sinus node dysfunction is present, the depression of automaticity is manifest by prolongation of the SNRT [3, 4, 89]. The resultant pause may be of several seconds duration in patients with sick sinus syndrome (❷ Fig. 4.7).

It is apparent that the duration of the pause following atrial pacing will also depend on the basic sinus cycle length (SCL): the slower the heart rate the longer the expected pause. The SNRT may be corrected for heart rate in a number of ways, the commonest being to subtract the mean SCL (corrected sinus node recovery time, CSNRT = SNRT – SCL) [90]. Different ranges of normal have been suggested by different investigators [85, 87], but a CSNRT > 550 ms is generally considered to be abnormal. Another commonly applied correction is the expression of the SNRT as a percentage of the SCL (normal SNRT/SCL × 100 < 150%) [85, 86].

In addition to the SNRT, further assessment of sinus function can be obtained by examining the atrial rhythm for several beats following pacing. While the first post-pacing pause is usually the longest, many patients with sinus dysfunction exhibit sudden prolongation of subsequent cycles [77]. Such "secondary pauses" are indicative of sinus node dysfunction and do not occur in normal individuals [91]. Pauses which are multiples of the basic SCL are a result of SA exit block. Secondary pauses may be the only manifestation of sinus dysfunction during electrophysiological study [77, 91]. The total recovery time (TRT) for the sinus cycle to return to stable prepacing values can also be taken as an indication of sinus function, and should be <5 s [77, 85].

4.3.5.2   Sinoatrial Conduction Time

An estimate of SA conduction may be obtained by examining the responses to atrial pacing, since a paced atrial activation must travel retrogradely into the sinus node and the subsequent sinus activity must then be conducted out to the atrium. Two methods of measuring the SA conduction time (SACT) are commonly used. The Strauss method [92] introduces atrial premature stimuli following successive runs of eight spontaneous sinus cycles (each impulse designated A_1). If the paced atrial extrastimulus (A_2) is introduced at an appropriate time in mid-diastole, it will penetrate the sinus node before it has fired spontaneously, and depolarize the pacemaker, which is then reset. The return cycle (the time from the paced atrial extrastimulus to the first spontaneous sinus beat, A_3) will be the sum of the time taken for the beat to conduct into the node, the basic SCL following reset and the SA exit conduction time. Thus $A_2A_3 = A_1A_1 + SACT$, where SACT is the total conduction time into and out of the node.

The method of Narula [93] is simpler, employing an 8-beat train of atrial pacing (A_p) at a slow rate (<10 bpm above the sinus rate). The return cycle to the first sinus beat (A) is then measured, and the total SACT calculated as A_pA-postpacing SCL. This method attempts to overcome one problem with the Strauss method – if there is any significant degree of sinus arrhythmia, then error will be introduced into the estimation of the SACT. The Narula method assumes that a short eight-beat train of slow atrial pacing effectively stabilizes the SCL, without significant suppression of automaticity.

The two methods for estimating SA conduction give similar, but not identical, values for SACT [83, 93, 94], and a fairly wide range of normal values for total SACT have been reported (from 200 to 344 ms, reviewed in [85]).

4.3.5.3   Sinus Node Refractoriness

Another technique which has been used for the assessment of sinus node function is the measurement of the retrograde sinus node effective refractory period (SNERP) [95]. Eight-beat trains of atrial pacing are followed by single extrastimuli of increasing prematurity and the return cycle A_2A_3 is plotted against the coupling interval A_1A_2. The SNERP is taken as the longest coupling interval that is followed by an interpolated beat. There appears to be clear separation between values of SNERP in normal individuals and in patients with sinus dysfunction (325 as opposed to 522 ms) [95]. A limitation of this technique is that the SNERP could only be measured in 75% of patients in one study [87].

4.3.5.4   Direct Sinus Node Recording

The development of catheter techniques to record directly from the region of the sinus node in humans [4, 82, 84] has allowed the validation of the indirect assessments of sinus node function [4, 83, 84]. The technique involves the placement of a multipole catheter in the proximity of the sinus node and, with appropriate amplification and filtering, a sinus node electrogram (SNE) can be recorded. The direct SNE parallels the membrane potential changes seen in sinus pacemaker cells, with a slow diastolic depolarization (phase 4) prior to the upstroke (phase 0) of the sinus action potential, which precedes the rapid upstroke of atrial depolarization. The SACT is measured from the onset of sinus node depolarization to the onset of atrial activation, and is less than around 120 ms in normal individuals [83, 84, 96]. An additional measurement, the duration of sinus node depolarization (SND_d), can be determined from direct sinus node recordings, and is usually <150 ms in normal subjects. A $SND_d \geq 200$ ms can indicate the presence of significant sinus node dysfunction [4].

The role of the SNE in the investigation of sinus node dysfunction is doubtful as the placement of the catheter is relatively time-consuming, and recordings can be obtained in only 80% of patients and are seldom stable [86]. The technique, however, has provided some fascinating insights into the interpretation of results from indirect assessment of sinus function. For example, many patients with long pauses after rapid atrial pacing, who are considered to have a prolonged SNRT, have in fact been found to have continuing sinus activity, as shown by the SNE, the pauses arising from SA exit block preventing atrial activation [97, 98].

4.3.5.5   Clinical Role of Electrophysiological Testing

The main limitations of electrophysiological assessment of sinus node dysfunction are the low sensitivity of the tests and the variable clinical significance of abnormalities if found. Abnormalities of the measurement of SNRT and SACT have sensitivities of only about 50% or less in symptomatic patients with sinus node dysfunction [8, 85, 99]. The sensitivity is improved if both tests are combined, and the specificity of the tests is good, being of the order of 75–95% [6, 8]. Autonomic blockade may increase the sensitivity of the electrophysiological tests [87, 100, 101], and particularly aids in the identification of those patients with intrinsic sinus dysfunction [81]. Both sensitivity and specificity are best in symptomatic patients, especially those with syncope, but are less helpful in asymptomatic patients [102]. Thus, with respect to establishing a diagnosis, electrophysiological testing may support the clinical suspicion of sinus node dysfunction if abnormalities are found, but cannot be used to exclude sinus node disease, given the limited sensitivity of the tests. In addition, since the prognosis of patients with sinus node dysfunction is good [66, 102, 103] and does not appear to be altered by pacemaker implantation [74, 103], the finding of sinus node dysfunction in itself does not mandate therapeutic intervention [74, 104].

The correlation of arrhythmia with symptoms is most important, but is not always possible to achieve even with ambulatory monitoring [69]. Invasive investigation of patients with syncope of undetermined origin reveals sinus node disease in about 10% of cases [8] and other electrophysiological abnormalities may be detected in up to 75% [105]. A presumed diagnosis of sick sinus syndrome can be made if major abnormalities of sinus node function (e.g., a SNRT > 3 s) are demonstrated in an electrophysiology study and other causes for the patient's symptoms have been ruled out [7, 21]. Other supporting findings on non-invasive testing include: persistent daytime HR < 40 bpm, often with little variation in HR; second degree SA block; prolonged sinus pauses (which are not vagally-mediated); abnormal intrinsic HR; and severe chronotropic incompetence [21].

In patients with the bradycardia-tachycardia syndrome, in whom monitoring may have failed to demonstrate significant pauses, there is good correlation between pauses observed after atrial pacing and those occurring on spontaneous termination of tachycardia [106]. Other patients with documented bradycardia-tachycardia syndrome may be symptomatic from the tachyarrhythmia rather than the bradycardia and antiarrhythmic therapy may be more appropriate than pacing. Electrophysiological testing can indicate whether drug therapy may worsen sinus dysfunction, meriting prophylactic pacemaker implantation. Full electrophysiological study may also demonstrate inducible tachyarrhythmias, such as ventricular tachycardia, as the true cause of symptoms in some patients with suspected sinus disease [105].

Finally, assessment of AV conduction is important in patients with sick sinus syndrome for whom a single-chamber atrial (AAI) pacemaker is planned. This is usually assessed at the time of pacemaker implantation, rather than in a separate electrophysiology study, and if AV conduction is normal, with 1:1 AV conduction at atrial pacing rates of ≥120 bpm, then AAI pacing is generally appropriate. It should be noted that serial electrophysiological studies after single-chamber atrial pacemaker implantation have shown that AV conduction may subsequently deteriorate in patients requiring additional antiarrhythmic therapy [107].

4.4   Atrial Arrhythmias

Atrial arrhythmias are common and may occur in patients without heart disease as well as being a feature of most cardiovascular conditions. They are of major clinical importance, and can be associated with significant morbidity, but are only rarely fatal in themselves. The majority may be diagnosed without invasive investigation on the basis of the surface ECG

[108–110]. Satisfactory pharmacological management is often achieved, although there is an increasing role for curative catheter ablation for several types of atrial arrhythmias (see ❷ Chap. 2, [108]).

4.4.1 Mechanisms of Atrial Arrhythmias

Tachyarrhythmias, in general, result from either abnormal impulse generation, such as abnormal automaticity and triggered activity, or abnormal impulse conduction, resulting in reentrant circuits [111].

Automatic atrial arrhythmias are a consequence of abnormal foci which have inherent pacemaker properties and thus generate arrhythmias spontaneously if their firing rate exceeds that of the sinus node. The pacemaker current, I_f, may contribute to this phenomenon in human atrial tissue [112]. Foci of abnormal automaticity can occur in a variety of sites, including within the vena cava and pulmonary veins [113, 114], and the arrhythmias they produce can be paroxysmal or incessant.

Triggered activity, by contrast, results from early or delayed afterdepolarizations which follow preceding action potentials [115]. These may reach threshold and result in further action potentials. Afterdepolarizations are a result of transient inward currents [116, 117] which are activated by oscillations of intracellular calcium in conditions of calcium overload, such as can be induced by cardiac glycosides or catecholamines. It is likely that triggered activity underlies arrhythmias caused by digoxin toxicity [118]. Intracellular calcium is also increased by repetitive stimulation which may induce afterdepolarizations.

Reentry is the commonest mechanism of cardiac arrhythmia generation, and can be dependent on a macro-reentrant circuit, such as in AV nodal reentrant tachycardia (AVNRT) and AV reciprocating tachycardia (AVRT), or on micro-rentrant circuits as in fibrillation (see ❷ Chaps. 2 and ❷ 5). Within the atria, structural or functional lines of block can exist which create the conditions necessary for macro-reentry [119]. The classic example is that of "typical" (cavo-tricuspid isthmus-dependent) flutter, as discussed in ❷ Sect. 4.8.

The underlying mechanisms of tachycardias may be differentiated electrocardiographically to some extent, but more particularly by the responses to pacing and premature stimulation. Characteristically, reentrant tachycardias are reproducibly initiated and terminated by premature stimuli, whereas automatic tachycardias are not [120]. The latter may display suppression and reset of the automatic focus in response to premature stimuli, followed by a noncompensatory pause. Triggered activity is more difficult to differentiate as it may be initiated and terminated by pacing [118].

Based on these mechanistic considerations, most regular atrial arrhythmias can be classified into two broad groups – *Focal atrial tachycardia*, where activation spreads from a central point and is due to an automatic, triggered, or micro-reentrant mechanism; and *Macro-reentrant atrial tachycardia*, where conduction is occurring around a defined circuit [119]. *Atrial fibrillation* is distinct and characterized by relatively chaotic atrial activation, driven by complex mechanisms including multiple circuit reentry [218], and irregular ventricular activity (when AV conduction is intact).

4.4.2 General Electrocardiographic Features of Atrial Arrhythmias

Focal atrial arrhythmias may originate at any site in the atria, frequently remote from the sinus node. The morphology of atrial activation usually differs from the P wave observed in sinus rhythm, and depends on the site of origin [121]. The P wave vector and morphology can be used to predict the site of origin of an ectopic rhythm [122] (see ❷ Sect. 4.6), although some limitations exist [121, 123, 124] and accurate localization can only be obtained with certainty by intracardiac mapping [125].

Reentrant atrial tachycardias are generally initiated by spontaneous atrial premature beats, the initial P wave usually differing from subsequent P waves during the tachycardia. Unlike the junctional reentrant tachycardias (i.e., AVNRT and AVRT), initiation of atrial tachycardia is independent of AV nodal conduction and may be initiated by atrial beats which block proximal to the His bundle [123].

Atrial arrhythmias have often been defined with respect to the atrial rate, distinguishing between atrial tachycardia (100–250 bpm), flutter (250–350 bpm) or fibrillation (400–600 bpm). However, atrial rate alone cannot be considered a rigid diagnostic criterion as exceptions may occur. For example, the atrial rate in atrial flutter may be slower, particularly in the presence of antiarrhythmic drugs, or faster, as rates of over 400 bpm have been documented [126]. Transition may occur between atrial arrhythmias, with atrial flutter or tachycardia converting to fibrillation [127, 128]. Intermediate forms may also be seen (termed "flutter fibrillation") where organized atrial activity can be recorded from some areas of the atrium but not others [129].

Focal and reentrant atrial arrhythmias can be incessant, defined as being present for at least 90% of the monitored time. The rate may vary during the day, increasing on exercise and slowing during sleep [130]. Incessant tachycardias can occur in young people with otherwise normal hearts and may cause heart failure due to "tachycardiomyopathy" [131]. In such cases, successful ablation of the arrhythmia can be curative and lead to a sustained improvement in cardiac function [132–134].

4.5   Atrial Premature Complexes

4.5.1   Overview

The commonest atrial arrhythmia is the atrial premature complex (APC), also known as an atrial extrasystole or atrial ectopic beat. These atrial impulses are characterized by their prematurity, occurring before the next expected sinus beat, and abnormal P-wave morphology, owing to their ectopic origin (❷ Fig. 4.8). With respect to terminology, the terms

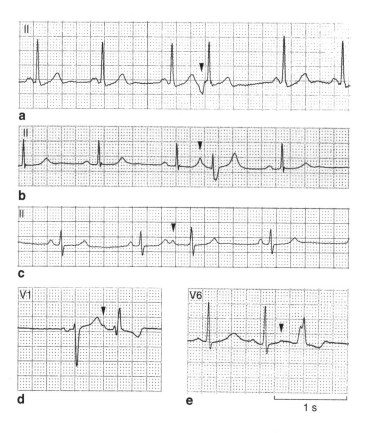

❑ Fig. 4.8

Atrial premature complexes (APCs, indicated by *arrowheads*). Part (**a**) shows an APC with a clearly abnormal P wave. Part (**b**) shows an APC superimposed on the preceding T wave, with aberrant conduction to the ventricles. In part (**c**), an APC occurs with a prolonged PR interval, and a less than compensatory pause. Parts (**d**) and (**e**) show APCs conducted with right bundle branch block, and left bundle branch block, respectively

atrial "premature complex" and "extrasystole" clearly refer to an extra, premature beat, whereas atrial "ectopic" defines the site of origin but not the timing of the beat. An atrial ectopic, for example, may occur as an escape beat following a sinus pause, and so the term includes both premature and escape rhythms. It is, therefore, a less specific term and thus the others are to be preferred.

Atrial premature complexes are common and occur in normal individuals of all ages [22, 23, 135, 136]. Their frequency increases with age, being found in 13% of healthy boys [22], 56% of male medical students [23] and in 75–88% of adult males, although frequent APCs occur only rarely (2–6%) [135, 136]. They are more common in patients with cardiac disease; for example APCs can be found in 94% of patients with mitral stenosis [137]. They are exacerbated by fatigue, stress, caffeine, tobacco and alcohol [135]. They rarely cause symptoms requiring treatment although, occasionally, frequent early or blocked APCs may cause an effective bradycardia – the extrasystolic beat has a low stroke volume owing to inadequate ventricular filling and is followed by a postectopic pause, or has no associated ventricular systole. In atrial bigeminy, for instance, the pulse rate may effectively be halved (❯ Fig. 4.9). In sick sinus syndrome, an APC may be followed by symptomatic sinus pauses owing to sinus node suppression. The more important clinical relevance of APCs, however, is their role in triggering other arrhythmias. Most reentrant supraventricular tachycardias, including atrial flutter, are initiated by APCs (❯ Fig. 4.10). Suppression of APCs may therefore be an important part of the prophylactic treatment of these arrhythmias, and can often be achieved with beta-blockers or calcium channel antagonists [108].

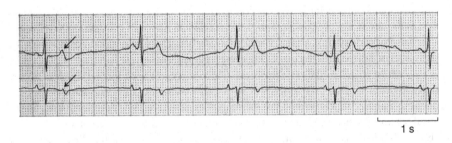

1 s

■ Fig. 4.9

Ambulatory monitor tracing showing atrial bigeminy, with blocked atrial premature complexes (*arrowed* for first complex). This results in effective bradycardia, with a ventricular rate of 39 bpm

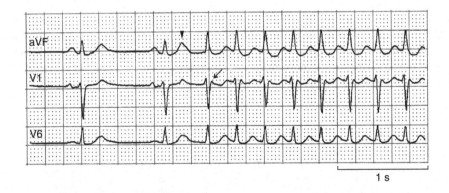

1 s

■ Fig. 4.10

Atrial premature complex initiating AV nodal reentrant tachycardia (AVNRT). The APC (*arrowhead*) is partly obscured by the preceding T wave and has a long PR interval due to conduction via the AV nodal slow pathway. Typical AVNRT occurs, with P waves almost coincident with the QRS complex. The presence of atrial activity can be inferred from the characteristic development of a "pseudo-R′ wave" (*arrowed*) in lead V1

4.5.2   Electrocardiographic Features

The relationship of an APC to ventricular activation will depend on its site of origin, its prematurity and the refractoriness of the AV node. The PR interval may be normal, or even short if the ectopic atrial activity is close to the AV node [138]. However, when an APC occurs early in diastole, close to the refractory period of the AV node, conduction may be delayed with resultant prolongation of the PR interval (❯ Fig. 4.8c). When the APC occurs even earlier, it may find that the AV node is refractory, preventing impulse conduction to the ventricles. Such a "blocked" atrial extrasystole may be obscured by the preceding T wave (❯ Fig. 4.9), and the following postextrasystolic pause may be incorrectly diagnosed as owing to sinus arrest.

The pause which follows an APC is most commonly a consequence of sinus resetting, as the premature atrial activity depolarizes not only the atria but also the sinus node. As a result, the pause is less than compensatory, the sinus node having fired earlier than expected. Thus the P-P interval flanking the APC is less than twice the basic cycle length (❯ Fig. 4.8a–c). This is in contrast to the pause following most ventricular premature complexes which do not interfere with sinus activity; the next sinus beat occurs as expected and the pause is fully compensatory, the P-P interval being equal to twice the basic cycle length. A compensatory pause can occasionally be seen after an APC when the atrial ectopic activity collides with the sinus impulse in the perinodal tissue, preventing the spread of the sinus beat to the atria but without resetting the pacemaker. Rarely, an APC may encounter SA entrance block in the perinodal tissue but the exit of the sinus beat is unaffected. The APC is thus interpolated between two consecutive sinus beats, although the sinus P-P interval is usually slightly prolonged.

While an APC produces abnormal atrial activation, conduction below the AV node is usually normal with a resultant narrow QRS complex, in the absence of preexisting bundle branch block. Aberrant conduction may occur, however, as the impulse may reach the His Purkinje system while it is still relatively refractory from the preceding beat. Refractoriness of the conducting system is related directly to the preceding cycle length, a slower rate being associated with a longer refractory period. This is in contrast to AV nodal refractoriness, which increases with increasing rate. Aberrant conduction is therefore most likely to occur when a premature beat with a short coupling interval follows a longer interval, owing either to bradycardia or to a pause. This is termed the Ashman phenomenon [139]. For this reason, aberrant conduction may be seen with atrial bigeminy, where every extrasystolic cycle is preceded by a postextrasystolic pause. The refractory period of the right bundle branch is generally longer than that of the left and so right bundle branch block (RBBB) is the commonest configuration seen when an APC is aberrantly conducted (❯ Fig. 4.8d). Less commonly, left bundle branch block (LBBB) may occur (❯ Fig. 4.8e), particularly at faster rates, since at shorter cycle lengths the refractory period of the left bundle may exceed that of the right [140].

In an individual with frequent APCs there is usually a relatively constant interval between the APC and the preceding sinus beat. Such a constant coupling interval may indicate a reentrant mechanism underlying the premature impulse, such as intra-atrial or AV nodal echoes. This is in contrast to the rarely seen atrial parasystole [141, 142] when an automatic focus produces atrial beats independent of the sinus activity. Since the rate of atrial parasystole differs from that of sinus rhythm, the APCs have no fixed relation to the sinus beats. Atrial premature complexes commonly occur singly and sporadically, but may occur following every second or third sinus beat, producing bigeminy and trigeminy, respectively (see ❯ Fig. 4.9). Multiple APCs may occur consecutively; the occurrence of six or more APCs is considered to be a burst of nonsustained atrial tachycardia (❯ Fig. 4.11).

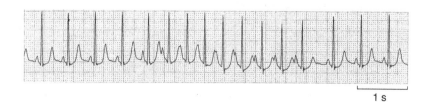

1 s

◾ Fig. 4.11

Ambulatory monitor tracing showing non-sustained atrial tachycardia

4.6   Focal Atrial Tachycardia

4.6.1   Overview

Focal atrial tachycardia is usually non-sustained and asymptomatic and is often an incidental finding on ambulatory monitoring. It has a prevalence of 0.34% in the general population and is higher in those with a history of palpitations [143]. Symptomatic sustained atrial tachycardia accounts for up to 17% of patients undergoing electrophysiology (EP) study for supraventricular tachycardia (SVT), with no sex preponderance [144–146]. There appears to be a bimodal distribution with peaks in the pediatric age group and in the elderly. This probably reflects different mechanisms of arrhythmogenesis in these groups, with AT due to increased automaticity being prevalent in the young and micro-reentry being more common with increasing age [146–148]. Pharmacological treatment is often unsuccessful, and curative radiofrequency ablation should be considered at an early stage. Ablation is associated with success rates of between 69% and 100% [146, 149–151], with recurrence rates of 7% [148].

4.6.2   The Electrocardiogram in the Diagnosis of Focal Atrial Tachycardia

Focal AT produces a narrow-complex tachycardia (or wide-complex in the presence of fixed or rate-related bundle branch block). The surface electrocardiogram provides clues to the diagnosis and helps differentiate it from sinus tachycardia and other causes of SVT. Important features are the mode of onset and termination, the R-P relationship and the P wave vector.

Abrupt onset or a short 4–5 beat "warm-up" period helps distinguish AT from sinus tachycardia, AVNRT and AVRT. Similarly, termination is usually abrupt (unlike sinus tachycardia) or displays a short "cool down phase" (unlike AVNRT or AVRT). Termination with block in the AV node (ending on a P wave) effectively excludes AT [152].

AT usually has a long RP interval (defined as >50% of RR interval), distinguishing it from typical AVNRT and most forms of AVRT. This is a useful indicator, but it is important to remember that there are exceptions to this rule. For example, delay in AV nodal conduction during rapid AT may cause prolongation of the PR interval producing a short-RP tachycardia. Similarly, atypical AVNRT, and AVRT utilizing a decremental accessory pathway as the retrograde limb, may produce a long-RP tachycardia. Other features of the RP relationship may help distinguish AT from other forms of SVT. In AT, AV nodal and ventricular activation are passive and not necessary for tachycardia maintenance. As such, the relationship between atrial and ventricular activity is not fixed and variation in the RP interval supports the diagnosis of AT [152–154] although multiple or decremental accessory pathways may display a similar variation in RP relationship. Higher degrees of AV block can also occur, for example in digoxin toxicity [155, 156] where the resulting arrhythmia is commonly referred to as "paroxysmal atrial tachycardia (PAT) with block."

Clues may also be gained from the P wave vector. A positive P wave in the inferior leads makes AT more likely, as a superiorly directed vector is characteristic in AVNRT and common in AVRT. However, a superior vector is seen in focal AT with origins from inferior structures such as the inferior annuli, CS os or low crista terminalis. All these features may aid in the diagnosis of AT, but ultimately, differentiation from other causes of supraventricular tachycardia may not be possible until the time of diagnostic EP study.

4.6.3   P Wave Morphology

P wave morphology is determined by point of origin and subsequent pattern of atrial activation. As such, analysis of the P wave provides information on the site of origin of focal AT, as activation spreads radially with the origin as the epicenter. However, the spatial resolution of the P wave is only 17 mm [124], and as such, P wave morphology can only be used to localize to a general region of interest. Fortunately, AT foci display characteristic anatomical distributions with clustering at several structures and therefore localizing to a general area is often sufficient to direct more detailed mapping at EP study. A useful algorithm has been developed to predict the site of origin of focal AT based on the P wave morphology, with a reported accuracy of 93% when compared to the anatomical site of successful ablation [157].

The P wave on the surface ECG is often obscured by fusion with the preceding T wave, in some cases giving the appearance of a junctional tachycardia [158]. Administration of adenosine or a short burst of ventricular pacing to induce

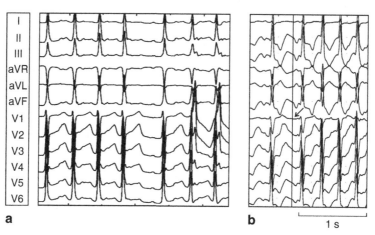

◘ Fig. 4.12
Assessment of P wave morphology in atrial tachycardia (AT). In part (**a**), intravenous adenosine has been administered. P wave morphology is clearly seen following transient AV block. The focus is right parahisian with a largely isoelectric P wave in lead V1 and positive P wave in the inferior leads. Part (**b**) illustrates the importance of assessing the initial P wave vector in determining the origin of an atrial tachycardia. The *vertical line* represents the onset of the P wave in the limb leads. The characteristic isoelectric component of V1 (*arrowed*) observed in AT from the os of the coronary sinus may have been missed if the P wave onset was not clearly defined. The ECG shows demonstrates the other features of AT from this site, with typical negative P wave in the inferior leads and a negative transition across the chest leads

transient AV block may be necessary to remove T-P fusion (❷ Fig. 4.12a). It is important to limit analysis to clearly defined P waves and to include the initial vector which may be isoelectric and easily missed (❷ Fig. 4.12b). Increasing the sweep speed to 50 or 75 mm/s and the amplitude to 50 mm/mV better defines small changes in vector and is a useful tool when analyzing P wave morphology. Characteristic features of P wave morphology have been described for most common foci and are a function of the anatomic relationship of these foci and normal propagation away from the focus. As such, the utility of the P wave in localization is limited in those with structural heart disease or previous atrial surgery or extensive atrial ablation.

4.6.4   Localizing Tachycardia Focus to the Left or Right Atrium

P wave morphology is useful in differentiating left from right atrial foci. This is a function of the anatomical relationship of the atria, with the left atrium being a more posterior and leftward structure than the right atrium. As such, leads V1 and aVL are useful discriminators [122]. Activation from right atrial foci spread leftwards, and a positive or biphasic P wave in aVL has a positive predictive accuracy of 83% and negative predictive value of 85%. In contrast, a positive P wave in V1 is a feature of left atrial foci as activation spreads anteriorly and rightward. It provides a sensitivity and specificity for a left atrial focus of 93% and 88% respectively [122]. Specificity is reduced by the virtue that foci arising from the high crista terminalis in the right atrium can display a positive P wave in this lead. Analysis of the sinus rhythm P wave can help in this situation. As the sinus node complex is located in the high crista [159], the tachycardia P wave morphology should be similar to the sinus P wave if site of origin is the high crista, but will be markedly different if tachycardia focus is of left atrial origin [122].

It is perhaps unsurprising that foci arising from septal structures provide exceptions to these rules, as activation wavefront progresses both left and rightward and a variety of P wave morphologies have been reported [160–163]. However, careful analysis of the initial vector may often help differentiate a right from left atrial origin. For example, tachycardias originating from the coronary sinus (CS) ostium [163] or right septal region [160, 161] often have an initial negative or isoelectric vector in lead V1, which is in keeping with a right atrial origin (❯ Fig. 4.12b). Missing this initial component may lead to misclassification of the P wave as positive, localizing the focus to the wrong chamber. It is therefore essential that careful analysis of the entire P wave is performed.

Using this simple tool, it is possible to define the focus to the left or right atrium with a high degree of accuracy. However, further localization is possible as specific anatomical locations are associated with characteristic P wave morphologies, which are discussed below.

4.6.5   Right Atrium

4.6.5.1   Crista Terminalis

Up to 50% of right atrial tachycardias arise from the crista terminalis [149]. This structure extends the entire length of the right atrium inserting supero-medially into the inter-atrial septum near Bachmann's bundle and being contiguous with the Eustachian ridge inferiorly. It is therefore not surprising that there is some variation in P wave morphology along its length. Low cristal sites are usually associated with an negative P wave in lead V1 [149]. However, high and mid-cristal foci often display a biphasic P wave morphology in V1 with an initial positive vector followed by a negative component (❯ Fig. 4.13a), although, as discussed above, a completely positive morphology is sometimes present and in this situation one should consider the morphology of the sinus P wave [122, 149, 164]. Lead aVL displays marked variation in morphology, but lead I is positive and aVR negative in the majority of cases [164]. The inferior leads display different vectors depending on the position of the tachycardia focus along the length of the crista. P waves are positive inferiorly in high cristal foci and isoelectric or negative in more inferior cristal sites.

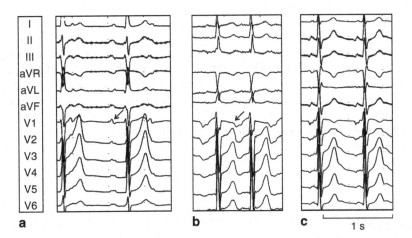

◼ **Fig. 4.13**
Surface electrocardiograms illustrating focal atrial tachycardias from different right atrial sites. Part (a) shows the characteristic P wave morphology of a high cristal focus being positive/negative biphasic in lead V1 (*arrowed*), negative in aVR and positive in lead I. A positive P wave vector in the inferior leads localizes the focus to the high crista terminalis. Part (b) illustrates an inferior tricuspid annulus (TA) focus. The P wave is negative in lead V1 (*arrowed*), and positive in lead I. P waves are isoelectric/negative inferiorly, localizing to the infero-anterior TA. Part (c) shows P wave morphology of a right atrial appendage focus, displaying a negative vector in lead V1, becoming increasingly positive across the precordial leads. P waves are positive in the inferior leads. Morphology from this site is similar to the superior TA, given its close anatomical proximity

4.6.5.2   Tricuspid Annulus

The tricuspid annulus (TA) is a less common site for focal AT, comprising 13% of right atrial tachycardias in a series by Morton et al. [165]. The TA is an anterior and a relatively rightward structure, and as such, the P wave is characteristically negative in lead V1 and positive in leads I and aVL [164, 165], except for the rare cases of tachycardia arising from the septal TA, where the P wave will have an isoelectric component. The majority of foci arise from the infero-anterior TA and negative or iso-electric P waves are usual in the inferior leads (❷ Fig. 4.13b). Positive P waves inferiorly indicate a superior TA focus.

4.6.5.3   CS Ostium

Tachycardias arising from the CS os account for 7% of all focal atrial tachycardia [163] and display a characteristic P wave morphology similar to that of the flutter wave of typical counter-clockwise isthmus dependent flutter. This is a function of the close proximity to the usual exit site of flutter with both displaying an initial negative or isoelectric component in lead V1 which is characteristic of foci arising from the septum. This initial negative vector is followed by a positive deflection which may become more negative across the precordial leads (❷ Fig. 4.12b). The CS os is an inferior structure, and atrial activation is therefore in a superior direction with resultant negative P waves in the inferior leads [160, 163].

4.6.5.4   Right Atrial Appendage

The right atrial appendage is an uncommon site for focal AT. Insights into P wave morphology can be gained from a series of seven patients by Roberts-Thomson and colleagues [166]. P waves were negative in lead V1 in all patients, in keeping with the relative anterior and rightward position of the appendage. P wave vector became progressively more positive across the precordial leads and generally displayed an inferior axis (❷ Fig. 4.13c).

4.6.5.5   The Inter-atrial Septum

Focal AT has been described from several septal structures other than the CS os both on the right and left sides. These include the triangle of Koch, the right and left perinodal regions and the septal insertion of the crista terminalis [149, 160–162]. In general, P wave duration is relatively short, reflecting a short total atrial activation time due to simultaneous activation of both the right and left atria. Lead V1 displays an initial negative or isoelectric component (❷ Fig. 4.12a), followed by a positive deflection with right septal sites, and is usually completely positive in left septal foci. The inferior leads help further localize right septal sites, with anteroseptal sites displaying a positive P wave, and negative P waves being a feature of mid-septal sites.

4.6.6   Left Atrium

4.6.6.1   Pulmonary Veins

The pulmonary veins are a common site for focal AT, especially the superior veins [167, 168]. The veins are a posterior and leftward structure and the P wave is characteristically positive in V1 and across the other chest leads. Left-sided veins are further from the septum and total atrial activation time is longer than for foci originating in the right-sided veins. As a result, the P wave in left atrial foci display a longer P wave duration and are characteristically notched in the inferior leads (❷ Fig. 4.14a) [167]. Given the relative anatomical relationship of the veins, the lateral limb leads help distinguish right from left pulmonary venous foci. Lead I is usually positive in right-sided veins and isoelectric or negative in the left veins. In contrast, lead aVL is a poor discriminator. The P wave vector in the inferior limb leads help discriminate between the upper and lower veins, being more positive in superior venous foci.

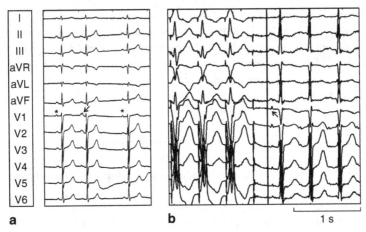

○ Fig. 4.14

Surface electrocardiograms illustrating focal atrial tachycardias from left atrial sites. Part (**a**) shows the characteristic P wave morphology from a left superior pulmonary vein focus (*arrowed*) between two sinus beats (*). Lead V1 is positive and notched. Note the notched positive P waves in the inferior leads. Part (**b**) illustrates an atrial tachycardia arising from the aorto-mitral continuity. A burst of ventricular pacing has produced transient AV block which allows clear definition of the P wave (*vertical line*). Note the initial negative deflection in lead V1 (*arrowed*)

4.6.6.2 Mitral Annulus

Focal AT arising from the mitral annulus is well described, with the most common area being the supero-medial aspect at the aorto-mitral continuity [169, 170]. In keeping with its fairly midline anatomical position, this site typically displays a short P wave duration. The P wave in lead V1 is biphasic with an initial negative deflection followed by a positive vector, which becomes progressively more isoelectric across the precordial leads (○ Fig. 4.14b). P waves are usually negative in leads I and aVL and weakly positive in the inferior leads [169, 170].

4.6.6.3 Other Left Atrial Foci

P wave morphology of tachycardia arising from the left septum has already been discussed. Other uncommon sites of tachycardia reported in the literature are the left atrial appendage [122, 168] and the body of the coronary sinus [171–173]. Foci arising from the left atrial appendage display a similar P wave morphology to left sided pulmonary vein foci given their close anatomical proximity, with the exception of deeply negative P waves in leads I and aVL. Tachycardias originating from the CS musculature display a positive P wave in lead V1 and across the precordial leads.

4.7 Multifocal Atrial Tachycardia

4.7.1 Overview

Multifocal atrial tachycardia (MAT), or "chaotic atrial tachycardia," is characterized by an atrial rate of greater than 100 bpm and discrete P waves of at least three different morphologies [174, 175]. The prevalence of MAT in hospitalized patients is 0.05–0.32%, and it characteristically occurs in severely ill elderly patients, in particular those with acute exacerbations of pulmonary disease [174–176]. Other associations include hypoxemia, pulmonary embolism, electrolyte disturbance, and administration of theophylline or beta-agonist therapy [175, 177–179]. There is a high associated mortality, related to the underlying disease [174, 175, 180]. Multifocal atrial tachycardia may also be found uncommonly in children, where it may occur in the absence of underlying disease [175, 181]. In children, it is rarely associated with atrial fibrillation and is commonly self-limiting in nature.

The cornerstones of management are treatment of the underlying condition, correction of hypoxia and electrolyte abnormalities (in particular, hypokalemia), and discontinuation of medications thought to exacerbate the arrhythmia. The arrhythmia generally resolves as the patient's condition improves, but if pharmacological treatment is required, then the agents with the most evidence of efficacy are metoprolol [182] and intravenous magnesium [183]. Several other drug treatments have been reported, but generally in small trials, often without adequate control groups (reviewed by McCord and Borzak [175]). If MAT is refractory to medical treatment, then the ventricular rate can be controlled by catheter ablation of the AV junction combined with ventricular pacing [184], or catheter ablation to modify AV conduction [185].

MAT is thought to be due to triggered activity caused by delayed afterdepolarizations [118, 177, 186]. Although direct evidence for this is lacking, the fact that MAT is seen in conditions of calcium overload (e.g., high catecholamine states, and in the presence of phosphodiesterase inhibition), and can be suppressed by magnesium, supports triggered activity as the underlying mechanism. Magnesium is thought to have membrane-stabilizing effects, reducing afterdepolarizations. MAT is not a manifestation of digoxin toxicity [174, 176, 180].

4.7.2 The Electrocardiogram in MAT

By definition, at least three different P wave morphologies are seen on the surface ECG, separated by isoelectric intervals, and there is irregular variation in the P–P interval [174]. The multiple P-wave morphologies suggest a multifocal atrial origin, although a single focus with multiple exit pathways or intra-atrial conduction disturbances cannot be excluded. The irregular rhythm of MAT may mimic atrial fibrillation. There is a relation between MAT and other atrial arrhythmias, since in about half of patients it is either preceded by atrial flutter or fibrillation, or these arrhythmias subsequently develop [176, 180].

4.8 Macro-Reentrant Atrial Tachycardia

4.8.1 Overview

In contrast to the point source origin of focal AT with passive activation of the rest of the atrium, macro-reentrant AT is defined as a re-entrant circuit which can be entrained from at least two sites > 2 cm apart [119]. Entrainment is the transient increase in the rate of the tachycardia to match that of the overdrive paced rate (see ❷ Chap. 2) [187–190]. On termination of pacing, the tachycardia reverts to its basic cycle length. Entrainment provides evidence of a reentrant circuit which has an excitable gap that can be penetrated by the paced impulse. The paced beat repeatedly resets the tachycardia resulting in a decrease in the tachycardia cycle length to that of the paced drive cycle. The morphology of the atrial complexes changes during entrainment owing to fusion beats resulting from collision of the paced impulse with the preceding tachycardia wavefront. When pacing ceases, the last entrained beat does not manifest fusion since there is no impulse collision. At a critical paced rate, the pacing wavefront blocks in both directions and the reentrant tachycardia is interrupted [187–190].

Macro-reentrant circuits usually have a central barrier to conduction and an area of slow conduction, producing the excitable gap necessary for macro-reentry. Historically, the classification of atrial macro-reentry, also commonly referred to as atrial flutter, has been conflicting, and recent attempts have been made to standardize nomenclature [119, 191]. Scheinman et al. [191], propose a classification with three main divisions – right atrial cavo-tricuspid isthmus (CTI) dependent flutter, right atrial non-CTI dependent flutter and left atrial flutter. The former is commonly referred to as typical flutter, with the latter two often called atypical flutters.

Typical flutter (right atrial CTI-dependent) accounts for around 90% of macro-reentrant atrial tachycardia, with an increasing prevalence with advancing age to a peak incidence of 0.6% in those over 80 years [192, 193]. Atrial fibrillation and flutter often co-exist, and share the same risk factors, both being more prevalent in the elderly, in males and those with structural heart disease, hypertension, chronic pulmonary disease or an acute illness [192, 194]. It may also be associated with toxic or metabolic conditions, such as alcohol excess or thyrotoxicosis. Right atrial non-CTI dependent flutter or left atrial flutter, often grouped together as the atypical flutters, are less common and usually patients have a prior history of atrial surgery, catheter ablation procedures, valvular heart disease or congenital heart disease [119, 195, 196], although spontaneous scarring causing a flutter circuit in the right atrial free wall has recently been reported in the absence of traditional risk factors [197].

The clinical significance of atrial flutter depends on the ventricular rate and the severity of underlying heart disease. In the acute setting, cardioversion can be achieved by external DC shock, atrial overdrive pacing or pharmacological agents (reviewed by Blomstrom-Lundqvist et al. [108], Wellens [198], Lee et al. [193]). Satisfactory pharmacological control of the ventricular rate in atrial flutter by blocking AV nodal conduction is often more difficult to achieve than it is in atrial fibrillation. Chronic therapy with Class Ia, Ic or III antiarrhythmic agents in an attempt to maintain sinus rhythm is only moderately successful and can be associated with proarrhythmia, such as torsades de pointes (with Class III agents) or 1:1 AV conduction during flutter (Class Ia and Ic agents) [108, 198].

The recognition of the anatomical substrates for macro-reentry and advances in catheter ablation have revolutionized the management of atrial flutter in the last 10–15 years. Linear ablation to interrupt the macro-reentrant circuit can be curative, with a high success rate for typical (CTI-dependent) flutter and a low rate of recurrence, particularly if bi-directional isthmus conduction block is demonstrated [108, 193]. Ablation should be considered early in the management of recurrent or persistent typical flutter. Indeed, a randomized comparison of first-line radiofrequency ablation with antiarrhythmic drug therapy has shown better maintenance of sinus rhythm, fewer hospitalizations, and better quality of life in those who underwent ablation [199]. Ablation is also having an increasing role in the management of "atypical" flutters, facilitated by the development of new endocardial mapping technologies [200–203].

4.8.2 The Electrocardiogram in the Differentiation of Macro-Reentrant from Focal Atrial Tachycardia

The rate of tachycardia does not help differentiate a focal from macro-reentrant mechanism. Although focal AT is usually associated with lower rates than macro-reentry [146], cycle length is highly variable in focal AT and rates can be as high as 340 bpm [204]. Similarly, although macro-reentrant tachycardia usually displays high rates, marked delay in conduction may produce much slower tachycardia cycle lengths.

Careful examination of the flutter or P wave and analysis of the intervening P-P interval may be of value. They may be obscured by the QRS or T wave and maneuvers to cause transient AV block may be required to unmask the atrial activity (❯ Fig. 4.15). Atrial activation is largely passive in focal AT, but, by definition, there is atrial activation over the whole tachycardia cycle length in atrial macro-reentry. As such, continuous activity is often seen in the 12 lead ECG, with no isoelectric period between the flutter waves ("saw-tooth" waveform, ❯ Fig. 4.16). However, there may be no obvious discernible isoelectric period in short cycle length focal AT and it is not always present in flutter. Despite these limitations, a high atrial rate or lack of an isoelectric component should alert the physician to the possibility of a macro-reentrant mechanism.

4.8.2.1 Electrocardiographic Features of Typical (CTI-Dependent) Flutter

Typical flutter is a macro-reentrant circuit confined to the right atrium. It is bounded by the tricuspid annulus anteriorly and by the caval veins, the Eustachian ridge and the crista terminalis posteriorly. An obligate part of the circuit is the cavo-tricuspid isthmus [205, 206]. Linear ablation within this isthmus by radiofrequency ablation is curative with a high success rate. In 90% of patients with typical flutter, activation is counterclockwise around this circuit [119], with

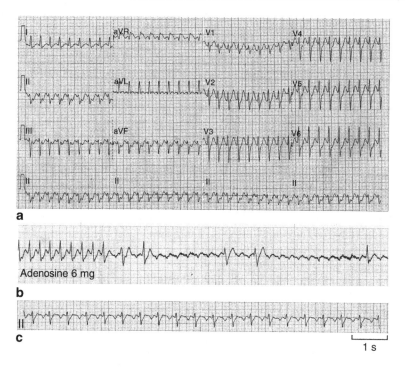

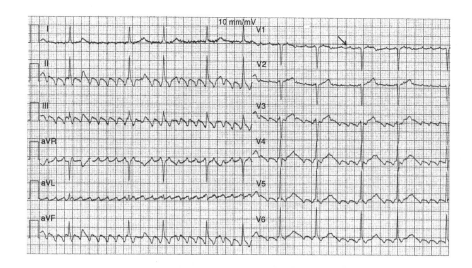

Fig. 4.15

Narrow-complex tachycardia (**a**), with a rate of 218 bpm. Intravenous adenosine (**b**) reveals flutter waves. After initial drug treatment, 2:1 AV conduction results, with a ventricular rate of 110 bpm (**c**)

Fig. 4.16

Typical counterclockwise cavotricuspid isthmus-dependent atrial flutter with isoelectric/positive P wave in lead V1 (*arrowed*) and negative "saw tooth" flutter waves in the inferior leads

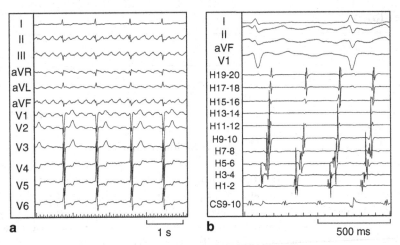

◘ Fig. 4.17

Characteristic flutter wave morphology of clockwise cavotricuspid isthmus-dependent atrial flutter. Part (**a**) shows negative flutter waves in lead V1 and positive flutter waves in the inferior leads. Part (**b**) shows surface leads I, II, aVF and V1, and intracardiac recordings from electrode pairs (H1-2 to H19-20) of a 20-pole "Halo" catheter lying around the tricuspid annulus (see ❷ Fig. 2.1c), and the proximal poles of a catheter lying in the coronary sinus (CS9-10). Atrial activation travels in a clockwise direction from the distal poles of the Halo catheter (H1-2) to the proximal poles (H19-20)

the activation wavefront exiting the CTI medially near the CS os [207], activating the posterior and septal aspects of the right atrium in a superior direction, with later inferior activation of the lateral wall. This gives rise to a characteristic appearance on the ECG with negative saw-tooth flutter waves in the inferior leads (❷ Fig. 4.16). Lead V1 displays a pattern similar to that seen in focal AT arising from the CS os [163], with an initial isoelectric component followed by a positive vector. The flutter waves become progressively more negative across the precordial leads. These features are highly specific for counterclockwise CTI-dependent flutter [119]. In 10% of patients with CTI-dependent flutter, activation is in the opposite direction (clockwise). Flutter wave morphology is reversed with positive saw tooth pattern in the inferior leads and lead V1 displaying a negative vector (❷ Fig. 4.17), although other morphologies have been reported [208].

The atrial rate in typical flutter ranges from 240 to 340 bpm, which is often almost exactly 300 bpm. The AV node rarely conducts as rapidly and so AV block is usually seen, commonly with 2:1 AV conduction, giving a ventricular rate of 150 bpm. The diagnosis of atrial flutter with 2:1 block should always be considered when a regular tachycardia of 150 bpm is identified. Higher degrees of AV conduction block can also be seen, for example in the presence of nodal blocking agents, with a ratio of 4:1, or rarely 3:1 (❷ Fig. 4.16). The preference for even multiples of conduction – 2:1 or 4:1 – may be due to two levels of block in the AV node [209]. Rarely, very rapid ventricular rates are found as a result of 1:1 AV conduction (❷ Fig. 4.15). This may arise because of the presence of an accessory pathway with a short refractory period, but may also occur with enhanced AV nodal conduction [210, 211], or because of slowing of the flutter rate by medication.

4.8.2.2 Electrocardiographic Features of Atypical (Non-CTI-Dependent) Flutter

The 12 lead ECG is of less use in localizing other forms of atrial macro-reentry. Flutter wave amplitude is often low in atypical flutter, regardless of the site of the circuit. Analysis of flutter wave morphology in leads V1 and V2 may be of some use, as left atrial flutters tend to display a positive flutter waves in these leads [212].

4.9   Atrial Fibrillation

4.9.1   Overview

Atrial fibrillation has been called the "grandfather of atrial arrhythmias" [213]. It was first described as a distinct rhythm in humans in the 1900s [214], but irregularities of the pulse associated with valvular heart disease had been recognized centuries before [215]. It is the commonest sustained arrhythmia in adults, may occur in normal hearts or as a feature of all types of cardiovascular diseases, and is associated with significant morbidity and mortality. A number of schemes for classifying AF have been proposed (e.g., [216]), but were of limited clinical utility. Current international guidelines recommend a simple classification, with paroxysmal, persistent and permanent AF [217]. It recognizes "*first detected*" AF, which may present itself in a number of ways – from a clearly defined, symptomatic episode, to an incidental finding on a routine ECG. If the arrhythmia is recurrent and each episode spontaneously reverts to sinus rhythm within 7 days, it is termed "*paroxysmal*". If it does not terminate spontaneously, AF is classed as "*persistent*" (usually lasting > 7 days). Persistent AF may respond to electrical or pharmacological cardioversion, or may go on to become "*permanent*" (e.g., lasting > 1 year) which is resistant to cardioversion. The classification also recognizes "*secondary*" AF, when the arrhythmia occurs as a consequence of another condition, for example acute myocardial infarction, pericarditis, cardiac surgery, or lower respiratory tract infection.

4.9.2   Mechanisms of Atrial Fibrillation

The electrophysiological mechanisms responsible for the initiation and maintenance of atrial fibrillation have been the subject of extensive experimental work [218]. Insights have been gained at single cell and whole tissue levels, as well as through computer modeling and clinical studies. Advancements in the understanding of the arrhythmia have led to novel therapeutic approaches that, in some cases, can offer the hope of a cure.

4.9.2.1   Focal Triggers of AF

Recent work has demonstrated that paroxysms of AF are frequently triggered by foci of ectopic activity in the sleeves of muscular tissue which extend into the proximal portions of the pulmonary veins [114]. This tissue is in electrical continuity with the left atrium, and it is proposed that a rapidly firing source within the vein can lead to fibrillatory conduction in the atrium ("focal trigger"). In some cases, continued activity of the focus may be required to sustain the arrhythmia ("focal driver"), whilst in others the fibrillation is self-sustaining within the atria. The underlying mechanism of the focal ectopic activity is as yet unclear, with possibilities including increased automaticity, triggered activity and micro-reentry, and indeed these mechanisms may not be mutually exclusive. The recognition of these focal initiators has led to the development of catheter ablation techniques for the treatment of AF. These were initially directed at ablating the ectopic focus itself, but have now evolved to aim for electrical isolation of all four pulmonary veins, with or without other lesions in the atria [219, 220] (see ❷ Chap. 2). Focal triggers have also been described in other venous structures, including the superior vena cava [113], the vein of Marshall [221] and the coronary sinus [172], and these may also be amenable to catheter ablation.

4.9.2.2   Tissue Substrate for Sustained AF

The mechanisms responsible for sustained fibrillatory conduction within the atria have also been the subject of much research. It has been proposed on the basis of experimental work and computer modeling that fibrillation develops when a wavefront becomes fractionated and produces multiple random reentrant wavelets [222, 223]. These wavelets would generate disorganized, chaotic atrial activity on the surface ECG. This theory requires a critical mass of atrial tissue to sustain several reentrant waves, and has been supported by the demonstration of such multiple wavelets resulting from intra-atrial reentry of the leading-circle type [224]. Further support comes from the observation that a surgical procedure to "compartmentalize" conduction in the left atrium (the Maze procedure) can cure chronic AF, presumably by preventing reentrant waves from being sustained [225]. However, more recent studies have proposed that in fact a single high frequency stably rotating spiral wave ("mother rotor"), usually in the left atrium, can lead to the activation pattern seen in AF (reviewed by Jalife et al. [226]).

4.9.2.3 Atrial Electrical Remodeling

It has been observed that the longer a patient has been in AF, the harder it is to restore and maintain sinus rhythm [227]. This observation has been confirmed in studies employing rapid atrial pacing in goats to induce AF – when AF was initially induced, it would self-terminate after a short time, but when repeatedly induced it would eventually lead to sustained fibrillation [228]. This has been encapsulated in the phrase "AF begets AF," and the underlying process is referred to as electrical remodeling. Studies have shown that AF leads to a marked shortening of the atrial effective refractory period, along with dispersion of refractoriness, and both factors may facilitate reentry within the atria. The underlying ionic mechanisms for these phenomena have been investigated in animal models and changes in a number of ion channel conductances have been implicated (reviewed by Nattel et al. [229]).

4.9.2.4 Influence of the Autonomic Nervous System on AF

There is a complex relationship between sympathetic and parasympathetic activity and atrial electrophysiology. The autonomic nervous system has been implicated in the triggering and maintenance of AF, and, by altering AV nodal conduction, can also affect the ventricular rate. Vagal stimulation can reduce markedly the action potential duration and effective refractory period of atrial cells [230], and this can occur in a spatially heterogeneous fashion [231]. This leads to increased dispersion of refractoriness and conditions which could facilitate wavelet reentry. In animal experiments, intense vagal stimulation can promote induction of AF by atrial extrastimuli [231, 232]. Adrenergic stimulation and high catecholamine states can increase atrial ectopy, which may trigger episodes of AF (reviewed by Olshansky [233]). This mechanism may be of particular relevance in postoperative patients who develop AF.

Clinical observations of patients with paroxysmal AF (PAF) lead Coumel to propose that some have "vagotonic" PAF, usually initiated during sleep or after meals; while some have "adrenergic" PAF, predominantly occurring after exercise or other high catecholamine states (e.g., see [234], reviewed by Olshansky [233]). Those classed as "vagotonic" appear less likely to benefit from catheter-based pulmonary vein isolation as a treatment for PAF [235]. Other studies of catheter ablation for AF have shown that in around a third of patients, delivery of radiofrequency energy to some areas of the posterior left atrium results in intense vagal stimulation (e.g., causing sinus bradycardia, asystole or AV block) and elimination of such reflexes correlates with increased freedom from AF recurrence [236]. These sites may correspond to areas of vagal innervation via ganglia lying within fat pads behind the left atrium [233].

4.9.3 Epidemiology of AF

Both the prevalence and incidence of AF double with every decade beyond the age of 50 years [2]. The prevalence rises from 0.5% in the 6th decade of life to just under 9% in the 9th decade [237], and the lifetime risk of developing AF in those over the age of 40 years is 1 in 4 [238]. At any age, the arrhythmia is commoner in men than in women, and other significant risk factors include heart failure, hypertension, valvular heart disease, coronary artery disease, diabetes mellitus and hyperthyroidism [2, 239–241]. Atrial fibrillation occurs in about 10–20% of patients with acute myocardial infarction and is associated with more extensive infarction and higher mortality [217, 242]. Long-term moderate alcohol intake does not appear to lead to AF, but higher levels of consumption do significantly increase its incidence [243], and an alcoholic binge can precipitate an acute episode [244, 245]. In a minority of cases, no associated medical condition is identified and these patients are considered to have "lone" AF [246, 247].

A number of the conditions which predispose to AF may do so through the "final common pathway" of increased left atrial pressure and consequent dilatation of that chamber [248, 249]. Given the proposed mechanisms for AF, this step may be crucial in providing the necessary substrate to sustain the arrhythmia. Several other echocardiographic findings are commoner in patients with AF (e.g., increased left ventricular size, mitral annular calcification), although often they are "markers" for other predisposing conditions, rather than risk factors in themselves. However, after correcting for other risk factors, reduced fractional shortening and left ventricular hypertrophy, as well as increased left atrial size, do appear to be independent predictors of AF [250].

Non-rheumatic atrial fibrillation is associated with a two- to seven-fold increase in the risk of stroke, and in the presence of rheumatic heart disease, this risk is even higher (around 17 times the risk of age-matched controls) [2, 217, 237]. AF is also associated with an increased incidence of heart failure [251] and overall mortality is doubled, although some of this increased risk can be attributed to underlying heart disease [217].

4.9.4 Electrocardiographic Features of Atrial Fibrillation

The atrial activity in atrial fibrillation is very rapid and irregular, and is seen on the surface ECG as chaotic fibrillatory ("f") waves at rates of up to 600 min^{-1} (❷ Fig. 4.18). P waves are absent as no coordinated atrial activity occurs. The amplitude of the atrial fibrillatory waves may vary, being described as "coarse" or "fine" fibrillation. There is no correlation between the fibrillatory wave amplitude and atrial size on echocardiography or etiology of heart disease [252].

The ventricular rate is dependent on the conduction properties of the AV node and is usually rapid, unless there is preexisting, or drug-induced, AV nodal conduction delay (❷ Fig. 4.18). The ventricular rhythm is characteristically irregularly irregular, which reflects not only the irregularities of the atrial activity, but also the conduction through the AV node. Some atrial impulses may penetrate the node but are blocked at different levels without being conducted to the ventricles. The consequent refractoriness influences the conduction of subsequent atrial impulses through the AV node, the extent of the delay depending on the degree of penetration of the preceding impulse. The effect of such concealed conduction on ventricular rate is demonstrated by the fact that the ventricular rate during rapid atrial pacing may be greater than the rate once atrial fibrillation is initiated [253]. Clinically, regularization of the ventricular rhythm may be

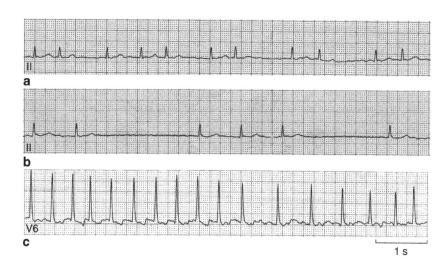

◘ Fig. 4.18

Ventricular rate in atrial fibrillation. In part (a) there is a controlled rate (66 bpm) due to treatment with a beta blocker. Part (b) shows AF with a slow ventricular response (36 bpm) in a patient on no cardioactive medication (suggestive of sick sinus syndrome). A rapid ventricular response (102 bpm) is seen in part (c)

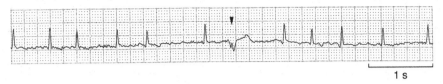

⬛ Fig. 4.19

Aberrant conduction in atrial fibrillation due to rate-dependent refractoriness of the conducting system (the Ashmann phenomenon). An aberrantly conducted beat (*arrowhead*) occurs close to a beat which was preceded by a long interval

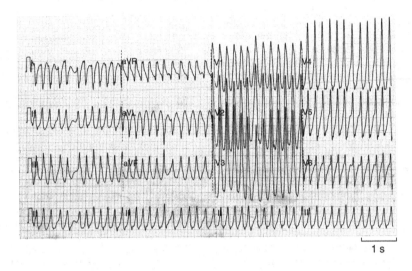

⬛ Fig. 4.20

Preexcited atrial fibrillation in the Wolff-Parkinson-White syndrome. The ventricular rate is rapid (282 bpm) and the complexes are broad and preexcited due to conduction down an accessory pathway

observed with third-degree AV block and a junctional or ventricular escape rhythm or in digoxin toxicity, owing to the development of a junctional rhythm.

The QRS complex is normally narrow, unless aberrant conduction is present. Intermittent aberrancy (sometimes called "phasic aberrant ventricular conduction") presents a particular diagnostic problem in atrial fibrillation since neither prematurity nor rate may distinguish between aberrancy and ventricular ectopics. Electrocardiographic criteria have been described to differentiate between aberrancy and ectopy based on QRS morphology and axis [254]. The aberrant morphology is usually RBBB, reflecting the relative refractory periods of the bundle, and it may exhibit the "Ashman phenomenon" (❯ Fig. 4.19, see ❯ Sect. 4.5.2). Less commonly, LBBB may occur, but at shorter cycles and independent of preceding cycle length [140]. A ventricular complex may be followed by a short "compensatory pause" even in atrial fibrillation, owing to retrograde penetration of the AV node inhibiting the next conducted beat [255].

An alternative, but less common, reason for broad complexes in atrial fibrillation is conduction via an accessory pathway in Wolff-Parkinson-White (WPW) syndrome (❯ Fig. 4.20). This diagnosis is important as the excessively rapid ventricular rate may lead to ventricular fibrillation, particularly if AV nodal blocking drugs are given which may enhance conduction down the bypass pathway [256]. Although reentrant tachycardia is the most common arrhythmia in such patients, there appears to be an increased incidence of atrial flutter and fibrillation [257]. Patients with WPW syndrome who exhibit preserved antegrade conduction via their accessory pathway at short cycle lengths (for example during exercise or rapid atrial pacing) are at particular risk of sudden death, and the treatment of choice is ablation of the pathway [217].

References

1. Kusumoto, F.M., and N. Goldschlager, Cardiac pacing. *N. Engl. J. Med.*, 1996;**334**: 89–97.

2. Kannel, W.B., P.A. Wolf, E.J. Benjamin, and D. Levy, Prevalence, incidence, prognosis, and predisposing conditions for atrial fibrillation: population-based estimates. *Am. J. Cardiol.*, 1998;**82**: 2N–9N.

3. Mandel, W., H. Hayakawa, R. Danzig, and H.S. Marcus, Evaluation of sino-atrial node function in man by overdrive suppression. *Circulation*, 1971;**44**: 59–66.

4. Reiffel, J.A. and M.J. Kuehnert, Electrophysiological testing of sinus node function: diagnostic and prognostic application-including updated information from sinus node electrograms. *Pace Clin. Electrophysiol.*, 1994;**17**: 349–365.

5. Callans, D.J., D. Schwartzman, C.D. Gottlieb, and F.E. Marchlinski, Insights into the electrophysiology of atrial arrhythmias gained by the catheter ablation experience: "learning while burning, Part II." *J. Cardiovasc. Electrophysiol.*, 1995;**6**: 229–243.

6. Brignole, M., P. Alboni, D.G. Benditt, L. Bergfeldt, J.J. Blanc, P.E.B. Thomsen, et al., Guidelines on management (diagnosis and treatment) of syncope – update 2004. The task force on syncope, European Society of Cardiology. *Europace*, 2004;**6**: 467–547.

7. Epstein, A.E., J.P. DiMarco, K.A. Ellenbogen, N.A.M. Estes III, R.A. Freedman, L.S. Gettes, et al, ACC/AHA/HRS 2008 guidelines for device-based therapy of cardiac rhythm abnormalities: a report of the American College of Cardiology/American Heart Association Task Force on Practice Guidelines (Writing Committee to revise the ACC/AHA/NASPE 2002 guideline update for implantation of cardiac pacemakers and antiarrhythmia devices). *J. Am. Coll. Cardiol.*, 2008;**51**: e1–e62.

8. Benditt, D.G., C.C. Gornick, D. Dunbar, A. Almquist, and S. Pool-Schneider, Indications for electrophysiologic testing in the diagnosis and assessment of sinus node dysfunction. *Circulation*, 1987;**75**: III93–102.

9. James, T.N., Structure and function of the sinus node, AV node and His bundle of the human heart: part I-structure. *Prog. Cardiovasc. Dis.*, 2002;**45**: 235–267.

10. Sanchez-Quintana, D., J.A. Cabrera, J. Farre, V. Climent, R.H. Anderson, and S.Y. Ho, Sinus node revisited in the era of electroanatomical mapping and catheter ablation. *Heart*, 2005;**91**: 189–194.

11. Irisawa, H., T. Nakayama, and A. Noma, Membrane currents of single pacemaker cells from rabbit S-A and A-V nodes, in D. Noble and T. Powell, Editors. London: Academic Press, 1987, pp. 167–186.

12. Mitsuiye, T., Y. Shinagawa, and A. Noma, Sustained inward current during pacemaker depolarization in mammalian sinoatrial node cells. *Circ. Res.*, 2000;**87**: 88–91.

13. Mangoni, M.E., B. Couette, E. Bourinet, J. Platzer, D. Reimer, J. Striessnig, et al., Functional role of L-type Cav1.3 Ca^{2+} channels in cardiac pacemaker activity. *Proc. Natl. Acad. Sci. U.S.A.*, 2003;**100**: 5543–5548.

14. Stieber, J., F. Hofmann, and A. Ludwig, Pacemaker channels and sinus node arrhythmia. *Trends Cardiovasc. Med.*, 2004;**14**: 23–28.

15. Cho, H.S., M. Takano, and A. Noma, The electrophysiological properties of spontaneously beating pacemaker cells isolated from mouse sinoatrial node. *J. Physiol. (Lond.)*, 2003;**550**: 169–180.

16. Vinogradova, T.M., V.A. Maltsev, K.Y. Bogdanov, A.E. Lyashkov, and E.G. Lakatta, Rhythmic Ca^{2+} oscillations drive sinoatrial nodal cell pacemaker function to make the heart tick. *Ann. N.Y. Acad. Sci.*, 2005;**1047**: 138–156.

17. Bleeker, W.K., A.J. Mackaay, M. Masson-Pevet, L.N. Bouman, and A.E. Becker, Functional and morphological organization of the rabbit sinus node. *Circ. Res.*, 1980;**46**: 11–22.

18. Morton, H.J. and E.T. Thomas, Effect of atropine on the heart-rate. *Lancet*, 1958;**2**: 1313–1315.

19. WHO/ISFC Task Force, Definition of terms related to cardiac rhythm. *Am. Heart J.*, 1978;**95**: 796–806.

20. Spodick, D.H., P. Raju, R.L. Bishop, and R.D. Rifkin, Operational definition of normal sinus heart rate. *Am. J. Cardiol.*, 1992;**69**: 1245–1246.

21. Brignole, M., Sick sinus syndrome. *Clin. Geriatr. Med.*, 2002;**18**: 211–227.

22. Scott, O., G.J. Williams, and G.I. Fiddler, Results of 24 hour ambulatory monitoring of electrocardiogram in 131 healthy boys aged 10 to 13 years. *Br. Heart J.*, 1980;**44**: 304–308.

23. Brodsky, M., D. Wu, P. Denes, C. Kanakis, and K.M. Rosen, Arrhythmias documented by 24 hour continuous electrocardiographic monitoring in 50 male medical students without apparent heart disease. *Am. J. Cardiol.*, 1977;**39**: 390–395.

24. Bjerregaard, P., Mean 24 hour heart rate, minimal heart rate and pauses in healthy subjects 40–79 years of age. *Eur. Heart J.*, 1983;**4**: 44–51.

25. Talan, D.A., R.A. Bauernfeind, W.W. Ashley, C. Kanakis Jr., and K.M. Rosen, Twenty-four hour continuous ECG recordings in long-distance runners. *Chest*, 1982;**82**: 19–24.

26. Adgey, A.A., J.S. Geddes, H.C. Mulholland, D.A. Keegan, and J.F. Pantridge, Incidence, significance, and management of early bradyarrhythmia complicating acute myocardial infarction. *Lancet*, 1968;**2**: 1097–1101.

27. Alpert, M.A. and G.C. Flaker, Arrhythmias associated with sinus node dysfunction. Pathogenesis, recognition, and management. *JAMA*, 1983;**250**: 2160–2166.

28. Adan, V. and L.A. Crown, Diagnosis and treatment of sick sinus syndrome. *Am. Fam. Physician*, 2003;**67**: 1725–1732.

29. Sheffield, L.T., J.H. Holt, and T.J. Reeves, Exercise graded by heart rate in electrocardiographic testing for angina pectoris. *Circulation*, 1965;**32**: 622–629.

30. Tanaka, H., K.D. Monahan, and D.R. Seals, Age-predicted maximal heart rate revisited. *J. Am. Coll. Cardiol.*, 2001;**37**: 153–156.

31. Yasuma, F. and J. Hayano, Respiratory sinus arrhythmia: why does the heartbeat synchronize with respiratory rhythm? *Chest*, 2004;**125**: 683–690.

32. Rosenbaum, M.B. and E. Lepeschin, The effect of ventricular systole on auricular rhythm in auriculoventricular block. *Circulation*, 1955;**11**: 240–261.

33. de Marchena, E., M. Colvin-Adams, J. Esnard, M. Ridha, A. Castellanos, and R.J. Myerburg, Ventriculophasic sinus arrhythmia in the orthotopic transplanted heart: mechanism of disease revisited. *Int. J. Cardiol.*, 2003;**91**: 71–74.

34. Bauernfeind, R.A., F. Amat-y-Leon, R.C. Dhingra, R. Kehoe, C. Wyndham, and K.M. Rosen, Chronic nonparoxysmal sinus

tachycardia in otherwise healthy persons. *Ann. Intern. Med.*, 1979;**91**: 702–710.

35. Brady, P.A., P.A. Low, and W.K. Shen, Inappropriate sinus tachycardia, postural orthostatic tachycardia syndrome, and overlapping syndromes. Pace Clin. Electrophysiol., 2005;**28**: 1112–1121.

36. Narula, O.S., Sinus node re-entry: a mechanism for supraventricular tachycardia. *Circulation*, 1974;**50**: 1114–1128.

37. Sperry, R.E., K.A. Ellenbogen, M.A. Wood, M.K. Belz, and B.S. Stambler, Radiofrequency catheter ablation of sinus node reentrant tachycardia. *Pace Clin. Electrophysiol.*, 1993;**16**: 2202–2209.

38. Gomes, J.A., D. Mehta, and M.N. Langan, Sinus node reentrant tachycardia. *Pace Clin. Electrophysiol.*, 1995;**18**: 1045–1057.

39. Gomes, J.A., R.J. Hariman, P.S. Kang, and I.H. Chowdry, Sustained symptomatic sinus node reentrant tachycardia: incidence, clinical significance, electrophysiologic observations and the effects of antiarrhythmic agents. *J. Am. Coll. Cardiol.*, 1985;**5**: 45–57.

40. Damato, A.N., Clinical evidence for sinus node reentry, in *The Sinus Node: Structure, Function and Clinical Relevance*, F.I.M. Bonke, Editor. The Hague: Nijhoff, 1978, pp. 379–388.

41. Bashour, T.T., Classification of sinus node dysfunction. *Am. Heart J.*, 1985;**110**: 1251–1256.

42. Thery, C., B. Gosselin, J. Lekieffre, and H. Warembourg, Pathology of sinoatrial node. Correlations with electrocardiographic findings in 111 patients. *Am. Heart J.*, 1977;**93**: 735–740.

43. Evans, R. and D.B. Shaw, Pathological studies in sinoatrial disorder (sick sinus syndrome). *Br. Heart J.*, 1977;**39**: 778–786.

44. Bharati, S., A. Nordenberg, R. Bauernfiend, J.P. Varghese, A.G. Carvalho, K. Rosen, et al., The anatomic substrate for the sick sinus syndrome in adolescence. *Am. J. Cardiol.*, 1980;**46**: 163–172.

45. Rosen, K.M., H.S. Loeb, M.Z. Sinno, S.H. Rahimtoola, and R.M. Gunnar, Cardiac conduction in patients with symptomatic sinus node disease. *Circulation*, 1971;**43**: 836–844.

46. Narula, O.S., Atrioventricular conduction defects in patients with sinus bradycardia. Analysis by His bundle recordings. *Circulation*, 1971;**44**: 1096–1110.

47. Kaplan, B.M., R. Langendorf, M. Lev, and A. Pick, Tachycardia-bradycardia syndrome (so-called "sick sinus syndrome"). Pathology, mechanisms and treatment. *Am. J. Cardiol.*, 1973;**31**: 497–508.

48. Demoulin, J.C. and H.E. Kulbertus, Histopathological correlates of sinoatrial disease. *Br. Heart J.*, 1978;**40**: 1384–1389.

49. Hwang, Y.T., C.D. Tseng, J.J. Hwang, K.L. Hsu, F.T. Chiang, Y.Z. Tseng, et al., Cardiac amyloidosis presenting as sick sinus syndrome and intractable heart failure: report of a case. *J. Formos. Med. Assoc.*, 1993;**92**: 283–287.

50. Wang, T.L., W.J. Chen, C.S. Liau, and Y.T. Lee, Sick sinus syndrome as the early manifestation of cardiac hemochromatosis. *J. Electrocardiol.*, 1994;**27**: 91–96.

51. Watt, A.H., Sick sinus syndrome: an adenosine-mediated disease. *Lancet*, 1985;**1**: 786–788.

52. Benedini, G., C. Cuccia, R. Bolognesi, A. Affatato, G. Gallo, E. Renaldini, et al., Value of purinic compounds in assessing sinus node dysfunction in man: a new diagnostic method. *Eur. Heart J.*, 1984;**5**: 394–403.

53. Benditt, D.G., D.W. Benson Jr., J. Kreitt, A. Dunnigan, M.R. Pritzker, L. Crouse, et al., Electrophysiologic effects of theophylline in young patients with recurrent symptomatic bradyarrhythmias. *Am. J. Cardiol.*, 1983;**52**: 1223–1229.

54. Alboni, P., C. Menozzi, M. Brignole, N. Paparella, G. Gaggioli, G. Lolli, et al., Effects of permanent pacemaker and oral theophylline in sick sinus syndrome the THEOPACE study: a randomized controlled trial. *Circulation*, 1997;**96**: 260–266.

55. Maisch, B., U. Lotze, J. Schneider, and K. Kochsiek, Antibodies to human sinus node in sick sinus syndrome. *Pace Clin. Electrophysiol.*, 1986;**9**: 1101–1109.

56. Lown, B., Electrical reversion of cardiac arrhythmias. *Br. Heart J.*, 1967;**29**: 469–489.

57. Ferrer, M.I., The sick sinus syndrome in atrial disease. *JAMA*, 1968;**206**: 645–646.

58. Bigger, J.T. Jr. and J.A. Reiffel, Sick sinus syndrome. *Annu. Rev. Med.*, 1979;**30**: 91–118.

59. Rubenstein, J.J., C.L. Schulman, P.M. Yurchak, and R.W. DeSanctis, Clinical spectrum of the sick sinus syndrome. *Circulation*, 1972;**46**: 5–13.

60. Short, D.S., The syndrome of alternating bradycardia and tachycardia. *Br. Heart J.*, 1954;**16**: 208–214.

61. Andersen, H.R., J.C. Nielsen, P.E. Thomsen, L. Thuesen, T. Vesterlund, A.K. Pedersen, et al., Atrioventricular conduction during long-term follow-up of patients with sick sinus syndrome. *Circulation*, 1998;**98**: 1315–1321.

62. Walter, P.F., I.S. Crawley, and E.R. Dorney, Carotid sinus hypersensitivity and syncope. *Am. J. Cardiol.*, 1978;**42**: 396–403.

63. Davies, A.B., M.R. Stephens, and A.G. Davies, Carotid sinus hypersensitivity in patients presenting with syncope. *Br. Heart J.*, 1979;**42**: 583–586.

64. Sutton, R. and R.A. Kenny, The natural history of sick sinus syndrome. *Pace Clin. Electrophysiol.*, 1986;**9**: 1110–1114.

65. Ferrer, M.I., The etiology and natural history of sinus node disorders. *Arch. Intern. Med.*, 1982;**142**: 371–372.

66. Simonsen, E., J.S. Nielsen, and B.L. Nielsen, Sinus node dysfunction in 128 patients. A retrospective study with follow-up. *Acta Med. Scand.*, 1980;**208**: 343–348.

67. Denes, P., L. Levy, A. Pick, and K.M. Rosen, The incidence of typical and atypical A-V Wenckebach periodicity. *Am. Heart J.*, 1975;**89**: 26–31.

68. Crook, B.R., P.M. Cashman, F.D. Stott, and E.B. Raftery, Tape monitoring of the electrocardiogram in ambulant patients with sinoatrial disease. *Br. Heart J.*, 1973;**35**: 1009–1013.

69. Reiffel, J.A., J.T. Bigger Jr., M. Cramer, and D.S. Reid, Ability of Holter electrocardiographic recording and atrial stimulation to detect sinus nodal dysfunction in symptomatic and asymptomatic patients with sinus bradycardia. *Am. J. Cardiol.*, 1977;**40**: 189–194.

70. Krahn, A.D., G.J. Klein, R. Yee, and C. Norris, Final results from a pilot study with an implantable loop recorder to determine the etiology of syncope in patients with negative noninvasive and invasive testing. *Am. J. Cardiol.*, 1998;**82**: 117–119.

71. Reiffel, J.A., R. Schwarzberg, and M. Murry, Comparison of autotriggered memory loop recorders versus standard loop recorders versus 24-hour Holter monitors for arrhythmia detection. *Am. J. Cardiol.*, 2005;**95**: 1055–1059.

72. Kantelip, J.P., E. Sage, and P. Duchene-Marullaz, Findings on ambulatory electrocardiographic monitoring in subjects older than 80 years. *Am. J. Cardiol.*, 1986;**57**: 398–401.

73. Molgaard, H., K.E. Sorensen, and P. Bjerregaard, Minimal heart rates and longest pauses in healthy adult subjects on two occasions eight years apart. *Eur. Heart J.*, 1989;**10**: 758–764.

74. Mazuz, M. and H.S. Friedman, Significance of prolonged electrocardiographic pauses in sinoatrial disease: sick sinus syndrome. *Am. J. Cardiol.*, 1983;**52**: 485–489.

75. Abbott, J.A., D.S. Hirschfeld, F.W. Kunkel, M.M. Scheinman, and G. Modin, Graded exercise testing in patients with sinus node dysfunction. *Am. J. Med.*, 1977;**62**: 330–338.

76. Dhingra, R.C., F. Amat-y-Leon, C. Wyndham, P. Denes, D. Wu, R.H. Miller, et al., Electrophysiologic effects of atropine on sinus node and atrium in patients with sinus nodal dysfunction. *Am. J. Cardiol.*, 1976;**38**: 848–855.

77. Strauss, H.C., J.T. Bigger, A.L. Saroff, and E.G. Giardina, Electrophysiologic evaluation of sinus node function in patients with sinus node dysfunction. *Circulation*, 1976;**53**: 763–776.

78. Cleaveland, C.R., R.E. Rangno, and D.G. Shand, A standardized isoproterenol sensitivity test. The effects of sinus arrhythmia, atropine, and propranolol. *Arch. Intern. Med.*, 1972;**130**: 47–52.

79. Jose, A.D. and D. Collison, The normal range and determinants of the intrinsic heart rate in man. *Cardiovasc. Res.*, 1970;**4**: 160–167.

80. Jordan, J.L., I. Yamaguchi, and W.J. Mandel, Studies on the mechanism of sinus node dysfunction in the sick sinus syndrome. *Circulation*, 1978;**57**: 217–223.

81. Szatmary, L.J., Autonomic blockade and sick sinus syndrome. New concept in the interpretation of electrophysiological and Holter data. *Eur. Heart J.*, 1984;**5**: 637–648.

82. Hariman, R.J., E. Krongrad, R.A. Boxer, M.B. Weiss, C.N. Steeg, and B.F .Hoffman, Method for recording electrical activity of the sinoatrial node and automatic atrial foci during cardiac catheterization in human subjects. *Am. J. Cardiol.*, 1980;**45**: 775–781.

83. Gomes, J.A., P.S. Kang, and N. El Sherif, The sinus node electrogram in patients with and without sick sinus syndrome: techniques and correlation between directly measured and indirectly estimated sinoatrial conduction time. *Circulation*, 1982;**66**: 864–873.

84. Reiffel, J.A., E. Gang, J. Gliklich, M.B. Weiss, J.C. Davis, J.N. Patton, et al., The human sinus node electrogram: a transvenous catheter technique and a comparison of directly measured and indirectly estimated sinoatrial conduction time in adults. *Circulation*, 1980;**62**: 1324–1334.

85. Josephson, M.E., *Sinus Node Function. Clinical Cardiac Electrophysiology: Techniques and Interpretations*, 4th edn. Philadelphia, PA: Lippincott Williams & Wilkins, 2008, pp. 69–92.

86. Reiffel, J.A., Electrophysiologic evaluation of sinus node function. *Cardiol. Clin.*, 1986;**4**: 401–416.

87. Yee, R. and H.C. Strauss, Electrophysiologic mechanisms: sinus node dysfunction. *Circulation*, 1987;**75**: III12–III18.

88. Vassalle, M., The relationship among cardiac pacemakers. Overdrive suppression. *Circ. Res.*, 1977;**41**: 269–277.

89. Narula, O.S., P. Samet, and R.P. Javier, Significance of the sinus-node recovery time. *Circulation*, 1972;**45**: 140–158.

90. Mandel, W.J., H. Hayakawa, H.N. Allen, R. Danzig, and A.I. Kermaier, Assessment of sinus node function in patients with the sick sinus syndrome. *Circulation*, 1972;**46**: 761–769.

91. Benditt, D.G., H.C. Strauss, M.M. Scheinman, V.S. Behar, and A.G. Wallace, Analysis of secondary pauses following termination of rapid atrial pacing in man. *Circulation*, 1976;**54**: 436–441.

92. Strauss, H.C., A.L. Saroff, J.T. Bigger Jr., and E.G. Giardina, Premature atrial stimulation as a key to the understanding of sinoatrial conduction in man. Presentation of data and critical review of the literature. *Circulation*, 1973;**47**: 86–93.

93. Narula, O.S., N. Shantha, M. Vasquez, W.D. Towne, and J.W. Linhart, A new method for measurement of sinoatrial conduction time. *Circulation*, 1978;**58**: 706–714.

94. Breithardt, G. and L. Seipel, Comparative study of two methods of estimating sinoatrial conduction time in man. *Am. J. Cardiol.*, 1978;**42**: 965–972.

95. Kerr, C.R. and H.C. Strauss, The measurement of sinus node refractoriness in man. *Circulation*, 1983;**68**: 1231–1237.

96. Juillard, A., F. Guillerm, H.V. Chuong, A. Barrillon, and A. Gerbaux, Sinus node electrogram recording in 59 patients. Comparison with simultaneous estimation of sinoatrial conduction using premature atrial stimulation. *Br. Heart J.*, 1983;**50**: 75–84.

97. Asseman, P., B. Berzin, D. Desry, D. Vilarem, P. Durand, C. Delmotte, et al., Persistent sinus nodal electrograms during abnormally prolonged postpacing atrial pauses in sick sinus syndrome in humans: sinoatrial block vs. overdrive suppression. *Circulation*, 1983;**68**: 33–41.

98. Asseman, P., B. Berzin, D. Desry, J.J. Bauchart, R. Reade, O. Leroy, et al., Postextrasystolic sinoatrial exit block in human sick sinus syndrome: demonstration by direct recording of sinus node electrograms. *Am. Heart J.*, 1991;**122**: 1633–1643.

99. Fujimura, O., R. Yee, G.J. Klein, A.D. Sharma, and K.A. Boahene, The diagnostic sensitivity of electrophysiologic testing in patients with syncope caused by transient bradycardia. *N. Engl. J. Med.*, 1989;**321**: 1703–1707.

100. Kang, P.S., J.A. Gomes, and N. El Sherif, Differential effects of functional autonomic blockade on the variables of sinus nodal automaticity in sick sinus syndrome. *Am. J. Cardiol.*, 1982;**49**: 273–282.

101. Bergfeldt, L., H. Vallin, M. Rosenqvist, P. Insulander, R. Nordlander, and H. Astrom, Sinus node recovery time assessment revisited: role of pharmacologic blockade of the autonomic nervous system. *J. Cardiovasc. Electrophysiol.*, 1996;**7**: 95–101.

102. Gann, D., A. Tolentino, and P. Samet, Electrophysiologic evaluation of elderly patients with sinus bradycardia: a long-term follow-up study. *Ann. Intern. Med.*, 1979;**90**: 24–29.

103. Shaw, D.B., R.R. Holman, and J.I. Gowers, Survival in sinoatrial disorder (sick-sinus syndrome). *Br. Med. J.*, 1980;**280**: 139–141.

104. Dhingra, R.C., F. Amat-y-Leon, C. Wyndham, P.C. Deedwania, D. Wu, P. Denes, et al., Clinical significance of prolonged sinoatrial conduction time. *Circulation*, 1977;**55**: 8–15.

105. Teichman, S.L., S.D. Felder, J.A. Matos, S.G. Kim, L.E. Waspe, and J.D. Fisher, The value of electrophysiologic studies in syncope of undetermined origin: report of 150 cases. *Am. Heart J.*, 1985;**110**: 469–479.

106. Gang, E.S., J.A. Reiffel, F.D. Livelli Jr., and J.T. Bigger Jr., Sinus node recovery times following the spontaneous termination of supraventricular tachycardia and following atrial overdrive pacing: a comparison. *Am. Heart J.*, 1983;**105**: 210–215.

107. van Mechelen, R., A. Segers, and F. Hagemeijer, Serial electrophysiologic studies after single chamber atrial pacemaker implantation in patients with symptomatic sinus node dysfunction. *Eur. Heart J.*, 1984;**5**: 628–636.

108. Blomstrom-Lundqvist, C., M.M. Scheinman, E.M. Aliot, J.S. Alpert, H. Calkins, A.J. Camm, et al., ACC/AHA/ESC guidelines for the management of patients with supraventricular arrhythmias – executive summary. A report of the American college

of cardiology/American heart association task force on practice guidelines and the European society of cardiology committee for practice guidelines (writing committee to develop guidelines for the management of patients with supraventricular arrhythmias) developed in collaboration with NASPE-Heart Rhythm Society. *J. Am. Coll. Cardiol.*, 2003;**42**: 1493–1531.

109. Chen, S.A., C.T. Tai, C.E. Chiang, and M.S. Chang, Role of the surface electrocardiogram in the diagnosis of patients with supraventricular tachycardia. *Cardiol. Clin.*, 1997;**15**: 539–565.

110. Obel, O.A. and A.J. Camm, Supraventricular tachycardia. ECG diagnosis and anatomy. *Eur. Heart J.*, 1997;**18**(Suppl. C): 2–11.

111. Hoffman, B.F. and M.R. Rosen, Cellular mechanisms for cardiac arrhythmias. *Circ. Res.*, 1981;**49**: 1–15.

112. Zorn-Pauly, K., P. Schaffer, B. Pelzmann, P. Lang, H. Machler, B. Rigler, et al., If in left human atrium: a potential contributor to atrial ectopy. *Cardiovasc. Res.*, 2004;**64**: 250–259.

113. Tsai, C.F., C.T. Tai, M.H. Hsieh, W.S. Lin, W.C. Yu, K.C. Ueng, et al., Initiation of atrial fibrillation by ectopic beats originating from the superior vena cava: electrophysiological characteristics and results of radiofrequency ablation. *Circulation*, 2000;**102**: 67–74.

114. Haissaguerre, M., P. Jais, D.C. Shah, A. Takahashi, M. Hocini, G. Quiniou, et al., Spontaneous initiation of atrial fibrillation by ectopic beats originating in the pulmonary veins. *N. Engl. J. Med.*, 1998;**339**: 659–666.

115. Wit, A.L. and M.R. Rosen, Afterdepolarizations and triggered activity: distinction from automaticity as an arrhythmogenic mechanism, in *The Heart and Cardiovascular System*, H.A. Fozzard, E. Haber, R.B. Jennings, A.M. Katz, and H.E. Morgan, Editors. New York: Raven Press, 1992, pp. 2113–2163.

116. Lederer, W.J. and R.W. Tsien, Transient inward current underlying arrhythmogenic effects of cardiotonic steroids in Purkinje fibres. *J. Physiol. (Lond.)*, 1976;**263**: 73–100.

117. Fedida, D., D. Noble, A.C. Rankin, and A.J. Spindler, The arrhythmogenic transient inward current iTI and related contraction in isolated guinea-pig ventricular myocytes. *J. Physiol. (Lond.)*, 1987;**392**: 523–542.

118. Rosen, M.R. and R.F. Reder, Does triggered activity have a role in the genesis of cardiac arrhythmias? *Ann. Intern. Med.*, 1981;**94**: 794–801.

119. Saoudi, N., F. Cosio, A. Waldo, S.A. Chen, Y. Iesaka, M. Lesh, et al., Classification of atrial flutter and regular atrial tachycardia according to electrophysiologic mechanism and anatomic bases: a statement from a joint expert group from the Working Group of Arrhythmias of the European Society of Cardiology and the North American Society of Pacing and Electrophysiology. *J. Cardiovasc. Electrophysiol.*, 2001;**12**: 852–866.

120. Wellens, H.J., Value and limitations of programmed electrical stimulation of the heart in the study and treatment of tachycardias. *Circulation*, 1978;**57**: 845–853.

121. MacLean, W.A., R.B. Karp, N.T. Kouchoukos, T.N. James, and A.L. Waldo, P waves during ectopic atrial rhythms in man: a study utilizing atrial pacing with fixed electrodes. *Circulation*, 1975;**52**: 426–434.

122. Tang, C.W., M.M. Scheinman, G.F. Van Hare, L.M. Epstein, A.P. Fitzpatrick, R.J. Lee, et al., Use of P wave configuration during atrial tachycardia to predict site of origin. *J. Am. Coll. Cardiol.*, 1995;**26**: 1315–1324.

123. Wu, D., P. Denes, F. Amat-y-Leon, R.C. Chhablani, and K.M. Rosen, Limitation of the surface electrocardiogram in diagnosis

of atrial arrhythmias. Further observations on dissimilar atrial rhythms. *Am. J. Cardiol.*, 1975;**36**: 91–97.

124. Man, K.C., Chan, K.K., P. Kovack, R. Goyal, F. Bogun, M. Harvey, et al., Spatial resolution of atrial pace mapping as determined by unipolar atrial pacing at adjacent sites. *Circulation*, 1996;**94**: 1357–1363.

125. Josephson, M.E., D.L. Scharf, J.A. Kastor, and J.G. Kitchen, Atrial endocardial activation in man. Electrode catheter technique of endocardial mapping. *Am. J. Cardiol.*, 1977;**39**: 972–981.

126. Wells, J.L. Jr., W.A. MacLean, T.N. James, and A.L. Waldo, Characterization of atrial flutter. Studies in man after open heart surgery using fixed atrial electrodes. *Circulation*, 1979;**60**: 665–673.

127. Killip, T. and J.H. Gault, Mode of onset of atrial fibrillation in man. *Am. Heart J.*, 1965;**70**: 172–179.

128. Bennett, M.A. and B.L. Pentecost, The pattern of onset and spontaneous cessation of atrial fibrillation in man. *Circulation*, 1970;**41**: 981–988.

129. Cosio, F.G., F. Arribas, and M. Lopez-Gil, Electrophysiologic findings in atrial fibrillation, in *Atrial Fibrillation: Mechanisms and Management*, R.H. Falk and P.J. Podrid, Editors. Philadelphia, PA: Lippincott-Raven, 1997, pp. 397–410.

130. Scheinman, M.M., D. Basu, and M. Hollenberg, Electrophysiologic studies in patients with persistent atrial tachycardia. *Circulation*, 1974;**50**: 266–273.

131. Shinbane, J.S., M.A. Wood, D.N. Jensen, K.A. Ellenbogen, A.P. Fitzpatrick, and M.M. Scheinman, Tachycardia-induced cardiomyopathy: a review of animal models and clinical studies. *J. Am. Coll. Cardiol.*, 1997;**29**: 709–715.

132. Walker, N.L., S.M. Cobbe, and D.H. Birnie, Tachycardiomyopathy: a diagnosis not to be missed. *Heart*, 2004;**90**: e7.

133. Calo, L., L. Sciarra, R. Scioli, F. Lamberti, M.L. Loricchio, C. Pandozi, et al., Recovery of cardiac function after ablation of atrial tachycardia arising from the tricuspid annulus. *Ital. Heart J.*, 2005;**6**: 652–657.

134. Raungratanaamporn, O., K. Bhuripanyo, R. Krittayaphong, C. Sriratanasathavorn, S. Raungratanaamporn, C. Kangkagate, et al., Reversibility of tachycardiomyopathy after successful radiofrequency catheter ablation: intermediate results. *J. Med. Assoc. Thai.*, 2001;**84**: 258–264.

135. Orth-Gomer, K., C. Hogstedt, L. Bodin, and B. Soderholm, Frequency of extrasystoles in healthy male employees. *Br. Heart J.*, 1986;**55**: 259–264.

136. Folarin, V.A., P.J. Fitzsimmons, and W.B. Kruyer, Holter monitor findings in asymptomatic male military aviators without structural heart disease. *Aviat. Space Environ. Med.*, 2001;**72**: 836–838.

137. Ramsdale, D.R., N. Arumugam, S.S. Singh, J. Pearson, and R.G. Charles, Holter monitoring in patients with mitral stenosis and sinus rhythm. *Eur. Heart J.*, 1987;**8**: 164–170.

138. Waldo, A.L., K.J. Vitikainen, G.A. Kaiser, J.R. Malm, and B.F. Hoffman, The P wave and P-R interval. Effects of the site of origin of atrial depolarization. *Circulation*, 1970;**42**: 653–671.

139. Gouaux, J.L. and R. Ashman, Auricular fibrillation with aberration simulating ventricular paroxysmal tachycardia. *Am. Heart J.*, 1947;**34**: 366–373.

140. Fisch, C., D.P. Zipes, and P.L. McHenry, Rate dependent aberrancy. *Circulation*, 1973;**48**: 714–724.

141. Chung, K.Y., T.J. Walsh, and E. Massie, Combined atrial and ventricular parasystole. *Am. J. Cardiol.*, 1965;**16**: 462–464.

142. Eliakim, M., Atrial parasystole. Effect of carotid sinus stimulation, Valsalva maneuver and exercise. *Am. J. Cardiol.*, 1965;**16**: 457–461.

143. Poutiainen, A.M., M.J. Koistinen, K.E. Airaksinen, E.K. Hartikainen, R.V. Kettunen, J.E. Karjalainen, et al., Prevalence and natural course of ectopic atrial tachycardia. *Eur. Heart J.*, 1999;**20**: 694–700.

144. Rodriguez, L.M., C. De Chillou, J. Schlapfer, J. Metzger, X. Baiyan, A. van den Dool, et al., Age at onset and gender of patients with different types of supraventricular tachycardias. *Am. J. Cardiol.*, 1992;**70**: 1213–1215.

145. Porter, M.J., J.B. Morton, R. Denman, A.C. Lin, S. Tierney, P.A. Santucci, et al., Influence of age and gender on the mechanism of supraventricular tachycardia. *Heart Rhythm*, 2004;**1**: 393–396.

146. Chen, S.A., C.E. Chiang, C.J. Yang, C.C. Cheng, T.J. Wu, S.P. Wang, et al., Sustained atrial tachycardia in adult patients. Electrophysiological characteristics, pharmacological response, possible mechanisms, and effects of radiofrequency ablation. *Circulation*, 1994;**90**: 1262–1278.

147. von Bernuth, G., W. Engelhardt, H.H. Kramer, H. Singer, P. Schneider, H. Ulmer, et al., Atrial automatic tachycardia in infancy and childhood. *Eur. Heart J.*, 1992;**13**: 1410–1415.

148. Chen, S.A., C.T. Tai, C.E. Chiang, Y.A. Ding, and M.S. Chang, Focal atrial tachycardia: reanalysis of the clinical and electrophysiologic characteristics and prediction of successful radiofrequency ablation. *J. Cardiovasc. Electrophysiol.*, 1998;**9**: 355–365.

149. Kalman, J.M., J.E. Olgin, M.R. Karch, M. Hamdan, R.J. Lee, and M.D. Lesh "Cristal tachycardias": origin of right atrial tachycardias from the crista terminalis identified by intracardiac echocardiography. *J. Am. Coll. Cardiol.*, 1998;**31**: 451–459.

150. Natale, A., L. Breeding, G. Tomassoni, K. Rajkovich, M. Richey, S. Beheiry, et al., Ablation of right and left ectopic atrial tachycardias using a three-dimensional nonfluoroscopic mapping system. *Am. J. Cardiol.*, 1998;**82**: 989–992.

151. Anguera, I., J. Brugada, M. Roba, L. Mont, L. Aguinaga, P. Geelen, et al., Outcomes after radiofrequency catheter ablation of atrial tachycardia. *Am. J. Cardiol.*, 2001;**87**: 886–890.

152. Knight, B.P., M. Ebinger, H. Oral, M.H. Kim, C. Sticherling, F. Pelosi, et al., Diagnostic value of tachycardia features and pacing maneuvers during paroxysmal supraventricular tachycardia. *J. Am. Coll. Cardiol.*, 2000;**36**: 574–582.

153. Benditt, D.G., E.L. Pritchett, W.M. Smith, and J.J. Gallagher, Ventriculoatrial intervals: diagnostic use in paroxysmal supraventricular tachycardia. *Ann. Intern. Med.*, 1979;**91**: 161–166.

154. Knight, B.P., A. Zivin, J. Souza, M. Flemming, F. Pelosi, R. Goyal, et al., A technique for the rapid diagnosis of atrial tachycardia in the electrophysiology laboratory. *J. Am. Coll. Cardiol.*, 1999;**33**: 775–781.

155. Lown, B., N.F. Wyatt, and H.D. Levine, Paroxysmal atrial tachycardia with block. *Circulation*, 1960;**21**: 129–143.

156. Storstein, O. and K. Rasmussen, Digitalis and atrial tachycardia with block. *Br. Heart J.*, 1974;**36**: 171–176.

157. Kistler, P.M., K.C. Roberts-Thomson, H.M. Haqqani, S.P. Fynn, S. Singarayar, J.K. Vohra, et al, P-wave morphology in focal atrial tachycardia - development of an algorithm to predict the anatomical site of origin. *J. Am. Coll. Cardiol.*, 2006;**48**: 1010–1017.

158. Zipes, D.P., W.E. Gaum, B.C. Genetos, R.D. Glassman, J. Noble, and C. Fisch, Atrial tachycardia without P waves masquerading as an A-V junctional tachycardia. *Circulation*, 1977;**55**: 253–260.

159. Boineau, J.P., T.E. Canavan, R.B. Schuessler, M.E. Cain, P.B. Corr, and J.L. Cox, Demonstration of a widely distributed atrial pacemaker complex in the human heart. *Circulation*, 1988;**77**: 1221–1237.

160. Chen, C.C., C.T. Tai, C.E. Chiang, W.C. Yu, S.H. Lee, Y.J. Chen, et al., Atrial tachycardias originating from the atrial septum: electrophysiologic characteristics and radiofrequency ablation. *J. Cardiovasc. Electrophysiol.*, 2000;**11**: 744–749.

161. Frey, B., G. Kreiner, M. Gwechenberger, and H.D. Gossinger, Ablation of atrial tachycardia originating from the vicinity of the atrioventricular node: significance of mapping both sides of the interatrial septum. *J. Am. Coll. Cardiol.*, 2001;**38**: 394–400.

162. Marrouche, N.F., A. SippensGroenewegen, Y. Yang, S. Dibs, and M.M. Scheinman, Clinical and electrophysiologic characteristics of left septal atrial tachycardia. *J. Am. Coll. Cardiol.*, 2002;**40**: 1133–1139.

163. Kistler, P.M., S.P. Fynn, H. Haqqani, I.H. Stevenson, J.K. Vohra, J.B. Morton, et al., Focal atrial tachycardia from the ostium of the coronary sinus: electrocardiographic and electrophysiological characterization and radiofrequency ablation. *J. Am. Coll. Cardiol.*, 2005;**45**: 1488–1493.

164. Tada, H., A. Nogami, S. Naito, M. Suguta, M. Nakatsugawa, Y. Horie, et al., Simple electrocardiographic criteria for identifying the site of origin of focal right atrial tachycardia. *Pace Clin. Electrophysiol.*, 1998;**21**: 2431–2439.

165. Morton, J.B., P. Sanders, A. Das, J.K. Vohra, P.B. Sparks, and J.M. Kalman, Focal atrial tachycardia arising from the tricuspid annulus: electrophysiologic and electrocardiographic characteristics. *J. Cardiovasc. Electrophysiol.*, 2001;**12**: 653–659.

166. Roberts-Thomson, K.C., P.M. Kistler, A.D. McGavigan, R.J. Hillock, I.H. Stevenson, S. Spence, et al., Focal atrial tachycardias arising from the right atrial appendage: electrocardiographic and electrophysiological characteristics and radiofrequency ablation. *J. Cardiovasc. Electrophysiol.*, 2007;**18**(4): 367–372.

167. Kistler, P.M., P. Sanders, S.P. Fynn, I.H. Stevenson, A. Hussin, J.K. Vohra, et al., Electrophysiological and electrocardiographic characteristics of focal atrial tachycardia originating from the pulmonary veins: acute and long-term outcomes of radiofrequency ablation. *Circulation*, 2003;**108**: 1968–1975.

168. Hachiya, H., S. Ernst, F. Ouyang, H. Mavrakis, J. Chun, D. Bansch, et al., Topographic distribution of focal left atrial tachycardias defined by electrocardiographic and electrophysiological data. *Circ. J.*, 2005;**69**: 205–210.

169. Kistler, P.M., P. Sanders, A. Hussin, J.B. Morton, J.K. Vohra, P.B. Sparks, et al., Focal atrial tachycardia arising from the mitral annulus: electrocardiographic and electrophysiologic characterization. *J. Am. Coll. Cardiol.*, 2003;**41**: 2212–2219.

170. Gonzalez, M.D., L.J. Contreras, M.R. Jongbloed, J. Rivera, T.P. Donahue, A.B. Curtis, et al., Left atrial tachycardia originating from the mitral annulus-aorta junction. *Circulation*, 2004;**110**: 3187–3192.

171. Tritto, M., M. Zardini, R. De Ponti, and J.A. Salerno-Uriarte, Iterative atrial tachycardia originating from the coronary sinus musculature. *J. Cardiovasc. Electrophysiol.*, 2001;**12**: 1187–1189.

172. Volkmer, M., M. Antz, J. Hebe, and K.H. Kuck, Focal atrial tachycardia originating from the musculature of the coronary sinus. *J. Cardiovasc. Electrophysiol.*, 2002;**13**: 68–71.

173. Badhwar, N., J.M. Kalman, P.B. Sparks, P.M. Kistler, M. Attari, M. Berger, et al., Atrial tachycardia arising from the coronary sinus musculature: electrophysiological characteristics and long-term outcomes of radiofrequency ablation. *J. Am. Coll. Cardiol.*, 2005;**46**: 1921–1930.

174. Shine, K.I., J.A. Kastor, and P.M. Yurchak, Multifocal atrial tachycardia. Clinical and electrocardiographic features in 32 patients. *N. Engl. J. Med.*, 1968;**279**: 344–349.

175. McCord, J. and S. Borzak, Multifocal atrial tachycardia. *Chest*, 1998;**113**: 203–209.

176. Lipson, M.J. and S. Naimi, Multifocal atrial tachycardia (chaotic atrial tachycardia). Clinical associations and significance. *Circulation*, 1970;**42**: 397–407.

177. Marchlinski, F.E. and J.M. Miller, Atrial arrhythmias exacerbated by theophylline. Response to verapamil and evidence for triggered activity in man. *Chest*, 1985;**88**: 931–934.

178. Strickberger, S.A., C.B. Miller, and J.H. Levine, Multifocal atrial tachycardia from electrolyte imbalance. *Am. Heart J.*, 1988;**115**: 680–682.

179. Levine, J.H., J.R. Michael, and T. Guarnieri, Multifocal atrial tachycardia: a toxic effect of theophylline. *Lancet*, 1985;**1**: 12–14.

180. Wang, K., B.L. Goldfarb, F.L. Gobel, and H.G. Richman, Multifocal atrial tachycardia. *Arch. Intern. Med.*, 1977;**137**: 161–164.

181. Bisset, G.S. III, S.F. Seigel, W.E. Gaum, and S. Kaplan, Chaotic atrial tachycardia in childhood. *Am. Heart J.*, 1981;**101**: 268–272.

182. Arsura, E., A.S. Lefkin, D.L. Scher, M. Solar, and S. Tessler, A randomized, double-blind, placebo-controlled study of verapamil and metoprolol in treatment of multifocal atrial tachycardia. *Am. J. Med.*, 1988;**85**: 519–524.

183. McCord, J.K., S. Borzak, T. Davis, and M. Gheorghiade, Usefulness of intravenous magnesium for multifocal atrial tachycardia in patients with chronic obstructive pulmonary disease. *Am. J. Cardiol.*, 1998;**81**: 91–93.

184. Tucker, K.J., J. Law, and M.J. Rodriques, Treatment of refractory recurrent multifocal atrial tachycardia with atrioventricular junction ablation and permanent pacing. *J. Invasive Cardiol.*, 1995;**7**: 207–212.

185. Ueng, K.C., S.H. Lee, D.J. Wu, C.S. Lin, M.S. Chang, and S.A. Chen, Radiofrequency catheter modification of atrioventricular junction in patients with COPD and medically refractory multifocal atrial tachycardia. *Chest*, 2000;**117**: 52–59.

186. Levine, J.H., J.R. Michael, and T. Guarnieri, Treatment of multifocal atrial tachycardia with verapamil. *N. Engl. J. Med.*, 1985;**312**: 21–25.

187. Watson, R.M. and M.E. Josephson, Atrial flutter. I. Electrophysiologic substrates and modes of initiation and termination. *Am. J. Cardiol.*, 1980;**45**: 732–741.

188. Waldo, A.L., W.A. MacLean, R.B. Karp, N.T. Kouchoukos, and T.N. James, Entrainment and interruption of atrial flutter with atrial pacing: studies in man following open heart surgery. *Circulation*, 1977;**56**: 737–745.

189. Greenberg, M.L., T.A. Kelly, B.B. Lerman, and J.P. DiMarco, Atrial pacing for conversion of atrial flutter. *Am. J. Cardiol.*, 1986;**58**: 95–99.

190. Waldo, A.L., Atrial flutter: entrainment characteristics. *J. Cardiovasc. Electrophysiol.*, 1997;**8**: 337–352.

191. Scheinman, M.M., Y. Yang, and J. Cheng, Atrial flutter: Part II Nomenclature. *Pace Clin. Electrophysiol.*, 2004;**27**: 504–506.

192. Granada, J., W. Uribe, P.H. Chyou, K. Maassen, R. Vierkant, P.N. Smith, et al., Incidence and predictors of atrial flutter in the general population. *J. Am. Coll. Cardiol.*, 2000;**36**: 2242–2246.

193. Lee, K.W., Y. Yang, and M.M. Scheinman, Atrial flutter: a review of its history, mechanisms, clinical features, and current therapy. *Curr. Probl. Cardiol.*, 2005;**30**: 121–167.

194. Vidaillet, H., J.F. Granada, P.H. Chyou, K. Maassen, M. Ortiz, J.N. Pulido, et al., A population-based study of mortality among patients with atrial fibrillation or flutter. *Am. J. Med.*, 2002;**113**: 365–370.

195. Kalman, J.M., G.F. VanHare, J.E. Olgin, L.A. Saxon, S.I. Stark, and M.D. Lesh, Ablation of "incisional" reentrant atrial tachycardia complicating surgery for congenital heart disease. Use of entrainment to define a critical isthmus of conduction. *Circulation*, 1996;**93**: 502–512.

196. Chugh, A., H. Oral, K. Lemola, B. Hall, P. Cheung, E. Good, et al., Prevalence, mechanisms, and clinical significance of macroreentrant atrial tachycardia during and following left atrial ablation for atrial fibrillation. *Heart Rhythm*, 2005;**2**: 464–471.

197. Stevenson, I.H., P.M. Kistler, S.J. Spence, J.K. Vohra, P.B. Sparks, J.B. Morton, et al., Scar-related right atrial macroreentrant tachycardia in patients without prior atrial surgery: electroanatomic characterization and ablation outcome. *Heart Rhythm*, 2005;**2**: 594–601.

198. Wellens, H.J., Contemporary management of atrial flutter. *Circulation*, 2002;**106**: 649–652.

199. Natale, A., K.H. Newby, E. Pisano, F. Leonelli, R. Fanelli, D. Potenza, et al., Prospective randomized comparison of antiarrhythmic therapy versus first-line radiofrequency ablation in patients with atrial flutter. *J. Am. Coll. Cardiol.*, 2000;**35**: 1898–1904.

200. Tai, C.T., T.Y. Liu, P.C. Lee, Y.J. Lin, M.S. Chang, and S.A. Chen, Non-contact mapping to guide radiofrequency ablation of atypical right atrial flutter. *J. Am. Coll. Cardiol.*, 2004;**44**: 1080–1086.

201. Della, B.P., A. Fraticelli, C. Tondo, S. Riva, G. Fassini, and C. Carbucicchio, Atypical atrial flutter: clinical features, electrophysiological characteristics and response to radiofrequency catheter ablation. *Europace*, 2002;**4**: 241–253.

202. Jais, P., M. Hocini, R. Weerasoryia, L. Macle, C. Scavee, F. Raybaud, et al., Atypical left atrial flutters. *Card. Electrophysiol. Rev.*, 2002;**6**: 371–377.

203. Olshansky, B., Advances in atrial flutter mapping: what goes around comes around. *J. Cardiovasc. Electrophysiol.*, 2004;**15**: 415–417.

204. Mehta, A.V. and L.L. Ewing, Atrial tachycardia in infants and children: electrocardiographic classification and its significance. *Pediatr. Cardiol.*, 1993;**14**: 199–203.

205. Olgin, J.E., J.M. Kalman, A.P. Fitzpatrick, and M.D. Lesh, Role of right atrial endocardial structures as barriers to conduction during human type I atrial flutter. Activation and entrainment mapping guided by intracardiac echocardiography. *Circulation*, 1995;**92**: 1839–1848.

206. Kalman, J.M., J.E. Olgin, L.A. Saxon, W.G. Fisher, R.J. Lee, and M.D. Lesh, Activation and entrainment mapping defines the tricuspid annulus as the anterior barrier in typical atrial flutter. *Circulation*, 1996;**94**: 398–406.

207. Schwartzman, D., D.J. Callans, C.D. Gottlieb, S.M. Dillon, C. Movsowitz, and F.E. Marchlinski, Conduction block in the inferior vena caval-tricuspid valve isthmus: association with

outcome of radiofrequency ablation of type I atrial flutter. *J. Am. Coll. Cardiol.*, 1996;**28**: 1519–1531.

208. Saoudi, N., M. Nair, A. Abdelazziz, H. Poty, A. Daou, F. Anselme, et al., Electrocardiographic patterns and results of radiofrequency catheter ablation of clockwise type I atrial flutter. *J. Cardiovasc. Electrophysiol.*, 1996;7: 931–942.

209. Besoain-Santander, M., A. Pick, and R. Langendorf, A-V conduction in auricular flutter. *Circulation*, 1950;2: 604–616.

210. Kennelly, B.M. and G.K. Lane, Electrophysiological studies in four patients with atrial flutter with 1:1 atrioventricular conduction. *Am. Heart J.*, 1978;**96**: 723–730.

211. Moleiro, F., I.J. Mendoza, V. Medina-Ravell, A. Castellanos, and R.J. Myerburg, One to one atrioventricular conduction during atrial pacing at rates of 300/minute in absence of Wolff-Parkinson-White Syndrome. *Am. J. Cardiol.*, 1981;**48**: 789–796.

212. Bochoeyer, A., Y. Yang, J. Cheng, R.J. Lee, E.C. Keung, N.F. Marrouche, et al., Surface electrocardiographic characteristics of right and left atrial flutter. *Circulation*, 2003;**108**: 60–66.

213. Selzer, A., Atrial fibrillation revisited. *N. Engl. J. Med.*, 1982;**306**: 1044–1045.

214. Lewis, T., Auricular fibrillation: a common clinical condition. *Br. Med. J.*, 1909;2: 1528.

215. McMichael, J., History of atrial fibrillation 1628–1819 Harvey – de Senac – Laennec. *Br. Heart J.*, 1982;**48**: 193–197.

216. Levy, S., G. Breithardt, R.W. Campbell, A.J. Camm, J.C. Daubert, M. Allessie, et al., Atrial fibrillation: current knowledge and recommendations for management. Working Group on Arrhythmias of the European Society of Cardiology. *Eur. Heart J.*, 1998;**19**: 1294–1320.

217. Fuster V., L.E. Rydén, D.S. Cannom, H.J. Crijns, A.B. Curtis, K.A. Ellenbogen, et al, ACC/AHA/ESC 2006 guidelines for the management of patients with atrial fibrillation: a report of the American College of Cardiology/American Heart Association Task Force on Practice Guidelines and the European Society of Cardiology Committee for Practice Guidelines (Writing Committee to Revise the 2001 Guidelines for the Management of Patients With Atrial Fibrillation). *J. Am. Coll. Cardiol.*, 2006;**48**:e149–246.

218. Nattel, S., New ideas about atrial fibrillation 50 years on. *Nature*, 2002;**415**: 219–226.

219. Quinn, F.R. and A.C. Rankin, Atrial fibrillation ablation in the real world. *Heart*, 2005;**91**: 1507–1508.

220. Oral, H., Mechanisms of atrial fibrillation: lessons from studies in patients. *Prog. Cardiovasc. Dis.*, 2005;**48**: 29–40.

221. Hwang, C., T.J. Wu, R.N. Doshi, C.T. Peter, and P.S. Chen, Vein of marshall cannulation for the analysis of electrical activity in patients with focal atrial fibrillation. *Circulation*, 2000;**101**: 1503–1505.

222. Moe, G.K., On the multiple wavelet hypothesis of atrial fibrillation. *Arch. Int. Pharmacodyn. Ther.*, 1962;**140**: 183–188.

223. Moe, G.K., W.C. Rheinboldt, and J.A. Abildskov, A computer model of atrial fibrillation. *Am. Heart J.*, 1964;**67**: 200–220.

224. Allessie, M.A., W.J.P. Lammers, and F.I.M. Bonke, Experimental evaluation of Moe's multiple wavelet hypothesis of atrial fibrillation, in *Cardiac Electrophysiology and Arrhythmias*, D.P. Zipes and J. Jalife, Editors. Orlando, FL: Grune and Statton, 1985, pp. 265–275.

225. Cox, J.L., R.B. Schuessler, and J.P. Boineau, The development of the Maze procedure for the treatment of atrial fibrillation. *Semin. Thorac. Cardiovasc. Surg.*, 2000;**12**: 2–14.

226. Jalife, J., O. Berenfeld, and M. Mansour, Mother rotors and fibrillatory conduction: a mechanism of atrial fibrillation. *Cardiovasc. Res.*, 2002;**54**: 204–216.

227. Ricard, P., S. Levy, J. Trigano, F. Paganelli, E. Daoud, K.C. Man, et al., Prospective assessment of the minimum energy needed for external electrical cardioversion of atrial fibrillation. *Am. J. Cardiol.*, 1997;**79**: 815–816.

228. Wijffels, M.C., C.J. Kirchhof, R. Dorland, and M.A. Allessie, Atrial fibrillation begets atrial fibrillation. A study in awake chronically instrumented goats. *Circulation*, 1995;**92**: 1954–1968.

229. Nattel, S., A. Shiroshita-Takeshita, B.J. Brundel, and L. Rivard, Mechanisms of atrial fibrillation: lessons from animal models. *Prog. Cardiovasc. Dis.*, 2005;**48**: 9–28.

230. Euler, D.E., B. Olshansky, and S.Y. Kim, Reflex vagal control of atrial repolarization. *Am. J. Physiol.*, 1996;**271**: H870–H875.

231. Alessi, R., M. Nusynowitz, J.A. Abildskov, and G.K. Moe, Nonuniform distribution of vagal effects on the atrial refractory period. *Am. J. Physiol.*, 1958;**194**: 406–410.

232. Euler, D.E. and P.J. Scanlon, Acetylcholine release by a stimulus train lowers atrial fibrillation threshold. *Am. J. Physiol.*, 1987;**253**: H863–H868.

233. Olshansky, B., Interrelationships between the autonomic nervous system and atrial fibrillation. *Prog. Cardiovasc. Dis.*, 2005;**48**: 57–78.

234. Coumel, P., Clinical approach to paroxysmal atrial fibrillation. *Clin. Cardiol.*, 1990;**13**: 209–212.

235. Oral, H., A. Chugh, C. Scharf, B. Hall, P. Cheung, S. Veerareddy, et al., Pulmonary vein isolation for vagotonic, adrenergic, and random episodes of paroxysmal atrial fibrillation. *J. Cardiovasc. Electrophysiol.*, 2004;**15**: 402–406.

236. Pappone, C., V. Santinelli, F. Manguso, G. Vicedomini, F. Gugliotta, G. Augello, et al., Pulmonary vein denervation enhances long-term benefit after circumferential ablation for paroxysmal atrial fibrillation. *Circulation*, 2004;**109**: 327–334.

237. Wolf, P.A., R.D. Abbott, and W.B. Kannel, Atrial fibrillation as an independent risk factor for stroke: the Framingham Study. *Stroke*, 1991;**22**: 983–988.

238. Lloyd-Jones, D.M., T.J. Wang, E.P. Leip, M.G. Larson, D. Levy, R.S. Vasan, et al., Lifetime risk for development of atrial fibrillation: the Framingham Heart Study. *Circulation*, 2004;**110**: 1042–1046.

239. Benjamin, E.J., D. Levy, S.M. Vaziri, R.B. D'Agostino, A.J. Belanger, and P.A. Wolf, Independent risk factors for atrial fibrillation in a population-based cohort. The Framingham Heart Study. *JAMA*, 1994;**271**: 840–844.

240. Tsang, T.S., Y. Miyasaka, M.E. Barnes, and B.J. Gersh, Epidemiological profile of atrial fibrillation: a contemporary perspective. *Prog. Cardiovasc. Dis.*, 2005;**48**: 1–8.

241. Forfar, J.C., H.C. Miller, and A.D. Toft, Occult thyrotoxicosis: a correctable cause of "idiopathic" atrial fibrillation. *Am. J. Cardiol.*, 1979;**44**: 9–12.

242. Rathore, S.S., A.K. Berger, K.P. Weinfurt, K.A. Schulman, W.J. Oetgen, B.J. Gersh, et al., Acute myocardial infarction complicated by atrial fibrillation in the elderly: prevalence and outcomes. *Circulation*, 2000;**101**: 969–974.

243. Djousse, L., D. Levy, E.J. Benjamin, S.J. Blease, A. Russ, M.G. Larson, et al., Long-term alcohol consumption and the risk of atrial fibrillation in the Framingham Study. *Am. J. Cardiol.*, 2004;**93**: 710–713.

244. Koskinen, P., M. Kupari, H. Leinonen, and K. Luomanmaki, Alcohol and new onset atrial fibrillation: a case-control study of a current series. *Br. Heart J.*, 1987;**57**: 468–473.

245. Thornton, J.R., Atrial fibrillation in healthy non-alcoholic people after an alcoholic binge. *Lancet*, 1984;**2**: 1013–1015.

246. Brand, F.N., R.D. Abbott, W.B. Kannel, and P.A. Wolf, Characteristics and prognosis of lone atrial fibrillation. 30-year follow-up in the Framingham Study. *JAMA*, 1985;**254**: 3449–3453.

247. Kopecky, S.L., B.J. Gersh, M.D. McGoon, J.P. Whisnant, D.R. Holmes Jr., D.M. Ilstrup, et al., The natural history of lone atrial fibrillation. A population-based study over three decades. *N. Engl. J. Med.*, 1987;**317**: 669–674.

248. Henry, W.L., J. Morganroth, A.S. Pearlman, C.E. Clark, D.R. Redwood, S.B. Itscoitz, et al., Relation between echocardiographically determined left atrial size and atrial fibrillation. *Circulation*, 1976;**53**: 273–279.

249. Aronow, W.S., K.S. Schwartz, and M. Koenigsberg, Prevalence of enlarged left atrial dimension by echocardiography and its correlation with atrial fibrillation and an abnormal P terminal force in lead V1 of the electrocardiogram in 588 elderly persons. *Am. J. Cardiol.*, 1987;**59**: 1003–1004.

250. Vaziri, S.M., M.G. Larson, E.J. Benjamin, and D. Levy, Echocardiographic predictors of nonrheumatic atrial fibrillation. The Framingham Heart Study. *Circulation*, 1994;**89**: 724–730.

251. Wang, T.J., M.G. Larson, D. Levy, R.S. Vasan, E.P. Leip, P.A. Wolf, et al., Temporal relations of atrial fibrillation and congestive heart failure and their joint influence on mortality: the Framingham Heart Study. *Circulation*, 2003;**107**: 2920–2925.

252. Morganroth, J., L.N. Horowitz, M.E. Josephson, and J.A. Kastor, Relationship of atrial fibrillatory wave amplitude to left atrial size and etiology of heart disease. An old generalization re-examined. *Am. Heart J.*, 1979;**97**: 184–186.

253. Cohen, S.I., S.H. Lau, W.D. Berkowitz, and A.N. Damato, Concealed conduction during atrial fibrillation. *Am. J. Cardiol.*, 1970;**25**: 416–419.

254. Wellens, H.J., F.W. Bar, and K.I. Lie, The value of the electrocardiogram in the differential diagnosis of a tachycardia with a widened QRS complex. *Am. J. Med.*, 1978;**64**: 27–33.

255. Pritchett, E.L., W.M. Smith, G.J. Klein, S.C. Hammill, and J.J. Gallagher, The "compensatory pause" of atrial fibrillation. *Circulation*, 1980;**62**: 1021–1025.

256. Klein, G.J., T.M. Bashore, T.D. Sellers, E.L. Pritchett, W.M. Smith, and J.J. Gallagher, Ventricular fibrillation in the Wolff-Parkinson-White syndrome. *N. Engl. J. Med.*, 1979;**301**: 1080–1085.

257. Campbell, R.W., R.A. Smith, J.J. Gallagher, E.L. Pritchett, and A.G. Wallace, Atrial fibrillation in the preexcitation syndrome. *Am. J. Cardiol.*, 1977;**40**: 514–520.

5 Clinical Electrophysiological Mechanisms of Tachycardias Arising from the Atrioventricular Junction

Demosthenes G. Katritsis · A. John Camm

P. W. Macfarlane et al. (eds.), *Cardiac Arrhythmias and Mapping Techniques*, DOI 10.1007/978-0-85729-877-5_5,

5.1 Atrioventricular Junctional Tachycardias

5.1.1 Definitions

Junctional tachycardias originate in the AV junction, i.e., the AV node and its approaches [1, 2]. Tachycardias originating in the AV junction can be classified into two types according to their underlying electrophysiological mechanism. The first type is caused by reentry movement in the region of the AV node and the adjacent perinodal tissue. It is therefore called atrioventricular nodal reentrant tachycardia (AVNRT). The second type comprises tachycardias that are caused by enhanced automaticity or triggered activity in the AV junction [1]. The term AV junction refers to a part of the atrioventricular specialized conducting system consisting of the transitional cell zone, the AV node and its extensions, and the penetrating part of the bundle of His [3–5]. Approximately one half of narrow QRS tachycardias are due to AV junctional reentry, and one third is due to reentry over accessory atrioventricular connections [1, 2]. In the absence of preexcitation during sinus rhythm, the most frequent cause of regular supraventricular tachycardia is reentry within the atrioventricular junction.

5.2 Atrioventricular Nodal Reentrant Tachycardia

5.2.1 Aetiology and Mechanism

Atrioventricular nodal reentrant tachycardia (AVNRT) is thought to result from reentry in the region of the AV junction. However, the precise anatomical site of the circuit and the pathways involved have not yet been established.

5.2.2 Conventional Concepts

The suggestion that circus movement in the atrioventricular node can be a mechanism for supraventricular tachycardia was made as early as 1913 [6]. The concept of dual AV nodal pathways dates from 1956 when Moe and colleagues [7] demonstrated evidence of a dual AV conduction system in dogs. They noted a sudden increase in the AV conduction time when a premature atrial impulse was delivered at a critical coupling interval after a regular extrastimuli series.

Denes et al. [8] in 1973 ascribed episodes of paroxysmal supraventricular tachycardia to AV node reentry due to the presence of dual atrioventricular nodal pathways. It was postulated that a dual conduction system was present, one having a faster conduction time and longer refractory period and the other having a slower conduction time and shorter refractory period (❯ Fig. 5.1). At a critical coupling interval, the premature impulse blocks in the faster pathway and conducts in the still excitable slow pathway, causing a sudden jump in the AV conduction time. Following this, the impulse returns to the atria, supposedly via the fast pathway, which has then recovered, and an atrial reciprocal response or "echo" beat or sustained tachycardia results (❯ Fig. 5.2) [8, 9]. Rosen et al. [10], using His bundle recordings and the atrial extrastimulus method, demonstrated sudden prolongation of the AH interval in a patient with dual atrioventricular nodal pathways. These discontinuities in AH conduction can be displayed by plotting A_2-H_2 conduction times or H_1-H_2 intervals against A_1-A_2 intervals giving the "antegrade conduction curve" (❯ Fig. 5.3) [11]. Normally, the AV node displays a gradual conduction time prolongation with atrial extrastimulation, thus resulting in smooth conduction curves with a progressive increment of the AH or HH intervals (❯ Fig. 5.4) [11]. A sudden increment of AV nodal conduction time results in a discontinuous curve. The portion of the curve to the right of the sudden increment was described as reflecting fast (or beta) pathway conduction time and that to the left as slow (or alpha) pathway conduction (❯ Fig. 5.3). An increase in H_1-H_2 of >50 ms for a decrease in A_1-A_2 of 10-20 ms was arbitrarily considered conduction "jump" reflecting the presence of dual AV nodal pathways [12–14].

Discontinuous refractory period curves, however, may not be present in all patients with AVNRT. Antegrade dual pathways are demonstrable in approximately 75% of patients with tachycardia [12, 14], and AVNRT may occur in the presence of continuous AV nodal conduction curves [15–17]. Conversely, antegrade dual pathways can be demonstrated in subjects without tachycardia [13, 18]. In children undergoing electrophysiological studies, up to 35% may have discontinuous curves [19, 20]. Similarly, people without tachycardia may exhibit discontinuous curves on antegrade or retrograde

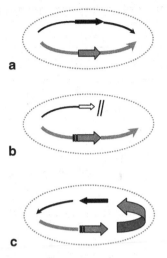

□ Fig. 5.1
Theoretical depiction of the AV nodal reentrant circuit. During sinus rhythm (a) the impulse penetrates both the fast and the slow pathway. A premature beat results in conduction block of the fast pathway and propagation through the slow (b). An earlier impulse encounters more delay in the slow pathway in a way that the blocked fast pathway has recovered when the now retrograde impulse arrives and tachycardia begins (c)

activation [21, 22]. It seems, therefore, that mere presence of AV nodal duality even in conjunction with AV echos is not enough to predispose to paroxysmal tachycardia.

In 5–10% of patients with AV nodal reentry, antegrade conduction is thought to proceed over the fast pathway and retrograde conduction over the slow pathway and may result in an incessant form of AVNRT [23, 24]. In these patients, antegrade conduction curves are not discontinuous. This pattern of conduction as well as the incessant nature can also be seen in the presence of concealed septal accessory pathways with decremental properties [25]. Depending on the orientation of the reentrant circuit, therefore, AVNRT has been traditionally classified into *slow-fast* or typical form and into *fast-slow* or atypical form.

5.2.3 Recent Developments

The concept of dual AV junctional pathways can provide explanations for many aspects of the electrophysiological behavior of these tachycardias, but several obscure points remain. These pathways have not been demonstrated histologically, and the exact circuit responsible for the reentrant tachycardia is unknown [26, 27]. Recently, exciting information from the ablation laboratory and the surgical theatre has appeared regarding the nature of the AVNRT circuit, although several questions still remain unsettled.

There has been considerable evidence that more than two pathways may be involved in the AVNRT circuit. Triple AV nodal pathways have been described [28, 29], and dual AV nodal conduction may persist in patients in whom AVNRT was abolished by catheter ablation [30]. Indeed, electrophysiologic demonstration of multiple discontinuities in the AV node conduction curve suggests the presence of multiple anterograde AV node pathways (❷ Fig. 5.5), although not all of them are involved in the initiation and maintenance of AVNRT [31]. In a series of 550 patients with AVNRT described by Tai et al., 36 patients had multiple anterograde and retrograde AV nodal pathways that constituted the substrates of multiple reentry circuits [32]. Hwang et al. [33] have also described 17 patients with the fast-slow or slow-slow forms of AVNRT in whom the slow-fast form was also inducible. This finding clearly suggests the potential existence of multiple slow pathways in certain patients in whom several different forms of AVNRT may coexist. There have also been reports of patients demonstrating evidence of multiple pathways following radiofrequency ablation of both the slow [33] and the fast pathway [34]. We have also reported on a patient with slow-fast AVNRT in whom, during radiofrequency ablation

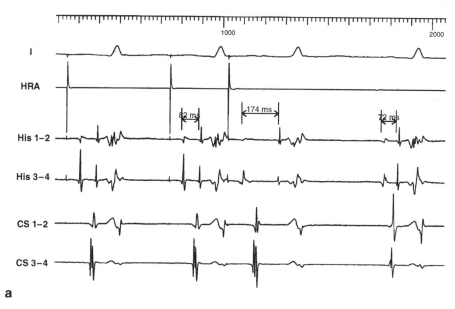

a

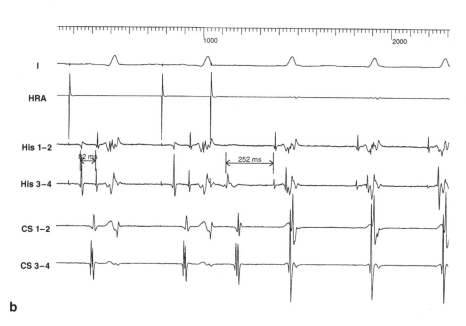

b

◘ Fig. 5.2

Anterograde jump and initiation of slow-fast AVNRT with atrial extrastimuli. At ventricular pacing cycle length of 500 s, a ventricular extrastimulus is delivered at 260 ms (**a**) with resultant decremental conduction through the fast pathway (AH = 174 ms). At a coupling interval of 240 ms (**b**) there is a conduction jump with AH = 252 ms and tachycardia is induced. Note that atrial electrograms are superimposed on the ventricular ones, but on His bundle 3–4 electrogram, the atrial electrogram preceeds the ventricular one. I: lead I of the surface ECG, *HRA*: high right atrium, *His*: His bundle, *CS*: coronary sinus

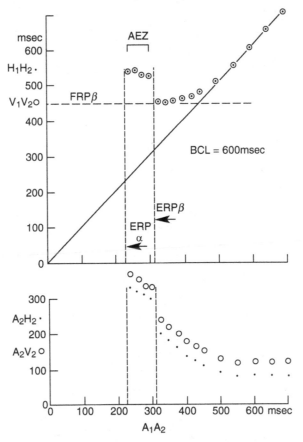

◻ Fig. 5.3

Anterograde conduction curves from a patient with "slow-fast" AVNRT. The sudden increase of AH (jump) indicates refractoriness of the fast (beta) pathway and conduction through the slow (alpha) pathway. Please see text for details (From Ward and Camm [11]. © Edward Arnold, London. Reproduced with permission)

of his slow pathway, retrograde activation was continuously alternating from a fast to a slow pathway producing alternating tachycardia cycles during both the anterior and posterior (or slow-slow) (❷ Fig. 5.6) forms of tachycardia [35]. In another report, the initiation of fast-slow AVNRT was dependent on sudden A-H prolongation, indicating antegrade conduction over a slow pathway that shortened during the ensuing beats [36]. It seems therefore that, at least according to conventional definitions, a group of such pathways may be involved in the reentrant circuit [31, 32, 37].

There has also been a long debate whether the adjacent atrial tissue constitutes an obligate part of the reentrant circuit or an "upper common pathway" is present within subatrial nodal structures in the triangle of Koch. Early studies have demonstrated dissociation of the atrium during AVNRT and provided evidence in favor of the presence of a common pathway [38, 39], with decremental conduction properties [40], without any participation of the atrium. High-resolution mapping of the triangle of Koch in canine hearts has demonstrated that reentrant ventricular echo beats did not require the perinodal tissue [41] and AVNRT has been recorded in a patient during atrial fibrillation [42]. However, observations based on conventional electrophysiology studies have questioned the confinement of the AVNRT circuit to the AV node and suggested that the retrograde fast pathway may not involve normal AV nodal tissue. Schuger et al. [43] have shown that after concealed antegrade impulse penetration, the retrograde fast pathway in AVNRT exhibits an abrupt transition from full excitability to absolute refractoriness unlike AV nodal tissue. This "all or none" type of conduction had also been described in other studies [44–46]. Experimental and clinical studies presented evidence of perinodal involvement in the tachycardia circuit [47, 48], and slow pathway radiofrequency ablation in patients with AVNRT also

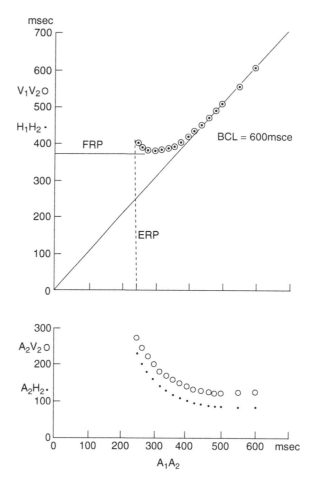

◻ Fig. 5.4

Normal anterograde conduction curves. Please note the gradual increase of AH intervals with shortening of the coupling intervals A₁A₂. ERP and FRP are the effective and functional refractory periods of the AV node (From Ward and Camm [11]. © Edward Arnold, London. Reproduced with permission)

resulted in persistent nondecremental retrograde conduction [49]. McGuire et al. [50] have demonstrated two types of presumed slow-fast AVNRT, corresponding to the A and B types previously described by the same group [51]. In the anterior type, the earliest atrial activity was recorded before ventricular activation and recorded near the His bundle, whereas in the posterior type, ventriculoatrial (VA) intervals were longer and the earliest atrial activity was recorded near the coronary sinus (CS) ostium. Although the different atrial activation sequences may be explained by intranodal circuits with different atrial exits, differences in ventriculoatrial intervals and tachycardia cycle lengths (TCLs) of the two tachycardias in each patient suggested different circuits for each tachycardia. This implies that a common pathway of AV nodal tissue is not present above the reentrant circuit and suggests that perinodal atrium forms part of the circuit. Recent observations have also documented that the majority of patients with AVNRT have multiple heterogenous sites of early atrial activation during the arrhythmia rather than a focal breakthrough site, thus arguing against the concept of an anatomically discrete pathway [52]. It has been therefore postulated that the so-called "proximal common pathway" is probably a broad area allowing fast and slow pathways to have different retrograde exit sites [52, 53]. A recent study with direct recording of the AV nodal electrograms and correlation with histology has showed that the AV nodal reentry occurs in the complex network of nodal and transitional cells and in the rim of surrounding atrial cells [54].

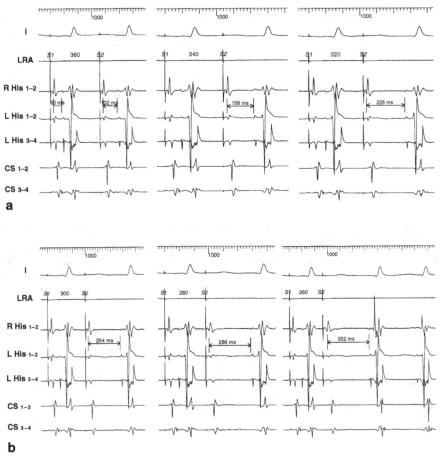

◻ Fig. 5.5
Multiple conduction jumps (a) and decrement before tachycardia initiation (b), indicating the presence of more than one "slow" pathway. *I*: ECG lead, *LRA*: low right atrium, *RHis*: His bundle recorded from the right septum, *LHis*: His bundle recorded from the left septum, *CS*: coronary sinus

Controversy also exists regarding the so-called lower common pathway, i.e., the tissue between the tachycardia circuit and the His bundle [40, 55, 56]. The conduction time over the lower common pathway has been usually estimated by subtracting the H-A interval during tachycardia from that during ventricular pacing at the same cycle length and considered a measurable interval in the majority of typical AVNRT cases [40]. Studies utilizing para-Hisian pacing, however, have failed to detect evidence of a lower common pathway in typical slow-fast AVNRT, as opposed to fast-slow or slow-slow AVNRT, and have actually used its presence to contribute toward the differential diagnosis between those forms of the tachycardia [55, 56].

Finally, the possibility of functional as opposed to anatomic reentry has also been raised. As already discussed, the demonstration of dual AV nodal characteristics is not a prerequisite for the induction of AVNRT, and successful ablation of the slow pathway does not necessitate changes in AV nodal duality characteristics and slow pathway electrophysiological parameters [57, 58]. The AV junction anatomical structure contains the conditions for the existence of functional pathways. A deep central portion is surrounded by successive layers of myocardium that gradually merge with atrial myocardium [59, 60]. In the region located anteriorly to the coronary sinus os, the terminal atrial tissue overlaps the AV node, showing a smooth rather than abrupt transition [61]. This area has the lowest velocity among cardiac tissues, including the node itself, demonstrates a high level of automaticity, and has characteristics of functional longitudinal

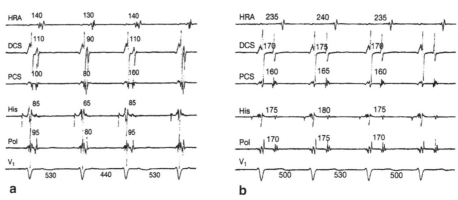

◻ Fig. 5.6

Anterior slow-fast AVNRT (**a**) and posterior slow-fast or slow-slow AVNRT (**b**) with alternating retrograde conduction intervals. This recording was obtained during slow pathway ablation and indicates AVNRT circuits alternatively using two different pathways in the retrograde direction. (From Katritsis et al. [35]. © John Wiley & Sons. Reproduced with permission.) V_1: ECG lead, *HRA*: high right atrium, *His*: His bundle, *Pol*: ablating catheter, *DCS*: distal coronary sinus, *PCS*: proximal coronary sinus

dissociation [3, 61, 62]. Jalife [63] has shown that conduction jump and reentry can occur in a nonhomogeneous linear structure if conduction occurs electrotonically across an area of block and has demonstrated dual pathway responses in isolated Purkinje fibers. It seems that tissue anisotropy, because of fiber orientation heterogenicity and consequent anisotropic conduction or spatial inhomogeneity of refractoriness, may contribute to different electrophysiological characteristics [64, 65] as well as pharmacological responses of functional pathways that, given the right conditions, might constitute the antegrade and retrograde limbs of the circuit [66, 67].

5.2.4   Proposed Models of the AVNRT Circuit

There is now evidence suggesting that AVNRT most probably results from reentry in various locations in the AV nodal and atrial perinodal area. The old model of the reentrant circuit comprised by two anatomically distinct limbs confined to the AV node is too oversimplified to represent reality. It is also debatable whether the two antegrade pathways seen in the majority of patients with AVNRT are the same two pathways used in the reentry circuit during tachycardia [68].

Wu and colleagues [69] have proposed that the slow pathway is the compact node and its posterior input of transitional cells, whereas the retrograde fast pathway is the anterior superficial group of transitional cells. Keim et al. [70] have proposed a more comprehensive model: the AV node, at least in patients with AVNRT, containing fibers capable of different conduction velocity. The fastest of the fast fibers and the slowest of the slow run at opposite edges of the AV node, superiorly and inferiorly, respectively, whereas the fibers between them are responsible for normal antegrade conduction without participation in the arrhythmia. Transitional nodal or atrial fibers constitute the upper connection of those two fiber sets. Patterson and Scherlag [68] have proposed a combined anatomic and functional model based on several hypotheses: transitional cells are the normal input for the fast pathway, AV Wenckebach behavior is due to another group of transitional cells (mid pathway), and fast pathway AV conduction during sinus rhythm and VA conduction during AVNRT are different. Spach and Josephson [71] have adopted a purely anisotropic model. The genesis of AVNRT is attributed to nonuniform anisotropy due to sparse side-to-side coupling between cells in the triangle of Koch. However, although anisotropic properties of the transitional cells do have a certain role in the genesis of this arrhythmia, anisotropic reentry as such cannot be accounted for the typical electrophysiologic characteristics of dual AV nodal conduction and AVNRT [72, 73].

5.2.5   The Role of Inferior Nodal Extensions

We have recently proposed a new model based on the description of the inferior nodal extensions [74, 75]. In 1906, Tawara described inferior extensions of the AV node in the human heart [76]. Later Becker and colleagues provided histological evidence of both rightward and leftward inferior extensions and speculated that they may be involved in slow pathway conduction [4, 77, 78]. The inferior nodal extensions are basically part of the AV node and facilitate atrial inputs that also contain transitional cells connecting atrial myocardium with the nodal extensions. Recent experimental studies in the rabbit heart have related the inferior (posterior) extension with slow pathway conduction properties [79–82], and histopathologic examination of the septum following successful ablation of the slow pathway in the human has demonstrated interruption of a long right inferior atrial extension [83]. We have shown that atrial inputs to the AV node can be studied in the human and have examined their electrophysiological properties in patients with and without discontinuous AV conduction curves [74, 75]. Fourteen patients without AVRT (atrioventricular reentrant tachycardia) or AV conduction jumps were studied by simultaneous recording of right- and left-sided His bundle electrograms during multisite atrial pacing. When atrial pacing resulted in conduction through the slow pathway, left inferoparaseptal pacing produced shorter stimulus to His intervals (St-H), as compared to low right atrial pacing. The difference between St-H at maximum decrement and St-H at constant pacing was significantly smaller during left inferoparaseptal than low right atrial pacing [74]. These findings are compatible with the observation that the leftward inferior extension is much shorter in length than the rightward inferior extension [78, 79], and suggest that the inferior atrial extensions are involved in "slow pathway" conduction. We have also studied ten patients with AV conduction jumps and inducible slow-fast AVNRT, before and after successful slow pathway ablation [75]. Simultaneous His bundle recordings from right and left sides of the septum were made during right and left inferoparaseptal pacing. Longer stimulus to His intervals was measured during right inferoparaseptal pacing compared to left inferoparaseptal pacing, at similar coupling intervals during AVNRT induction. Post-ablation, St-H intervals at maximum AV nodal conduction decrement were similar during right inferoparaseptal and left inferoparaseptal pacing, at similar coupling intervals. Pre-ablation, differences between St-H intervals at AVNRT induction or maximum AV conduction decrement (indicating slow pathway conduction) and constant cycle length pacing (indicating fast pathway conduction) for right His recordings with right inferoparaseptal pacing were significantly greater than differences measured with left His during left inferoparaseptal pacing. Post-ablation, these differences disappeared. Resetting of AVNRT with a left inferoparaseptal extrastimulus was achieved in seven of ten patients and indicated the presence of an atrio-nodal connection that is operating on the left side of the septum and allows the advancement of the next His bundle electrogram.

Thus, the electrophysiologic characteristics of the right and left inferior atrial inputs to the human AV node in patients with AVNRT and their response to slow-pathway ablation provide further evidence that the inferior nodal extensions represent the anatomic substrate of the slow pathway. Nodal decremental conduction might represent a fusion between a decrementally conducting AV node as well as activation through the inferior inputs. The demonstration of a jump indicates a shift of activation through the inferior extensions that now act as the "slow pathway." Whether other superior extensions or the compact node itself [79, 80] might be responsible for the "fast pathway" is not known. Superior atrial inputs to the node have not been histologically demonstrated. However, the existence of multiple atrial inputs to the node is now established [84], and one might speculate that yet undefined superior extensions may also play a role in initial "fast pathway" conduction. There has been now considerable evidence that the right and left inferior extensions of the human AV node and the atrio-nodal inputs they facilitate may provide the anatomic substrate of the slow pathway, and a comprehensive model of the tachycardia circuit for all forms of atrioventricular nodal reentrant tachycardia based on the concept of atrio-nodal inputs has been proposed (❯ Fig. 5.7) [85].

5.3   The Electrocardiogram

Typically, AVNRT is a narrow, complex tachycardia, i.e., QRS duration is less than 120 ms (❯ Fig. 5.8), unless aberrant conduction, usually of the RBBB type, or a previous conduction defect exists. The QRS is normal in contour, but tachycardia-related ST depression may be seen during and after the event. The RR interval is regular, although some

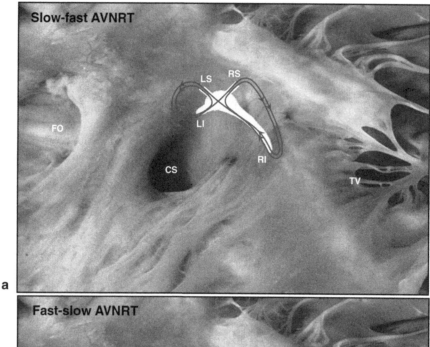

a

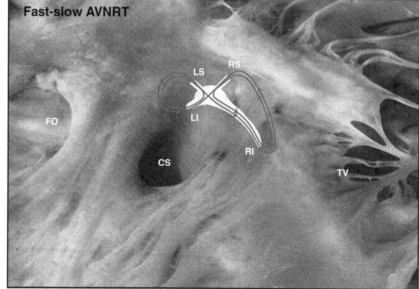

b

◘ Fig. 5.7

(a) Proposed circuit of slow-fast AVNRT. Right- or left-sided circuits may occur with antegrade conduction through the inferior inputs (slow pathway conduction) and retrograde conduction through the superior inputs (fast pathway conduction). Theoretical possibilities are for a *right-sided* circuit, a *left-sided* circuit, simultaneous right and left circuits, and figure-of-eight reentry. *Overlapping lines* indicate possibilities of alternating operating circuits. The site of earliest retrograde atrial activation also depends on the relative length of left and right superior atrial inputs. (b) Proposed circuit of fast-slow AVNRT. Circuits may occur with antegrade conduction through the superior inputs (fast pathway conduction), and retrograde conduction through the inferior inputs (slow pathway conduction). Possibilities are as in slow-fast but in the opposite direction. The site of earliest retrograde atrial activation depends on the relative length of left and right inferior atrial inputs. (c) Proposed circuit of slow-slow AVNRT. The circuit travels antegradely through the right inferior input and retrogradely through the left inferior input, although theoretically the opposite might also occur (please see text for details). (Adapted with kind permission from Katritsis and Becker.[85]) *RS*: right superior input, *LS*: left superior input, *RI*: right inferior input, *LI*: left inferior input, *CS*: coronary sinus, *TV*: tricuspid valve, *FO*: foramen ovale

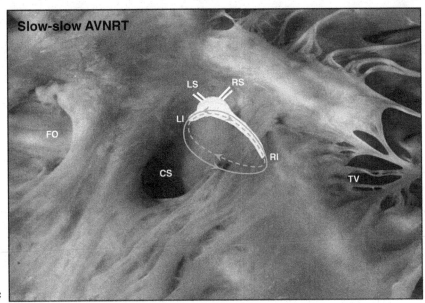

c

◘ Fig. 5.7 (Continued)

variation due to changes in AV nodal conduction time (as mainly determined by the slow pathway conduction characteristics) may be seen.

Abnormal (retrograde) P' waves are constantly related to the QRS and, in the majority of cases, are indiscernible or very close to the QRS complex ($RP'/RR < 0.5$). Thus P' waves are either masked by the QRS complex or seen as a small terminal P' wave that is not present during sinus rhythm (❷ Figs. 5.8 and ❷ 5.9). In the atypical form of AVNRT (fast-slow), P' waves are clearly visible before the QRS, i.e., $RP'/P'R > 0.75$ (❷ Fig. 5.10), denoting a "*long RP tachycardia*," and are negative in leads II, III, aVF, and V_6 but positive in V_1. P' waves are shallow in the inferior leads in the rare form of anterior fast-slow AVNRT [86]. Although AV dissociation is usually not seen, it can occur since neither the atria (or, more precisely, the majority of atrial tissue) nor the ventricles are necessary for the reentry circuit. If the tachycardia is initiated by atrial ectopic beats, the initial (ectopic) P' wave usually differs from the subsequent (retrograde) P' waves.

5.4 Electrophysiologic Study

5.4.1 Antegrade and Retrograde AV Conduction Curves

Discontinuous AV conduction curves (A_1-A_2/H_1-H_2 or A_1-A_2/A_2-H_2) are suggestive of the presence of antegrade dual AV junction pathway [12]. As previously discussed, discontinuous refractory period curves may not be necessarily demonstrated in all patients with AVNRT. In addition, the mere presence of AV nodal duality is not enough to predispose to paroxysmal tachycardia. Conventionally, an increase of at least 50 ms (conduction jump) in the AH interval for a decrease of 10 ms in the coupling interval (A_1-A_2) is considered to reflect dual AV nodal (or, more precisely, junctional) pathways. Failure to demonstrate dual pathways in patients with AVNRT may occur due to several factors as follows.

1. The functional refractory period of the atrium limits the prematurity with which extrastimuli can encounter the AV node [13], or the refractory periods of the slow and fast pathways are similar. Stimulation at faster rates or the introduction of multiple extrastimuli is required in these cases in order to decrease atrial refractoriness or merely dissociate the two pathways [16].

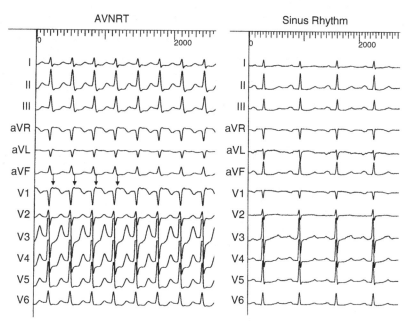

◘ Fig. 5.8
12-lead ECG during "slow-fast" AVNRT. Note that small P′ waves that are seen during tachycardia (*arrows*) are not present during sinus rhythm

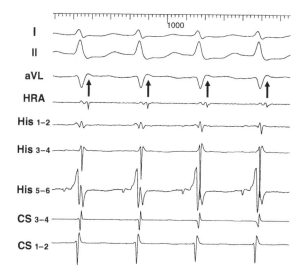

◘ Fig. 5.9
Slow-fast AVNRT from the same patient as in ❷ Fig. 5.8. Small P′ waves at the end of QRS correspond to retrograde atrial conduction (*arrows*). I: ECG lead, II: lead II of the surface ECG, *aVL*: lead aVL of the surface ECG, *HRA*: high right atrium, *His*: His bundle, *CS*: coronary sinus

2. The slow pathway has a longer antegrade refractory period than the fast one, thus preventing the demonstration of a jump, as happens with the fast-slow variety of AVNRT. Retrograde stimulation curves in these patients may demonstrate a jump if the retrograde refractory period of the fast pathway exceeds the retrograde refractory period of the slow one [23].

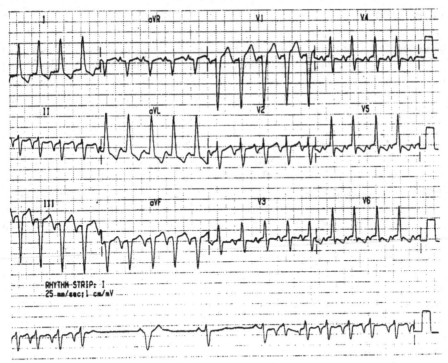

◘ Fig. 5.10
12-lead ECG during fast-slow AVNRT. Note the prolonged R-P′ and the incessant nature of the tachycardia

Ventricular extrastimulation frequently demonstrates continuous VA conduction curves with either fixed or minimal prolongation of the VA interval in patients with typical slow-fast AVNRT [87–89]. This has been traditionally accepted to reflect retrograde fast pathway conduction [90]. Decremental conduction or retrograde jumps may also occur. During retrograde stimulation curves, it is often difficult to obtain recordings of the retrograde His bundle potential. In the literature, retrograde conduction properties of the fast and slow pathways have been derived indirectly by analyzing the conduction curves (V_1-V_2/A_1-A_2). Thus, in case of discontinuous retrograde curves, the longest V_1-V_2 interval in which conduction fails in the fast pathway is assumed to be the retrograde effective refractory period of the fast pathway, and the shortest attainable A_1-A_2 interval on the fast pathway conduction curves (i.e., to the right of discontinuity) is assumed to be its functional refractory period. Similarly, the analysis of the curves on the left of discontinuity, which represent a slow pathway conduction, provides the refractory periods of the slow pathway [24, 53]. This method assumes that no other causes of discontinuities in VA conduction, such as intraventricular conduction delays, exist.

As a rule, at least two cycle lengths (usually 600 and 400 ms) should be studied both antegradely and retrogradely. On certain occasions, the application of two or three extrastimuli may be necessary to expose slow pathway conduction or to induce critical conduction delay required for the initiation of reentry.

5.4.2 Initiation of Tachycardia

The initiation of AVNRT in the electrophysiology laboratory can be accomplished by atrial or ventricular extrastimulation. These modes of induction have been explained according to the conventionally accepted mechanism, although, as previously discussed, this may not be the case.

5.4.2.1 Slow-Fast AVNRT

According to conventionally accepted mechanisms, the requirements for the induction of AVNRT are blocked in an antegrade fast pathway conduction with continued conduction in a slow pathway with critical AV nodal (AH) delay, followed by retrograde conduction over the fast pathway [91]. A critical AV node conduction is necessary in order to allow the antegradely blocked fast pathway to recover and resume retrograde conduction, leading to the occurrence of an atrial echo beat. Depending, therefore, on both critical antegrade delay and retrograde conduction properties, the echo zones may not coincide with the entire slow pathway conduction curves. Sustained reentry requires the ability for repetitive antegrade slow pathway and repetitive retrograde fast pathway conduction.

A *single atrial extrastimulus* can initiate the slow-fast form of tachycardia by producing antegrade block in the fast pathway while conducting through the slow one (❯ Fig. 5.2). If the tachycardia is induced during the conduction of antegrade AV conduction curves, usually a typical decrement (jump) precedes the initiation of tachycardia, but this is not always seen. If the atrial pacing length has already reached antegrade fast pathway refractoriness, with resultant antegrade AV conduction exclusively over the slow pathway, tachycardia initiation is associated by smooth rather than discontinuous AV node conduction curves. *Double or triple atrial extrastimuli* or *incremental atrial pacing* may occasionally be required for tachycardia induction [16]. At critical atrial pacing rates, either a jump or an atypical Wenckebach periodicity or even both can be seen [92]. At faster pacing cycle lengths, the conduction time of one pathway may be prolonged with simultaneous lengthening of the refractoriness of the other pathway. Consequently, the resultant atrial echo zone is widened, and self-initiation (i.e., without an atrial extrastimulus) of sustained reentry may become possible at shorter pacing lengths. Rarely, atrial extrastimuli or even sinus beats may produce simultaneous fast and slow pathway conduction, resulting in double ventricular responses [93]. Repetition of such a phenomenon produces a paroxysmal form of non-reentrant tachycardia [94, 95].

Ventricular extrastimuli or *incremental ventricular pacing* may also initiate slow-fast reentry, but much less commonly than atrial stimulation. In one third of patients, tachycardia can be initiated by ventricular extrastimuli [90]. This mode of tachycardia initiation requires that the slow pathway has a retrograde refractory period longer than that of the fast pathway. Consequently, the ventricular extrastimulus blocks in the slow pathway and is conducted over the fast one, thus preventing the demonstration of any retrograde jump. Retrograde refractoriness of the His–Purkinje system appears to be an important limiting factor with respect to initiation by ventricular pacing.

5.4.2.2 Fast-Slow AVNRT

Ventricular extrastimuli may cause initiation of tachycardia after blocking the fast pathway and conducted retrogradely over the slow pathway. After the attainment of a critical VA conduction delay (H_2-A_2), the impulse is conducted through the fast pathway in the antegrade direction and produces a ventricular echo. The ventricular echo zone may or may not coincide with the entire retrograde slow pathway conduction curves since the ventricular or the His–Purkinje tissue may exhibit conduction delay in response to ventricular extrastimulation, thereby precluding maintenance of critical H_2-A_2 delay. When tachycardia is induced during retrograde curves, its initiation is usually preceded by a sudden jump in ventriculoatrial conduction times. If, however, the ventricular pacing length has already reached retrograde fast pathway refractoriness with resultant retrograde VA conduction exclusively over the slow pathway, tachycardia initiation is associated by smooth rather than discontinuous VA conduction curves. *Incremental ventricular pacing* can also induce tachycardia of this form with a mechanism analogous to the one described previously for the slow-fast form.

Atrial extrastimuli can initiate tachycardia of this form only if the slow pathway has an antegrade refractory period longer than that of the fast pathway being incapable of antegrade conduction. Sudden increment of AV conduction, therefore, is not noted in this case. The critical AV node conduction delay required for the initiation of an atrial echo or sustained reentry is minimal, since the A_1-H_2 interval is within the range of antegrade fast pathway conduction times. When the slow pathway has markedly prolonged antegrade refractoriness relative to that of the fast pathway (wide window), late atrial premature beats or spontaneous acceleration of the sinus rate can easily induce AV node reentry of the fast-slow form. This may explain the incessant nature of this tachycardia.

The initiation of an AV junctional reentry tachycardia of any form is therefore dependent on several factors such as the effective refractory periods of the two pathways, the functional refractory periods of the atrium or the ventricle, and the number of the delivered extrastimuli or the cycle length of the basic pacing drive. Both atrial and ventricular incremental pacing may facilitate initiation of AV node reentry tachycardia of either form [12]. In certain occasions, isoprenaline infusion or atropine may be necessary to modulate the autonomic tone and allow the induction and sustenance of tachycardia [96].

5.4.3 Effect of Stimulation During Tachycardia

A late single atrial extrastimulus may fail to depolarize the entire atria or, if the atria are depolarized, may fail to penetrate the reentrant circuit causing a compensatory pause without affecting the cycle length of the tachycardia. Earlier extrastimuli may penetrate the reentrant circuit, resulting in premature depolarization of the atria and termination of the tachycardia. Resetting of the tachycardia may also occur, although rarely, because atrial refractoriness usually does not allow adequately early extrastimuli. The latter usually happens in AVNRTs with cycle lengths more than 300 ms, unless the stimulation is carried out very close to the AV node (❯ Fig. 5.11). Faster AVNRTs usually require two extrastimuli or rapid atrial pacing to stop.

Ventricular extrastimuli behave in a similar manner. A very important point typical of AVNRTs is the inability of His-synchronous ventricular extrastimuli to capture the atrium and advance or delay the subsequent atrial activation or reset the whole tachycardia cycle. Ventricular extrastimulation is very important for the differential diagnosis, as will be discussed later.

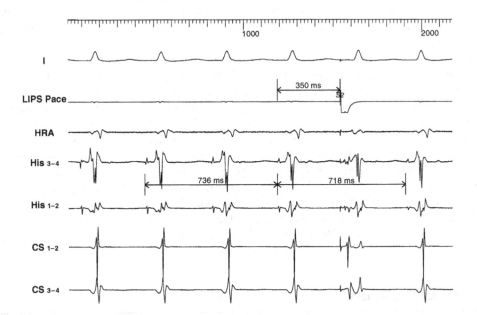

☐ Fig. 5.11
Resetting of slow-fast AVNRT. The tachycardia cycle length is 365 ms. An atrial extrastimuli is delivered from the left inferoparaseptal area very close to the His area, 350 ms following the His bundle activation, and results in resetting of the next His bundle electrogram. I: ECG lead, *HRA*: high right atrium, *His*: His bundle, *CS*: coronary sinus, *LIPS*: left inferoparaseptal pacing

5.5   Electrophysiologic Forms of AVNRT

According to the conventional description of a dual AV junctional pathway, AVNRT has been traditionally classified as slow-fast or typical AVNRT, and fast-slow or atypical AVNRT. The fast pathway of the reentry circuit runs superiorly and anteriorly in the triangle of Koch, whereas the slow pathway runs inferiorly and posteriorly close to the coronary sinus ostium [70]. Indeed, detailed endocardial mapping in patients with AVNRT has demonstrated that in the majority of slow-fast cases of AVNRT, the site of earliest atrial activation is close to the apex of Koch's triangle, near the AV node–His bundle junction, i.e., anterior to the node [44, 97]. Thus, the earliest retrograde A, whenever atrial electrograms are separated from ventricular ones, occurs in the His bundle electrogram, followed by the ostium of the coronary sinus, distal coronary sinus, and high right atrium [14, 97]. Depolarization of the distal coronary sinus may also be simultaneous or slightly later than in the high right atrium. However, the recognition of the fact that all forms of AVNRT may present with atypical retrograde atrial activation has made classification attempts more complicated, and a universally accepted scheme does not exist. Most authors, however, would accept the following classification:

1. In *typical or slow-fast form* of AVNRT, the onset of atrial activation appears prior, at the onset, or just after the QRS complex, thus maintaining an atrial-His/His-atrial ratio A-H/H-A > 1 (❂ Fig. 5.2). In particular, the following criteria are considered as diagnostic for the slow-fast form of AVNRT: an A-H/H-A ratio > 3 [44], a VA interval measured from the onset of ventricular activation on the surface ECG to the earliest deflection of the atrial activation in the His bundle electrogram < 60 ms, or a VA interval measured at the high right atrium < 95 ms [98]. Although, typically, the earliest retrograde atrial activation is being recorded at the His bundle electrogram, cases of posterior retrograde fast pathways, i.e., with posterior earliest retrograde atrial activation at the CS [99] have been described.

2. In *atypical or fast-slow form* of AVNRT (approximately 5–10% of all AVNRT cases), retrograde atrial electrograms begin well after ventricular activation with an A-H/H-A ratio < 1, indicating that retrograde conduction is slower than antegrade conduction [24]. The VA interval measured from the onset of ventricular activation on surface ECG to the earliest deflection of the atrial activation in the His bundle electrogram is > 60 ms, and in the high right atrium > 100 [100]. In the majority of fast-slow cases, the site of earliest atrial activation is posterior to the AV node near the orifice of the coronary sinus [49, 101]. However, anterior and mid-forms of fast-slow AVNRT have also been described [33, 86].

3. In the *slow-slow form*, the A-H/H-A ratio is > 1 but the VA interval is > 60 ms, suggesting that two slow pathways are utilized for both anterograde and retrograde activation [33, 102]. Usually, but not always, earliest atrial activation is at the posterior septum (coronary sinus ostium) [33, 102]. The so-called *posterior or type B* AVNRT can be demonstrated in approximately 2% of patients with the anterior form of slow-fast AVNRT [50]. In posterior tachycardia, the VA times (as measured from the onset of ventricular activity to the onset of atrial activity by whichever electrode recorded the earliest interval) may be prolonged, ranging from 76 to 168 ms [50]. The atrial-His/His-atrial ratio, however, remains more than one. Some cases of posterior slow-fast AVNRT may actually represent the slow-slow form [26, 99]. Since conduction times are sensitive to autonomic changes, attempts to classify the AVNRT forms according to retrograde atrial activation sequence and the possibility of demonstrating a lower common pathway, have appeared [56]. We know now that all forms of AVNRT (slow-fast, fast-slow, and slow-slow) may display anterior, posterior, and middle retrograde activation patterns [86]. Heterogeneity of both fast and slow conduction patterns has been well described, and in certain patients all forms of AVNRT may be inducible [33, 86].

5.6   Differential Diagnosis

5.6.1   Narrow-QRS Tachycardia

In the presence of a narrow QRS tachycardia, AVNRT should be differentiated from atrial tachycardia or orthodromic atrioventricular reentrant tachycardia (AVRT) due to an accessory pathway, i.e., tachycardia using the AV node for antegrade conduction and the accessory pathway for retrograde conduction.

5.6.1.1 AVNRT versus Atrial Tachycardia

Simple pacing maneuvers can be utilized in order to exclude reentrant or triggered atrial tachycardias. If there is demonstration of change in (1) AA interval when a ventricular extrastimulus is delivered during tachycardia, (2) tachycardia termination by a ventricular extrastimulus that did not conduct to the atrium, (3) constant His-atrial interval of the return cycle after the introduction of a premature atrial impulse with a wide range of coupling intervals during tachycardia, and (4) ventricle to atrium to His sequence during retrograde initiation of tachycardia, then the aetiology is other than atrial tachycardia [103–105]. In particular, the atrial response upon cessation of ventricular pacing associated with 1:1 ventriculoatrial conduction during tachycardia can distinguish between atrial tachycardia and AVNRT or AVRT. Atrial tachycardia is associated with an A-A-V response, whereas AVNRT or AVRT produce an A-V response [104]. The difference in the AH interval between atrial pacing and the tachycardia may also allow differentiation of AVNRT from atrial tachycardia. A Δ A-H >40 ms indicates AVNRT, whereas in atrial tachycardia this difference is <10 msec [105]. This concept is discussed later under the differential diagnosis of AVNRT vs. AVRT.

5.6.1.2 AVNRT versus AVRT due to Accessory Pathways

The eccentric retrograde atrial activation during ventricular stimulation or tachycardia and the demonstration of continuous AV or VA conduction curves usually characterizing nonseptal concealed accessory pathways, differentiate this form of atrioventricular reentry from AVNRT. Care is needed, however, since AVNRT is now known to occur with eccentric atrial activation and, in addition, decremental septal pathways may mimic AVNRT especially of the fast-slow or slow-slow forms (❷ Fig. 5.12). Septal pathways may have the property of decremental conduction [106, 107] and normal atrial retrograde activation during tachycardia. These tachycardias tend to be incessant [108, 109]. The documentation of preexcited beats as well as AV dissociation and the induction of bundle branch block (BBB) during tachycardia may assist the differential diagnosis. The demonstration of AV block or AV dissociation during tachycardia is characteristic of AVNRT excluding the presence of an accessory pathway [110, 111]. Similarly, the development of bundle branch block either spontaneously or after the introduction of ventricular extrastimuli during AVNRT does not change the AA or HH intervals. Although the first VV interval may be prolonged for one cycle due to HV prolongation associated with the development of BBB, the subsequent cycles of tachycardia are identical to the basic tachycardia cycle length. A significant change in the VA interval with the development of bundle branch block is diagnostic of orthodromic AVRT and localizes the pathway to the same side as the block [112].

In general, septal ventriculoatrial interval < 70 ms is diagnostic of slow-fast AVNRT provided that atrial tachycardia has been excluded [113, 114]. In the case of relatively delayed retrograde conduction that allows the identification of retrograde P waves, ECG criteria can be applied for diagnosis. The presence of a pseudo r′ wave in lead V1 or a pseudo S wave in leads II, III, and aVF was indicative of anterior AVNRT with an accuracy of 100%. A difference of RP′ intervals in lead V_1 and III > 20 ms was indicative of posterior AVNRT rather than AVRT due to a posteroseptal pathway [115].

In septal decremental pathways, ventricular extrastimuli introduced while the His bundle is refractory during tachycardia may advance or delay subsequent atrial activation (extranodal capture), whereas in slow-fast AVNRT, either anterior or posterior, atrial activity is not perturbed. Atrial capture at a time when the His bundle is refractory implies the presence of an accessory pathway (❷ Fig. 5.13) [116]. In practice, the extrastimulus has to be delivered coincident with the His potential or up to 50 ms before this [117]. Failure to reset the atria (❷ Fig. 5.14) suggests, but does not prove, that an accessory pathway is not present or that it is relatively far from the site of premature stimulation (e.g., right ventricular stimulation in the presence of a left free wall pathway) [118]. Theoretically, it is possible that resetting of the atrium might be a result of an increase in conduction time over such a pathway of a magnitude equal to the interval by which the extrastimulus preceded atrial activation, but such a coincidence is rare. In addition, at the time of His bundle activation, the accessory pathway may be refractory and resetting by ventricular extrastimuli may not be seen. Failure to demonstrate resetting, therefore, does not exclude an anomalous septal pathway with decremental properties. Thus,

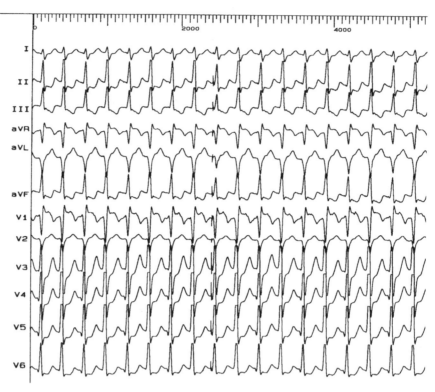

◘ Fig. 5.12

12-lead ECG during atrioventricular reentrant tachycardia due to a posteroseptal accessory pathway

resetting or termination of the tachycardia with His-refractory ventricular extrastimuli is a specific but not highly sensitive criterion for differential diagnosis. Additional criteria have therefore been suggested. Using ventricular-induced atrial preexcitation, Miles et al. [119] devised a preexcitation index for the differentiation of AVNRT and AVRT using an accessory pathway. Progressively premature right ventricular extrastimuli (V_2) were introduced during tachycardia, and the difference between the tachycardia cycle length and the longest V_1V_2 at which atrial preexcitation occurred defined the preexcitation index. Atrial preexcitation occurred in 10% of 22 patients with AVNRT compared with 89% of 55 patients with AVRT. A preexcitation index of 100 ms or greater characterized AVNRT, whereas an index less than 45 ms characterized AVRT using a septal pathway. Left free wall pathways had indices of 75 ms or greater. In another report of 16 patients with AVNRT and 23 patients with AVRT studied at St. George's Hospital in London, the ratio between the minimum ventriculoatrial interval during tachycardia and ventricular pacing was 0.32–0.27 in AVNRT, 0.48–0.71 in AVRT using a left free wall pathway, 0.91–1.08 in posteroseptal pathways, 0.94–1.29 in anteroseptal pathways, and 1.53–1.68 in right free wall pathways [114]. A difference in the VA interval during tachycardia and right apical ventricular pacing > 90 ms has also been reported to differentiate patients with AVNRT from those with AVRT [120]. The difference between the ventriculoatrial interval obtained during apical pacing and that obtained during posterobasal pacing (ventriculoatrial index) can also discriminate between patients with posteroseptal pathways (> 10 ms) and patients with nodal retrograde conduction (< 5 ms) [121].

Miller et al. [122] found the His to atria (HA) intervals to offer more precise discrimination. Their criterion is the difference between His to atrial intervals during pacing and during tachycardia (ΔHA). In 84 patients, a retrograde His was present in 93% of them and the ΔHA was > 0 ms in AVNRT and < −27 ms in orthodromic AVRT incorporating a septal accessory pathway. Thus, an intermediate value of ΔHA = −10 ms had 100% sensitivity, specificity, and predictive accuracy in differentiating the two forms of tachycardia. Parahisian pacing and the change in timing and sequence of retrograde atrial activation between His and proximal right bundle branch capture and noncapture has also been

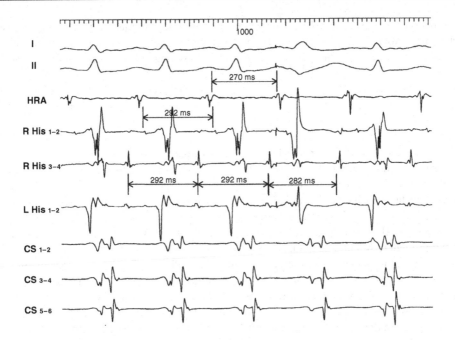

◘ Fig. 5.13
Resetting of atrioventricular reentrant tachycardia due to a left posteroseptal accessory pathway. The tachycardia cycle length is 292 ms. At 270 ms, a ventricular extrastimulus is delivered at a time when the His bundle is expected to be refractory and resets the next atrial electrogram (from 292 to 282 ms). I, II: ECG leads, *HRA*: high right atrium, *RHis*: His bundle recorded from the right septum, *LHis*: His bundle recorded from the left septum, *CS*: coronary sinus

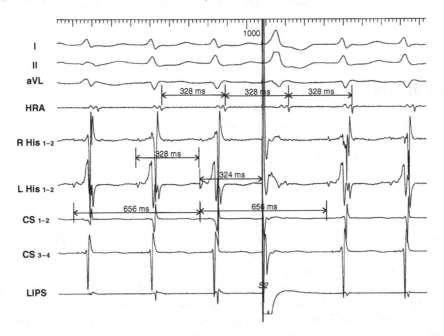

◘ Fig. 5.14
No resetting of AVNRT. Absence of resetting with para-Hisian pacing from the right septum. I, II, aVL: ECG leads, *HRA*: high right atrium, *RHis*: His bundle recorded from the right septum, *LHis*: His bundle recorded from the left septum, *CS*: coronary sinus, *RIPS*: right inferoparaseptal area

used for differentiation between AV nodal and septal pathway retrograde conduction [123]. The response is considered extranodal when the retrograde atrial activation during His bundle capture is the same as during ventricular capture without His bundle capture. These techniques, however, require recording of both antegrade and retrograde His bundle activation.

The difference in the AH interval between atrial pacing and the tachycardia may also allow differentiation of atypical AVNRT from other types of long RP tachycardias. A ΔA-H > 40 ms indicates AVNRT, whereas in atrial tachycardia, this difference is <10 ms [105].

Right apical stimulation is relatively close to the insertion of a septal accessory pathway as opposed to the AV junction. Thus, ventricular fusion during resetting or entrainment of tachycardia has been reported to occur in patients with AVRT due to septal pathways but not with AVNRT [124]. Michaud et al. [100] have proposed two additional criteria for differential diagnosis. The ventriculoatrial (VA) interval and tachycardia cycle length (TCL) were measured during tachycardia, and entrainment of the tachycardia was accomplished with right apical ventricular pacing. The intervals between the last ventricular pacing stimulus and the last entrained atrial depolarization during tachycardia (SA) as well as the post-pacing interval were considered. All patients with AVNRT had SA-VA intervals > 85 ms and PPI-TCL intervals > 114 ms [100]. Conventional entrainment techniques do not take into account pacing induced incremental AV nodal conduction (ie in the post-pacing A-H) that may alter the PPI. Thus, Gonzalez-Torrecilla et al [126], "corrected" the PPI-TCL difference by subtracting from it the difference: postpacing AH interval minus basic AH interval. The presence of a corrected PPI-TCL < 110 ms indicated AVRT. Entrainment through basal RV pacing away from the septum may produce prolonged PPI-TCL intervals in the absence of a septal pathway due to the distance of the RV base from the AV node (activation occurs retrogradely through the distal His-Purkinje system) and has been found superior to apical entrainment for diagnostic purposes [127]. A differential (between base and apex) corrected PPI-TCL >30 ms or a differential VA interval > 20 ms has been reported to predict AVNRT very reliably [128]. The main advantage of this technique is that the differential VA interval could be calculated from the last paced beat in case the tachycardia was terminated after transient entrainment.

It should be noted that in clinical practice, pacing or other maneuvers cannot be applied to all cases and multiple criteria have to be used for the differential diagnosis of narrow complex tachycardias with atypical characteristics [113].

5.6.2   Wide-WRS Tachycardia

In the presence of wide-QRS tachycardia, when ventricular tachycardia is excluded, antidromic atrioventricular reentrant tachycardia should be differentiated from AVNRT with a bystanding accessory pathway, and the possibilities of AVNRT or atrial tachycardia with aberrant conduction due to bundle branch block should also be considered.

5.6.2.1   AVNRT with a bystanding Accessory Pathway versus Antidromic AVRT

Antidromic AVRT, i.e., tachycardia utilizing the accessory pathway for antegrade conduction and the AV node for retrograde conduction, may be induced in approximately 6% of the patients with accessory pathways located in the left or right free wall, or the anterior septum at an adequate distance from the AV node [125]. In some cases, atrioventricular junctional reentry may be the underlying mechanism of the preexcited tachycardia and the possibility of AVNRT conducting over a bystanding accessory pathway should be considered in the presence of transition from narrow to wide complex tachycardia of a similar cycle length and without disturbing the HH intervals [129]. In this case, atrial extrastimuli fail to induce advancement of the following preexcited QRS complex, the next retrograde His bundle deflection where apparent, and the subsequent atrial deflection, as may happen in the presence of a macroreentrant loop [130].

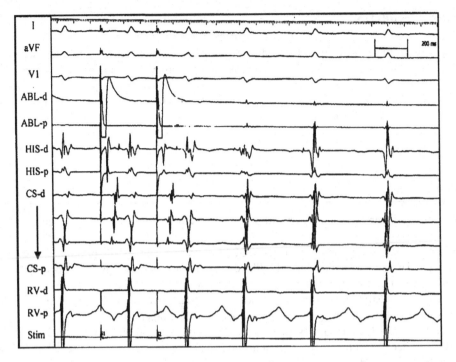

◘ Fig. 5.15

Junctional tachycardia initiated with atrial pacing. Although there is a prolonged AH interval during tachycardia, the first tachycardia beat conducts without AH delay. (Reproduced from Hamdan et al. [136] with kind permission.) I, aVF, V₁: ECG leads, *ABL*: ablation catheter, *His*: His bundle, *CS*: coronary sinus, *RV*: right ventricle, *Stim*: stimulation channel

5.7 Non-Reentrant AV Junctional Tachycardias

5.7.1 Non-Paroxysmal Junctional Tachycardias

The term *non-paroxysmal junctional tachycardia was* initially used to denote junctional rhythms of gradual onset and termination with a rate between 70 and 130 beats/min [131]. This tachycardia was frequently diagnosed in the past, and considered to be a typical example of a digitalis-induced arrhythmia [132]. Non-paroxysmal junctional tachycardia usually occurs in patients with underlying heart disease, such as myocardial infarction, or after open-heart surgery, although it can occur rarely in apparently normal persons [133, 134].

Most cases of non-paroxysmal junctional tachycardia, especially the digitalis-induced, are caused by delayed afterdepolarizations and triggered activity in the AV node [135]. In these patients, tachycardia can be induced by atrial ectopics or atrial pacing. Enhanced automaticity can also occur however, as suggested by the ability of this tachycardia in some patients to accelerate with enhanced sympathetic tone.

5.8 Focal Junctional Tachycardia

Focal junctional tachycardias have been also called automatic junctional tachycardias since the dominant (but not the only) mechanism is enhanced automaticity [136].

5.8.1 Pediatric Population

These tachycardias were first described in the pediatric population as junctional ectopic tachycardias [137] or His bundle tachycardias [138]. They may occur as a congenital arrhythmia [138–140] or early after infant open-heart surgery [141, 142]. The focus of the tachycardia seems to be localized in the lower part of the AV junction or, most probably, within the His bundle. They are dangerous forms of arrhythmia refractory to medical therapy, overdrive pacing, and DC cardioversion. Diagnosis is made on the ECG, which shows a narrow QRS tachycardia with slower and dissociated P waves. In electrophysiology study, there is a normal HV interval and normal AV conduction curves [139, 143].

5.8.2 Adults

In adult patients, the tachycardia is associated with a structurally normal heart and the prognosis is usually benign [144, 145].

The usual electrocardiographic finding is a narrow QRS tachycardia with AV dissociation. Occasionally, the tachycardia might be irregular, thus resembling atrial fibrillation. In the electrophysiology laboratory, the arrhythmia is not inducible by programmed electrical stimulation, thus making reentry an unlikely mechanism. It is, however, sensitive to isoproterenol administration, and in some cases, rapid atrial or ventricular pacing may result in tachycardia induction, suggesting abnormal automaticity or triggered activity as the other possible mechanism. During tachycardia, there is a normal or increased HV interval with atrioventricular dissociation that is interrupted by frequent episodes of ventriculoatrial conduction with earliest atrial activation in the posteroseptal, anteroseptal, or midseptal regions. At times, the mode of tachycardia induction resembles a double AV nodal response that is characteristic of AVNRT (❯ Fig. 5.15) [136].

References

1. Camm, A.J. and D. Katritsis, The diagnosis of tachyarrhythmias, in *Heart Disease*, 2 edn., D.G. Julian, A.J. Camm, K.M. Fox, R.J.C. Hall, and P.A. Poole-Wilson, Editors. Philadelphia, PA: Saunders, 1996, pp. 6606–6621.

2. Josephson, M.E. and H.J. Wellens, Electrophysiologic evaluation of supraventricular tachycardia. *Cardiol. Clin.*, 1997;**15**: 567–586.

3. Anderson, R.H., M.J. Janse, F.J.L. Van Capelle, et al., A combined morphological and electrophysiological study of the atrioventricular node of the rabbit heart. *Circulation* 1974;**35**: 909–922.

4. Becker, A.E. and R.H. Anderson, Morphology of the human atrioventricular junctional area, in *The Conduction System of the Heart. Structure, Function and Clinical Implications*, H.J.J. Wellens, K.I. Lie, and M.J. Janse, Editors. Leiden: HE Stenfert Kroese BV, 1976; pp. 263–286.

5. Racker, D.K., Atrioventricular node and input pathways: A correlated gross anatomical and histological study of canine atrioventricular junctional region. *Anat. Rec.*, 1989;**224**: 336–354.

6. Mines, G.R., On dynamic equilibrium of the heart. *J. Physiol.*, 1913;**46**: 349–354.

7. Moe, G.K., J.B. Preston, and H. Burlington, Physiologic evidence of a dual AV transmission system. *Circ. Res.*, 1956;**4**: 357–375.

8. Denes, P., R.C. Dhingra, R. Chuquimia, et al., Demonstration of dual AV nodal pathways in patients with paroxysmal supraventricular tachycardia. *Circulation*, 1973;**48**: 549–555.

9. Mendez, C., J. Han, P.D. Carcia de Jalon, et al., Some characteristics of ventricular echoes. *Circ. Res.*, 1965;**16**: 561–581.

10. Rosen, K.M., A. Mehta, and R.A. Miller, Demonstration of dual atrioventricular nodal pathways in man. *Am. J. Cardiol.*, 1974;**33**: 13–18.

11. Ward, D.E. and A.J. Camm, *Clinical Electrophysiology of the Heart*. London: E Arnold, 1987.

12. Katritsis, D.G. and A.J. Camm, Classification and differential diagnosis of atrioventricular nodal re-entrant tachycardia. *Europace*, 2006;**8**: 29–36.

13. Denes, P., D. Wu, R. Dhingra, et al., Dual atrioventricular nodal pathways. A common electrophysiological response. *Br. Heart J.*, 1975;**37**: 1069–1076.

14. Josephson, M.E. and J.A. Kastor, Supraventricular tachycardia: Mechanisms and management. *Ann. Intern. Med.*, 1977;**87**: 346–358.

15. Tai, C.T., S.A. Chen, C.E. Chiang, et al., Complex electrophysiological characteristics in atrioventricular nodal re-entrant tachycardia with continuous atrioventricular node function curves. *Circulation*, 1997;**95**: 2541–2547.

16. Kuo, C.T., K.H. Lin, N.J. Cheng, et al., Characterization of atrioventricular nodal reentry with continuous atrioventricular node conduction curve by double atrial extrastimulation. *Circulation*, 1999;**99**: 659–665.

17. Sheahan, R.G., G.J. Klein, R. Yee, C.A. Le Feuvre, and A.D. Krahn, Atrioventricular node reentry with 'smooth' AV

node function curves: A different arrhythmia substrate? *Circulation*, 1996;**93**: 969–972.

18. Levites, R. and J.I. Haft, Evidence suggesting dual AV nodal pathways in patients without supraventricular tachycardias. *Chest*, 1975;**67**: 36–42.

19. Thapar, M.K. and P.C. Gillette, Dual atrioventricular nodal pathways: A common electrophysiologic response in children. *Circulation*, 1979;**60**: 1369–1374.

20. Casta, A., G.S. Wolff, A.V. Mehta, et al., Dual atrioventricular nodal pathways: A benign finding in arrhythmia-free children with heart disease. *Am. J. Cardiol.*, 1980;**46**: 1013–1018.

21. Brugada, P., B. Heddle, M. Green, et al., Initiation of atrioventricular nodal reentrant tachycardia in patients with discontinuous anterograde atrioventricular nodal conduction curves with and without documented supraventricular tachycardia: Observations on the role of discontinuous retrograde conduction curve. *Am. Heart J.*, 1984;**107**: 685–697.

22. Reyes, W., S. Milstein, A. Dunnigan, et al., Indications for modification of coexisting dual atrioventricular node pathways in patients undergoing surgical ablation of accessory atrioventricular connections. *J. Am. Coll. Cardiol.*, 1991;**17**: 1561–1567.

23. Wu, D., P. Denes, F. Amay-y-Leon, et al., An unusual variety of atrioventricular nodal re-entry due to retrograde dual atrioventricular nodal pathways. *Circulation*, 1977;**56**: 50–59.

24. Sung, R.J., J.L. Styperek, R.J. Myerburg, and A. Castellanos, Initiation of two distinct forms of atrioventricular nodal reentrant tachycardia during programmed ventricular stimulation in man. *Am. J. Cardiol.*, 1978;**42**: 404–415.

25. Coumel, P., P. Attuel, and J.F. Leclercq, Permanent form of junctional reciprocating tachycardia: Mechanism, clinical and therapeutic implications, in *Cardiac Arrhythmias: Electrophysiology, Diagnosis and Management*, O.S. Narula, Editors. Baltimore, MD: Williams and Wilkins, 1979, pp. 347–363.

26. Otomo, K., Z. Wang, R. Lazzara, and W.M. Jackman, Atrioventricular nodal reentrant tachycardia: Electrophysiological characteristics of four forms and implications for the reentrant circuit, in *Cardiac Electrophysiology: From Cell to Bedside*, 3rd edn., D.P. Zipes and J. Jalife, Editors. Philadelphia, PA: WB Saunders Company, 1999, pp. 504–521.

27. Kwaku, K.F. and M.E. Josephson, Typical AVNRT. An update on mechanisms and therapy. *Card. Electrophysiol. Rev.*, 2002;**6**: 414–421.

28. Swiryn, S., R. Bauernfeind, E. Palileo, B. Strasberg, C.E. Duffy, and K.M. Rosen, Electrophysiologic study demonstrating triple antegrade AV nodal pathways in patients with spontaneous and/or induced supraventricular tachycardia. *Am. Heart J.*, 1982;**103**: 168–174.

29. Sublettt, K.L. and O. Fujimura, Atrioventricular node reentry that utilizes triple nodal pathways. *Am. Heart J.*, 1992;**124**: 777–779.

30. Lee, M.A., F. Morady, A. Kadish, et al., Catheter modification of the atrioventricular junction with radiofrequency energy for control of atrioventricular nodal reentry tachycardia. *Circulation*, 1991;**83**: 827–835.

31. Tai, C.T., S.A. Chen, C.E. Chiang, et al., Multiple anterograde atrioventricular node pathways in patients with atrioventricular node reentrant tachycardia. *J. Am. Coll. Cardiol.*, 1996;**28**: 725–731.

32. Tai, C.T., S.A. Chen, C.E. Chiang, et al., Electrophysiologic characteristics and radiofrequency catheter ablation in patients with multiple atrioventricular nodal reentry tachycardias. *Am. J. Cardiol.*, 1996;**77**: 52–58.

33. Hwang, C., D.J. Martin, J.S. Goodman, et al., Atypical atrioventricular node reciprocating tachycardia masquerading as tachycardia using a left-sided accessory pathway. *J. Am. Coll. Cardiol.*, 1997;**30**: 218–225.

34. Mitrani, R.D., L.S. Klein, F.K. Hackett, D.P. Zipes, W.M. Miles, Radiofrequency ablation of atrioventricular node reentrant tachycardia: Comparison between fast (anterior) and slow (posterior) pathway ablation. *J. Am. Coll. Cardiol.*, 1992;**21**: 432–435.

35. Katritsis, D., A. Slade, A.J. Camm, E. Rowland, Atrioventricular junctional reentrant tachycardia utilising multiple retrograde fibres during ablation of the slow pathway. *Clin. Cardiol.*, 1993;**16**: 889–891.

36. Fujiki, A., S. Yoshida, K. Mizumaki, and S. Sasayama, Fast-slow type of atrioventricular nodal reentrant tachycardia: Horizontal dissociation of the AV node during tachycardia. *Pacing Clin. Electrophysiol.*, 1988;**11**: 1559–1565.

37. Ward, D.E. and C. Garratt, Atrioventricular nodal reentrant tachycardia. Is there a third pathway? *J. Electrophysiol.*, 1993;**4**: 62–67.

38. Bauernfeind, R.A., D. Wu, P. Denes, and K.M. Rosen, Retrograde block during dual pathway atrioventricular nodal reentrant paroxysmal tachycardia. *Am. J. Cardiol.*, 1978;**42**: 499–505.

39. Ko, P.T., G.V. Naccarelli, S. Gulamhusein, E.N. Prystowski, D.P. Zipes, and G.J. Klein, Atrioventricular dissociation during paroxysmal junctional tachycardia. *PACE*, 1981;**4**: 670–678.

40. Miller, J.M., M.E. Rosenthal, J.A. Vassalo, and M.E. Josephson, Atrioventricular nodal reentrant tachycardia: Studies on upper and lower "common pathways". *Circulation*, 1987;**75**: 930–940.

41. Loh, P., J.M. de Bakker, B. Hocini, M. Thibault, R.N. Hauer, and M.J. Janse, Reentrant pathway during ventricular echoes is confined to the atrioventricular node: High-resolution mapping and dissection of the triangle of Koch in isolated, perfused canine hearts. *Circulation*, 1999;**100**: 1346–1353.

42. Chen, J. and M.E. Josephson, Atrioventricular nodal tachycardia occurring during atrial fibrillation. *J. Cardiovasc. Electrophysiol.*, 2000;**11**: 812–815.

43. Schuger, C.D., R.T. Steinman, and M.H. Lehmann, Recovery of retrograde fast pathway excitability in the atrioventricular node reentrant circuit after concealed antegrade impulse penetration. *J. Am. Coll. Cardiol.*, 1991;**17**: 1129–1137.

44. Akhtar, M., A.N. Damato, J. Ruskin, et al., Antegrade and retrograde conduction characteristics in three patterns of paroxysmal atrioventricular junctional reentrant tachycardia. *Am. Heart J.*, 1978;**95**: 22–42.

45. Gomes, J.A.C., M.S. Dhatt, N.S. Rubenson, and A.N. Damato, Electrophysiologic evidence for selective retrograde utilization of a specialized conducting system in atrioventricular nodal reentry tachycardia. *Am. J. Cardiol.*, 1979;**43**: 687–698.

46. Wu, D., J.S. Hung, C.T. Kuo, K.S. Hsu, and W.B. Shieh, Effects of quinidine on atrioventricular nodal reentrant paroxysmal tachycardia. *Circulation*, 1981;**64**: 823–831.

47. Yamabe, H., Y. Shimasaki, O. Honda, Y. Kimura, and Y. Hokamura, Demonstration of the exact anatomic tachycardia circuit

in the fast-slow form of atrioventricular nodal reentrant tachycardia. *Circulation*, 2001;**104**: 1268–1273.

48. Iinuma, H., L.S. Dreifus, T. Mazgalev, R. Price, and E.L. Michelson, Role of the perinodal region in atrioventricular nodal reentry: Evidence in an isolated rabbit heart preparation. *J. Am. Coll. Cardiol.*, 1983;**2**: 465–473.

49. Kay, G.N., A.E. Epstein, S.M. Dailey, and V.J. Plumb, Selective radiofrequency ablation of the slow pathway for the treatment of atrioventricular nodal reentrant tachycardia. Evidence for involvement of perinodal myocardium within the reentrant circuit. *Circulation*, 1992;**85**: 1675–1688.

50. McGuire, M.A., K.-C. Lau, D.C. Johnson, D.A. Richards, J.B. Uther, and D.L. Ross, Patients with two types of atrioventricular junctional (AV nodal) reentrant tachycardia. Evidence that a common pathway of nodal tissue is not present above the reentrant circuit. *Circulation*, 1991;**83**: 1232–1246.

51. Ross, D.L., D.C. Johnson, A.R. Dennis, M.J. Cooper, D.A. Richards, and J.B. Uther, Curative surgery for atrioventricular junctional ("AV nodal") reentrant tachycardia. *J. Am. Coll. Cardiol.*, 1985;**6**: 1383–1392.

52. Anselme, F., B. Hook, K. Monahan, et al., Heterogeneity of retrograde fast-pathway conduction pattern in patients with atrioventricular nodal reentry tachycardia: Observations by simultaneous multisite catheter mapping of Koch's triangle. *Circulation*, 1996;**93**: 960–968.

53. Sung, R.J., H.L. Waxman, S. Saksena, and Z. Juma, Sequence of retrograde atrial activation in patients with dual atrioventricular nodal pathways. *Circulation*, 1981;**64**: 1059–1067.

54. Loh, P., S.Y. Ho, T. Kawara, et al., Reentrant circuits in the canine atrioventricular node during atrial and ventricular echoes: Electrophysiological and histological correlation. *Circulation*, 2003;**108**: 231–238.

55. Heidbuchel, H., H. Ector, and F. Van de Werf, Prospective evaluation of the length of the lower common pathway in the differential diagnosis of various forms of AV nodal reentrant tachycardia. *Pacing Clin. Electrophysiol.*, 1998;**21**: 209–216.

56. Heidbuchel, H. and W.M. Jackman, Characterization of subforms of AV nodal reentrant tachycardia. *Europace*, 2004;**6**: 316–329.

57. Gianfranchi, L., M. Brignole, P. Delise, et al., Modification of antegrade slow pathway is not crucial for successful catheter ablation of common atrioventricular nodal reentrant tachycardia. *Pacing Clin. Electrophysiol.*, 1999;**22**: 263–267.

58. Manolis, A.S., P.J. Wang, and N.A. Estes 3rd., Radiofrequency ablation of slow pathway in patients with atrioventricular nodal reentrant tachycardia. Do arrhythmia recurrences correlate with persistent slow pathway conduction or site of successful ablation? *Circulation*, 1994;**90**: 2815–2819.

59. Zipes, D.P., C. Mendez, and G.K. Moe, Evidence for summation and voltage dependency in rabbit atrioventricular nodal fibers. *Circ. Res.*, 1973;**32**: 170–177.

60. Efimov, I.R. and T.N. Mazgalev, High-resolution, three-dimensional fluorescent imaging reveals multilayer conduction pattern in the atrioventricular node. *Circulation*, 1998;**98**: 54–57.

61. Spach, M.S., M. Lieberman, J.G. Scott, R.C. Barr, E.S. Johnson, and J.M. Kootsey, Excitation sequences of the atrial septum and the AV node in isolated hearts of the dog and rabbit. *Circulation*, 1971;**29**: 156–172.

62. Tse, W.W., Transmembrane potentials of canine AV junctional tissues. *Am. Heart J.*, 1986;**11**: 1100–1105.

63. Jalife, J., The sucrose gap preparation as a model of AV nodal transmission: Are dual pathways necessary for reciprocation and AV nodal "echoes"? *PACE*, 1983;**6**: 1106–1110.

64. Spach, M.S., Anisotropic structural complexities in the genesis of reentrant arrhythmias. *Circulation*, 1991;**84**: 1447–1450.

65. Malik, M. and A.J. Camm, Complexity of AV nodal function: Complex nodal structure or complex behavior of nodal elements? *PACE*, 1998;**11**: 425–433.

66. Spach, M.S., W.T. Miller, D.B. Geselowitz, R.C. Barr, J.M. Kootsey, E.A. Johnson, The discontinuous nature of propagation in normal canine cardiac muscle: Evidence for recurrent discontinuities of intracellular resistance that affect the membrane currents. *Circ. Res.*, 1981;**48**: 39–54.

67. Paes de Carvallho, A. and D.F. de Almeida, Spread of activity through the atrioventricular node. *Circ. Res.*, 1960;**8**: 801–809.

68. Patterson, E. and B.J. Scherlag, Anatomic and functional fast atrioventricular conduction pathway. *J. Cardiovasc. Electrophysiol.*, 2002;**13**: 945–949.

69. Wu, D., S.-J. Yeh, C.-C. Wang, M.-S. Wen, H.-J. Chang, F.-C. Lin, Nature of dual atrioventricular node pathways and the tachycardia circuit as defined by radiofrequency ablation technique. *J. Am. Coll. Cardiol.*, 1992;**20**: 884–895.

70. Keim, S., P. Werner, M. Jazayeri, M. Akhtar, and P. Tchou, Localization of the fast and slow pathways in atrioventricular nodal reentrant tachycardia by intraoperative ice mapping. *Circulation*, 1992;**86**: 919–925.

71. Spach, M.S. and M.E. Josephson, Initiating reentry: The role of nonuniform anisotropy in small circuits. *J. Cardiovasc. Electrophysiol.*, 1994;**5**: 182–209.

72. Hocini, M., P. Loh, S.Y. Ho, et al., Anisotropic conduction in the triangle of Koch of mammalian hearts: Electrophysiologic and anatomic correlations. *J. Am. Coll. Cardiol.*, 1998;**31**: 629–636.

73. Patterson, E. and B.J. Scherlag, Decremental conduction in the posterior and anterior AV nodal inputs. *J. Interv. Card. Electrophysiol.*, 2002;**7**: 137–148.

74. Katritsis, D.G., A.E. Becker, K.A. Ellenbogen, E. Giazitzoglou, S. Korovesis, and A.J. Camm, The right and left inferior extensions of the atrioventricular node may represent the anatomic substrate of the slow pathway in the human. *Heart Rhythm*, 2004;**1**: 582–586.

75. Katritsis, D.G., A.E. Becker, K.A. Ellenbogen, E. Giazitzoglou, S. Korovesis, and A.J. Camm, Effect of slow pathway ablation in atrioventricular nodal reentrant tachycardia on the electrophysiologic characteristics of the inferior atrial inputs to the human atrioventricular node. *Am. J. Cardiol.* 2006;**97**: 860–865.

76. Tawara, S., *Das Reitzleitungssystem des Säugetierherzens: Eine anatomisch-histologische Studie über das Atrioventrikularbundel und die Purkinjeschen Fäden*. Jena, Germany: Gustav Fischer, 1906; pp. 135–136.

77. Inoue, S. and A.E. Becker, Posterior extensions of the human compact atrioventricular node: A neglected anatomic feature of potential clinical significance. *Circulation*, 1998;**97**: 188—193.

78. Waki, K., J.S. Kim, and A.E. Becker, Morphology of the human atrioventricular node is age dependent: A feature of potential clinical significance. *J. Cardiovasc. Electrophysiol.*, 2000;**11**: 1144—1151.

79. Khalife, K., J. Billette, D. Medkour, et al., Role of the compact node and its posterior extension in normal atrioventricular nodal conduction, refractory, and dual pathway properties. *J. Cardiovasc. Electrophysiol.*, 1999;**10**: 1439–1451.

80. Lin, L.J., J. Billette, D. Medkour, M.C. Reid, M. Tremblay, and K. Khalife, Properties and substrate of slow pathway exposed with a compact node targeted fast pathway ablation in rabbit atrioventricular node. *J. Cardiovasc. Electrophysiol.*, 2001;**12**: 479–486.

81. Reid, M.C., J. Billette, K. Khalife, and R. Tadros, Role of compact node and posterior extension in direction-dependent changes in atrioventricular nodal function in rabbit. *J. Cardiovasc. Electrophysiol.*, 2003;**14**: 1342–1350.

82. Dobrzynski, H., V.P. Nikolski, A.T. Sambelashvili, et al., Site of origin and molecular substrate of atrioventricular junctional rhythm in the rabbit heart. *Circ. Res.*, 2003;**93**: 1102–1110.

83. Inoue, S., A.E. Becker, R. Riccardi, and F. Gaita, Interruption of the inferior extension of the compact atrioventricular node underlies successful radio frequency ablation of atrioventricular nodal reentrant tachycardia. *J. Interv. Card. Electrophysiol.*, 1999;**3**: 273–277.

84. Antz, M., B.J. Scherlag, K. Otomo, et al., Evidence for multiple atrio-AV nodal inputs in the normal dog heart. *J. Cardiovasc. Electrophysiol.*, 1998;**9**: 395–408.

85. Katritsis, D.G. and A. Becker, The Circuit of Atrioventricular Nodal Reentrant Tachycardia: a Proposal. *Heart Rhythm.* 2007;**4**: 1354–1360.

86. Nawata, H., N. Yamamoto, K. Hirao, et al., Heterogeneity of anterograde fast-pathway and retrograde slow-pathway conduction patterns in patients with the fast-slow form of atrioventricular nodal re-entrant tachycardia: Electrophysiologic and electrocardiographic considerations. *J. Am. Coll. Cardiol.*, 1998;**32**: 1731–1740.

87. Gomes, J.A.C., M.S. Dhatt, A.N. Damato, M. Akhtar, and C.A. Holder, Incidence, determinants and significance of fixed retrograde conduction in the region of the atrioventricular node: Evidence for retrograde atrioventricular nodal bypass tracts. *Am. J. Cardiol.*, 1979;**44**: 1089–1098.

88. Wu, D., Dual atrioventricular nodal pathway: A reappraisal. *PACE*, 1982;**5**: 72–77.

89. Wu, D., P. Denes, F. Amat-Y-Leon, et al., Clinical electrocardiographic and electrophysiological observations in patients with paroxysmal supraventricular tachycardia. *Am. J. Cardiol.*, 1978;**41**: 1045–1051.

90. Wu, D., H.C. Kou, S.J. Yeh, F.C. Lin, and J.S. Hung, Determinants of tachycardia induction using ventricular stimulation in dual pathway atrioventricular nodal reentrant tachycardia. *Am. Heart J.*, 1984;**108**: 44–55.

91. Denes, P., D. Wu, F. Amat-y-Leon, R. Dhingra, C. Wyndham, and K.M. Rosen, The determinants of atrioventricular nodal reentrance with premature atrial stimulation in patients with dual AV nodal pathways. *Circulation*, 1977;**56**: 253–259.

92. Wu, D., P. Denes, R. Dhingra, et al., Determinants of fast and slow pathway conduction in patients with dual AV nodal pathways. *Circ. Res.*, 1975;**36**: 782–790.

93. Wu, D., P. Denes, R. Dhingra, R. Pietras, and K.M. Rosen, New manifestations of dual AV nodal pathways. *Eur. J. Cardiol.*, 1975;**2**: 459–466.

94. Csapo. G., Paroxysmal nonrentrant tachycardia due to simultaneous conduction in dual atrioventricular nodal pathways. *Am. J. Cardiol.*, 1979;**43**: 1033–1045.

95. Kim, S.S., R. Lal, and R. Ruffy, Paroxysmal nonrentrant supraventricular tachycardia due to simultaneous fast and slow pathway conduction in dual atrioventricular nodal pathways. *J. Am. Coll. Cardiol.*, 1987;**10**: 456–461.

96. Huycke, E.C., W.T. Lai, N.X. Nguyen, E.C. Keung, and R.J. Sung, Role of intravenous isoproterenol in the electrophysiologic induction of atrioventricular node reentrant tachycardia in patients with dual atrioventricular nodal pathways. *Am. J. Cardiol.*, 1989;**64**: 1131–1137.

97. Amat-y-Leon, F., R. Dhingra, D. Wu, P. Denes, C. Wyndham, and K.M. Rosen, Catheter mapping of retrograde atrial activation. Observations during ventricular pacing and AV nodal re-entrant paroxysmal tachycardia. *Br. Heart J.*, 1976;**38**: 355–362.

98. Benditt, D.G., E.L.C. Pritchett, W.M. Smith, and J.J. Gallagher, Ventriculoatrial intervals: Diagnostic use in paroxysmal supraventricular tachycardias. *Ann. Intern. Med.*, 1979;**91**: 161–166.

99. Engelstein, E.D., K.M. Stein, S.M. Markowitz, and B.B. Lerman, Posterior fast atrioventricular node pathways: Implications for radiofrequency catheter ablation of atrioventricular node reentrant tachycardia. *J. Am. Coll. Cardiol.*, 1996; **27**: 1098–1105.

100. Michaud, G.F., H. Tada, S. Chough, et al., Differentiation of atypical atrioventricular node re-entrant tachycardia from orthodromic reciprocating tachycardia using a septal accessory pathway by the response to ventricular pacing. *J. Am. Coll. Cardiol.*, 2001;**38**: 1163–1167.

101. Jazayeri, M.R., S.L. Hempe, J.S. Sra, et al., Selective transcatheter ablation of the fast and slow pathways using radiofrequency energy in patients with atrioventricular nodal reentrant tachycardia. *Circulation*, 1992;**85**: 1318–1328.

102. Goldberger, J., R. Brooks, and A. Kadish, Physiology of "atypical" atrioventricular junctional reentrant tachycardia occurring following radiofrequency catheter modification of the atrioventricular node. *Pacing Clin. Electrophysiol.*, 1992;**15**: 2270–2282.

103. Taniguchi, Y., S.J. Yeh, M.S. Wen, C.C. Wang, and D. Wu, Atypical atrioventricular nodal reentry tachycardia with atrioventricular block mimicking atrial tachycardia: Electrophysiologic properties and radiofrequency ablation therapy. *J. Cardiovasc. Electrophysiol.*, 1997;**8**: 1302–1308.

104. Knight, B.P., A. Zivin, J. Souza, et al., A technique for the rapid diagnosis of atrial tachycardia in the electrophysiology laboratory. *J. Am. Coll. Cardiol.*, 1999;**33**: 775–781.

105. Man, K.C., M. Niebauer, E. Daoud, et al., Comparison of atrial-His intervals during tachycardia and atrial pacing in patients with long RP tachycardia. *J. Cardiovasc. Electrophysiol.*, 1995;**6**: 700–710.

106. Farre, J., D.L. Ross, I. Wiener, F.W. Bar, E.J. Vanagt, H.J.J. Wellens, Reciprocal tachycardias using accessory pathways with long conduction times. *Am. J. Cardiol.*, 1979;**44**: 1099–1109.

107. Atie, J., P. Brugada, J. Brugada, et al., Longitudinal dissociation of atrioventricular accessory pathways. *J. Am. Coll. Cardiol.*, 1991;**17**: 161–166.

108. Sung, R.J., Incessant supraventricular tachycardia. *PACE*, 1983;**6**: 1306–1326.

109. Coumel, P., Functional reciprocating tachycardias. The permanent and paroxysmal forms of AV nodal reciprocating tachycardias. *J. Electrocardiol.*, 1975;**8**: 79–90.

110. Vassalo, J.A., D.M. Cassidy, and M.E. Josephson, Atrioventricular nodal supraventricular tachycardia. *Am. J. Cardiol.*, 1985;**56**: 193–195.

111. Yeh, S.-J., T. Yamamoto, F.-C. Lin, and D. Wu, Atrioventricular block in the atypical form of junctional reciprocating tachycardia: Evidence supporting the atrioventricular node as the site of reentry. *J. Am. Coll. Cardiol.*, 1990;**15**: 385–392.

112. Kerr, C.R., J.J. Gallagher, and L.D. German, Changes in ventriculoatrial intervals with bundle branch block aberration during reciprocating tachycardia in patients with accessory atrioventricular pathways. *Circulation*, 1982;**66**: 196–201.

113. Knight, B.P., M. Ebinger, H. Oral, et al., Diagnostic value of tachycardia features and pacing maneuvers during paroxysmal supraventricular tachycardia. *J. Am. Coll. Cardiol.*, 2000;**36**: 574–582.

114. Crozier, I., S. Wafa, D. Ward, and J. Camm, Diagnostic value of comparison of ventriculoatrial interval during junctional tachycardia and right ventricular apical pacing. *PACE*, 1989;**12**: 942–953.

115. Tai, C.T., S.A. Chen, C.E. Chiang, et al., A new electrocardiographic algorithm using retrograde P waves for differentiating atrioventricular node reentrant tachycardia from atrioventricular reciprocating tachycardia mediated by concealed accessory pathway. *J. Am. Coll. Cardiol.*, 1997;**29**: 394–402.

116. Spurrell, R.A.J., D.M. Krikler, and E. Sowton, Concealed bypass of the atrioventricular node in patients with supraventricular tachycardia revealed by intracardiac electrical stimulation and verapamil. *Am. J. Cardiol.*, 1974;**33**: 590–595.

117. Ross, D.L. and J.B. Uther, Diagnosis of concealed accessory pathways in supraventricular tachycardia. *PACE*, 1983;**7**: 1069–1085.

118. Benditt, D.G., D.W. Benson, A. Dunnigan, et al., Role of extrastimulus site and tachycardia cycle length in inducibility of atrial preexcitation by premature ventricular stimulation during reciprocating tachycardia. *Am. J. Cardiol.*, 1987;**60**: 811–819.

119. Miles, W.M., R. Yee, G.J. Klein, D.P. Zipes, and E.N. Prystowsky, The preexcitation index: An aid in determining the mechanism of supraventricular tachycardia and localizing accessory pathways. *Circulation*, 1986;**74**: 493–500.

120. Tai, C.T., S.A. Chen, C.E. Chiang, and M.S. Chang, Characteristics and radiofrequency catheter ablation of septal accessory atrioventricular pathways. *Pacing Clin. Electrophysiol.*, 1999;**22**: 500–511.

121. Martinez-Alday, J.D., J. Almendral, A. Arenal, et al., Identification of concealed posteroseptal Kent pathways by comparison of ventriculoatrial intervals from apical and posterobasal right ventricular sites. *Circulation*, 1994;**89**: 1060–1067.

122. Miller, J.M., M.E. Rosenthal, C.D. Gottlieb, J.A. Vassalo, and M.E. Josephson, Usefulness of the ΔHA interval to accurately distinguish atrioventricular nodal reentry from orthodromic septal bypass tract tachycardias. *Am. J. Cardiol.*, 1991;**68**: 1037–1044.

123. Hirao, K., K. Otomo, X. Wang, et al., Para-Hisian pacing. A new method for differentiating retrograde conduction over an accessory AV pathway from conduction over the AV node. *Circulation*, 1996;**94**: 1027–1035.

124. Ormaetxe, J.M., J. Almendral, A. Arenal, et al., Ventricular fusion during resetting and entrainment of orthodromic supraventricular tachycardia involving septal accessory pathways. Implications for the differential diagnosis with atrioventricular nodal reentry. *Circulation*, 1993;**88**: 2623–2631.

125. Packer, D.L., J.J. Gallagher, and E.N. Prystowsky, Physiological substrate for antidromic reciprocating tachycardia. Parequisite characteristics of the accessory pathway and atrioventricular conduction system. *Circulation*, 1992;**85**: 574–588.

126. González-Torrecilla, E., A. Arenal, F. Atienza, J. Osca, J. García-Fernández, A. Puchol, A. Sánchez, and J. Almendral, First post-pacing interval after tachycardia entrainment with correction for atrioventricular node delay: a simple maneuver for differential diagnosis of atrioventricular nodal reentrant tachycardias versus orthodromic reciprocating tachycardias. *Heart Rhythm.* 2006;**3**: 674–679.

127. Veenhuyzen, G.D., K. Coverett, F.R. Quinn, J.L. Sapp, A.M. Gillis, R. Sheldon, D.V. Exner, and L.B. Mitchell, Single diagnostic pacing maneuver for supraventricular tachycardia. *Heart Rhythm.* 2008;**5**: 1152–1158.

128. Segal, O.R., L.J. Gula, A.C. Skanes, A.D. Krahn, R. Yee, and G.J. Klein, Differential ventricular entrainment: a maneuver to differentiate AV node reentrant tachycardia from orthodromic reciprocating tachycardia. *Heart Rhythm.* 2009;**6**: 493–500.

129. Smith, W.M., A. Broughton, M.J. Reiter, D.W. Benson, A.O. Grant, J.J. Gallagher, Bystander accessory pathway during AV node reentrant tachycardia. *PACE*, 1983;**6**: 537–543.

130. Atie, J., P. Brugada, J. Brugada, et al., Clinical and electrophysiologic characteristics of patients with antidromic circus movement tachycardia in the Wolff-Parkinson-White syndrome. *Am. J. Cardiol.*, 1990;**66**: 1082–1091.

131. Pick, A. and P. Dominguez, Nonparoxysmal A-V nodal tachycardia. *Circulation*, 1967;**16**: 1022–1031.

132. Dreifus, L.S., M. Katz, Y. Watanabe, et al., Clinical significance of disorders of impulse formation and conduction in the atrioventricular junction. *Am. J. Cardiol.*, 1963;**11**: 384–391.

133. Rosen, K.M., Junctional tachycardia: Mechanisms, diagnosis, differential diagnosis and management. *Circulation*, 1973;**67**: 654–664.

134. Palileo, E.V., R.A. Brauernfeind, S.P. Swiryn, C.R. Wyndham, K.M. Rosen, Chronic nonparoxysmal junctional tachycardia. *Chest*, 1981;**80**: 106–108.

135. Rosen, M.R., C. Fisch, B.F. Hoffman, P. Danilo, D.E. Lovelace, J.B. Knoebel, Can accelerated atrioventricular junctional escape rhythms be explained by delayed afterdepolarizations? *Am. J. Cardiol.*, 1980;**45**: 1272–1284.

136. Hamdan, M.H., N. Badhwar, and M.M. Scheinman, Role of invasive electrophysiologic testing in the evaluation and management of adult patients with focal junctional tachycardia. *Card. Electrophysiol. Rev.*, 2002;**6**: 431–435.

137. Garson, A. and P.C. Gillette, Junctional ectopic tachycardia in children: Electrocardiography, electrophysiology and pharmacologic response. *Am. J. Cardiol.*, 1979;**44**: 298–302.

138. Coumel, P., J.E. Fifelle, P. Attuel, et al., Tachycardia focale hissiennes congenitales. Etudes cooperative de sept cas. *Arch. Mal. Coeur.*, 1976;**69**: 899–909.

139. Villain, E., V.L. Vetter, J.M. Garcia, J. Herre, A. Cifarelli, A. Garson Jr., Evolving concepts in the management of congenital junctional ectopic tachycardia. A multicenter study. *Circulation*, 1990;**81**: 1544–1549.

140. Wren, C. and R.W. Campbell, His bundle tachycardia-arrhythmogenic and antiarrhythmic effects of therapy. *Eur. Heart J.*, 1987;**8**: 647–650.

141. Walsh, E.P., J.P. Saul, G.F. Sholler, et al., Evaluation of a staged treatment protocol for rapid automatic junctional tachycardia after operation for congenital heart disease. *J. Am. Coll. Cardiol.*, 1997;**29**: 1046–1053.

142. Gillette, P.C., Diagnosis and management of postoperative junctional ectopic tachycardia. *Am. Heart J.*, 1989;**118**: 192–194.

143. Wren, C., Incessant tachycardias. *Eur. Heart J.*, 1998;**19**(Suppl E): E32–E36.

144. Ruder, M.A., J.C. Davis, M. Eldar, J.A. Abbott, J.C. Griffin, J.J. Seger, and M.M. Scheinman, Clinical and electrophysiologic characterization of automatic junctional tachycardia in adults. *Circulation*, 1986;**73**: 930–937.

145. Scheinman, M.M., R.P. Gonzalez, M.W. Cooper, M.D. Lesh, R.J. Lee, and L.M. Epstein, Clinical and electrophysiologic features and role of catheter ablation techniques in adult patients with automatic atrioventricular junctional tachycardia. *Am. J. Cardiol.*, 1994;**74**: 565–572.

6 Atrioventricular Dissociation

Anton P.M. Gorgels · Frits W. Bär · Karel Den Dulk† · Hein J.J. Wellens

---

†Deceased

P. W. Macfarlane et al. (eds.), *Cardiac Arrhythmias and Mapping Techniques*, DOI 10.1007/978-0-85729-877-5_6,

6.1 Introduction

6.1.1 Definitions

The atrioventricular (AV) conduction system has the property of anterograde AV conduction in case of supraventricular activation of the heart, and in many instances of retrograde VA conduction, in case the heart is dominated by ventricular activation. AV dissociation is the phenomenon of independent activation of the atria and the ventricles. Different mechanisms for its occurrence exist, but the common denominator is the absence of the usual antegrade AV relation or retrograde VA relation. AV dissociation can be (1) complete or incomplete, (2) continuous or intermittent, and (3) structural or functional. When AV dissociation is incomplete, occasional AV or VA conducted beat is termed a capture beat (❷ Fig. 6.1). AV dissociation is not synonymous to AV block, the latter being just one of the mechanisms for AV dissociation [1].

6.1.2 Types

Three types of AV dissociation can be differentiated.

(a) AV dissociation may be found in the presence of a slow sinus or atrial rhythm, where the atrial rate is below the AV junctional or ventricular escape rhythm in combination with second-degree or incomplete block in the anterograde and retrograde direction. If the AV dissociation is incomplete, this could be the result of intermittent anterograde capture of sinus (or atrial) impulses or of intermittent capture of retrogradely conducted ventricular (❷ Fig. 6.2) or AV junctional escape beats. Complete AV dissociation is diagnosed when complete block in both directions is present.

(b) The second type is found in the presence of an AV junctional or ventricular rhythm with rate above the sinus (or atrial) rate in combination with second (❷ Fig. 6.3) or third (❷ Fig. 6.4) degree block in the retrograde direction. In

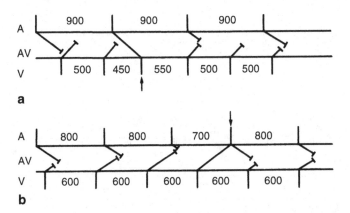

❏ Fig. 6.1
The ladder diagrams illustrate incomplete AV dissociation during ventricular tachycardia. Part (**a**) demonstrates occasional atrial capture of the ventricle (*arrow*), while part (**b**) shows occasional ventricular capture of the atrium (*arrow*). In (**a**), there is retrograde block of the atrioventricular conduction system (AV) during ventricular tachycardia (cycle length 500 ms). The second atrial impulse from the left is able to capture the ventricle, because at that time there is no retrograde invasion of the AV conduction system. Part (**b**) shows the opposite. Anterograde conduction of atrial impulses is not possible during the existing ventricular tachycardia. However, a retrograde capture (fourth ventricular impulse) can arise if concealed anterograde penetration of the atrial impulse is absent. In this illustration, it can be seen that this impulse gives an echo beat back to the ventricle due to a dual AV nodal pathway

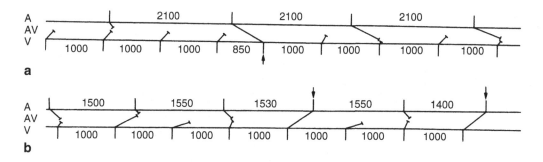

a

b

■ Fig. 6.2

The ladder diagrams illustrate intermittent capture (*arrows*) during sinus bradycardia: (**a**), anterograde capture and (**b**), retrograde capture. In (**a**), the ventricular escape rhythm is not able to conduct in the retrograde direction. Because of the feasibility of anterograde conduction, the second beat from the left of the slow atrial rhythm captures the ventricle. In (**b**), anterograde conduction of the slow atrial rhythm is not possible. No retrograde conduction is present in the third and sixth ventricular escape beats. The fifth and eighth ventricular beats from the left are able to capture the atrium (*arrows*) because at that time anterograde concealed penetration from the atrium is absent. No echo beat is seen, because there is no dual AV nodal pathway as was present in ❷ Fig. 6.1

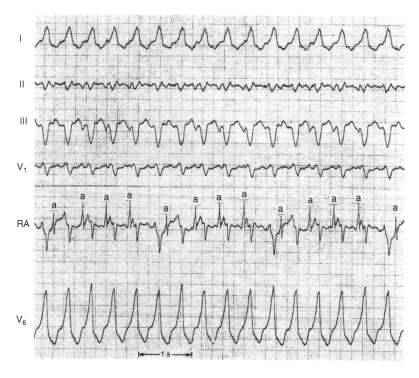

■ Fig. 6.3

Simultaneously recorded five-channel ECG and a right-atrial endocavitary recording illustrating a rather rare example of 5:4 retrograde VA conduction in a patient with ventricular tachycardia. As can be seen in this case, leads II and V$_1$ are often helpful in detecting P waves on the surface ECG (*RA*: right atrium, *a*: atrial endocavitary signal)

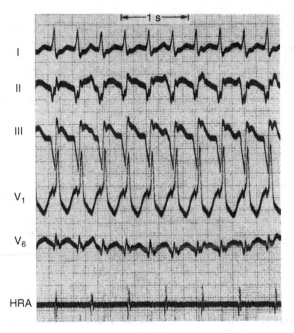

◘ Fig. 6.4
This five-channel ECG shows a tachycardia with a rate of 150 beats min^{-1} (bmp). The endocavitary atrial recording (*HRA*) indicates complete AV dissociation with a ventricular rate higher than the atrial rate. The P waves are also clearly visible in lead II. The finding of complete AV dissociation is extremely suggestive of the presence of ventricular tachycardia

the presence of normal anterograde conduction, capture beats can frequently be seen at lower rates of the accelerated ventricular (or AV junctional) rhythm (❯ Fig. 6.5). Higher ventricular (or AV junctional rates usually do not allow anterograde conduction (complete AV dissociation). This form of AV dissociation is clinically important in tachycardias with a wide QRS complex. It helps to differentiate a supraventricular tachycardia with aberrant conduction from a ventricular tachycardia [1]. AV dissociation in wide QRS tachycardias is diagnostic of ventricular tachycardia. Approximately 50% of ventricular tachycardias have complete AV dissociation. In the other 50%, 1:1, 2:1, or Wenckebach type, VA conduction is present [2–5]. Capture or fusion beats are also of help in differentiating supraventricular tachycardia with aberrant conduction from ventricular tachycardia. However, their occurrence is rare (6%) [2].

(c) The third and most important type of AV dissociation is AV block. Block describes delay or failure of impulse propagation. Varying degrees of block exist. AV block is usually classified as first-, second-, or third-degree block according to the severity of the conduction disturbance [6]. AV block will be discussed in detail, because it is the most frequent cause of AV dissociation and its presence has important clinical implications.

6.2 History of Atrioventricular Block

In 1827, Robert Adams [7] opposed Morgagni's hypothesis [8] that the brain was the cause of seizures in patients with bradycardia. He stated that perhaps the heart was the cause of the bradycardia and the neurological symptoms were the subsequent result. Many disagreed with Adams, but William Stokes [9] concluded in 1846 that Adams' concept was correct. The term heart block was introduced by Gaskell [10, 11] in 1882. Einthoven [12] demonstrated the first case of AV block on an electrocardiogram. Wenckebach [13], Hay [14], and Mobitz [15] described and classified several types of AV

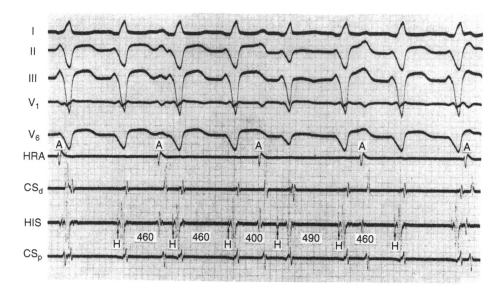

◘ Fig. 6.5
Recording of a ventricular tachycardia with a rate of approximately 135 bmp. The HH intervals are 460 ms. The fifth beat from the left is a little earlier than expected with an HH interval of 400 ms. The QRS configuration is also different. The intracardiac recordings indicate that this premature beat is a fusion between an anterogradely conducted (capture) beat and impulse formation in the ventricle (HRA, high right atrium; CS$_d$, distal coronary sinus; HIS, His bundle; CS$_p$, proximal coronary sinus)

block. In the following years, many other clinical and experimental studies were published [16–19]. The introduction of intracardiac recordings [20] made possible more precise determination of location of block in humans.

6.3   Classification of Atrioventricular Block

6.3.1   First-Degree AV Block

This represents a prolongation of the AV conduction time (PR interval) beyond 0.2 s. However, every atrial impulse is conducted to the ventricle. Therefore the term block should be avoided. These criteria can be applied only in the presence of a regular sinus or atrial rhythm. The normal PR interval is age-dependent. In younger patients, the PR interval is shorter due to sympathetic tone. The PR interval is also shortened during exercise.

6.3.2   Second-Degree AV Block

This is diagnosed when some of the atrial impulses are not conducted to the ventricle. Second-degree block can be subdivided into the following categories.

6.3.2.1   Mobitz Type I (Wenckebach) Block

In this form of second-degree AV block, the PR interval in several successive beats becomes progressively prolonged, resulting in the dropping on one ventricular depolarization due to failure of conduction. The subsequent PR interval is shortened (❯ Fig. 6.6) [13, 15, 21].

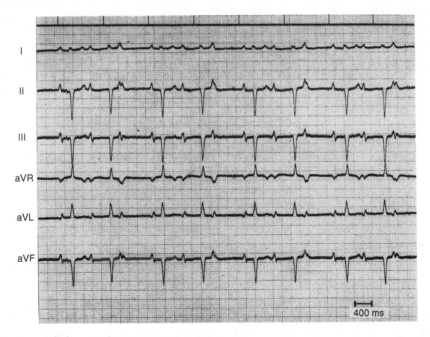

⊡ Fig. 6.6
Six-channel ECG recording illustrating a Mobitz type I AV block in the AV node or His bundle (narrow QRS complex). Statistically, there is an 8:1 chance that the block is situated in the AV node

6.3.2.2 Mobitz Type II Block

In this type of second-degree AV block, there is a sudden failure of one or more atrial impulses to be conducted during maintenance of a constant PR interval (❷ Fig. 6.7) [15–21].

6.3.2.3 Higher Degree AV Block

In 2:1 AV block, every second atrial impulse is not propagated to the ventricle (❷ Fig. 6.8). High-degree or advanced AV block, such as 3:1 or 4:1 block, or occasional conducted impulses can exist [22].

6.3.2.4 Third-Degree (Complete) AV Block

In third-degree (complete) AV block, no atrial impulses are propagated to the ventricle (❷ Fig. 6.9).

6.4 Methodology for Determining the Site of a Block

The conduction defect can be present in the AV node, His bundle, bundle branches, or at multiple sites. Determination of the location of the type of block has important consequences in terms of prognosis and treatment.

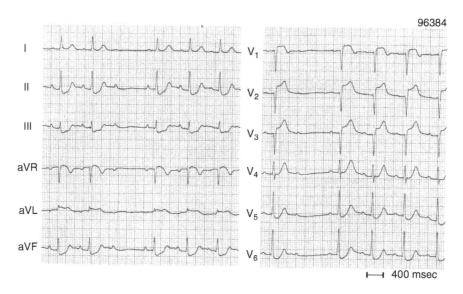

96384

⊢⊣ 400 msec

□ Fig. 6.7
Twelve-lead ECG of a patient with Mobitz II block in acute anteroseptal infarction. The third P wave in the left panel and the second P wave in the right panel are suddenly blocked. The QRS width is narrow, suggesting a conduction problem within the His bundle

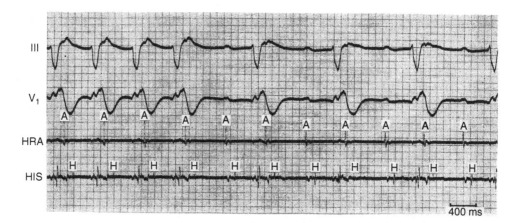

400 ms

□ Fig. 6.8
In this recording, leads III, V₁, high rate atrium (HRA), and His-bundle lead (HIS) are shown. On the left side of the figure, sinus tachycardia at a rate of 105 bpm with 1:1 conduction is present. First-degree AV block is seen with an AH interval of 120 ms (normal 50–120 ms) and an HV interval of 260 ms (normal 35–55 ms). The sudden change from 1:1 to 2:1 AV block develops without further prolongation of the preceding HV interval. The His recording proves that AV block is located distal to His, because every atrial activation is followed by a His signal. The presence of block in the bundle branches is suggested by the QRS width (±220 ms) in the surface ECG. The configuration in lead V₁ indicates the presence of a right bundle branch block and the negative QRS complex in lead III is in favor of a left anterior fascicular block

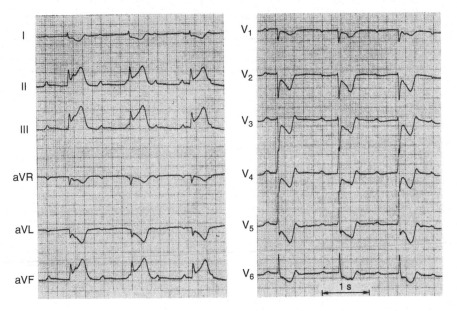

🗖 Fig. 6.9
This ECG shows an extensive acute infero posterior wall myocardial infarction with third-degree block situated in the AV node and an AV nodal escape rhythm (narrow QRS complexes) of 38 bpm. In acute inferior myocardial infarction, AV block can occur due to vagal stimulation. Usually, the sinus rate is then also low. In this illustration, the sinus rate is approximately 100 bpm, which makes it unlikely that the AV conduction disturbance is caused by vagal influences

6.4.1   The Value of the Electrocardiogram

6.4.1.1   PR Interval

The PR interval is the time between the beginning of the P wave and the beginning of the QRS complex, and as such, gives an indication of AV conduction.

AV conduction delay or block can be present in the atrium, AV node, His bundle, bundle branches or Purkinje fibers, but the actual site cannot be determined from the surface ECG. PR prolongation of more than 0.3 s is very suggestive of conduction delay in the AV node, but a PR interval between 0.2 and 0.3 s has no indicative value as to the site of block. Block can also be simultaneously present at different levels of the conduction system.

6.4.1.2   QRS Complex

Puech et al. [23], Narula [24], and Schuilenburg [25] found in their studies that the width of the conducted QRS complex gives an indication of the site of block.

6.4.1.3   Conducted Beats: Narrow QRS Complexes

QRS complexes of less than 0.12 s usually signify that the block is located in the AV node or His bundle (❯ Fig. 6.10). A rare exception of a narrow, conducted QRS complex in the presence of trifascicular disease is the coincidence of identical conduction delay in both bundle branches, resulting in PR prolongation and a narrow QRS complex.

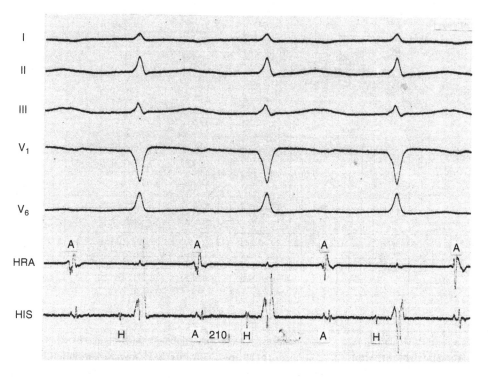

⬛ Fig. 6.10

Leads I, II, III, V₁, and V₆ are shown in combination with the intracardiac recordings from high right atrium (HRA) and His bundle (HIS). Paper speed is 100 mm/s. First-degree AV block is present. Because of the prolonged AH time of 210 ms, the conduction delay is located in the AV node. This might have been expected from the surface ECG because of the narrow QRS complexes (0.09 s)

6.4.1.4   Conducted Beats: Widened QRS Complexes

QRS complexes ⩾0.12 s do not allow any conclusions to be drawn as to the site of block. A significant group of patients has a combination of AV nodal or intra-Hisian block associated with an intraventricular conduction defect (❷ Fig. 6.11), while others have block in the bundle branches (❷ Fig. 6.8). However, AV block with widened QRS complexes in the setting of an extensive anterior wall infarction is frequently associated with bilateral bundle branch block (❷ Fig. 6.12) [26–28].

6.4.1.5   Escape Rhythm

In patients with third-degree block situated in the AV node, 65% have an escape rhythm with a narrow QRS complex, while 35% have a wide QRS complex [29–31]. All patients with trifascicular block have a wide QRS escape rhythm.

Although Adams–Stokes attacks cannot be predicted on the ECG, patients having wide QRS complexes with a slow escape rate are most prone to syncopal attacks, because distal block has a slow (25–45 bpm) and unreliable escape rhythm with long periods of asystole (❷ Fig. 6.13) [32]. The escape rate in the AV node is usually higher and reliable (40–60 bpm). Sometimes the escape rhythm is faster than expected (❷ Fig. 6.14). These accelerated idioventricular rhythms (AIVR) have rates between 60 and 125 bpm, and are commonly seen in the reperfusion phase of an acute myocardial infarction. AIVR is a very specific reperfusion arrhythmia with a specificity of more than 80% and a positive predictive value of more than 90% [33–35]. AIVR is probably caused by reperfusion damage. It is a transient, self-terminating arrhythmia that does not need treatment. It usually has no major hemodynamic consequences, and it is not a precursor of more malignant

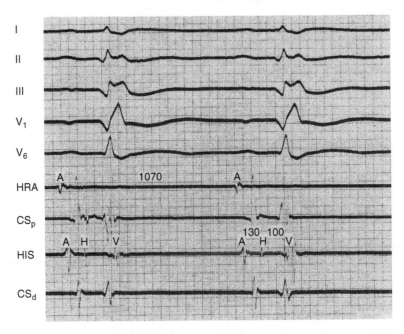

◘ Fig. 6.11
Five surface and four intracardiac recordings illustrating that the first-degree AV block arises from conduction delay at two levels. The AH interval is slightly prolonged (130 ms). The most important delay is present in the distal conduction system (HV interval = 100 ms). This last finding is an indication for pacemaker implantation

arrhythmias. Engelen et al. [36] showed a relation between the number and duration of AIVR's and the recovery of left ventricular function following reperfusion. In that study, it was also found that after percutaneous coronary intervention, AIVR was less frequent than after reperfusion due to fibrinolytic treatment.

6.4.2 The Value of Diagnostic Interventions

6.4.2.1 Noninvasive Methods

Noninvasive interventions can be useful for detecting the location of block. These interventions include the following.

Atropine
Atropine, when given intravenously in a dosage of 0.5–1 mg, has an accelerating effect on the sinus rate, which can produce further deterioration of AV conduction. On the other hand, the drug improves impulse conduction through the AV node [24]. Because of the delicate balance of these two effects, it is not surprising that the outcome of atropine administration is not completely predictable, since it depends on the variable responses of impulse formation and conduction (❷ Fig. 6.15). When given to patients with AV nodal conduction problems, atropine can shorten the PR interval or diminish the degree of block. In patients with a conduction problem below the AV node, no effect on conduction is seen although sometimes a more severe degree of block is provoked by the increase of the sinus rate.

Ajmaline
A latent conduction defect, present in the bundle branches, can be uncovered by ajmaline (50 mg intravenously) because this drug depresses conduction below the AV node [37–39].

This test is dangerous, however, because it can result in ventricular asystole (for explanation see ❷ Sect. 6.4.1.5). Ajmaline should be given only after introducing an external ventricular pacemaker. The second rare, but more serious,

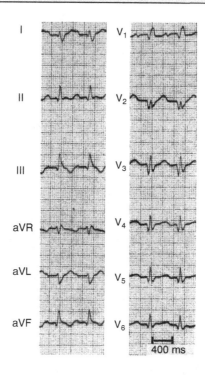

◘ Fig. 6.12

Twelve-lead ECG of a patient with an extensive anteroseptal myocardial infarction and trifascicular conduction problems which were acquired during the infarction. Lead V_1 shows a QR pattern typical of septal involvement of the infarct in combination with a complete right bundle branch block. Right axis deviation suggests block in the posterior fascicle of the left bundle, while the PR prolongation (0.26 s) is most likely caused by additional block in the third bundle – the anterior fascicle of the left bundle. Intracardiac recordings showed a normal AH interval and a prolonged HV interval indicating that conduction delay indeed was located below the His bundle. Mortality is extremely high (86%) due to the extensive muscle damage, which can be indirectly derived from the above-mentioned conduction defects

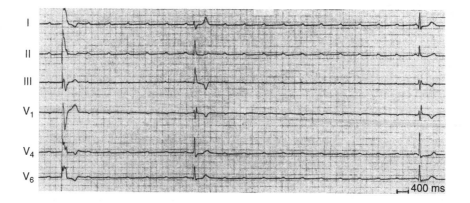

◘ Fig. 6.13

ECG recording demonstrating third-degree AV block in a patient with Lev's disease. The external pacemaker rate was gradually turned down and switched off. After the last paced beat, long periods of ventricular asystole can be seen

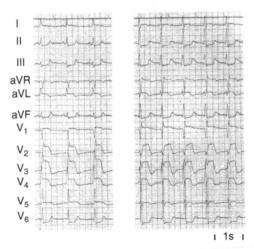

⬛ Fig. 6.14

Left panel. Twelve-lead ECG of a patient with an acute anteroseptal infarction. Right panel. Accelerated idioventricular rhythm (AIVR) with a configuration suggesting an origin in the basal septal part of the left ventricle, that is, the infarcted area. Typically, AIVR in this setting starts with a long coupling interval and has regular R–R intervals

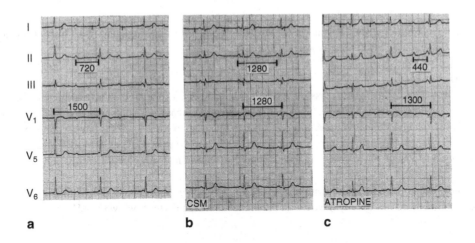

⬛ Fig. 6.15

Six surface ECG leads of a patient with distal AV conduction disturbance. In (a) third-degree block is present. Because of the narrow QRS escape rhythm, the conduction problem is located in the AV node or the His bundle. P–P interval is 720 ms and R–R interval 1500 ms. In (b) carotid sinus massage (CMS) is performed. In proximal AV block, further depression of AV nodal conduction would therefore be expected. However, the significant slowing of the sinus rate allows the AV node to propagate every P wave to the ventricle and to restore normal conduction. In (c) atropine was given. In proximal AV block, atropine improves AV nodal conduction. In this case, the important decrease in P–P interval (440 ms) prevents normal conduction. The two opposite effects result in second-degree AV block. It can be deduced that the second beat from the left is conducted because it comes earlier than expected and its configuration is identical to that in the conducted beats in (b) and different from the escape beats in (a). The rate of the escape rhythm has increased slightly with the R–R interval shortening from 1500 to 1300 ms

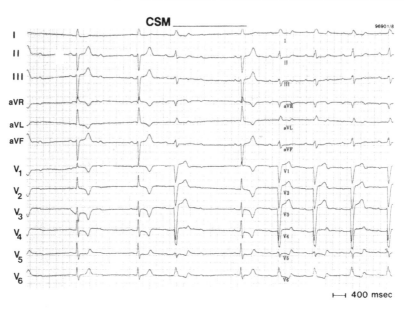

■ Fig. 6.16

Twelve-lead ECG showing a complex arrhythmia due to distal conduction disease in a patient after aortic valve replacement. Advanced AV block present with the first 2 QRS complexes show incomplete right bundle branch block and left axis deviation (anterior fascicular block). The 3^d QRS complex is conducted with a prolonged PR interval and shows left bundle branch block. A fourth beat with the initial configuration is seen, followed, due to carotid sinus massage (CSM)–induced mild slowing of the sinus rate, by 1:1 conduction with prolonged PR intervals and left bundle branch block

complication that has been described is ventricular fibrillation. Therefore, sound advice is to restrict this test to special cases only.

Vagal maneuvers

Vagal maneuvers, such as carotid sinus massage, have the opposite effect to atropine and produce further prolongation of the PR interval or provoke second-degree block in the AV node, whereas no effect is seen in distal block [24]. However, the vagal maneuver can give concomitant AV nodal conduction delay in those patients having conduction problems in the His–Purkinje system [40]. Furthermore, conduction may be restored in both types of block because of slowing of the sinus rate (❷ Figs. 6.15 and ❷ 6.16). Therefore, vagal maneuvers are of less value for differentiation among various sites of block.

Vagal maneuvers can depress, and atropine or exercise can accelerate, the escape rhythm in the AV node during third-degree block. They do not usually have much influence on escape rhythm below the AV node.

Exercise

Exercise has an adrenergic effect on the heart, which is comparable to atropine. During exercise, sinus rate increases and AV nodal conduction improves. In patients with conduction problems in the His bundle or bundle branches, exercise may enhance the degree of block due to increase of the sinus rate (❷ Fig. 6.17). Occasionally, in patients with bridging of one of the coronary arteries, block can also develop during exercise [41].

6.4.2.2   Invasive Methods

Atrial pacing

Atrial pacing will produce further prolongation of the PR interval, and can result in a higher degree of AV nodal block in patients with AV nodal disease. In contrast to this, the effect of atrial pacing on infranodal block is

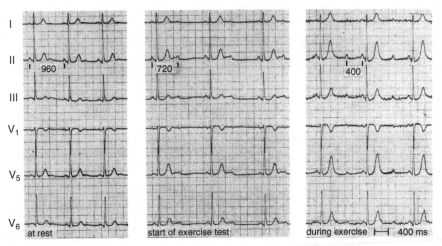

◼ Fig. 6.17

Six-lead ECG of a 54-year-old male, who exercised on a treadmill. A sudden change from 1:1 to 2:1 AV conduction was found at sinus rates more than 65 bpm, as well as a change to 3:1 AV conduction at sinus rates above 145 bpm. In this patient, the His bundle is the most likely location of block, because the PR interval of the (probably) conducted P wave remained constant (0.15 s) and the QRS complex was narrow (0.09 s)

minor. Patients with first-degree block in the His–Purkinje system will usually maintain 1:1 conduction at high atrial rates [24].

The escape rhythm can be suppressed by ventricular stimulation in patients with third-degree AV block in or distal to the His bundle (❷ Fig. 6.13). The escape rhythm in AV nodal block is not so easily suppressed by ventricular pacing.

There is no difference in respect of the reaction to atropine, exercise, and artificial pacing of the atrium in a normal heart [42–44]. The same holds also for the diseased heart. This is true for first-degree as well as for second-degree block [45–48].

The His-bundle ECG

The most appropriate method for determining the site of block is His-bundle recording [20, 25, 49–58]. Using this approach, the intra-atrial (PA) conduction time can be measured. This is the time between the onset of the P wave on the surface ECG (or the intracavitary high right-atrial ECG) and the first rapid deflection of the atrial wave in the His-bundle recording (see ❷ Fig. 6.5) AV nodal conduction is measured as the AH time (the time between the atrial wave and the beginning of the His-bundle spike on the His-bundle recording). The HV time is the time from the beginning of the His-bundle spike to the earliest onset of activation of the ventricle. PA time varies between 25 and 45 ms, AH time between 50 and 120 ms and HV time between 35 and 55 ms. The width of the His-bundle potential is 15–20 ms [46, 54, 55, 59–65]. A full discussion on His-bundle ECG recording is presented in ❷ Chap. 2.

Electrophysiological investigations are of great help in the presence of AV block and widened QRS complexes. Such recordings allow us to find the exact location of block (❷ Figs. 6.11 and ❷ 6.18), to predict the likelihood of asystole, and to determine the reliability of the escape rhythm. His-bundle recordings may be required to identify those patients at risk of developing complete block, because in patients with bifascicular block, abnormal conduction of the remaining fascicle may also be present. It has been shown that AV conduction delays may exist in the absence of PR prolongation or other electrocardiographic abnormalities [46].

A His-bundle recording is, however, not a routine procedure because it is a time-consuming and invasive investigation [66]. The level of the conduction defect can roughly be estimated by studying the PR interval, QRS duration, and AV relationship on the surface ECG in the majority of cases [67–69].

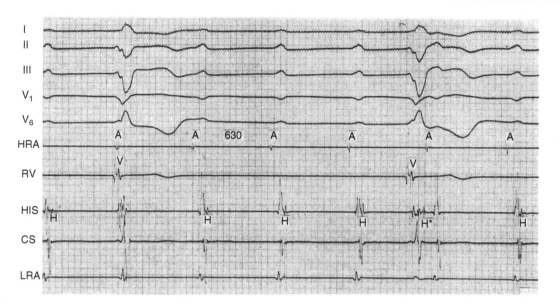

◘ Fig. 6.18

This recording is taken from a patient with Adams–Stokes attacks due to paroxysmal complete AV block. It shows five surface leads and five intracardiac recordings. The His-bundle electrogram shows that every atrial signal is followed by a His deflection, indicating that block is located distal to His. The rate of the ventricular escape rhythm is only 26 bpm. The second escape beat is retrogradely conducted to the His bundle. The next atrial event is blocked proximal to the His bundle because of retrograde concealed penetration of the AV node (HRA, high right atrium; RV, right ventricle; HIS, His bundle; CS; coronary sinus; LRA, low right atrium; interval given in milliseconds)

For the clinician, a knowledge of whether the site of the block is above or below the His bundle is probably sufficient. Invasive and noninvasive methods for determining the site of block will be discussed in detail for all three types of conduction disturbances.

6.5   Incomplete Block

6.5.1   First-Degree AV Conduction Delay

In the following discussion, the term first-degree AV "block" will be avoided, as there is no block but rather delay in conduction.

In first-degree AV conduction delay, the site of the delay is most frequently located in the AV node, but can also be found infranodally (❷ Table 6.1). Some patients have PR prolongation due to intra-atrial conduction delay. The P wave will then be widened and markedly diminished in voltage [70]. In these cases there may be no impaired conduction in the AV nodal or His–Purkinje system. However, intra-atrial conduction delay is often related to atrial arrhythmia [70].

PR prolongation greater than 0.2 s has no value as far as locating the site of block is concerned. However, a PR interval greater than 0.3 s is very suggestive of a delay within the AV node. Narula et al. [24] stated that in 79% of all cases with prolonged PR interval, the conduction delays were located at more than one site, although the AV node was the dominant site of delay (83%). Delay at a single site was noted in the atrium in 3%, in 11% in the AV node, and in the His–Purkinje system in 7%. Puech et al. [29] reported conduction disturbances at multiple sites in only 20% of their cases.

A narrow QRS complex suggests that block is located in the AV node (❷ Fig. 6.10). First-degree AV conduction delay in combination with a wide QRS complex is most commonly associated with a conduction defect in the bundle branches

◘ Table 6.1

Incidence of the location of block in first degree AV-block [29]

	AV node	Intra-Hisian	Bundle branches
Narrow WRS compex (< 0.12 s)	87%	13%	
Wide QRS complex (⩾ 0.12 s)	22%	12%	66%

(❷ Figs. 6.8 and ❷ 6.11). However, frequently (66%) block is present at two levels, especially in those with left bundle branch block [29, 30, 68, 69, 71, 72]. When PR prolongation and left bundle branch block are found together, block is predominantly located in the common bundle (❷ Fig. 6.7) [29, 71, 72]. Complete right bundle branch block with first-degree AV conduction delay, without extreme right or left axis deviation, is associated with conduction delay in the left bundle branch in only 40% of the cases. All other patients have additional conduction problems in the AV node or His bundle. The combination of first-degree AV conduction delay and bifascicular block (right bundle branch block and left anterior or posterior fascicular block) is commonly a result of a conduction delay in the third bundle branch (❷ Fig. 6.12), although in rare cases the conduction delay can be located in the AV node [71, 72].

In patients where the ECG shows a PR prolongation and a wide QRS complex, His-bundle studies should be performed. HV intervals of more than 75 ms are an indication for pacemaker implantation [73, 74], because in patients with these findings, total AV block and syncope will probably shortly appear due to progressive disease of the conduction system. In contrast to this, first-degree AV nodal delay carries a good prognosis. In such cases, pacing is not indicated.

It has to be realized that occasional prolongation of PR time is found in apparently normal subjects [43, 75, 76]. PR intervals up to 0.28 s were found in 1.6% of 19,000 healthy aviators [3, 77]. A 10-year follow-up study showed that none of these people had progression of their first-degree AV block [78].

Interventions such as atropine (❷ Fig. 6.15) and exercise will decrease PR interval in patients with AV nodal conduction delay. On the other hand, carotid sinus massage produces further prolongation of the PR interval, or can give second-degree block when the conduction delay is present in the AV node. Carotid sinus massage, when performed in patients with first-degree block in the His–Purkinje system, does not generate second-degree block. In patients with AV nodal disease, atrial pacing at rates above 130 bpm will either produce further prolongation of the PR interval or second-degree block. In the presence of HV prolongation, atrial pacing at rapid rates usually maintains 1:1 AV conduction without further prolongation of the HV interval. Only occasionally does second-degree infranodal block develop.

6.5.2 Second-Degree AV Block

❷ Table 6.2 presents the incidence of second-degree block at the various sites.

6.5.2.1 Mobitz Type I (Wenckebach) Block

The classic type I second-degree block is characterized by a progressive lengthening of the PR interval until a P wave is blocked. The PR interval is longest in the beat preceding the blocked P wave and the shortest after the dropped beat. The maximum PR increment occurs between the first and second conducted beat. In the following conducted cycles, the increment of PR interval gradually diminishes, resulting in a lessening of the PR interval increment (❷ Figs. 6.6 and ❷ 6.18).

The explanation for this type of conduction defect is probably that the progressive delay is caused by increasing fatigue of the AV node or distal conduction system until a block occurs. Presumably, each impulse arrives earlier in the relative refractory phase of the conduction system (see ❷ Chap. 3). Therefore, the impulse is conducted more slowly, until it reaches the absolute refractory phase. After the dropped beat, the conduction system has partially recovered, resulting in a shorter PR interval. The Wenckebach phenomenon can be observed in any portion of depressed conduction system [13, 67, 79–82]. However, this classic pattern of Wenckebach block is seen infrequently (14%) [83, 84]; it is seen more often in patients with higher conduction ratios such as 4:3 or 5:4. Conduction ratios such as 7:6 are normally associated

☐ Table 6.2

Incidence of the location in second-degree AV block [29]

	AV node	Intra-Hisian	Bundle branches
Mobitz type I (Wenckebach)	72%	9%	19%
Mobitz type II		20%	80%
2:1 block	27%	23%	50%

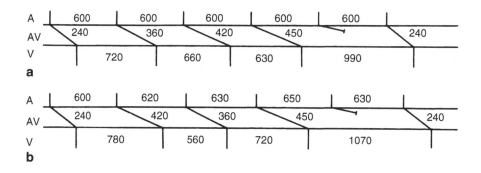

☐ Fig. 6.19

Part (a) represents a typical 5:4 Wenckebach sequence. Progressive lengthening of the AV interval is present. The increment of the AV interval becomes smaller from beat to beat, decreasing from 120 to 30 ms over the first four cycles. This results in shortening of the R–R intervals. Part (b) also shows a Wenckebach sequence. The behavior of this block is atypical. In other words, although there is a gradual prolongation, the AV interval changes unpredictably from beat to beat. The atypical behavior of the Wenckebach sequence is in this case caused by the change in atrial rate

with an atypical behavior. They show progressive PR prolongation with unpredictable changes in increment. This is called atypical Wenckebach (❷ Fig. 6.19).

The explanations for the atypical Wenckebach behavior have been described by Langendorf and others [83–93], and are as follows.

(a) Changes in sinoatrial rate which influence the PR interval. This is probably the most important explanation. The change in sinoatrial rate could be caused by a change in cardiac output caused by the Wenckebach sequence.

(b) Interpolated atrial premature contractions causing changes in AV conduction [89].

(c) Reentry or premature impulses giving rise to concealed premature depolarization of conduction tissue [86–88, 90–93]. Concealed conduction may lead to an unanticipated prolongation of PR interval or blocked P waves after a Wenckebach pause, because partial penetration of an impulse into the conduction system influences the subsequent impulse conduction. The degree of penetration of a blocked impulse can sometimes be inferred from its effect on subsequent events. Atypical Mobitz type I block is seen intranodally as frequently as infranodally [94].

Location of type I block is rather unpredictable and requires His-bundle studies, especially when the conduction disturbance is associated with wide QRS complexes [94, 95]. Minimal increment in the PR interval suggests distal block, but it is not diagnostic.

Significant prolongation of the PR interval during the Wenckebach cycles suggests AV nodal block. Second-degree block located in the AV node has a relatively benign course in patients without organic heart disease and does not produce syncope [96, 97]. In contrast to this, distal second-degree block requires pacemaker implantation [98].

First-degree and second-degree type I block can be present in normal subjects especially during sleep [75, 99–104]. A 6% incidence of spontaneous Wenckebach periods during sleep has been reported in healthy students without apparent heart disease. In none of these subjects were symptoms or progression of block observed in a 6-year follow-up period [101]. The same was found in athletes, where there was a 9% incidence of Wenckebach periods [76, 100–103, 105]. However, the benign prognosis of this type of block is not confirmed in all studies. During prospective analysis of 16 infants with second-degree type I AV block, seven of them had progression to third-degree block, and one of these seven experienced syncopal attacks [102].

Intervention procedures are not helpful for the differential diagnosis between normal and diseased subjects [45–48].

6.5.2.2 Mobitz Type II Block

Mobitz type II second-degree AV block is characterized by a sudden failure of a P wave to be conducted to the ventricle without PR prolongation in the preceding beats (❷ Fig. 6.7 and ❷ 6.20). This type of block is always located below the AV node (❷ Table 6.1). The nonconducted P wave will be followed by a His-bundle signal. Sometimes a "split" His can be seen in the His-bundle recording in the presence of His-bundle disease. In the rare case of a proximal His-bundle defect, the His signal will not be seen after the P wave, but preceding every QRS complex thereby fallaciously simulating AV nodal block [46, 106, 107]. In patients having disease of the bundle branches, widened QRS complexes are present [24], while the PR interval is usually normal or slightly prolonged [79]. One-third of the cases of chronic second-degree block have the typical behavior of Mobitz type II AV block. A finding of Mobitz type II block is always an indication for pacemaker implantation, because it is usually permanent and often progresses to complete AV block [108].

With respect to interventions during second-degree Mobitz type I or II AV block, atropine and exercise can enhance AV conduction and restore 1:1 conduction. Such a finding is suggestive of AV nodal block. If distal block is present, sometimes the reverse effect can be seen and progression of block will appear because of an increase in sinus rate without improvement of conduction of the His–Purkinje system [40]. The opposite is seen after carotid sinus massage.

In AV nodal block, atrial pacing will produce further progression of AV block, while in His–Purkinje system block, minor changes are seen in PR and HV intervals.

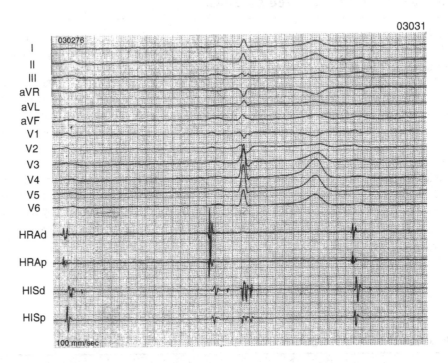

⬛ Fig. 6.20

Twelve-lead surface ECG combined with intracavitary recordings from the same patient, as in ❷ Fig. 6.7, shows the location of the block distal from the His bundle

Differentiation between type I and II is important with respect to management, because type II block is always indicative of distal disease. Distinction between types of block can be difficult if there is only a minimal increment in PR interval before and after a dropped beat or in the presence of 2:1 block. In these patients, exercise or atropine may clarify the situation by provoking Wenckebach periods due to higher sinus rates. Vagal maneuvers may produce a higher degree of block and indicate which is the underlying type of block.

6.5.2.3   2:1 or Higher Degree AV Block

Several terms are used for this type of block such as advanced AV block [22] and severe or high-degree block [109]. In 2:1 block, every second P wave is conducted to the ventricle (❷ Fig. 6.8). These cases cannot be distinguished as type I or type II unless two consecutively conducted beats are seen, such as during temporary 3:2 block or 1:1 conduction (❷ Fig. 6.8) [96]. Changes in conduction can be secondary to slight alterations of the vagal tone [30].

With respect to interventions in this group, carotid sinus massage, if applied with caution, may be clinically useful in indicating the site of block. Increase of block in the AV node is suggestive of an AV nodal conduction problem, while decrease of block indicates distal block because of slowing of the sinus rate. In rare cases with bradycardia-dependent distal block (phase 4 block – see ❷ Chap. 1), carotid sinus massage aggravates block [56, 110]. Atropine and exercise have the opposite effect to vagal stimulation [30, 47, 48, 111].

The interesting phenomenon of ventriculophasic arrhythmias in digitalis intoxication should be mentioned. Excess of digitalis can produce all three types of block in the AV node [112, 113]. Second-degree AV block as a manifestation of digitalis intoxication most commonly shows the Wenckebach type of block or a constant type of 2:1, 3:1, or 4:1 block. During 2:1 AV conduction, the P–P interval embracing the QRS complex [114] differs from the P–P interval without a QRS complex [114]. This is possibly the result of a change in autonomic tone during the cardiac cycle [115, 116].

6.6   Complete Block (Third-Degree AV Block)

In complete block, no atrial impulses are propagated to the ventricle. Third-degree or complete AV block can be located at all three sites of the conduction system [61, 72, 117] (❷ Table 6.3). The location of block cannot be predicted from the escape rhythm. However, during the acute phase of a myocardial infarction the site of infarction provides indirect information as to the site of block. Myocardial infarction located in the inferior wall can give AV nodal block (❷ Fig. 6.9), while damage located in the anteroseptal wall indicates that the conduction disorders are in the bundle branches (❷ Fig. 6.12) [26, 28, 118]. If the rate of the escape rhythm is more or less the same as the atrial rate, it can be difficult to distinguish this "isorhythmic dissociation" from sinus rhythm with 1:1 conduction to the ventricle. An example of such a problem is given in ❷ Fig. 6.21.

Interventions can be performed in patients where the origin of block is unclear. In contrast to findings during distal block, exercise and atropine [47, 48] can increase rate in the AV node significantly or can restore first- or second-degree AV block [30, 32, 60, 118–120]. Atrial pacing does not help in further differentiation between sites of block. Ventricular pacing has to be carried out with caution because subsidiary pacemakers are readily suppressed by ventricular stimulation and can produce long episodes of asystole. Such a finding is suggestive of distal block. Carotid sinus massage may slow the AV nodal escape rhythm, but can produce second-degree block instead of third-degree block in distal conduction disturbances due to slowing of the sinus rate with late arrival of the impulses at the distal conduction system, giving them more time to recover [121, 122].

◻ Table 6.3

Incidence and location of block in third-degree AV block [29]

Escape rhythm	AV node	Intra-Hisian	Bundle branches
Narrow QRS complex (<0.12 s)	48%	52%	
Wide QRS complex (⩾0.12 s)	11%	5%	84%

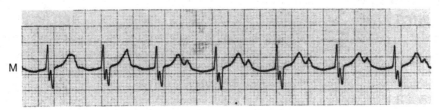

◘ Fig. 6.21
The rhythm in this tracing is either sinus rhythm with first-degree AV block or "isorhythmic dissociation," that is, a situation where, in the presence of complete block, rates at atrial and ventricular level are more or less identical. In this registration, careful measurement will show that the PR intervals of the first two beats are longer than the other PR intervals, which could fit with an isorhythmic dissociation. However, the sinus rate of the first two beats is higher, causing further lengthening of PR interval. The key for making the correct diagnosis is that the R–R interval of the first beats is also shorter. Therefore, a relation between atrium and ventricle must be present. If complete block were present, the ventricular rate would not have been influenced. This proves that sinus rhythm with first-degree AV block is the correct diagnosis

6.7 Etiology of Atrioventricular Block

Multiple pathological processes can affect the conduction system. The common causes of AV block are the following.

6.7.1 Fibrosis

The most frequent cause of AV block (40–50%) [123] is fibrosis of the specialized conduction system due to progressive sclerosis of the ventricular septum and the surrounding tissues [16, 123–126]. This is also called Lenègre and Lev disease. It is a typical disease of the elderly. These patients can have normal coronary arteries [127–131].

6.7.2 Ischemic Heart Disease

The second important cause of AV block (40%) is ischemic heart disease. Two out of five occurrences are chronic [130] and three out of five can be found in the setting of an acute myocardial infarction (❷ Figs. 6.9 and ❷ 6.13) [132–135]. In approximately 19% of patients having an acute myocardial infarction, AV block develops (8% first degree, 5% second degree and 6% third degree) [136–138]. Only a few patients have exercise-related ischemic AV block.

6.7.3 Drugs

Digitalis [112, 114, 139–141] can create different degrees of AV nodal block, especially when given in a toxic dosage (❷ Fig. 6.22). Other drugs which can create AV nodal block are verapamil, amiodarone, diphenylhydantoin [142], and beta-blocking agents [143]. Quinidine and other class I drug [144] can produce block in the His–Purkinje system.

6.7.4 Vagal Influences

Not uncommonly, vagal reactions, for example, due to pain (❷ Fig. 6.9) or during carotid sinus massage, can produce complete AV block, sometimes with longer ventricular asystole [145–148]. In elderly patients, the presence of hypersensitive carotid sinus syndrome can produce profound fall in arterial pressure and marked slowing in heart rate either by slowing of the sinus rate and/or the development of second-degree or third-degree AV block [147, 149, 150]. This may or may not be combined with a vagal vasodilatory effect.

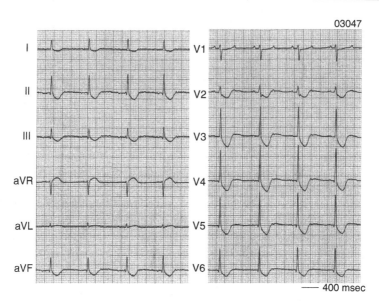

◘ Fig. 6.22
Atrial tachycardia with 2:1 AV conduction in digitalis intoxication. After dissipation of the digitalis compound from the blood, sinus rhythm with normalization of the AV conduction and the ST segments reoccurred

6.7.5   Valvular Disease

Disease of the aortic or mitral valve with a calcified valve ring (rheumatic, congenital bicuspid, or other) can give rise to block in the His bundle. This is frequently seen in aortic stenosis. When the aortic valve is severely calcified, the deposits can extend down into the ventricular septum and advanced or complete block may develop (❷ Fig. 6.16) [125, 130, 151].

6.7.6   Postsurgery

Replacement of a calcified aortic or mitral valve [5], closure of a ventricular septal defect, or other surgical traumas can result in AV block [19, 134, 152–156].

6.7.7   Congenital Disease

Complete AV block may also be congenital occurring as an isolated finding or, in half of the patients, in association with congenital malformations of the heart [152, 154, 157–167]. Most patients with congenital block have their conduction disturbance in the AV node and some of them in the His bundle [72, 153, 159, 168]. Microscopic studies suggest that there is a failure of the atrial myocardium to contact the AV region or a congenital separation between the AV node and the His–Purkinje system caused by an alteration in the development of the AV node [19, 120, 125, 130, 153, 169–175].

6.7.8   Cardiomyopathy

Any type of block can coexist with any type of cardiomyopathy as in amyloidosis, sarcoidosis (❷ Fig. 6.23) [176], and hypertrophic obstructive cardiomyopathy [125, 130, 177–179].

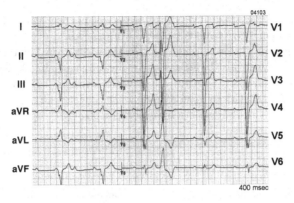

Fig. 6.23
Twelve-lead ECG of a male with documented cardiac sarcoidosis, involving the distal conduction system. Sinus rhythm is present with complete AV block and a slow escape rhythm suggesting an origin in the inferior part of the right ventricle

6.7.9 Myocarditis

Myocarditis can be bacterial, like acute rheumatic fever, diphtheria or Lyme disease, or viral [180–192]. AV block developing in this setting is a sign of a poor prognosis in the evolution of the disease [125, 130].

6.7.10 Potassium

High potassium levels [193, 194] can create AV block at plasma levels above 6.5 mEql^{-1}.

6.7.11 Others

An association of AV block with muscular and neuromuscular heredodegenerative syndromes is known [124, 125, 195–197]. In myotonic muscular dystrophy, Kearns–Sayre syndrome [198], Erb's dystrophy (limb-girdle), and peroneal muscular atrophy with or without symptoms of pacemaker implantation should be considered because there may be unpredictable progression of AV conduction disease [199, 200]. Cardiac tumors, primary [201] or metastatic [202], after chemotherapy [203] and radiation [204], cysts [125, 205], myocardial bridging [41], and traumas [125, 206] have been described as rare causes of AV block. Also in the congenital long QT syndrome the conduction system may be involved and functional 2:1 block and bundle branch block was described [207].

6.8 Age and Sex

Campbell [208] found in patients with chronic third-degree AV block that age varied between 50 and 70 years and that males predominated in a ratio of 4:1. In Ide's series [209], peak incidence occurred between 70 and 80 years of age and the ratio of males to females was 5:2. Elderly women are predilected to distal lesions due to degenerative calcified infiltrations in that area. They are three times more likely to have block in that region compared to men [210, 211].

6.9 Clinical Features

Clinical features are dependent on ventricular rate during the presence of AV block. First-degree and most types of second-degree AV block do not produce symptoms. An exception is the Mobitz type II second-degree AV block, where sudden longer episodes of ventricular asystole can produce syncope. Higher degrees of second-degree block (3:1 or 4:1 AV block) with lower ventricular rates may give symptoms similar to those of third-degree block. These patients can develop dizziness or syncopal attacks (Adams–Stokes attacks). Syncope is usually caused by transient ventricular asystole, but ventricular tachycardia or fibrillation can also be the etiology of the complaints [29, 52, 56, 212–215]. Fatigue, dyspnea or cardiac asthma, and angina can be present in patients with marginal myocardial reserve or coronary circulation at rates of 40–50 bpm or lower [71, 72, 216–218]. Generally, in contrast to the patients with chronic and stable third-degree block, those with paroxysmal episodes of third-degree block have most complaints.

6.10   Therapy

Only in those patients who are symptomatic, or who will have a high chance of becoming symptomatic, is therapy needed. This can be atropine, isoproterenol, or artificial pacing. Atropine and isoproterenol are useful for short-term treatment. Atropine can be given to patients having a severe vagal reaction which, for example, is not uncommon in the acute stage of an inferior wall infarction (❷ Fig. 6.9). In the other patients, a temporary or permanently implanted pacemaker may be indicated. When drugs play a role in the presence of the AV block, the drug should be discontinued, or at least the dosage should be lowered or a pacemaker implanted if it is important to continue the use of the drug. Isoproterenol is sometimes helpful as an acute temporary treatment prior to insertion of a temporary pacemaker in patients having bock in the His–Purkinje system.

AV block located below the AV node, that is, in the His bundle or bundle branches, is associated with a high incidence of sudden asystole [219–223]. Most investigators agree that patients with bifascicular block with HV prolongation and neurological symptoms should be paced [224–226]. If the HV interval exceeds 75 ms, pacing is indicated even without the presence of neurological complaints [227].

Each patient should be evaluated individually. If any doubt exists, other possible causes of syncope must be excluded prior to pacemaker implantation [215]. In patients with syncopal attacks due to AV conduction problems, long term ambulatory rhythm monitoring is very useful to confirm the diagnosis (see ❷ Chap. 7 of *Specialized Aspects of Electrocaridiography*)

Approaches to treatment of patients with chronic AV conduction disturbances can be summarized as follows [228].

6.10.1   Normal PR Interval

The HV interval can be prolonged in patients with a normal PR interval. The HV interval should be measured in symptomatic patients with bifascicular block. If the HV interval is prolonged, pacemaker implantation should be considered. The incidental finding at electrophysiological study of a markedly prolonged HV interval (greater than or equal to 100 ms) in asymptomatic patients is a class IIa indication for pacemaker implantation.

6.10.2   First-Degree AV Delay

Asymptomatic first-degree AV delay is treated conservatively. Even asymptomatic conduction delay with bifascicular block is considered a class III indication for pacemaker insertion. First-degree AV delay with symptoms suggestive of pacemaker syndrome and documented alleviation of symptoms with temporary AV pacing is a class IIa indication for pacemaker treatment [229, 230].

6.10.3   Second-Degree AV Block

No pacemaker is indicated in asymptomatic type I second-degree AV block at the supra-Hisian (AV nodal) level not known to be intra or infra-Hisian. Type II second-degree AV block is a pacemaker indication. Also the non-physiological induction of distal AV block at electrophysiological study is a class IIa indication. After the acute phase of myocardial infarction, transient advanced second-degree AV block and associated bundle branch block should be treated with a pacemaker. If the site of block is uncertain, an electrophysiological study may be necessary. Persistent second-degree block at the AV nodal level is considered a class IIb indication for a pacemaker.

6.10.4 Third-Degree AV Block

A pacemaker must be used in case of intermittent or permanent third-degree AV block and also in alternating bundle branch block. Also, after the acute phase of myocardial infarction, distal AV block is a pacemaker indication.

6.11 Prognosis

The prognosis of heart block depends on the causative factor. Before the existence of artificial pacemakers, the average life expectancy following discovery of complete chronic heart block varied between 2.5 and 7 years [136, 138, 208]. Since restoration of the heartbeat by artificial pacing was made possible, the prognosis of patients having chronic AV block is much better [231]. At the present time, pulse generators last well beyond 5–10 years. The prognosis of patients with serious underlying cardiac or other diseases is therefore related to this disease [135, 232–236] while the pacemaker patient without serious underlying disease has the same mortality rate as the general population [232].

In patients with ischemic heart disease, inferior wall infarction is the most frequent cause of AV block; less often it can be found in extensive anterior wall infarctions. In patients with an inferior infarct, block is located in the AV node [118, 237]. When third-degree AV nodal block develops, the patients usually have a reliable escape rhythm and are not threatened by asystole. In nearly all cases, the conduction disturbance disappears within 1–2 weeks. In the prereperfusion era the in-hospital mortality of patients with inferior wall infarction in combination with second- or third-degree AV block was 22% compared to 9% in patients with an inferior infarct and normal AV conduction or first-degree AV block [26, 238–245]. This difference in mortality is probably a result of larger infarct size.

Patients with an extensive anterior wall infarction have a conduction problem in the bundle branches. This is associated with a poor prognosis. Block can be fatal, because of long periods of asystole due to an unreliable escape rhythm arising in the ventricle when third-degree block is present [18, 133, 238, 246]. However, the major cause of death is the extent of the myocardial damage [26, 238, 243, 245]. Cardiac pacing will, therefore, not change the mortality but it can prevent Adams–Stokes attacks [133, 241]. In the prereperfusion era development of right bundle branch block in setting of such an infarct had an in-hospital mortality of 67%, right bundle branch block in combination with left anterior fascicular block 72%, and in combination with left posterior fascicular block 86% (❷ Fig. 6.12). Ninety-five percent of the patients with trifascicular block died [241]. The incidence rates of complete heart block resulting from AMI have not changed over time [247, 248]. Early reperfusion either by thrombolytic therapy or percutaneous coronary intervention can reverse ischemia related conduction disturbances, but they remain an indicator of higher risk [247–254].

In the general population, asymptomatic subjects with bifascicular block statistically carry little risk of developing total block and dying. Conduction studies are not necessary [255, 256]. In the selected group of hospital inpatients with this phenomenon, however, prognosis is compromised. This is probably related to the prognosis of the underlying disease. In a retrospective study, McAnulty et al. [257] found a 5-year morality of 55%. Narula [258] and Gupta [259] also stated in their prospective studies that there was a positive correlation with both mortality and complete block inpatients with bifascicular block.

In another prospective study, Kulbertus recorded in 32% progression to complete block in 5 years [260]. He found that although bifascicular block is related to a high incidence of death, it is not related to the conduction disturbance itself, but to other (e.g., cardiac) causes.

References

1. WHO/ISFC Task Force, Definition of terms related to cardiac rhythm. *Am. Heart J.*, 1978;**95**: 796–806.
2. Wellens, H.J.J., F.W. Bär, E.J. Vanagt, P. Brugada, and J. Farré, The differentiation between ventricular tachycardia and supraventricular tachycardia with aberrant conduction: the value of the 12-lead electrocardiogram, in *What's New in Electrocardiography?* H.J.J. Wellens and H.E. Kulbertus, Editors. The Hague: Nijhoff, 1981, pp. 184–199.

3. Touboul, P., C. Clément, J. Magrina, Y. Tessier, and J.P. Delhaye, Enregistrement de l'activité électrique du tissue de conduction auriculo-ventriculaire au cours des tqchycqrdies ventriculaires. *Arch. Mal. Coeur Vaiss.*, 1972;**65**: 1409–1421.

4. Carcia Civera, R., R. Sanjuan, J.A. Ferrero, R. Blanquer, R. Llacer, and J. Llavador, Valor del Hisiograma en el diagnostico deferencial de las taquicardias ventriculares. *Rev. Esp. Cardiol.*, 1975;**28**: 191.

5. Wellens, H.J.J, D.R. Düren, E. Downar, and K.I. Lie, Mechanism, V-A conduction and QRS configuration in ventricular tachycardia in man. *Circulation*, 1975;**51–52**(Suppl. II): 137.

6. Kastor, J.A., Atrioventricular block. *N. Engl. J. Med.*, 1975;**292**: 462–465, 572–574.

7. Adams, R., Cases of diseases of the heart, accompanied with pathological observations. *Dublin Hosp. Rep.*, 1827;**4**: 353–453.

8. Morgagni, J.B,. *De Sedibus et Causis Morborum*, 2nd edn. Padua: Remondini, 1765.

9. Stokes, W., Observations on some cases of permanently slow pulse. *Dublin Q. J. Med. Sci.*, 1846;**2**: 73–85.

10. Gaskell, W.H., On the rhythm of the heart of the frog, and on the nature of the action of the vagus nerve. *Philos. Trans. R. Soc. Lond.*, 1882;**173**: 993–1033.

11. Gaskell, W.H., On the innervation of the heart, with especial reference to the heart of the tortoise. *J. Physiol. (London)*, 1883;**4**: 43–127.

12. Einthoven, W., Le télécardiogramme. *Arch. Int. Physiol.*, 1906–1907;**4**: 132–164.

13. Wenckebach, K.F., Zur Analyse des unregelmässigen Pulses. *Z. Klin. Med.*, 1899;**37**: 475–488.

14. Hay, J., Bradycardia and cardiac arrhythmia produced by depression of certain of the functions of the heart. *Lancet*, 1906;**1**: 139–143.

15. Mobitz, W., Über die unvollständige Störung der Erregungsüberleitung zwischen Vorhof und Kammer des menschlichen Herzens. *Z. Gesamte Esp. Med.*, 1924;**41**: 180–237.

16. Yater, W.M. and V.H. Cornell, Heart block due to calcareous lesions of the bundle of His: review and report of a case with delaited histopathologic study. *Ann. Intern. Med.*, 1935;**8**: 777–789.

17. Besoain-Santander, M., A. Pick, and R. Langendorf, AV conduction in auricular flutter. *Circulation*, 1950;**2**: 604–616.

18. Julian, D.G., P.A. Valentine, and G.G. Miller, Disturbances of rate, rhythm and conduction in acute myocardial infarction. *Am. J. Med.*, 1964;**37**: 915–927.

19. Lev, M., The pathology of complete atrioventricular block. *Prog. Cardiovasc. Dis.*, 1964;**6**: 317–326.

20. Scherlag, B.J., S.H. Lau, R.H. Helfant, W.D. Berkowitz, E. Stein, and A.N. Damato, Catheter technique for recording His bundle activity in man. *Circulation*, 1969;**39**: 13–18.

21. Mobitz, W., Über den partiellen Herzblock. *Z. Klin. Med.*, 1928;**107**: 449–462.

22. Watanabe, Y. and L.S. Dreifus, Levels of concealment in second degree and advanced second degree AV-block. *Am. Heart J.*, 1972;**84**: 330–347.

23. Puech, P. and R. Grolleau, Localization of AV block, in *The Cardiac Arrhythmias*, P. Peuch and R. Slama, Editors. Paris: Roussel UCLAF, 1979, p. 139.

24. Narula, O.S., Atrioventricular block, in *Cardiac Arrhythmias: Electrophysiology, Diagnosis and Management*, O.S. Narula, Editors. Baltimore, MD: Williams and Wilkins, 1979, pp. 85–113.

25. Schuilenburg, R.M. and D. Durrer, Conduction disturbances located within the His bundle. *Circulation*, 1972;**45**: 612–628.

26. Lie, K.I., H.J. Wellens, R.M. Schuilenburg, A.E. Becker, and D. Durrer, Factors influencing prognosis of bundle branch block complicating acute antero-septal infarction. The value of His bundle recordings. *Circulation*, 1974;**50**: 935–941.

27. Sutton, R. and M. Davies, The conduction system in acute myocardial infarction complicated by heart block. *Circulation*, 1968;**38**: 987–992.

28. Rosen, K.M., H.S. Loeb, R. Chuquimia, M.Z. Sinno, S.H. Rahimotoola, and R.M. Gunnar, Site of heart block in acute myocardial infarction. *Circulation*, 1970;**42**: 925–933.

29. Puech, P., R. Grolleau, and C. Guimond, Incidence of different types of A-V block and their localization by His bundle recordings, in *The Conduction System of the Heart*, H.J.J. Wellens, K.I. Lie, and M.J. Janse, Editors. Leiden: Stenfert Kroese, 1976, pp. 467–484.

30. Narula, O.S., Current concepts of atrioventricular block, in *His Bundle Electrocardiography and Clinical Electrophysiology*, A.S. Narula, Editor. Philadelphia, PA: Davis, 1975, pp. 139–175.

31. Rosen, K.M., R.C. Dhingra, H.S. Loeb, and S.H. Rahimtoola, Chronic heart block in adults. Clinical and electrophysiological observations. *Arch. Intern. Med.*, 1973;**131**: 663–672.

32. Levy, A.M., A.J. Camm, and J.F. Keane, Multiple arrhythmias detected during nocturnal monitoring in patients with congenital complete heart block. *Circulation*, 1977;**55**: 247–253.

33. Goldberg, S., A.J. Greenspon, P.L. Urban, B. Muza, B. Berger, P. Walinsky, P. Maroko, Reperfusion arrhythmia: a marker of restoration of antegrade flow during intracoronary thrombolysis for acute myocardial infarction. *Am. Heart J.*, 1983;**105**: 26–32.

34. Gorgels, A.P., M.A. Vos, I.S. Letsch, E.A. Verschuuren, F.W. Bar, J.H. Janssen, and H.J.J. Wellens, Usefulness of the accelerated idioventricular rhythm as a marker for myocardial necrosis and reperfusion during thrombolytic therapy in acute myocardial infarction. *Am. J. Cardiol.*, 1988;**61**: 231–235.

35. Gressin, V., Y. Louvard, M. Pezzano, and H. Lardoux, Holter recording of ventricular arrhythmias during intravenous thrombolysis for acute myocardial infarction. *Am. J. Cardiol.*, 1992;**69**: 152–159.

36. Engelen, D.J., V. Gressin, M.W. Krucoff, D.A. Theuns, C. Green, E.C. Cheriex, P. Maison-Blanche, W.R. Dassen, H.J. Wellens, and A.P. Gorgels, Usefulness of frequent arrhythmias after epicardial recanalization in anterior wall acute myocardial infarction as a marker of cellular injury leading to poor recovery of left ventricular function. *Am. J. Cardiol.*, 2003;**92**: 1143–1149.

37. Puech, P., M. Blondeau, P. Bohyn, et al., L'évolution des blocs de branche vers le bloc auriculo-ventriculair complet. *Acta Cardiol.*, 1976;**21**(Suppl.): 33–66.

38. Slama, R., G. Motté, and R. Grolleau, Paroxysmal atrioventricular block, in *The Cardiac Arrhytmias*, P. Puech and R. Slama, Editors. Paris: Roussel UCLAF, 1979, p. 151.

39. Guérot, C.L., A. Coste, P.E. Valère, and R. Tricot, Lé'preuve à l'Ajmaline dans le diagnostic du bloc auriculo-ventriculaire paroxistyque. *Arch. Mal. Cœur Vaiss.*, 1973;**66**: 1241–1253.

40. Schuilenberg, R.M. and D. Durrer Rate-dependency of functional block in the human His bundle and bundle branch-Purkinje system. *Circulation*, 1973;**48**: 526–540.

41. Den Dulk, K., P. Brugada, S. Braat, B. Heddle, and H.J.J. Wellens, Myocardial bridging as a cause of paroxysmal atrioventricular block. *J. Am. Coll. Cardiol.*, 1983;**1**: 965–969.

42. Manning, G.W. and G.A. Sears, Postural heart block. *Am. J. Cardiol.*, 1962;**9**: 558–563.

43. Scherf, D. and J.H. Dix, The effects of posture on A-V conduction. *Am. Heart J.*, 1952;**43**: 494–506.

44. Lister, J.W., E. Stein, B.D. Kosowsky, S.H. Lau, and A.N. Damato, Atrioventricular conduction in man: effect of rate, exercise, isoproterenol and atropine on the P-R interval. *Am. J. Cardiol.*, 1965;**16**: 516–523.

45. Gupta, P.K., E. Lichtstein, and K. Chadda, Electrophysiological features of complete AV block within the His bundle. *Br. Heart J.*, 1973;**35**: 610–615.

46. Narula, O.S., Conduction disorders in the AV transmission system, in *Cardiac Arrhythmias*, L.S. Dreifus and W. Likoff, Editors. New York: Grune and Stratton, 1973, pp. 259–291.

47. Schweitzer, P. and H. Mark, The effect of atropine on cardiac arrhythmias and conduction. Part 1., *Am. Heart J.*, 1980;**100**: 119–127.

48. Schweitzer, P. and H. Mark, The effect of atropine on cardiac arrhythmias and conduction. Part 2., *Am. Heart J.*, 1980;**100**: 255–261.

49. Mahaim, I., *Les Maladies Organiques du Faisceau de His-Tawara*. Paris: Masson, 1931.

50. Yater, W.M., V.H. Cornell, and T. Claytor, Auriculoventricular heart block due to bilateral bundle-branch lesions. *Arch. Intern. Med.*, 1936;**57**: 132–173.

51. Lenègre, J., Bilateral bundle branch block. *Cardiologia*, 1966;**48**: 134–147.

52. Schuilenburg, R.M. and D. Durrer, Observations on atrioventricular conduction in patients with bilateral bundle branch block. *Circulation*, 1970;**41**: 967–979.

53. Rosen, K.M., Evaluation of cardiac conduction in the cardiac catheterisation laboratory. *Am. J. Cardiol.*, 1972;**30**: 701–703.

54. Dhingra, R.C., K.M. Rosen, and S.H. Rahimtoola, Normal conduction intervals and responses in sixty-one patients using His bundle recording and atrial pacing. *Chest*, 1973;**64**: 55–59.

55. Schuilenburg, R.M., *Observations on atrioventricular conduction in man using intracardiac electrocardiography and stimulation*, thesis. Amsterdam: Swado Offset, 1974.

56. Schuilenburg, R.M. and D. Durrer, Problems in the recognition of conduction disturbances in the His bundle. *Circulation*, 1975;**51**: 68–74.

57. Wellens, H.J.J., Value and limitations of programmed electrical stimulation of the heart in the study and treatment of tachycardias. *Circulation*, 1978;**57**: 845–853.

58. Ohkawa, S.-I., Sugiura, M., Itoh, Y., et al., Electrophysiologic and histologic correlations in chronic complete atrioventricular block. *Circulation*, 1981;**64**: 215–231.

59. Damato, A.N. and S.H. Lau, Clinical value of the electrogram of the conduction system. *Prog. Cardiovasc. Dis.*, 1970;**13**: 119–140.

60. Narula, O.S., B.J. Sherlag, P. Samet, and R.P. Javier, Atrioventricular block. Localization and classification by His bundle recordings. *Am. J. Med.*, 1971;**50**: 146–165.

61. Narula, O.S., R.P. Javier, P. Samet, and L.C. Maramba, Significance of His and left bundle recordings from the left heart in man. *Circulation*, 1970;**42**: 385–396.

62. Damato, A.N., J.J. Gallagher, R.N. Schnitzler, and S.H. Lau, Use of His bundle recordings in understanding A-V conduction disturbances. *Bull. N. Y. Acad. Med.*, 1971;**47**: 905–922.

63. Castellanos, A. Jr., C.A. Castillo, and A.S. Agha, Contribution of His bundle recordings to the understanding of clinical arrhythmias. *Am. J. Cardiol.*, 1971;**28**: 499–508.

64. Puech, P. and R. Grolleau, *L'Activité du Faisceau de His Normale et Pathologique*. Paris: Sandoz, 1972.

65. Bekheit, S., P. Morton, J.G. Murtagh, and E. Fletcher, Comparison of sinoventricular conduction hn children and adults using bundle of His electrograms. *Br. Heart J.*, 1973;**35**: 507–515.

66. Ross, D.L., J. Farre, F.W.H.M. Bär, et al., Comprehensive clinical electrophysiologic studies in the investigation of documented or suspected tachycardias. Time, staff, problems and costs. *Circulation*, 1980;**61**: 1010–1016.

67. Narula, O.S., L.S. Cohen, P. Samet, J.W. Lister, B.J. Scherlag, and F.J. Hildner, Localization of A-V conduction defects in man by recording of the His bundle electrogram. *Am. J. Cardiol.*, 1970;**25**: 228–237.

68. Narula, O.S. and P. Samet, Significance of first degree A-V block. *Circulation*, 1971;**43**: 772–773.

69. Levites, R. and J.I. Haft, Significance of first degree heart block (prolonged P-R interval) in bifascicular block. *Am. J. Cardiol.*, 1974;**34**: 259–264.

70. Narula, O.S., M. Runge, and P. Samet, Second degree Wenckebach type AV block due to block within the atrium *Br. Heart J.*, 1972;**34**: 1127–1136.

71. Puech, P., Atrioventricular block: the value in intracardiac recordings, in *Cardiac Arrhythmias*, D.M. Krikler and J.F. Goodwin, Editors. Philadelphia, PA: Saunders, 1975, p. 81.

72. Guimond, C. and P. Puech, Intra-His bundle blocks (102 cases). *Eur. J. Cardiol.*, 1976;**4**: 481–493.

73. Fisher, J.D., H.L. Cohen, M.M. Kay, and D. Seinfeld, The complete His bundle study. *Clin. Res.*, 1977;**25**: 648A.

74. Dhingra, R.C., E. Palileo, B. Strasberg, et al., Significance of the HV interval in 517 patients with chronic bifascicular bloc. *Circulation*, 1980;**64**: 1265–1271.

75. Johnson, R.L., K.H. Averill, and L.E. Lamb, Electrocardiographic findings in 67,375 asymptomatic subjects: VII. Atrioventricular block. *Am. J. Cardiol.*, 1960;**6**: 153–177.

76. Viitasalo, M.T., R. Kala, and A. Eisalo, Ambulatory electrocardiographic recording in endurance athletes. *Br. Heart J.*, 1982;**47**: 213–220.

77. Graybiel, Q., R.A. McFarland, D.C. Gates, and V.A. Webster, Analysis of the electrocardiograms obtained from 1000 young healthy aviators. *Am. Heart J.*, 1944;**27**: 524–549.

78. Packard, J.M., J.S. Graettinger, and A. Gaybiel, Analysis of the electrocardiograms obtained from 1000 young healthy aviators: ten year follow-up. *Circulation*, 1954;**10**: 384–400.

79. Narula, O.S. and P. Samet, Wenckebach and Mobitz type II A-V block due to block within the His bundle and bundle branches. *Circulation*, 1970;**41**: 947–965.

80. Dreifus, L.S., Y. Watanabe, R. Haiat, and D. Kimbiris, Atrioventricular block. *Am. J. Cardiol.*, 1971;**28**: 371–380.

81. Kretz, A. and H.O. DaRuos, Experimental Luciani-Wenckebach phenomenon in the anterior and posterior divisions of the left bundle branch of the canine heart. *Am. Heart J.*, 1972;**84**: 513–524.

82. Wennemark, J.R. and J.P. Bandura, Microelectrode study of Wenckebach periodicity in canine Purkinje fibers. *Am J. Cardiol.*, 1974;**33**: 390–398.

83. Friedman, H.S., J.A.C Gomes, and J.I. Haft, An analysis of Wenckebach periodicity. *J. Electrocardiol.*, 1975;**8**: 307–315.

84. Denes, P., L. Levy, A. Pick, and K.M. Rosen, The incidence of typical and atypical A-V Wenckebach periodicity. *Am. Heart J.*, 1975;**89**: 26–31.

85. Wenckebach, K.F. and H. Winterberg, *Die Unregelmässige Hertztätigkeit*. Leipzig: Wilhelm Engelmann, 1927, p. 305.

86. Langendorf, R. and J.S. Mehlman, Blocked (nonconducted) A-V nodal premature systoles imitating first and second degree A-V block. *Am. Heart J.*, 1947;**34**: 500–506.

87. Rosen, K.M., S.H. Rahimtoola, and R.M. Gunnar, Pseudo A-V block secondary to premature nonpropagated His bundle depolarizations. Documentation by His bundle electrocardiography. *Circulation*, 1970;**42**: 367–373.

88. Lindsay, A.E. and L. Schamroth, Atrioventricular junctional parasystole with concealed conduction simulating second degree atrioventricular block. *Am. J. Cardiol.*, 1973;**31**: 397–399.

89. Watanabe, Y., Atrioventricular block (in Japanese). *Saishin Igaku*, 1970;**25**: 799–805.

90. Watanabe, Y. and L.S. Dreifus, Inhomogeneous conduction in the A-V node. A model for re-entry. *Am. Heart J.*, 1965;**70**: 505–514.

91. Watanabe, Y. and L.S. Dreifus, Second degree atrioventricular block. *Cardiovasc. Res.*, 1967;**1**: 150–158.

92. Fisch, C., D.P. Zipes, and P.L. McHenry, Electrocardiographic manifestations of concealed junctional ectopic impulses. *Circulation*, 1976;**53**: 217–223.

93. Littmann, L. and R.H. Svenson, Concealed re-entry: a mechanism of atrioventricular nodal alternating Wenckebach periodicity. *Circulation*, 1982;**65**: 1269–1275.

94. El-Sherif, N., J. Aranda, B. Befeler, and R. Lazzara, Atypical Wenckebach periodicity simulating Mobitz II AV block. *Br. Heart J.*, 1978;**40**: 1376–1383.

95. Scherlag, B.J., N. El-Sherif, and R. Lazarra, Experimental model for study of Mobitz type II and paroxysmal atrioventricular block. *Am. J. Cardiol.*, 1974;**34**: 309–317.

96. Langendorf, R. and A. Pick, Atrioventricular block, type II (Mobitz)—Its nature and clinical significance. *Circulation*, 1968;**38**: 819–821.

97. Strasberg, B., F. Amat-Y-Leon, R.C. Dhingra, et al., Natural history of chronic second-degree atrioventricular nodal block. *Circulation*, 1981;**63**: 1043–1049.

98. Donoso, E., L.N. Adler, and C.K. Friedberg, Unusual forms of second-degree atrioventricular block, including Mobitz type-II block, associated with the Morgagni-Adams-Stokes syndrome. *Am. Heart. J.*, 1964;**67**: 150–157.

99. Grossman, M., Second degree heart block with Wenckebach phenomenon: its occurrence over a period of several years in a young healthy adult. *Am. Heart J.*, 1958;**56**: 607–610.

100. Meyles, I., E. Kaplinsky, J.H. Yahini, N. Hanne-Paparo, and H.N. Neufeld, Wenckebach A-V block: a frequent feature following heavy physical training. *Am. Heart J.*, 1975;**90**: 426–430.

101. Brodsky, M., D. Wu, P. Denes, C. Kanakis, and K.M. Rosen, Arrhythmias documented by 24 hour continuous electrocardiographic monitoring in 50 male medical students without apparent heart disease. *Am. J. Cardiol.*, 1977;**39**: 390–395.

102. Young, D., R. Eisenberg, B. Fish, and J.D. Fisher, Wenckebach atrioventricular block (Mobitz type I) in children and adolescents. *Am. J. Cardiol.*, 1977;**40**: 393–399.

103. Otsuka, K., Y. Ichimaru, and T. Yanaga, Studies of arrhythmias by 24 hour polygraphic recordings: relation between atrioventricular block and sleep states. *Am. Heart J.*, 1983;**105**: 934–940.

104. Dickinson, D.F. and O. Scott, Ambulatory electrocardiographic monitoring in 100 healthy teenage boys. *Br. Heart J.*, 1984;**51**: 179–183.

105. Zeppilli, P., R. Fenici, M. Sassara, M.M. Pirrami, and G. Gaselli, Wenckebach second degree A-V block in top-ranking athletes: an old problem revisited. *Am. Heart J.*, 1980;**100**:281–294.

106. Langendorf, R., H. Cohen, and E.G. Gozo Jr., Observations on second degree atrioventricular block, including new criteria for the differential diagnosis between type I and type II block. *Am. J. Cardiol.*, 1972;**29**: 111–119.

107. Goodfriend, M.A. and S.S. Barold, Tachycardia-dependent and bradycardia-dependent Mobitz type II atrioventricular block within the bundle of His. *Am. J. Cardiol.*, 1974;**33**: 908–913.

108. Gilchrist, A.R., Clinical aspects of high-grade heart-block. *Scott. Med. J.*, 1958;**3**: 53–75.

109. Friedberg, C.K., Disturbance in conduction: heart block and bundle branch block, in *Diseases of the Heart*, C.K. Friedberg, Editor. Philadelphia, PA: Saunders, 1966, pp. 583–639.

110. Jonas, E.A., B.D. Kosowsky, and K. Ramaswamy, Complete His-Purkinje block produced by carotid sinus massage: report of a case. *Circulation*, 1974;**50**: 192–197.

111. Narula, O.S., Wenckebach type I and type II atrioventricular block (revisited), in *Complex Electrocardiography*, vol. 2, C. Fisch, Editor, Philadelphia, PA: Davis, 1974, pp. 137–136.

112. Gaultier, M., E. Fournier, M.L. Efthymiou, J.P. Frejaville, P. Jouannot, and M. Dentan, Intoxication digitalique aigue (70 observations). *Bull. Soc. Med. Hop. Paris*, 1968;**119**: 247–274.

113. Smith, T.W. and J.T. Willerson, Suicidal and accidental digoxin ingestion. Report of five cases with serum digoxin level correlations. *Circulation*, 1971;**44**: 29–36.

114. Vanagt, E.J. and H.J.J. Wellens, The electrocardiogram in digitalis intoxication, in *What's New in Electrocardiography?* H.J.J. Wellens and H.E. Kulbertus, Editors. The Hague: Nijhoff, 1981, pp. 315–343.

115. Roth, I.R. and B. Kisch, The mechanism of irregular sinus rhythm in auriculoventricular heart block. *Am. Heart J.*, 1947;**36**: 257–276.

116. Rosenbaum, M.B. and E. Mepeschkin, The effects of ventricular systole on auricular rhythm in auriculoventricular block. *Circulation*, 1955;**11**: 240–261.

117. Narula, O.S., B.J. Sherlag, R.P. Javier, F.J. Hildner, and P. Samet, Analysis of the Q-V conduction defect in complete heart block utilizing His bundle electrograms. *Circulation*, 1970;**41**: 437–448.

118. Lie, K.I., H.J.J. Wellens, R.M. Schuilenburg, and D. Durrer Mechanism and significance of widened QRS complexes during complete atrioventricular block in acute inferior myocardial infarction. *Am. J. Cardiol.*, 1974;**33**: 833–889.

119. Narula, O.S. and P. Samet, Effect of atropine and glucagons on A-V nodal and His bundle pacemakers in man. *Circulation*, 1971;**44** (Suppl. II): 205.

120. Kelly, D.T., S.J. Brodsky, M. Mirowski, L.J. Krovetz, and R.D. Rowe, Bundle of His recording in congenital complete heart block. *Circulation*, 1972;**45**: 277–281.

121. Tavazzi, L., J.A. Salerno, M. Chimienti, M. Ray, and P. Bobba, Electrophysiological mechanisms of the paroxysmal atrioventricular block, in *Diagnosis, and Treatment of Cardiac Arrhythmias*, A. Bayes and J. Cosin, Editors. Oxford: Pergamon, 1980, pp. 415–430.

122. Narula, O.S. and N. Shantha, Atrioventricular block: clinical concepts and His bundle electrocardiography, in *Cardiac Arrhythmias: Their Mechanisms, Diagnosis, and Management*, W.J. Mandel, Editor. Philadelphia, PA: Lippencott, 1980, p. 437.

123. Zoob, M. and K.S. Smith, The aetiology of complete heart-block. *Br. Med. J.*, 1963;**2**: 1149–1153.

124. Lenègre, J., Etiology and pathology of bilateral bundle branch block in relation to complete heart block. *Prog. Cardiovasc. Dis.*, 1964;**6**: 409–444.

125. Lev, M., Anatomic basis for atrioventricular block. *Am. J. Med.*, 1964;**37**: 742–748.

126. Lev, M., P.N. Unger, K.M. Rosen, and S. Bharati The anatomic substrate of complete left bundle branch block. *Circulation*, 1974;**50**: 479–486.

127. Lenégre, J., Les blocks auriculo-ventriculaires complets chroniques. Etude des causes et des lesions à propos de 37 cas. *Mal. Cardiol. Vasc.*, 1962;**3**: 311–343.

128. Davies, M.J., A histological study of the conduction system in complete heart block. *J. Pathol.*, 1967;**94**: 351–358.

129. Rosenbaum, M.B., M.V. Elizari, J.O. Lazzari, G.J. Nau, R.J. Levi, and M.S. Halpern, Intraventricular trifascicular blocks. Review of the literature and classification. *Am. Heart J.*, 1969;**78**: 450–459.

130. Harris, A., M. Davies, D. Redwood, A. Leatham, and H. Siddons, Aetiology of chronic heart bock: a clinico-pathological correlation in 65 cases. *Br. Heart J.*, 1969;**31**: 206–218.

131. Rosenbaum, M.B., The hemiblocks: diagnostic and clinical significance. *Mod. Concepts Cardiovasc. Dis.*, 1970;**39**: 141–146.

132. Begg, F.R., G.J. Margovern, W.J. Cushing, E.M. Kent, and D.L. Fisher, Selective cine coronary arteriography in patients with complete heart block. *J. Thorac. Cardiovasc. Surg.*, 1969;**57**: 9–16.

133. Escher, D.J.W., The use of artificial pacemakers in acute myocardial infarction, in *Controversy in Cardiology: The Practical Clinical Approach*, E.K. Chung, Editor. New York: Springer, 1976, p. 51.

134. Furman, S., Cardiac pacing and pacemakers I. Indications for pacing bradyarrhythmias. *Am. Heart J.*, 1977;**93**: 523–530.

135. Simon, A.B. and A.E. Zloto, Atrioventricular block: natural history after permanent ventricular pacing. *Am. J. Cardiol.*, 1978;**41**: 500–507.

136. Penton, G.B., H. Miller, and S.A. Levine, Some clinical features of complete heart block. *Circulation*, 1956;**13**: 801–824.

137. Wright, J.C., M.R. Hejtmancik, G.R. Herrmann, and A.H. Shields, A clinical study of complete heart block. *Am. Heart J.*, 1956;**52**: 369–378.

138. Rowe, J.C. and P.D. White, Complete heart block: a follow-up study. *Ann. Intern. Med.*, 1958;**49**: 260–270.

139. Mason, D.T., R. Zelis, G. Lee, J.L. Hughes, J.F. Spann Jr., and E.A. Amsterdam, Current concepts and treatment of digitalis toxicity. *Am. J. Cardiol.*, 1971;**27**: 546–559.

140. Przybyla, A.C., K.L. Paulay, E. Stein, and A.N. Damato, Effects of digoxin on atrioventricular conduction patterns in man. *Am. J. Cardiol.*, 1974;**33**: 344–350.

141. Rosen, M.R., A.L. Wit, and B.F. Hoffman, Electrophysiology and pharmacology of cardiac arrhythmias. IV. Cardiac antiarrhythmic and toxic effects of digitalis. *Am. Heart J.*, 1975;**89**: 391–399.

142. Wit, A.L., M.R. Rosen, and B.F. Hoffmann, Electrophysiology an pharmacology of cardiac arrhythmias. VIII. Cardiac effects of diphenylhydantoin B. *Am. Heart J.*, 1975;**90**: 397–404.

143. Wit, A.L., B.F. Hoffman, and M.R. Rosen, Electrophysiology and pharmacology of cardiac arrhythmias. IX. Cardiac electrophysiologic effects of beta arenergic receptor stimulation and blockade. Part B. *Am. Heart J.*, 1975;**90**: 665–675.

144. Hoffman, B.F., M.R. Rosen, and A.L. Wit, Electrophysiology and pharmacology of cardiac arrhythmias. VII. Cardiac effects of quinidine and procaine amide. B. *Am. Heart J.*, 1975;**90**: 117–122.

145. Mackenzie, J., Definition of the term "heart-block". *Br. Med. J.*, 1906;**2**: 1107–1021.

146. Weiss, S. and E.B. Ferris Jr., Adams-Stokes syndrome with transient heart block of vagovagal reflex origin: mechanism and treatment. *Arch. Intern. Med.*, 1934;**54**: 931–951.

147. Weiss, S. and J.P. Baker, The carotid sinus reflex in health and disease: its rôle in the causation of fainting and convulsions. *Medicine*, 1933;**12**: 297–354.

148. Strasberg, B., W. Lam, S. Swiryn, et al., Symptomatic spontaneous paroxysmal AV nodal block due to localized hyperresponsiveness of the AV node to vagotonic reflexes. *Am. Heart J.*, 1982;**103**: 795–801.

149. Lown, B. and S.A. Levine, The carotid sinus: clinical value of its stimulation. *Circulation*, 1961;**23**: 766–789.

150. Lesser, L.M. and N.K. Wenger, Carotid sinus syncope. *Heart Lung*, 1976;**5**: 453–456.

151. Sanoudos, G. and G.E. Reed, Late heart block in aortic valve replacement. *J. Cardiovasc. Surg.*, 1974;**15**: 475–478.

152. Griffiths, S.P., Congenital complete heart block. *Circulation*, 1971;**43**: 615–617.

153. Rosen, K.M., A. Metha, S.H. Rahimtoola, R.A. Miller, Sites of congenital and surgical heart block as defined by His bundle electrocardiography. *Circulation*, 1971;**44**: 833–841.

154. Furman, S. and D. Young, Cardiac pacing in children and adolescents. *Am. J. Cardiol.*, 1977;**39**: 550–558.

155. Hofshire, P.J., D.M. Nicoloff, and J.H. Moller, Postoperative complete heart block in 64 children treated with and without cardiac pacing. *Am. J. Cardiol.*, 1977;**39**: 559–562.

156. Kim, M.H., G.M. Deeb, K.A. Eagle, D. Bruckman, F. Pelosi, H. Oral, C. Sticherling, R.L. Baker, S.P. Chough, K. Wasmer, G.F. Michaud, B.P. Knight, S.A. Strickberger, and F. Morady, Complete atrioventricular block after valvular heart surgery and the timing of pacemaker implantation. *Am. J. Cardiol.*, 2001;**87**: 649–651, A10.

157. Yabek, S.M., R.E. Swensson, and J.M. Jarmakani, Electrocardiographic recognition of sinus node dysfunction in children and young adults. *Circulation*, 1977;**56**: 235–239.

158. Williams, W.G., T. Izukawa, P.M. Olley, G.A. Trusler, and R.D. Rowe, Permanent cardiac pacing in infants and children. *PACE*, 1978;**1**: 439–447.

159. Reid, J.M., E.N. Coleman, and W. Doig, Complete congenital heart block. Report of 35 cases. *Br. Heart J.*, 1982;**48**: 236–239.

160. Blake, R.S., E.E. Chung, H. Wesley, and K.A. Hallidie-Smith, Conduction defects, ventricular arrhythmias, and late death after surgical closure of ventricular septal defect. *Br. Heart J.*, 1982;**47**: 305–315.

161. Furman, S. and G. Robinson, The use of an intracardiac pacemaker in the correction of total heart block. *Surg. Forum*, 1958;**9**: 245–248.

162. Paul, M.H., A.M. Rudolph, and A.S. Nadas, Congenital complete atrioventricular block: problems of clinical assessment. *Circulation*, 1958;**18**: 183–190.

163. Elmqvist, R. and A. Senning, An implantable pacemaker for the heart, in *Medical Electronics Proceedings of the 2nd International Conference on Medical Electronics*, C.N. Smyth, Editor. London: Iliffe, 1960, pp. 253–254.

164. Zoll, P.M., H.A. Frank, L.R.N. Zarsky, A.J. Linenthal, and A.H. Belgard, Long-term electrical stimulation of the heart for Stokes-Adams disease. *Ann. Surg.*, 1961;**154**: 330–346.

165. Kantrowitz, A., R. Cohen, H. Raillard, J. Schmidt, and D.S. Feldman, The treatment of complete heart block with an implanted controllable pacemaker. *Surg. Gynecol. Obstet.*, 1962;**115**: 415–420.

166. Nakamura, F.F. and A.S. Nada, Complete heart block in infants and children. *N. Engl. J. Med.*, 1964;**270**: 1261–1268.

167. Lemberg, L., A. Castellanos Jr., and B. Berkovits, Pacemaking on demand in AV block. *J. Am. Med. Assoc.*, 1965;**191**: 12–14.

168. Nasrallah, A.T., P.C. Gillette, and C.E. Mullins, Congenital and surgical atrioventricular block within the His bundle. *Am. J. Cardiol.*, 1975;**36**: 914–920.

169. Feldt, R.H., J.W. DuShane, and J.L. Titus, The atrioventricular conduction system in persistent common atrioventricular canal defect. Correlation with electrocardiogram. *Circulation*, 1970;**42**: 437–444.

170. Lev, M., J. Silverman, F.M. Fitzmaurice, M.H. Paul, D.E. Cassels, and R.A. Miller Lack of connection between the aria and the more peripheral conduction system in congenital atrioventricular block. *Am. J. Cardiol.*, 1971;**27**: 481–490.

171. Ferris, J.A.J. and W.A. Aherne, Cartilage in relation to the conduction tissue of the heart in sudden death. *Lancet*, 1971;**9**: 64–66.

172. Lev, M., Cuadros, H., and M.H. Paul, Interruption of the atrioventricular bundle with congenital atrioventricular block. *Circulation*, 1971;**43**: 703–710.

173. Anderson, R.H., A.E. Becker, R. Arnold, and J.L. Wilkinson, The conducting tissues in congenitally corrected transposition. *Circulation*, 1974;**50**: 911–923.

174. James, T.N., M.S. Spencer, and J.C. Kloepfler, De subitaneis mortibus, XXI. Adult onset syncope with comments on the nature of congenital heart block and the morphogenesis of the human atrioventricular septal junction. *Circulation*, 1976;**54**: 1001–1009.

175. Anderson, R.H., A.C.G. Wenick, T.G. Losekoot, and A.E. Becker, Congenitally complete heart block: developmental aspects. *Circulation*, 1977;**56**: 90–101.

176. Smedema, J.P., G. Snoep, M.O. van Kroonenburgh, R.J. van Geuns, E.C. Cheriex, A.P. Gorgels, and H.J. Crijns, The additional value of gadolinium-enhanced MRI to standard assessment for cardiac involvement in patients with pulmonary sarcoidosis. *Chest*, 2005;**128**: 1629–1637.

177. Rosen, K.M., S.H. Rahimtoola, S. Bharati, and M. Lev, Bundle branch block with intact atrioventricular conduction. Electrophysiologic and pathologic correlations in three cases. *Am. J. Cardiol.*, 1973;**32**: 783–793.

178. Matlof, H.J., J.C. Zener, and D.C. Harrison, Idiopathic hypertrophic subaortic stenosis and heart block. Cycle-to-cycle variation as a function of alteration in preload and afterload. *Am. J. Cardiol.*, 1973;**32**: 719–722.

179. Bashour, F.A., T. MacConnel, W. Skinner, and M. Hanson, Myocardial sarcoïdosis. *Dis. Chest*, 1968;**53**: 413–420.

180. Bernstein, M., Auriculoventricular dissociation following scarlet fever: report of a case. *Am. Heart J.*, 1938;**16**: 582–586.

181. Menon, T.B. and C.K.P. Rao, Tuberculosis of the myocardium causing complete heart block. *Am. J. Pathol.*, 1945;**21**: 1193–1196.

182. Logue, R.B. and J.F. Hanson, Complete heart block in German measles. *Am. Heart J.*, 1945;**30**: 205–207.

183. Rosenberg, D.H., Electrocardiographic changes in epidemic parotitis (mumps). *Proc. Soc. Exp. Biol. Med.*, 1945;**58**: 9–11.

184. Rantz, L.A., W.W. Spink, and P.J. Boisvert, Abnormalities in the electrocardiogram following haemolytic streptococcus sore throat. *Arch. Intern. Med.*, 1946;**77**: 66–79.

185. Clark, N.S., Complete heart block in children. Report of three cases possibly attributable to measles. *Arch. Dis. Child*, 1948;**23**: 156–162.

186. Engle, M.A., Recovery from complete heart block in diphtheria. *Pediatrics*, 1949;**3**: 222–233.

187. Kaindl, F. and K. Rummelhardt, Zur Therapie rezidivierender Adams-Stokes-Anfälle. *Wien. Klin. Wochenschr.*, 1956;**68**: 583–584.

188. Shee, J.C., Stokes-Adams attacks due to toxoplasma myocarditis. *Br. Heart J.*, 1964;**26**: 151–153.

189. Kleid, J.J., E.S. Kim, B. Brand, S. Eckles, and G.M. Gordon, Heart block complicating acute bacterial endocarditis. *Chest*, 1972;**61**: 301–303.

190. Lim, C.-H., C.C.S Toh, B.-L. Chia, and L.-P. Low, Stokes-Adams attacks due to acute non-specific myocarditis. *Am. Heart J.*, 1975;**90**: 172–178.

191. Wray, R. and M. Iveson, Complete heart block and systemic lupus erythematosus. *Br. Heart J.*, 1975;**37**: 982–983.

192. Lev, M., S. Bharati, F.G. Hoffman, and L. Leight, The conduction system in rheumatoid arthritis with complete atrioventricular block. *Am. Heart J.*, 1975;**90**: 78–83.

193. Surawicz, B., Relationship between electrocardiogram and electrolytes. *Am. Heart J.*, 1967;**73**: 814–834.

194. Fisch, C., Relation of electrolyte disturbances to cardiac arrhythmias. *Circulation*, 1973;**47**: 408–419.

195. Clark, D.S., R.J. Myerburg, A.R. Morales, B. Befeler, F.A. Hernandez, and H. Gelband, Heart block in Kearns-Sayre syndrome. Electrophysiologic-pathologic correlation. *Chest*, 1975;**68**: 727–730.

196. Sanyal, S.K. and W.W. Johnson, Cardiac conduction abnormalities in children with Duchenne's progressive muscular dystrophy: electrocardiographic features and morphologic correlates. *Circulation*, 1982;**66**: 853–863.

197. Komajda, M., R. Frank, J. Vedel, G. Fontaine, J.-C. Petitot, and Y. Grosgogeat Intracardiac conduction defects in dystrophia myotonica: electrophysiological study of 12 cases. *Br. Heart J.*, 1980;**43**: 315–320.

198. Schwartzkopff, B., H. Frenzel, B. Losse, M. Borggrefe, K.V. Toyka, W. Hammerstein, R. Seitz, M. Deckert, and G. Breithardt, Heart involvement in progressive external ophthalmoplegia (Kearns-Sayre syndrome): electrophysiologic, hemodynamic and morphologic findings, *Z. Kardiol.*, 1986;**75**: 161–169.

199. Hiromasa, S., T. Ikeda, K. Kubota, et al., Myotonic dystrophy: ambulatory electrocardiogram, electrophysiologic study, and echocardiographic evaluation. *Am. Heart J.*, 1987;**113**: 1482–1488.

200. Stevenson, W.G., J.K. Perloff, J.N. Weiss, and T.L. Anderson Facioscapulohumeral muscular dystrophy: evidence for selective, genetic electrophysiologic cardiac involvement. *J. Am. Coll. Cardiol.*, 1990;**15**: 292–299.

201. Arai, T., C. Kurashima, S. Wada, K. Chida, and S. Ohkawa, An unusual site for the AV node tumor: report of two cases. *Cardiovasc. Pathol.*, 1999;**8**: 325–328.

202. Van Hare, G.F., C.K. Phoon, F. Munkenbeck, C.R. Patel, D.L. Fink, and N.H. Silverman, Cardiac involvement by non-Hodgkin's lymphoma: an unusual presentation of heart conduction disturbances. *Pacing Clin. Electrophysiol.*, 1994;**17**: 1561–1564.

203. Ando, M., T. Yokozawa, J. Sawada, Y. Takaue, K. Togitani, N. Kawahigashi, M. Narabayashi, K. Takeyama, R. Tanosaki, S. Mineishi, Y. Kobayashi, T. Watanabe, I. Adachi, and K. Tobinai, Cardiac conduction abnormalities in patients with breast cancer undergoing high-dose chemotherapy and stem cell transplantation. *Bone Marrow Transplant.*, 2000;**25**: 185–189.

204. Kaplan, B.M., A.J. Miller, S. Bharati, M. Lev, and I. Martin Grais, Complete AV block following mediastinal radiation therapy: electrocardiographic and pathologic correlation and review of the world literature. *J. Interv. Card. Electrophysiol.*, 1997;**1**: 175–188. Review.

205. James, T.N., D.J.L. Carson, and T.K. Marshall, De subitaneis mortibus, I, Fibroma compressing His bundle. *Circulation*, 1973;**48**: 428–433.

206. Rosen, K.M., R. Heller, A. Ehsani, and S.H. Rahimtoola, Localization of site of traumatic heart block with His bundle recordings. Electrophysiologic observations regarding the nature of "split" H potentials. *Am. J. Cardiol.*, 1972;**30**: 412–417.

207. Gorgels, A.P., F. Al Fadley, L. Zaman, M.J. Kantoch, and Z. Al Halees, The long QT syndrome with impaired atrioventricular conduction: a malignant variant in infants. *J. Cardiovasc. Electrophysiol.*, 1998;**9**: 1225–1232.

208. Campbell, M., Complete heart block. *Br. Heart J.*, 1944;**6**: 69–92.

209. Ide, L.W., The clinical aspects of complete auriculoventricular heart block: a clinical analysis of 71 cases. *Ann. Intern. Med.*, 1950;**32**: 510–523.

210. Pomerance, A., Pathological and clinical study of calcification the mitral valve ring. *J. Clin. Pathol.*, 1970;**23**: 354–361.

211. Narula, O.S. and P. Samet, Predilection of elderly females for intra-His bundle (BH) blocks. *Circulation*, 1974;**50**(Suppl. III): 195.

212. Escher, D.J.W. and S. Furman, Pacemaker therapy for chronic rhythm disorders. *Prog. Cardiovasc. Dis.*, 1972;**14**: 459–474.

213. Conklin, E.F., S. Giannelli Jr., and T.F. Nealon Jr., Four hundred consecutive patients with permanent transveneous pacemakers. *J. Thorac. Cardiovasc. Surg.*, 1975;**69**: 1–7.

214. Wellens, H.J.J., P. Brugada, and F.W.H.M. Bär, The role of intraventricular conduction disorders in precipitating sudden death. *Ann. N. Y. Acad. Sci.*, 1982;**382**: 136–142.

215. Ezri, M., B.B. Lerman, F.E. Marchlinski, A.E. Buxton, and M.E. Josephson, Electrophysiologic evaluation of syncope in patients with bifascicular block. *Am. Heart J.*, 1983;**106**: 693–697.

216. Concklin, E.F. and S. Giannelli Jr., Four hundred consecutive patients with permanent transveneous pacemakers. *J. Thorac. Cardiovasc. Surg.*, 1975;**69**: 1.

217. Havia, T., M. Arstila, H. Wendelen, and R. Heinonen, Permanent endocardial pacing. An analysis of 90 patients. *Acta med. Scand.*, 1976;**596**: 7–11.

218. Sixth semi-annual clinical evaluation report to the United States Nuclear Regulatory Commission, Medtronic Inc. Medtronic implantable demand isotopic pulse generator, Laurens-Alcatel model 9000. 1976.

219. Ranganathan, N., R. Dhurandhar, J.H. Phillips, and E.D. Wigle, His bundle electrogram in bundle-branch block. *Circulation*, 1972;**45**: 282–294.

220. Hunt, D., J.T. Lie, J. Vohra, and G. Sloman, Histopathology of heart block complicating acute myocardial infarction: correlation with the His bundle electrogram. *Circulation*, 1973;**48**: 1252–1261.

221. Lichstein, E., P.K. Gupta, K.D. Chadda, H.-M. Liu, and M. Sayeed, Findings of prognostic value in patients with incomplete bilateral bundle branch block complicating acute myocardial infarction. *Am. J. Cardiol.*, 1973;**32**: 913–918.

222. Nasrallah, A.T. and E.F. Beard, Intra-his bundle block complicating acute inferior myocardial infarction. *Chest*, 1976;**69**: 420–422.

223. Kourtesis, P., E. Lichstein, K.D. Chadda, and P.K. Gupta, Incidence and significance of left anterior hemiblock complicating acute inferior wall myocardial infarction. *Circulation*, 1976;**53**: 784–787.

224. Lichstein, E., P.K. Gupta, and K.D. Chadda, Indications for pacing in patients with chronic bifascicular block. *PACE*, 1978;**1**: 540–543.

225. Kastor, J.A., Cardiac electrophysiology: hemiblocks and stopped hearts. *N. Engl. J. Med.*, 1978;**299**: 249–251.

226. Fisher, J.D., H.E. Kulbertus, and O.S. Narula, Panel discussion: the prognostic value of the H-V interval. *PACE*, 1978;**1**: 132–139.

227. McAnulty, J.H, S.H. Rahimtoola, E.S. Murphy, et al., A prospective study of sudden death in "high-risk" bundle branch block. *N. Engl. J. Med.*, 1978;**299**: 209–215.

228. Gregoratos, G., J. Abrams, A.E. Epstein, R.A. Freedman, D.L. Hayes, M.A. Hlatky, R.E. Kerber, G.V. Naccarelli, M.H. Schoenfeld, M.J. Silka, S.L. Winters, R.J. Gibbons, E.M. Antman, J.S. Alpert, G. Gregoratos, L.F. Hiratzka, D.P. Faxon, A.K. Jacobs, V. Fuster, and S.C. Smith Jr., American College of Cardiology/American Heart Association Task Force on Practice Guidelines/North American Society for Pacing and Electrophysiology Committee to Update the 1998 Pacemaker Guidelines.

229. Connelly, D.T. and D.M. Steinhaus, Mobitz type I atrioventricular block: an indication for permanent pacing? *Pacing Clin. Electrophysiol.*, 1996;**19**: 261–264.

230. Barold, S.S., Indications for permanent cardiac pacing in firstdegree AV block: class I, II, or III? *Pacing Clin. Electrophysiol.*, 1996;**19**: 747–751.

231. Glikson, M., J.A. Dearani, L.K. Hyberger, H.V. Schaff, S.C. Hammill, and D.L. Hayes, Indications, effectiveness, and long-term dependency in permanent pacing after cardiac surgery. *Am. J Cardiol.*, 1997;**80**: 1309–1313.

232. Wohl, A.J., N.J. Laborde, J.M. Atkins, C.G. Blomqvist, and C.B. Mullins, Prognosis of patients permanently paced for sick sinus syndrome. *Arch. Intern. Med.*, 1976;**136**: 406–408.

233. Lichstein, E., C. Ribas-Meneclier, D. Naik, K.D. Chadda, P.K. Gupta, and H. Smith Jr., The natural history of trifascicular disease following permanent implantation: significance of continuing changes in atrioventricular conduction. *Circulation*, 1976;**54**: 780–783.

234. Furman, S., V. Parsonnet, M. Bilitch, and D. Escher, Fate of patients with permanent pacemakers. *Circulation*, 1977;**56**(Suppl. III): 12.

235. Nolan, S.P., R.S. Crampton, L.B. McGuire, R.C. McGann, H.C. Holz, and W.H. Muller Jr., Factors influencing survival of patients with permanent cardiac pacemackers. *Ann. Surg.*, 1977;**185**: 122–127.

236. Ginks, W., R. Sutton, H. Siddons, and A. Leatham, Unsuspected coronary artery disease as cause of chronic atrioventricular block in middle age. *Br. Heart J.*, 1980;**44**: 699–702.

237. Resnekov, L., Pacemaking and acute myocardial infarction. *Impulse*, 1978;**11**: 1.

238. Col, J.J. and S.L. Weinberg, The incidence and mortality of intraventricular conduction in acute myocardial infarction. *Am. J. Cardiol.*, 1972;**29**: 344–350.

239. Atkins, J.M., S.J. Leshin, G. Blomqvist, and C.B. Mullins, Ventricular conduction blocks and sudden death in acute myocardial infarction. Potential indications for pacing. *N. Engl. J. Med.*, 1973;**288**: 281–284.

240. Waugh, R.A., G.S. Wagner, T.L. Haney, R.A. Rosati, and J.J. Morris, Jr., Immediate and remote prognostic significance of fascicular block during myocardial infarction. *Circulation*, 1973;**47**: 765–775.

241. Lie, K.I., *Acute myocardial infarction in the coronary care unit: Factors influencing its immediate prognosis*, thesis. Amsterdam: Peco, 1974.

242. Lie, K.I., H.J.J. Wellens, and R.M. Schuilenberg, Bundle branch block and acute myocardial infarction, in *The Conduction System of the Heart: Structure, Function and Clinical Implications*, H.J.J. Wellens, K.I. Lie, and M.J. Janse, Editors. Leiden: Stenfert Kroese, 1976, pp. 662–672.

243. Mullins, C.B. and J.M. Atkins, Prognoses and management of ventricular conduction blocks in acute myocardial infarction. *Mod. Concepts Cardiovasc. Dis.*, 1976;**45**: 129–133.

244. Tans, A.C., K.I. Lie, and D. Durrer, Clinical setting and prognostic significance of high degree atrioventricular block in acute inferior myocardial infarction: a study of 144 patients. *Am. Heart J.*, 1980;**99**: 4–8.

245. Juma, Z., A. Castellanos, and R.J. Myerburg, Prognostic significance of the electrocardiogram in patients with coronary heart disease, in *What's New in Electrocardiography?* H.J.J. Wellens and H.E. Kulbertus, Editors. The Hague: Nijhoff, 1981, pp. 1–22.

246. Meltzer, L.E. and J.B. Kitchell, The incidence of arrhythmias associated with acute myocardial infarction. *Prog. Cardiovasc. Dis.*, 1966;**9**: 50–63.

247. Goldberg R. J., J.C. Zevallos, J. Yarzebski, J.S. Alpert, J.M. Gore, Z. Chen, and J.E. Dalen, Prognosis of Acute Myocardial Infarction Complicated by Complete Heart Block (the Worcester Heart Attack Study. *Am. J. Cardiol.*, 1992;**69**: 1139–1141.

248. Archbold R.A., J.W. Sayer, S. Ray, P. Wilkinson, K. Ranjadayalan, and A.D. Timmis, Frequency and prognostic implications of conduction defects in acute myocardial infarction since the introduction of thrombolytic therapy. *Eur. Heart J.*, 1998;**19**: 893–898.

249. Sgarbossa E.B., S.L. Pinski, E.J. Topol, R.M. Califf, A. Barbagelata, S.G. Goodman, K.B. Gates, C.B. Granger, D.P. Miller, D.A. Underwood, and G.S. Wagner, Acute myocardial infarction and complete bundle branch block at hospital admission: clinical characteristics and outcome in the thrombolytic era. GUSTO-I Investigators. Global Utilization of Streptokinase and t-PA [tissue-type plasminogen activator] for Occluded Coronary Arteries *J. Am. Coll. Cardiol.*, 1998;**31**: 105–110.

250. Harpaz D., S. Behar, S. Gottlieb, V. Boyko, Y. Kishon, and M. Eldar, for the SPRINT Study Group and the Israeli Thrombolytic Survey Group, Complete atrioventricular block complicating acute myocardial infarction in the thrombolytic era. *J. Am. Coll. Cardiol.*, 1999;**34**: 1721–1728.

251. Spencer F.A., S. Jabbour, D. Lessard, J. Yarzebski, S. Ravid, V. Zaleskas, M. Hyder, J.M. Gore, and R.J. Goldberg, Two-decade-long trends (1975–1997) in the incidence, hospitalization, and long-term death rates associated with complete heart block complicating acute myocardial infarction: A community-wide perspective. *Am. Heart J.*, 2003;**145**: 500–507.

252. Aplin M., T. Engstrøm, N.G. Vejlstrup, P. Clemmensen, C. Torp-Pedersen, L. Køber, and on behalf of the TRACE Study Group, Prognostic importance of complete atrioventricular block complicating acute myocardial infarction. *Am. J. Cardiol.*, 2003;**92**: 853–856.

253. Meine T.J., S.M. Al-Khatib, J.H. Alexander, C.B. Granger, H.D. White, R. Kilaru, K. Williams, E.M. Ohman, E. Topol, and R.M. Califf, Incidence, predictors, and outcomes of high-degree atrioventricular block complicating acute myocardial infarction treated with thrombolytic therapy. *Am. Heart J.*, 2005;**149**: 670–674.

254. Ho K.W., T.H. Koh, P. Wong, S.L. Wong, Y.T. Lim, S.T. Lim, and L.F. Hsu, Complete atrioventricular block complicating acute anterior myocardial infarction can be reversed with acute coronary angioplasty. *Ann. Acad. Med. Singapore*, 2010;**39**: 254–257.

255. Lister, J.W., R.S. Kline, and M.E. Lesser, Chronic bilateral bundle branch block. Long-term observations in ambulatory patients. *Br. Heart J.*, 1977;**39**: 203–207.

256. Kulbertus, H.E., F. de Leval-Rutten, M. Dubois, and J.M. Petit, Prognostic significance of left anterior hemiblock with right bundle branch block in mass screening. *Am. J. Cardiol.*, 1978;**41**: 385.

257. McAnulty, J.H., S. Kauffman, E. Murphy, D.G. Kassebaum, and S.H. Rahimtoola, Survival in patients with intraventricular conduction defects. *Arch. Intern. Med.*, 1978;**138**: 30–35.

258. Narula, O.S., D. Gann, and P. Samet, Prognostic value of H-V interval in patients with right bundle branch block (RBBB) and left axis deviation (LAD): follow-up observations from one to six years. *Circulation*, 1974;**50**(Suppl. III): 56.

259. Gupta, P.K., E. Lichstein, and K.D. Chadda, Follow-up studies in patients with right bundle branch block and left anterior hemiblock: significance of H-V interval. *J. Electrocardiol.*, 1977;**10**: 221–224.

260. Kulbertus, H.E., The magnitude of risk of developing complete heart block in patients with LAD-RBBB. *Am. Heart J.*, 1973;**86**: 278–279.

7 Ventricular Tachycardia

Guy Fontaine · Alain Coulombe · Jèrôme Lacotte · Robert Frank

P. W. Macfarlane et al. (eds.), *Cardiac Arrhythmias and Mapping Techniques*, DOI 10.1007/978-0-85729-877-5_7,

7.1 Introduction

Ventricular arrhythmias are an important topic in cardiology and are frequently observed in clinical practice. They present in different forms ranging from benign ventricular extrasystoles to ventricular tachycardia and fibrillation which may lead to sudden death.

The latter group has been the focus of major interest in recent years. Such arrhythmias are usually observed as a complication of coronary artery disease and are responsible for about 500,000 deaths a year in North America. Autopsy findings often show minimal lesions or chronic scars, which suggest that some of these deaths are entirely the result of an arrhythmia and that the treatment of these severe ventricular arrhythmias should be one of the major objectives of modern electrophysiology. This is especially true now that significant advances have been made in the following areas:

- The synthesis of new antiarrhythmic drugs
- The effectiveness of implantable defibrillators
- The benefit of catheter ablation techniques

This chapter on ventricular arrhythmias has been arbitrarily divided into two parts: the first deals with ventricular extrasystoles and the second, with ventricular tachycardia and fibrillation. This is, of course, an artificial distinction and the same pathological situations may be discussed according to whether they present clinically as a form of isolated ventricular extrasystoles or ventricular tachycardia. This latter form is not necessarily a sign of disease's progression, as patients may show one or the other arrhythmia from the beginning.

It might be necessary to consider first the electrophysiological mechanisms of these arrhythmias. It should be emphasized that there are probably significant differences between those observed in an electrophysiological bath with microelectrodes in normal animal tissues placed in artificial electrophysiological conditions, and those which are the substrate of human pathology. Although the relationship between these two approaches remains uncertain, both the cellular electrophysiological and clinical aspects will be discussed.

7.1.1 Cellular Electrophysiological Mechanisms of Arrhythmias

The electrophysiological mechanisms of cardiac arrhythmias at cellular level can be divided into three main groups; namely, increased automaticity, triggered activity, and reentry.

7.1.2 Increased Automaticity

Increased automaticity corresponds with an increase in the normal phenomena of automaticity, and is the result of a slow diastolic depolarization in phase 4 of the action potential [1]. The activation of the adjacent nonspecific myocardium is the result of an electrotonic effect occurring when the resting potential of the automatic cells reaches its threshold. In abnormal automaticity, the resting potential is less negative (-60 mV) than in normal His-Purkinje fibers (-90 mV). In pathological conditions, every ventricular myocardial fiber [2] may exhibit this abnormal rapid automaticity. At these low potentials, which correspond to partial depolarization, the rapid sodium channel is inactivated. The ionic mechanism on which this abnormal activity is most dependent may be influenced by a number of factors. In particular, myocardial ischemia, which increases the extracellular potassium concentration, may lead to this type of abnormal automaticity when a certain level of myocardial depolarization is reached.

In addition, the partial depolarization which inactivates the rapid sodium channel can cause a conduction defect which suppresses the physiological inhibition of automatic activity by a more rapid rhythm arising from the sinus node. This is the case in complete atrioventricular block [1].

7.1.3 Triggered Activity

Triggered activity is the term used to describe a possible mechanism whereby, a cardiac arrhythmia does not occur spontaneously in resting fibers, but arises only after electrical stimulation [3]. It is immediately apparent that this cellular electrophysiological phenomenon, which is distinct from re-entry, may pose a diagnostic problem in clinical electrophysiology where the same property of triggering and termination is considered to be a criterion of re-entry.

Two types of triggered activity have been described [4, 5] and have been restudied and developed in cellular electrophysiology [6, 7]. One is the result of early after-depolarization occurring on the plateau phase of the action potential, or in phase 3, corresponding to the T wave of the surface ECG [6, 8]. The other is owing to delayed after-depolarization occurring at the end of phase 3 or the beginning of phase 4 of the action potential, corresponding to the end of the T wave, or the remaining part of the diastolic period. The latter has been particularly well studied in atrial tissues [9].

Early after-depolarization has also been observed in myocardial ischemia as a result of hypoxia or increase in the partial pressure of carbon dioxide. It is characterised by an abrupt "hump" in the action potential at the end of phase 2, which may trigger another action potential. This action potential therefore may occur at a low or at a high membrane potential level although the initial potential of the first stimulated beat had a normal resting potential (-75 to $-80\,mV$). Early after-depolarization is, however, considered as being "triggered" because it is only observed if a stimulated potential which initiates the sequence is present. This phenomenon is facilitated by slow pacing while fast pacing can abolish it. After the triggered action potential at a low resting membrane potential, repetitive activity, known as oscillatory after-depolarization becomes possible [6].

Low level early after-depolarization occurs at low membrane potentials suggesting intervention of the calcium window current underlie by L-type Ca^{2+} channel, triggering slowly conducted action potential. High level early after-depolarization occurring at high membrane potentials are triggered by an increase of the window sodium current often giving rise to bursts of fast conducted re-excitations [10, 11]. Following the formation of thrombus in cardiac cavities or coronaries, the serine protease thrombin is formed and can reach the myocardial tissue by the active process of extravasation. It was recently shown that thrombin markedly increases the window sodium current, and thus may induce high level EAD that underlies Torsades de pointes [12].

Sodium channel mutations (E1295K and ΔKPQ) responsible for a familial form of long QT syndrome (LQTS-3) result in notable increase in window sodium current [13]. Activity arising from low level early after-depolarisations is generally short-lived as the fibers return to a normal potential after a few oscillations.

Delayed after-depolarization is observed at the end of repolarization of the stimulated potentials in fibers placed under special electrophysiological conditions in which the presence of steroid or glucoid cardiotonics seem to play an important role (❷ Fig. 7.1). The stimulated action potential is first followed by depolarization, but it then returns to an even more negative value of resting potential than the basal resting membrane potential (hyperpolarization). This is followed by a wave which comprises the delayed after-potential or several oscillatory potentials and which has a less-negative value that may return to the value of the fiber's resting potential if its amplitude is small. If the amplitude is large enough, the peak of the wave created by the delayed after-depolarization will reach the threshold level and an action potential will be initiated. Depending on local conditions, these potentials may fade away, after having initiated a new depolarization and another delayed after-depolarization which is unable to reach the threshold of depolarization. However, if the threshold of depolarization is reached, a second action potential will be triggered and so on. Once triggered, this repetitive activity can continue for a long period of time (several hours). A warming-up phenomenon is often observed with an acceleration of the rate of depolarization. It is the activity related to this delayed after-depolarization which can cause diagnostic difficulties with tachycardia resulting from re-entry.

There are different means by which a delayed after-depolarization may reach threshold level. It may result from the rate of stimulation; that is, if the first stimulus induces an after-depolarization which does not attain the threshold value, there will be no propagation. However, the following stimulation, if sufficiently early in the cycle, will produce an increase in the amplitude of its after-depolarization which may or may not reach the threshold value. The next stimulus will again increase the amplitude of its after-depolarization, until eventually it reaches the threshold value, thereby generating a propagated action potential. That is to say that acceleration of the pacing rate will increase the amplitude of the delayed after-depolarization and the number of the propagated triggered action potentials, and will decrease their coupling interval: the faster the pacing rate, the faster the rate of the triggered rhythm.

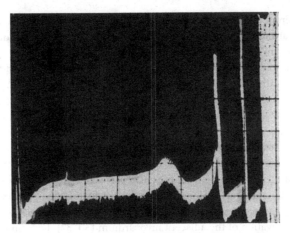

■ Fig. 7.1

Delayed after-depolarization occurring in sheep Purkinje fibers following hypokalemia (2.7 µmol l⁻¹) and the addition of a toxic amount of ouabain. The first oscillation is subthreshold, the second one reaches threshold and is followed by the beginning of triggered action potentials (Courtesy of Dr F. Fillette)

The same sequence of events may be observed after a premature stimulation during an artificially driven rhythm. The amplitude of the delayed depolarization and its prematurity both increase when the stimulus is delivered earlier in the cycle. This is a notable feature and will be referred to later in the discussion on the mechanism of arrhythmias in clinical electrophysiology. It explains the warming-up phenomenon; its action potential gives rise to a new delayed after-depolarization earlier in the cycle and of greater amplitude, which then plays the same role as an extrastimulus for the following potential.

At the cellular level, delayed-after-depolarizations are favoured by high intracellular calcium load and are due to the activation of calcium-dependent transient inward current (Iti). Various ionic conductances can underlie Iti [14, 15]. It can be a calcium-activated nonselective cationic channel [16], or calcium-dependent chloride current [17] but in most cases it is the Na-Ca exchanger when it removes calcium from the cytosol that generated Iti [18, 19]. The molecular nature of Iti takes into account that both the occurrence and amplitude of delayed-after-depolarization increase in conditions characterized by an enhanced intracellular calcium load such as rapid stimulation rate or beta-adrenergic stimulation. In failing myocardium, the altered excitation-contraction coupling process results in an abnormal intracellular calcium homeostasis that can favour delayed-after-depolarization [20].

7.1.4 Re-entry

The third fundamental mechanism of arrhythmias is the re-entry phenomenon [21]. Well known in clinical studies of the Wolff-Parkinson-White (WPW) syndrome, it has been extended to the field of ventricular tachycardia, as the myocardium behaves in a similar way during programmed pacing [22]. There are three essential conditions for the initiation of re-entry, as follows:

- The presence of two separate conduction pathways with different functional electrophysiological properties.
- Unidirectional block (usually induced by the preceding beat and located at the junction between healthy and pathological myocardium).
- A conduction delay hindering the activation front from encountering excitable myocardium beyond the site of the block.

Reentry phenomena have different clinical expressions, depending on whether they have microreentry (between Purkinje fibers and healthy myocardium), or macroreentry circuits (involving the bundle branches in case of dilated cardiomyopathy and/or a larger amount of myocardium) [23–25].

At that time, it was difficult to accept that conduction could be sufficiently delayed for the propagation time of the activation front to exceed the duration of the refractory period of the tissues located distal to the block. This was because calculations showed that it required delays about 100 times the normal value for this phenomenon to be possible [26]. In fact, this was only demonstrated partially by the recording of delayed potentials occurring in the diastolic period 250 ms after the onset of QRS complexes in experimental acute ischemic tissue [27]. These delayed potentials were observed in the animal and later in humans in diverse pathological conditions, and their behavior during premature stimulation showed unusual phenomena commonly observed in the nodo-Hisian conduction system [28, 29]. These time-dependent properties support the explanation of the mechanism of ventricular tachycardia initiation; that is, the prematurity of the extrastimulus increases the conduction time in abnormally slow conducting fibers, so allowing the most delayed potentials to transmit the activation to adjacent myocardium in the same way that stimulation of fibers in a zone of markedly delayed conduction enables reactivation of the adjacent myocardium [30–33]. Experimental studies have demonstrated the phenomenon of reentry by mapping the first cycles of an ischemic ventricular tachycardia [34, 35].

These mechanisms are important in clinical arrhythmias because ventricular tachycardia can be initiated and terminated by programmed pacing, or by bursts of rapid pacing. However, the demonstration of triggered activity unrelated to reentry has raised the problem of distinguishing between these two mechanisms.

It has also been demonstrated that programmed pacing is able to initiate ventricular arrhythmias in only a small number of cases in the acute phase of myocardial infarction, a situation in which it was thought that both increased automaticity and reentry could play a role.

On the other hand, intraventricular reentry is probably the only operative mechanism in sustained chronic ventricular tachycardia in the chronic phase after myocardial infarction. In clinical practice, the phenomena of extrasystoles, and even ventricular tachycardia can be triggered by pacing methods in severe digitalis overdose. However, pacing methods are often used to prevent bradycardias or atrioventricular blocks induced by digitalis [36].

Finally, focal reexcitation phenomena may be observed when the repolarization of adjacent fibers is asynchronous, a condition favored by beta-adrenergic stimulation or acute ischemia [35].

A delayed activation of normal myocardium after pacing in a zone where late potentials were recorded was reported in 1978 by Fontaine et al [31]. This again reinforced the concept of reentrant phenomenon in heart muscle and definitely excluded the mechanism of triggered activity. In patients at the chronic phase of myocardial infarction, De Bakker demonstrated the presence of a "zig-zag" slow conduction pattern, in which wave fronts could travel perpendicular to the fiber direction ensheathed by collagenous septa [37].

7.1.5   Criteria for Discriminating Between Cellular Electrophysiological and Clinical Mechanisms of Tachycardia

The main difficulty concerning the respective mechanisms of reentry and phenomena of triggered activity is the paucity of discriminating methods which can be used both in cellular and clinical electrophysiology. It was noted above that the induction and termination of tachycardia by programmed stimulation may be observed in both situations, but there is one way of differentiating the two mechanisms. In tachycardias triggered by delayed after-depolarization, the coupling interval of the first propagated potential decreases with increasing prematurity of the initiating extrasystole. Indeed, the moment at which delayed after-depolarization reaches the threshold becomes more premature as the coupling interval of the extrastimulus decreases. Conversely, in reentry, the coupling interval of the first propagated potential which initiates the tachycardia increases as the prematurity of the extrastimulus increases. This is owing to the conduction-time increase in the zone of delayed conduction.

Using these criteria, a retrospective study of 425 patients investigated in the authors' clinical electrophysiological laboratory in which tachycardia could be initiated and terminated by programmed pacing, showed that in 33 patients tachycardia originated in the atrium, whilst in 79 patients the point of origin was ventricular. Seven patients with atrial tachycardia and only one with ventricular tachycardia had positive evidence in favor of a mechanism of triggered activation. In addition, in five of the patients with atrial tachycardia and in the patient with ventricular tachycardia, the administration of intravenous verapamil terminated the tachycardia and prevented its reinitiation.

These results suggest that the role played by a triggered activity in the clinical situation is quite modest especially as far as the ventricular arrhythmias are concerned [38].

7.2 Ventricular Extrasystoles

Ventricular extrasystoles (VES) result from premature depolarization of the myocardium distal to the atrioventricular junction; that is, below the bifurcation of the His bundle. They may, therefore, arise from either of the two ventricles or from the interventricular septum. Recently, triggers of VES and of ventricular fibrillation (VF) were found in various locations within the Purkinje network in patients presenting with recurrent VF without underlying cardiac disease and were successfully treated by radiofrequency catheter ablation [39].

7.2.1 Clinical Features

From the clinical standpoint it is useful to distinguish between asymptomatic VES detected during clinical examination and confirmed by ECG, and symptomatic VES which are not necessarily the most dangerous, but which can have important effects on the quality of life.

Ventricular extrasystoles may be totally asymptomatic, but often they cause symptoms such as palpitations, a sensation of a missed beat, of cardiac arrest or of strong beats. Less commonly, when VES are frequent or in salvos, the patient may experience dizziness, angina, hypotension and finally tachyarrhythmia cardiomyopathy.

It is important to inquire about the patient's general health and lifestyle, in order to assess as accurately as possible the functional disturbance and the frequency of symptoms, as well as to detect any predisposing factors such as exercise, anxiety, stimulants (tobacco, alcohol, coffee, and so on), sleep disturbances, hypoxia, physical stress, drug administration, and so forth.

On examination, VES cause an irregular heart beat and changes in the intensity of the heart sounds. A systolic murmur may be detected. Organic aortic systolic murmurs decrease in intensity during the extra systolic beat but are accentuated during the following systole (contraction produced by the strong normal beat following the compensatory pause).

The hemodynamic effects of VES include the following [40]:

- Reduction in left ventricular systolic pressures (prematurity dependent)
- Increase in the length of diastole (postextrasystolic compensatory pause) resulting in an increase of stroke volume of the following systole (❷ Fig. 7.2)
- Abnormal valve motion (premature closure, mitral valve prolapse, decreased valve opening, and so on) clearly demonstrated by echocardiography

7.2.1.1 Relationship to the P Wave

Diagnosis and study of VES depend on the analysis of the ECG. Ventricular extrasystoles are premature, wide QRS complexes (usually > 120 ms) followed by a T wave with an axis opposite to that of the QRS. Characteristically, VES are not preceded by P waves. As the P wave is not easily detected in some leads, simultaneous multichannel recordings are useful in distinguishing VES from atrial and junctional extrasystoles with aberrant conduction. As a rule, VES are completely dissociated from the preceding atrial activity but they may be followed by a retrograde P wave (❷ Fig. 7.3).

A bipolar sternal lead recording with the "right arm" electrode on the manubrium and "left arm" electrode on the xiphoid process may help to show the P waves. Another more sensitive method of recording the atrial activity is to use an esophageal or an endocardial lead (❷ Fig. 7.2).

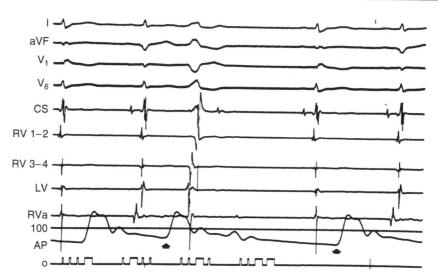

⬛ Fig. 7.2
Left ventricular extrasystole recorded during an endocardial study: CS, coronary sinus showing the atrial and the ventricular component of the ECG; RV 1–2, RV 3–4, Quadripolar catheter positioned in the infundibular area; LV, left ventricle showing that the activation commences first in this ventricle; RVa, apex of the right ventricle; AP, arterial pressure recorded on the radial artery. The second arrow indicates the drop of end-diastolic blood pressure

7.2.1.2 Morphology

It is often difficult to distinguish VES from supraventricular or junctional extrasystoles with ventricular aberration resulting from a decrease in conduction in the intraventricular conduction system. Conversely, VES arising just above the division of the His bundle will give rise to narrow QRS complexes, suggesting supraventricular activity [41]. In addition, an extrasystole occurring at the appropriate time may lead to a narrow QRS complex in the case of fusion with a normal ventricular activation, but showing bundle branch block ipsilateral to the site of origin of the extrasystole.

The morphology of VESs may generally indicate their site of origin. Appearances of right bundle branch block are observed in left ventricular extrasystoles. The arrhythmia arises within the right ventricle or septum when left bundle branch block appearances are recorded, the site being apical when the QRS is negative in leads I, II and III, and basal when positive in these leads [42]. Right-sided VES always give rise to appearances of left-sided delay whilst left-sided VES (base of interventricular septum) could show appearances of right- or left-sided delay [43].

The morphology of VES may be unchanged from one extrasystole to the next (❷ Fig. 7.3), or they may vary (❷ Fig. 7.4), in an unpredictable manner (polymorphic extrasystoles). Polymorphism must be distinguished from possible fusion between very late VES and normal depolarization (QRS complex preceded by a normal P wave with shortened PR interval and an intermediate QRS morphology).

7.2.1.3 Chronology

Ventricular extrasystoles may be divided into two types according to their relationship to the preceding QRS complex; namely, those with a short coupling interval occurring near to or on the peak of the T wave (R-on-T phenomenon) and late VES with long coupling intervals (❷ Fig. 7.5). These intervals may be fixed (varying less than 80 ms) suggesting parasystole (❷ Fig. 7.6) [41, 44]; that is, the interectopic interval is approximately a multiple (>1) of a fixed interval.

The following types of VES may be distinguished from the analysis of their relationship to the sinus beats.

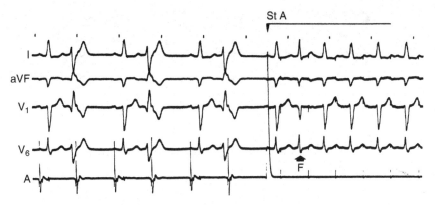

◧ Fig. 7.3
Bigeminy is visible at the beginning of the tracing. Tracing A represents the endocardial atrial electrogram. In this case, atrial activity is not modified by the extrasystoles which are therefore followed by a full compensatory pause. On the right, there is atrial pacing (St A) at a period longer than the coupling interval of extrasystoles, resulting in complete disappearance of extrasystoles. A fusion beat F is observed at the beginning of atrial pacing

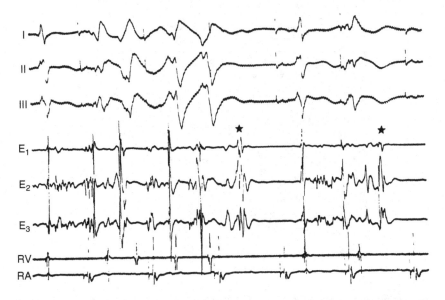

◧ Fig. 7.4
Polymorphic ventricular extrasystoles recorded during open chest surgery. Note the existence of multiple fragmented potentials on the epicardial leads E_1-E_3 preceding runs of extrasystoles which end with highly fragmented complexes (stars). RV is the potential recorded from the epicardium of the right ventricle. Note the major asynchrony between the two ventricles. RA is the atrial endocardial lead. Each atrial activity is preceded by the stimulation artifact

- VES with a compensatory pause (❯ Fig. 7.3) is the most common type. The interval between the sinus beat preceding the extrasystole, and the VES itself added to that following the VES, corresponds to two normal periods (retrograde conduction to the atrium and normal anterograde depolarization are blocked).
- In VES with retrograde conduction which recycles the sinus node, the pause following the VES is equal to the normal sinus period (❯ Fig. 7.7b).
- Interpolated VES do not affect the normal period. These VES are not conducted to the atrium and the normal sinus depolarization which follows is not blocked in refractory, junctional tissues (❯ Fig. 7.7a).

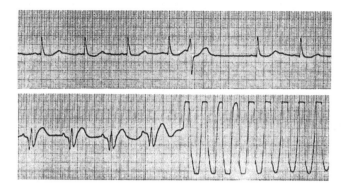

Fig. 7.5

The top panel illustrates an extrasystole with a relatively short coupling interval. The bottom panel shows an extrasystole with a relatively long coupling interval initiating a run of sustained ventricular tachycardia

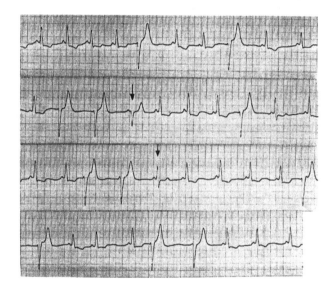

Fig. 7.6

Parasystolic focus interfering with sinus rhythm. The interval measurements demonstrate that this focus is not completely protected from the supraventricular beats. The strips are continuous running from top to bottom. The arrows indicate fusion beats

Other ECG appearances may also be observed [41]:

- The VES may be followed by AV junctional escape (> Fig. 7.7c).
- The VES may have a visible retrograde conduction. In this case, a P′ wave, usually negative in lead II, is situated in the ST segment or T wave.
- The VES may have a ventricular echo. Here, the abnormal activation is conducted retrogradely to the atrium and then returns to the ventricle without the intervention of sinus node activity. Ventricular extrasystoles are followed by either a normal or widened (aberration) ventricular complex with a fixed coupling interval which may be preceded by a P′ wave and is often followed by a compensatory pause.

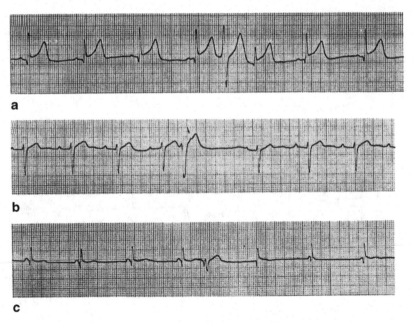

◘ Fig. 7.7
Part (a) illustrates an interpolated extrasystole; part (b) shows an extrasystole with an atrial retrograde conduction (arrow) and part (c) shows an extrasystole followed by a junctional escape

Finally, when VES are repeated with a fixed coupling interval, it is possible to record the following:

- Ventricular bigeminy when one ventricular extrasystole follows each normal complex (❷ Fig. 7.3).
- Ventricular trigeminy when one ventricular extrasystole occurs following every two normal beats (in fact, trigeminy literally corresponds to one normal complex following every two VES).
- A salvo defined as three or more successive VES (❷ Fig. 7.2).
- When more than three successive VES are recorded, it is sometimes called ventricular tachycardia (VT), or a burst of VT (❷ Fig. 7.8).

7.2.2 Endocavitary Studies

Electrophysiological investigations (❷ Chap. 2) are rarely indicated for the study of VES in themselves, but the latter could be undertaken during electrophysiological studies indicated for other reasons. Ventricular extrasystoles always precede the H potential on His-bundle recordings. In case of ventriculoatrial conduction, they are followed by a retrograde atrial electrogram.

However, it could be important to study the behavior of VES during atrial pacing. In some, cases, the VES are suppressed beyond a critical pacing rate. This rate is not stable with time, but an appropriate level could be found in certain patients and this could be used to prevent VES in the long-term, using an atrial pacemaker system (❷ Fig. 7.3).

Pace mapping [45] is a technique of endocavitary pacing, which may be carried out in sinus rhythm (and sometimes during tachycardia). Its object is to duplicate the configuration of VT and so define its site of origin. However, this technique also has its limitations [46].

7.2.3 Management

Management is the major problem of VES. The prognosis is closely related to the presence of underlying cardiac disease, especially ischemic cardiomyopathy. Although the vast majority of VES are benign, even in cases with underlying cardiac

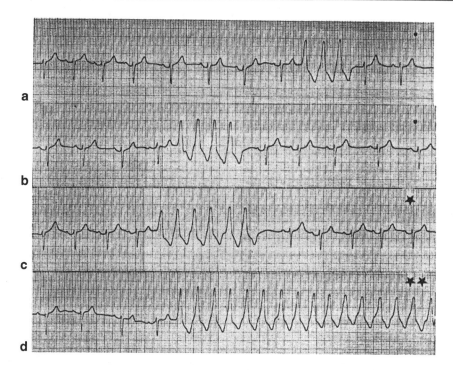

□ Fig. 7.8

Difficulties in the definition of ventricular tachycardia are exemplified in these ECGs. There are salvos of three (a) or four (b) ectopic ventricular beats; a burst of extrasystoles, alternatively regarded as a short run of ventricular tachycardia is seen in (c) and the beginning of a sustained episode of ventricular tachycardia in (d)

disease, others are markers of potentially dangerous arrhythmias and indicate a high risk of sudden death. Investigation and treatment must take these two facts into consideration.

Some investigations provide information about the arrhythmia itself, whilst other, mainly noninvasive, techniques (echocardiography, angiography, exercise-stress testing, Holter monitoring and scintigraphy) may provide clues to the underlying cause of the arrhythmia. As a general rule, only cases of potentially lethal arrhythmias, or patients with history of cardiac arrest or "resuscitated sudden deaths" are referred for electrophysiological investigation and coronary angiography for evaluation of the risks of ventricular tachycardia or ventricular fibrillation (VF).

7.2.4   VES in Normal Subjects with Apparently Healthy Hearts

Ventricular extrasystoles in "normal" persons are often called "idiopathic." The widespread use of Holter monitoring (❷ Chap. 1 of Specialized Aspects of Electrocardiography) has shown that this arrhythmia is very common and may be observed in nearly all cases when the period of observation is long enough (73% in 48 h monitoring) [47–51]. The frequency of VES increases with age and other factors which must be considered when assessing the prognosis.

A number of workers, including Rosenbaum [42] have described the following characteristic features of "benign" VES: vertical axis, left bundle branch block pattern, large R waves in leads II and III, fixed, long coupling intervals, secondary ST-T wave changes (sloping ST depression and T wave of opposite polarity to the QRS), isolated and infrequent VES.

Electrophysiological studies and epicardial mapping have shown that these VES arise in the upper part of the right side of the interventricular septum (❷ Fig. 7.9), also called right ventricular outflow tract VES. They usually disappear on exercise and are only recorded on Holter monitoring when the spontaneous rhythm slows [47, 52].

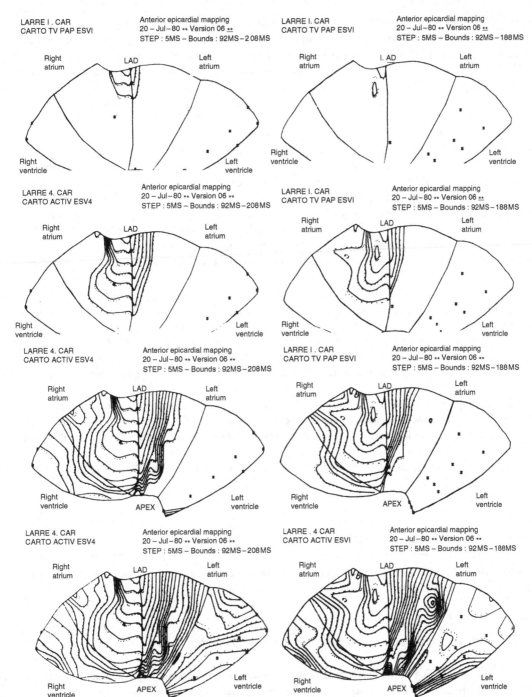

◘ Fig. 7.9

Spread of activation is shown on epicardial maps during normal sinus rhythm on the right, and on the left during an extrasystole arising from the upper part of the septum. The latter could lead to paroxysmal episodes of extrasystoles or runs of ventricular tachycardia, which could in some very rare cases be treated by a surgical approach if antiarrhythmic therapy had failed. In sinus rhythm, epicardial activation is first seen in the free wall of the right ventricle in the anteroparaseptal area. On the left, the earliest epicardial activation is noted at the origin of the left anterior descending (LAD) coronary artery. In all maps, the time interval between isochrones is 5 ms

This concept of "benign" VES must be interpreted with caution but it remains useful when the arrhythmia is totally asymptomatic in patients without apparent cardiac disease. Treatment is unnecessary [53] in most cases but therapy may be required for psychological reasons in some patients. These VES are particularly common in women and may be poorly tolerated. To complicate matters, most classic antiarrhythmic drugs are ineffective. This explains the use of drugs aimed more at relieving symptoms than at treating the arrhythmia; formerly, patients were prescribed sedatives, or usually, as second-line therapy, relatively weak antiarrhythmic agents such as beta blockers or verapamil. Nowadays, the use of radiofrequency ablation [54] or powerful antiarrhythmic drugs (class I, like flecainide) which are easy to use in healthy hearts, has completely transformed the lives of these patients.

Identical VES have been reported to come more rarely from the left ventricular outflow tract, the aortic sinus of Valsalva or the trunk of the pulmonary artery [55]. The VES morphology in precordial leads, especially the presence of a transition complex, is a good first approximation regarding the location of the successful ablation site [56].

Ventricular extrasystoles observed during the period of awakening, or during or immediately after exercise in apparently normal patients, are also very common. The autonomic nervous system is thought to play a major role in their initiation [57–59]. The frequency of this type of VES varies with age [57]. They are observed on Holter recording when the patient awakes, and tend to become more frequent on exercise but disappear during sleep. This arrhythmia does not seem to be a marker for a latent coronary artery disease and is not associated with an increased risk of sudden death [52, 57, 59, 60].

Treatment is based on the underlying physiopathogenic mechanism of the arrhythmia and so beta blockers are considered appropriate first-line drugs. As most patients require long-term therapy, beta blocker with a 24 h duration of action, some of which also have weak class I antiarrhythmic effects, are to be preferred.

Even in patients with "normal" hearts, short coupling intervals [61], changing morphologies, complex interaction (bigeminy, ventricular tachycardia) and predisposing factors (sleep, exercise, postexercise) may be observed without higher risk of potentially lethal arrhythmia or sudden death [62], especially when the VES are infrequent and the patients are young [47–49, 52, 63].

Nevertheless, frequent (over 5/h or 10/1,000 sinus beats) and/or polymorphic VES, aggravated by exercise in patients over 40 years old are suggestive of coronary artery disease, even in the absence of cardiovascular risk factors. They appear to be associated with a higher risk of sudden death and coronary events [49, 50, 58, 63–65] although this premise is not universally accepted [60, 66].

The presence of cardiovascular risk factors increases the predictive value of these VES especially that of complex VES [58–60, 63–67].

7.2.5   VES and Coronary Artery Disease

It is useful to distinguish VES occurring in the acute phase of myocardial infarction (the first 10 days) from those observed in chronic coronary insufficiency (with or without previous infarction).

7.2.5.1   Acute Phase of Myocardial Infarction (Lown's Classification)

Electrocardiogram monitoring in the coronary care unit has shown that VES are very common and are nearly always present [68–70]. Different classifications have been proposed for assessing the prognosis but the best known is that of Lown [53, 71], as shown in ❷ Table 7.1.

This classification distinguishes dangerous arrhythmias (grade 2 and over) from apparently benign arrhythmias. Although some points are debatable, especially the significance of grade 5, this classification is still used [68, 72, 73].

High-grade VES (that is, frequent and repetitive VES) do not seem to be related to the site of infarction but are related to its size [74, 75]. These VES (especially grade 5) seem to increase the risk of VT [68], but effective treatment of them has not been shown to prevent VT or VF as these particular arrhythmias seem to have different triggering factors.

No significant correlation has been found between ventricular arrhythmias (VES, VT and VF) observed in the acute phase and those observed after hospital discharge (after 3 weeks) [76], probably because they have different mechanisms;

■ Table 7.1

Lown's classification of ventricular extra-systoles (VES) [53, 71]

Grade	Type of VES
0	no VES
1a	isolated, rare VES (>1 mn-1 or >30 h)
1b	infrequent VES (>1 mn-1 but <30 h)
2	frequent monomorphic VES (>30 h)
3	frequent polymorphic VES
4a	Couplets
4b	triplets or salvos > 3
5	R-on-T phenomenon

namely, reentry in the chronic phase and increased automaticity in the acute phase [77]. However, the more serious repetitive VES observed in the acute phase are also probably as a result of reentry [74].

The treatment in the acute phase is now well established. When the arrhythmia exceeds grade 1 (l b for some authors) treatment with intravenous (IV) lidocaine is recommended [71, 78]. This drug is effective and has only a slightly depressive effect on contractility and conduction. In addition, its time of action is short. Therefore, this drug is easier to handle in the case of negative inotropic effects. On the other hand, IV administration with an electric pump is mandatory in order to have a constant infusion rate.

In the rare cases of complete or relative inefficacy or major side effects (usually owing to overdosage), drugs with the least-negative inotropic effects are to be preferred. In the authors' experience IV amiodarone is very useful as it has both an antianginal and powerful antiarrhythmic action without depression of the activation process or myocardial contractility. It may be administered intravenously by continuous infusion (2 g in 24 h). Bolus injection is dangerous because of the hypotensive effect of the excipient. Oral administration with high loading doses (1.2 g per day for the first 4 days) is also well tolerated and reduces the delay of onset of action [79].

Other antiarrhythmic agents, especially the class I drugs were used in the 80s but their negative inotropic effects must not be overlooked. They are best administered by slow IV infusion, preferably with an electric syringe, again to ensure a constant infusion rate.

7.2.5.2 The Chronic Phase

The problem of management of VES is more difficult at the chronic phase of myocardial infarction.

There is a need to determine the following:

- The best means of detecting the VES and assessing their severity;
- The most appropriate moment after infarction at which to perform the study;
- The prognosis of the arrhythmia detected and the risks of sudden death or progression of the coronary artery disease;
- The best treatment and effective prophylaxis against more serious arrhythmias.

Some of these questions have now been answered. Most workers agree that all patients at risk should undergo at least one 24 h Holter ECG before hospital discharge, sometimes associated with an exercise test. If repeated or performed after the third week postinfarction, the test does not seem to provide any additional information [80] despite the fact that the frequency and complexity of VES may increase up to the sixth month [81].

It is more difficult to assess the severity and prognosis. Lown's classification remains useful: grade 2 or more complex arrhythmias must be carefully managed while complex VES are associated with a higher risk of sudden death [53] [82–85] or cardiac death [63, 86, 87].

Holter monitoring seems to be more useful than exercise-stress testing in the evaluation of these arrhythmias but the two methods are complementary [80, 88]. Exercise testing may show an increase in the number of VES as well as changes in the ST segment.

In order to assess the prognosis, the arrhythmias must be interpreted in a wider context, taking into account a number of other factors. First, factors related to the cardiac rhythm must be considered. These are as follows.

- Low ejection fraction and raised left ventricular end diastolic pressure [53, 89–94];
- The frequency of VES appears to be proportional to the mean sinus rate [47, 95];
- Aggravation during exercise has been known to be a poor prognostic factor for a long time [47] but is not a constant finding in uncomplicated myocardial infarction without global left ventricular dysfunction [80];
- Second, cardiac factors should be considered: the severity of coronary artery disease is difficult to dissociate from ventricular arrhythmias. The following factors play a role;
- Previous myocardial infarction;
- ST changes on exercise-stress testing have been shown to be more sensitive than Holter monitoring [80, 95, 96];
- Segmental abnormalities of wall motion [84, 92, 93, 97];
- The number of diseased vessels [92], although this factor is not universally accepted [84, 93].

On the other hand, the site of infarction does not seem to be important [51] although some workers do not agree [53]. Finally, the clinical context and the patient's mental condition have to be taken into consideration. The roles of the autonomic nervous system and of certain hormonal and humoral factors, though not fully understood, are certainly not completely divorced from the mechanism of some arrhythmias [53].

The presence of complex and frequent VES after myocardial infarction seems to be associated with higher mortality, especially as a result of sudden arrhythmic death, and also appears to be independent of other factors [83, 86, 87, 90, 93, 94, 98]. The risk is maximal during the first six months and then gradually decreases [81, 99].

A cooperative study on a group of 804 cases [100] studied by Holter monitoring was able to indicate, after univariate analysis, that it was possible to classify these patients into three groups at risk of sudden death over a two-year period. Two electrocardiographic markers are considered: number of VES per hour and the presence or absence of runs (i.e., three or more VES in a row). In the first grade, defined as patients having less than three VES per hour and no runs, the two-year mortality rate is 8%; in the second, which consisted of patients having more than three VES per hour, or having runs, the mortality rate increases to 16%; in the third group, composed of patients having more than three VES per hour and runs, the mortality rate increases to 37%.

Other investigators have proposed electrophysiological studies shortly after the acute phase of myocardial infarction for these high-risk patients. The recording of repetitive ventricular responses to a single extrastimulus may help identify the subgroup with a high risk of sudden arrhythmic death [91].

About 90% of complex VES can now be effectively controlled by antiarrhythmic drugs, the number of which is continually increasing [94]. However, the role of VES in the induction of more severe arrhythmias is still not clear, and the suppression of VES has not been shown to protect patients from sudden death [53, 70, 94, 97]. Some drugs suppress VES without reducing the risk of sudden arrhythmic death. Other drugs seem to reduce the risk with only a partial but perhaps adequate, effect on the VES [41, 51, 53, 82]. Beta blockers belong to this latter group.

It is, nevertheless, rational to treat patients with complex, frequent, repetitive VES at rest or at exercise, irrespective of whether they are associated with other bad prognostic factors such as previous infarction and poor ventricular function [51, 86, 89, 90]. The benefits of treatment are less obvious in patients who have suffered small, uncomplicated infarcts and who have rare, monomorphic VES [47, 53, 89].

Patients in whom an effective antiarrhythmic treatment is most useful are included in the subgroup with salvos or short coupled VES [101]. In a study of 140 patients including two thirds with coronary artery disease, the suppression of salvos and most of the isolated extrasystoles led to a marked decrease in the annual rate of sudden arrhythmic death from 40% to 2.8%. This result was even more impressive in the subgroup of patients with a reduced ejection fraction in which

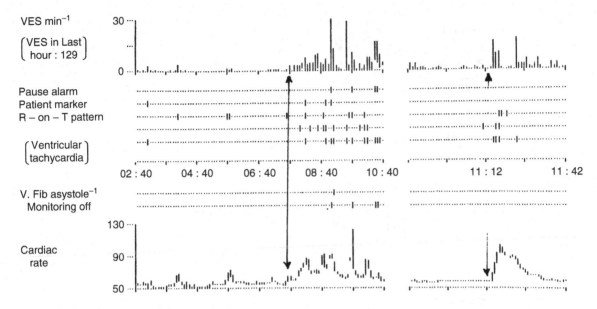

◘ Fig. 7.10
Computerized bedside monitoring report showing premature ventricular contraction (VES min⁻¹), in a patient with ventricular extrasystoles after myocardial infarction. The vertical arrows indicate that during the awakening period (7.40 a.m.), the basic cardiac rate (lower curve) increases, to be followed by a concomitant increase in the frequency of premature ventricular contractions (V.Fib, ventricular fibrillation)

the control of ventricular arrhythmias led to a decrease in the annual risk of sudden arrhythmic death from 80 to less than 5%.

Several methods of evaluating the efficacy of treatment have been proposed, all based to a certain degree on repeated bedside or Holter monitoring and/or exercise-stress testing (❯ Fig. 7.10). These investigations are used to determine the most effective drug with least side effects. Beta blockers in combination with amiodarone have the advantage of associating an antianginal and an antiarrhythmic effect (❯ Fig. 7.11) [79].

7.2.6 Chronic Coronary Insufficiency Without Infarction

Spontaneous or exercise-induced VES are generally recognized as having an important predictive value in patients with coronary artery disease. VES induced or aggravated by exercise are usually associated with more severe, multivessel disease [78, 96, 102] often associated with abnormalities of regional-wall function [59]. The risk of sudden death or of further ischemic events is higher. A reduction in the frequency of VES on exercise also seems to have the same significance [58]. It is, therefore, logical to treat these arrhythmias especially when they are complex and associated with ST changes on exercise-stress testing. Infrequent monomorphic VES, on the other hand, require only regular follow-up.

7.2.7 Other Cardiac Diseases

Most cardiac diseases are associated with a higher risk of ventricular arrhythmias and sudden death. The relationship between these two factors has often been studied and the efficacy of antiarrhythmic therapy evaluated. Three main types of cardiac disease may be distinguished: cardiomyopathies, mitral valve prolapse, and aortic valve disease.

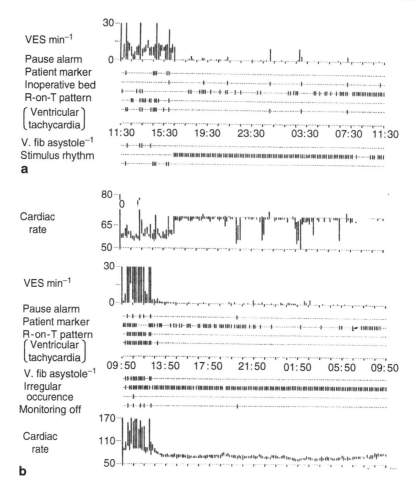

◻ Fig. 7.11

A study of the effect of two opposite antiarrhythmic methods in the treatment of premature ventricular contraction (VES min⁻¹) in two patients in the chronic phase of myocardial infarction. In (a), ventricular extrasystoles are suppressed by increasing the patients cardiac rate from 55 to 70 min⁻¹ by a temporary pacemaker. In (b), sinus tachycardia related extrasystoles (on the left) are suppressed after administration of acebutolol which produces a decrease in the cardiac rate from 120 to 65 min⁻¹, with complete disappearance of the premature ventricular contractions

7.2.7.1   VES and Cardiomyopathies

The study of ventricular arrhythmias in cardiomyopathy is difficult because of the poor definition of the frontiers of this condition. Cardiomyopathy may, however, be broadly divided into three subgroups: hypertrophic cardiomyopathy (HCM), dilated cardiomyopathy (DCM), and restrictive cardiomyopathy (RCM).

Hypertrophic cardiomyopathy has been studied in more depth than the other forms. The incidence and prognosis of arrhythmias seem to be the same, whether the hypertrophy is diffuse or localized to the interventricular septum (asymmetric septal hypertrophy), with or without obstruction (HOCM). Ventricular extrasystoles are common, especially on Holter monitoring, and the incidence varies from 80 to 90% [103–105]. The arrhythmia is severe (frequent and/or polymorphic, grade 2 or more in Lown's classification) in about half the patients [104–106]. There is little correlation between symptoms and the severity of the arrhythmia. Ventricular arrhythmias are commonly asymptomatic and often occur at night [103–105]. Holter monitoring is the investigation of choice for detecting these arrhythmias, the presence of which, in the experience of most workers increases the risk of sudden death [103, 104, 107, 108]. A family history of sudden death, especially in young patients, and asymptomatic VT on Holter monitoring are two factors which help identify a subgroup of patients at high risk [103, 106, 109] requiring antiarrhythmic therapy or a prophylactic implantation of an ICD [110]. The classical treatment of HCM is beta-blocker therapy but it is not 100% effective in preventing sudden death [106, 111]. Of note, verapamil is the gold standard treatment of atrial fibrillation in hypertrophic cardiomyopathy [112].

Ventricular extrasystoles are also more frequent and complex in DCM and RCM than in so-called "normal" hearts. They become more severe as the disease progresses in association with the increased risk of sudden death. However, the presence of ventricular arrhythmias does not appear to be an independent prognostic criterion [113–115], and its treatment remains subject to caution. Numerous mutations have been reported, encoding for sarcomeric protein genes, some conveying either favorable or adverse prognosis [116].

7.2.7.2 Mitral Valve Prolapse

Mitral valve prolapse is the most common form of valvular disease (5 – 15% of the general population) and is easily diagnosed by echocardiography. Ventricular arrhythmias are commonly observed in association (60 to 70% of cases) and they may be complex. In the majority of subjects this is an obviously benign condition, but a small number are at high risk from of severe arrhythmias. Holter monitoring is a more sensitive means of identifying these patients than the standard ECG [117, 118]. There is no correlation between the severity of the arrhythmia and the clinical symptoms or the valvular lesions [117–119]. High-risk patients may show ST-T wave changes in the posterior and/or lateral leads [119, 120] and frequent VES (over 400 per 24 h) [117]. The clinical context seems to play an important role.

The arrhythmias often seem to be influenced by the sympathetic nervous system, with a reduction of the number of VES during the night and an increase on exercise [119]. Considering the high incidence of mitral valve prolapse, it is probable that a number of cases of sudden death in young asymptomatic patients are the result of high-grade ventricular arrhythmias, especially VF [121], but this hypothesis has never been clearly demonstrated [122] and no consistent predictor of sudden cardiac death (SCD) has been found. However, the presence of a myocardial dysfunction or a severe mitral regurgitation is correlated with a poor outcome.

Antiarrhythmic treatment is logical in high-risk patients. Beta-blockers are indicated in obvious adrenergic-induced arrhythmias.

7.2.7.3 Aortic Valve Disease

The frequency and complexity of VES in aortic stenosis or regurgitation without associated coronary artery disease are comparable with those in HCM. Ventricular extrasystoles are usually asymptomatic [123], and unrelated to the transvalvular pressure gradient in aortic stenosis, or to the severity of the leak in aortic regurgitation [124]. Arrhythmias seem to be more common in dilated ventricles [125] when the ejection fraction is low and the peak systolic stress increases [73, 126]. The frequency of these VES seems to paradoxically increase after valve replacement. This behavior is not related to any preoperative feature of the disease.

Myocardial dysfunction is thought to be an important causal factor [73], but the treatment of these arrhythmias remains controversial. Some authors believe antiarrhythmic therapy to be mandatory [126] while others question its efficacy in this type of pathology [73].

In conclusion, the management of VES is clearly dependent on the type and severity of the underlying cardiac disease. An accurate assessment of the risk of "degeneration" of the arrhythmia is essential in each condition and each patient. This remains difficult and further study of the mechanisms involved in the initiation of life-threatening arrhythmias, the cause of most sudden deaths, is required.

7.3　Ventricular Tachycardias

Ventricular tachycardia is defined as a tachycardia originating below the bifurcation of the His bundle and consisting of at least three successive complexes, occurring with a frequency between 100 and 250 per minute (❷ Fig. 7.8) [127, 128].

7.3.1　Diagnosis

The diagnosis of ventricular tachycardia is generally established by study of the ECG recording. In most cases, this diagnosis is relatively simple. However, at times, it can be extremely difficult or misleading even for experts. The most common problem is distinguishing ventricular tachycardia from supraventricular tachycardia with aberration or more complex situations like the involvement of an accessory pathway. As the consequences of these alternative diagnoses may be very different from a therapeutic point of view, it may sometimes be necessary to confirm the diagnosis by esophageal recordings, or by endocavitary investigation [128–131] without delaying the DC shock in case of poorly tolerated arrhythmia.

7.3.1.1　Electrocardiographic Features

The characteristic features of VT are the following:

- Regular tachycardia with a rate usually between 100 and 200 beats/min,
- Wide deformed monomorphic ventricular complexes (QRS > 0.12 s), and
- Anterograde atrioventricular dissociation.

Atrial activity

The atrial rhythm depends on the sinus node and is usually slower than rapid rhythm of the VT (❷ Fig. 7.12). However, retrograde ventriculoatrial conduction is often observed with the ventricular activation conducted 1:1 to the atrium, or with retrograde block of different degrees.

In order to confirm VT, the P waves capable of capture or fusion must be carefully identified. This may be difficult using classical surface recordings and a bisternal lead or an esophageal recording may help in the diagnosis. This occurrence of fusion indicates that a ventricular focus has been modified by an external influence, usually supraventricular, but which may also be of ventricular origin. Capture of the ventricle by the supraventricular rhythm with a normal QRS complex implies an atrial origin of the activation. However, extrasystoles arising from the contralateral site of origin of the VT can also normalize the QRS width.

There are exceptions to the above. Atrial rhythm is not always slower and dissociated from the ventricular rhythm. This may be the case in two situations:

- There may be retrograde conduction. Therefore, ventricular tachycardia should be differentiated from atrial or junctional tachycardia with 1:1 conduction with either functional bundle branch block or preexcitation.
- The atrial activity may be atrial fibrillation or an isorhythmic atrial tachycardia.

Conversely atrial activation at a slower rate dissociated during tachycardia with wide QRS complexes, is not always a ventricular tachycardia. A tachycardia originating in the His bundle associated with bundle branch block and retrograde block may also give the same appearances.

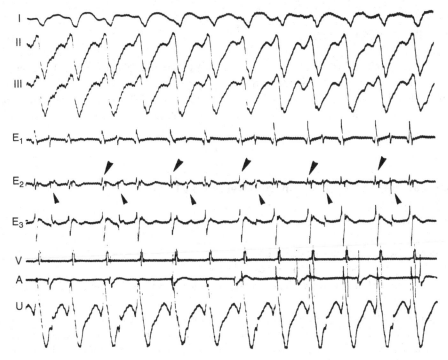

◐ Fig. 7.12
An episode of sustained ventricular tachycardia recorded during epicardial mapping. E_I, E_2, E_3 are the epicardial leads. The atrial rhythm (A) is completely dissociated from the ventricular rhythm (V) recorded on the anterior aspect of the right ventricle. In this patient with arrhythmogenic right ventricular dysplasia, the moving epicardial probe (E) records a phenomenon of 2: 1 Mobitz II block in the ventricle. The delayed potential stressed by the upward directed arrows appears on one of the other beats, and follows a normal synchronous beat indicated by the downward oriented arrow. U is the unipolar recording from the bipolar roving probe

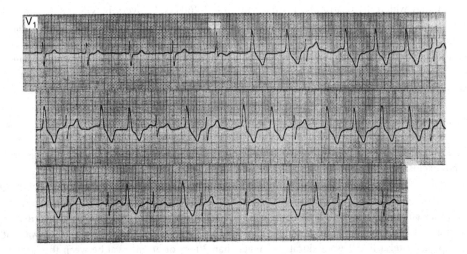

◐ Fig. 7.13
Accelerated idioventricular rhythm with a fusion beat owing to simultaneous activation between the supraventricular activity and the ventricular rhythm. The strips are recorded continuously, beginning with the top panel

Ventricular activity

The ventricular rhythm may be as follows:

- Irregular (ventricular tachyarrhythmia), posing the difficult differential diagnosis of a Kent bundle with a short refractory period in atrial fibrillation (pseudoventricular tachycardia);
- Slower (< 100 beats/min), in cases of accelerated idioventricular rhythm (❯ Fig. 7.13) or on account of treatment; or
- Faster (> 200 beats/min), with a regular large-amplitude sinusoidal wave called "ventricular flutter."

7.3.1.2   Electrocardiographic Discrimination Between VT and SVT

In the case of a wide complex tachycardia (WCT), a SVT may simulate a VT because of:

- A rate dependent bundle branch block aberration
- An accessory pathway with fast atrioventricular conduction
- Some electrolyte disorders (i.e. hyperkalemia) or antiarrhythmic drugs widening the QRS complex (especially class I).

Many algorithms based on ECG features have been published in the last two decades [140, 141] to improve the differential diagnosis between SVT and VT when major criteria like capture and fusion phenomenon or atrioventricular dissociation are missing or dubious. Before using these complex algorithms, the first step of clinical evaluation is to look for the presence of the following abnormalities on previously recorded ECGs (in sinus rhythm) if available:

- LBBB or RBBB
- Ventricular preexcitation
- VES with the same morphology as the WCT.

Other criteria like QRS axis and QRS duration generally provide a small contribution to the diagnosis. However, a QRS axis rotation between $-90°$ and $-180°$ is considered as very specific of a ventricular origin, whereas other deviations can be achieved by both VT and SVT. Concerning QRS duration, a value above 140ms was found to have a very high specificity for VT, even if antiarrhythmic drug administration (class Ia and Ic especially) during SVT or conduction through an accessory pathway may widen the ventricular complex up to 140–160 ms. Conversely, VT arising from the ventricular septum or from the His-Purkinje system in patients without structural heart disease is known to give relatively "narrow" WCT. These data suggest that there is no reliable measure able to discriminate SVT from VT, even if a QRS duration of more than 140 ms has a high specificity in the absence of antiarrhythmic drugs or Wolff-Parkinson-White syndrome.

The main step in the differential diagnosis is ultimately based on the analysis of QRS morphology during WCT, which can be divided into LBBB or RBBB pattern according to the polarity of QRS in lead V_1:

- When V_1 has a RBBB morphology, monophasic R wave or biphasic qR and Rs patterns are very suggestive of VT whereas a triphasic ventricular complex like rSr', rsr', rSR' or rsR' is more consistent with an aberration in conduction. At the same time, an R/S ratio < 1 in V_6 is expected during a WCT related to SVT. Classical patterns for VT in V_6 are rS, QS or an R exclusive wave (❯ Fig. 7.14).
- When V_1 has an LBBB morphology, the discrimination criteria are mainly based on the beginning of the QRS complex. When the depolarization is transmitted from the atrium to the ventricle through the His-Purkinje network, the QRS complex keeps a sharp onset even in the presence of aberrant conduction. Conversely, the ventricular depolarization of a VT through undifferentiated or scar tissue is supposed to give a slow rising or descending wave at the onset of the QRS complex. Criteria like R wave duration longer than 30 ms or an interval between the onset of the QRS to the S wave nadir of at least 60 ms in V_1, are highly correlated with a ventricular origin [142]. In V_6, the common pattern encountered during SVT is R exclusive or RR', with the lack of an initial q wave. In the case of VT, the usual morphologies are QR or QS (❯ Fig. 7.15).

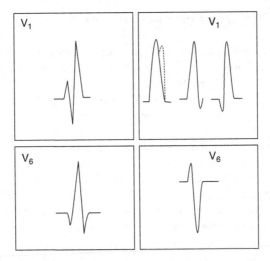

■ Fig. 7.14

Classical morphologies of QRS in V_1 and V_6 encountered in case of SVT (left patterns) and VT (right patterns) with a RBBB pattern

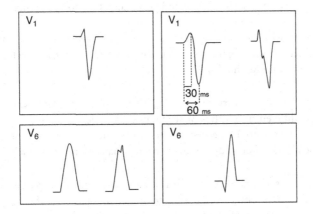

■ Fig. 7.15

Classical morphologies of QRS in V_1 and V_6 encountered in case of SVT (left patterns) and VT (right patterns) with a LBBB pattern. R duration above 30 ms and interval between the onset of the QRS to the S wave nadir of at least 60 ms in V_1 suggest VT

This analysis of QRS morphology during WCT may seem so difficult to carry out that some authors have suggested to look for more simple features like:

- lack of RS complex in precordial leads, highly suggestive of a VT according to Brugada [140], especially in the presence of a long interval between the onset of the QRS to the S wave nadir of at least 60 ms in V_1 (specificity = 100%);
- negative or positive concordance from V_1 to V_6 (all precordial leads predominantly positive or negative) is very uncommon in SVT except in the presence of an accessory pathway.

In case of an uncertain diagnosis, especially during administration of antiarrhythmic drugs (given the risk of false positive criteria for VT), the ultimate step for WCT discrimination is the use of vagal maneuvers (carotid sinus massage or valsalva maneuver for instance) of parasympathomimetic drugs.

7.3.1.3 Results of Endocavitary Investigations During VT

Endocavitary electrophysiological investigations can be of diagnostic and therapeutic value when the VT is well tolerated and does not require immediate cardioversion. Electrophysiological studies usually confirm the diagnosis of VT, and in addition define the atrial rhythm (sinus, retrograde, ectopic).

In the His-bundle recording in VT, the His potential H' is dissociated from P waves and related to the QRS complex. The timing of H' with respect to the QRS is variable, but it is usually situated within or just after the QRS complex. This is an argument in favor of VT. However, a WPW syndrome with reciprocating tachycardia involving Mahaim fibers in the retrograde direction may pose a difficult differential diagnosis with VT.

A programmable stimulator is used to deliver 2 ms pulse duration stimuli at twice the diastolic threshold (around 2 mA), this amplitude being sometimes increased up to five times the threshold value. The stimuli can be directed to any of the three catheters through a remote-controlled switch box. Two stimulators should be available, one preset for tachycardia interruption and the other for programmed pacing during the investigation.

Ventricular tachycardia may be initiated by either atrial or ventricular pacing. In the former, the maneuvers involve introducing two or three atrial extrastimuli with increasing prematurity into a basal sinus cycle. When this is ineffective, coupled extrastimuli at increasing prematurity are introduced on a fixed atrial paced rhythm. Finally, overdrive pacing up to the Wenckebach point can be used. Ventricular pacing, includes the following:

- Asynchronous ventricular pacing at an increasing rate, from 70 to 200 beats/min;
- Coupled ventricular stimulation, then paired ventricular extrastimuli during sinus rhythm at increasing prematurity until the effective refractory period (erp) is reached and eventually three to five premature stimulations up to the erps (❯ Fig. 7.16);
- Paired ventricular stimulation which is repeated at fixed basic ventricular rate at 100, 130 and 150 beats/min;
- Bursts of rapid ventricular pacing with each stimulus eliciting a ventricular response for a period of 3–7 s;
- Pharmacological injection of isoproterenol [143].

In fact, protocols and definitions of VT vary from group to group. Selected protocols have been summarized in ❯ Table 7.2. Some groups use different intensities of stimulation or different sites of stimulation [144, 145]. However, these protocols are very controversial [146, 147] especially as some groups use them to test the effectiveness of treatment.

Different sorts of response may be elicited by the above pacing maneuvers. These include the following:

- Simple repetitive ventricular responses with an identical configuration to the paced beat. This type of response is physiological and corresponds to re-entry from branch to branch and has no pathological significance [148].
- Initiation of sustained (≥30 s) or nonsustained (<30 s) VT that comprises at least three successive complexes. The frequency, configuration and electrical axis enable VT to be classified as "clinical" when identical to the spontaneous recorded VT, or "nonclinical" when otherwise. However, nonclinical VT may in fact correspond to a clinical VT which has not been recorded.
- Rapid and poorly tolerated VT or ventricular fibrillation must be defibrillated when the patient has lost consciousness.

7.3.2 Etiologies

The cause of VT may be deduced from clinical examination of the patient and from the results of different complementary investigations. In patients without clinically obvious cardiac disease, investigations may be limited to standard electrocardiography, stress testing, echocardiography, and eventually myocardial scintigraphy. In patients with obvious underlying cardiac disease, it may be necessary to perform right and left ventriculography, as well as coronary arteriography. The most common pathologies are outlined in the following subsections.

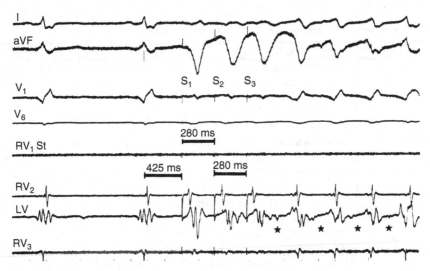

⬛ Fig. 7.16
Induction of sustained ventricular tachycardia by three premature stimuli S_1, S_2, S_3 during sinus rhythm, in a patient in the chronic phase of myocardial infarction. RV_1, RV_2, RV_3 are recorded from the right ventricle. LV indicates the endocardial bipolar lead in an abnormal zone of the left ventricle showing fragmentation, both during sinus rhythm and during programmed pacing. When ventricular tachycardia is elicited, note the fragmentation of delayed potential bridging diastole (stars)

7.3.2.1 Coronary Artery Disease

Coronary artery disease occurs in about 80% of cases. Acute myocardial infarction is often complicated by polymorphic ventricular arrhythmias which explained the high mortality previously associated with acute myocardial infarction [149]. Ventricular arrhythmias may also be observed after a delay of 10 to 15 years following the initial infarct and may be the only clinical sign of a ventricular aneurysm [150, 151]. In this group of patients, the association with cardiac failure is a poor prognostic factor.

During the last decade, several major studies have clearly demonstrated the benefit of the ICD in the secondary [152–154] and primary prevention [155–157] of sudden cardiac death compared with an optimal treatment including ACE and beta-blockers, sometimes completed with an antiarrhythmic drug strategy guided by an electrophysiologic testing. A major challenge in the management of patients with CAD remains the definition of subgroups at high risk of SCD. Major criteria in this risk stratification strategy are, a previous history of SCD or spontaneous sustained VT, and left ventricular ejection fraction of 30% or less one month after an acute coronary syndrome. Conversely, prevention of ventricular arrhythmias by ICD or drugs in patients with preserved systolic function still remains unclear.

During the early phase after myocardial infarction (40 days), ICD shows no benefit in terms of survival among high risk patients with reduced left ventricular ejection fraction of 35% or less and depressed heart-rate variability.

According to these trials, indications for ICD implantation [110] in patients with a coronary heart disease are:

- Spontaneous sustained VT with impaired left ventricular ejection fraction,
- Syncope of undetermined origin with clinically relevant, hemodynamically significant sustained VT or VF induced at electrophysiological study when drug therapy is ineffective, not tolerated, or not preferred (bad compliance on long term),
- Coronary disease, prior myocardial infarction, left ventricular dysfunction, and inducible VF or sustained VT at electrophysiological study that is not controlled by a Class I antiarrhythmic drug,
- Spontaneous sustained VT that is not amenable to other treatments,

◘ Table 7.2

Protocols of programmed pacing and definition of ventricular tachycardia (VT)

Study	Programmed pacing	Definition of VT
Mason and Winkle [134]	A1 atrial stimulation V1 ventricular stimulation extrastimulus V2, V2-V3, V2-V3-V4, V2-V3-V4-V5 V1,V2,V3 stimulation burst of VT RV1 + LV2 isoproterenol	Sustained for > 15 s Nonsustained: 6–15 complexes.
Mann et al [135]	ventricular stimulation (apex + septum) extrastimulus V2, V2-V3, V2-V3-V4, V2-V3-V4-V5 stimulation (500 ms) + extrastimulus burst of VT.	sustained for > 1 min or necessitating intervention for termination (poor hemodynamic tolerance) nonsustained > 6 beats, spontaneous termination within one minute.
Doherty and Josephson [136]	atrial A1, A1-A2, A1-A2-A3, stimulation extrastimulus V2, V2-V3, V2-V3-V4 ventricular pacing V2, V2-V3 other site isoproterenol	
Ruskin et al [137]	atrial A1, A1-A2, stimulation V1 ventricular stimulation extrastimulus V2, V2-V3 burst (RV) of VT	sustained VT: 100 narrow nonspontaneous complexes nonsustained VT > 5 complexes and < 100 complexes repetitive ventricular response, 3 or 4 extrasystoles.
Vandepol et al [138]	V2, V1-V2, V1-V2-V3 during sinus rhythm burst (multiple site) of VT	sustained VT > 1 min, nonspontaneous termination nonsustained VT > 3 complexes < 1 min, spontaneous termination
Perrot et al [131]	A1-A2, A1-A2, -A3 atrial stimulation ventricular stimulation with V1-V2, V1-V2-V3 extrastimuli pacing from 70 to 100 min-1.	nonsustained VT > 5 complexes at a rate of > 100 min-1 for < 1 min, spontaneous termination, sustained VT > 1 min, frequency > 100 min-1.
Livelli et al [139]	A1-V2, A1-V2-V3 atrial stimulation V1-V2, V1-V2-V3 during sinus rhythm burst (apex, infundibulum RV) of VT.	sustained VT: nonspontaneous termination (necessitate intervention) nonsustained VT > 3 complexes, but spontaneous termination.
Fisher [132]	A1-A2, A1-A2-A3 atrial stimulation + V1-V2-V3, V1-V2-V3-V4 burst of VT isoproterenol	VT > 3 ventricular complexes with a frequency > 100 min-1.
Josephson et al [2]	A1-A2, V1-V2-V3 during sinus rhythm and pacing (multiple sites, sometimes right sided, sometimes left sided).	sustained VT > 30 s or termination by extrastimuli or shock (when poorly tolerated) nonsustained VT: spontaneous termination before 10 complexes.
Breithardt et al [215]	V1-V2, V1-V2-V3 during sinus rhythm and ventricular pacing (120, 140, 160, 180 min-1) burst of VT from 10 to 20 s (180 to 220 min-1).	sustained VT > 30 s or necessitating intervention for termination nonsustained VT: spontaneous termination within 30 s.

- Patients with left ventricular ejection fraction ≤30%, at least one month post myocardial infarction and three months post coronary artery revascularization surgery.

7.3.2.2   Dilated Cardiomyopathy

Dilated cardiomyopathy (4% of cases) is generally associated with normal coronary arteriography [158]. Ventricular arrhythmias, especially VT and ventricular fibrillation, are some of the lethal complications of this condition. These arrhythmias may be very varied, usually polymorphic, and have a poor prognosis. Sudden death is commonly observed an average of three years after the clinical onset of the arrhythmias, unless the natural outcome is shortened by other complications of this condition such as embolism and chronic heart failure. However, some cases of dilated cardiomyopathy (DCM) progress very slowly, with some patients surviving more than ten years. Some of these cases of dilated cardiomyopathy may be of viral origin [159]. In patients with DCM, primary prevention of SCD is more and more based on ICD, often combined with a resynchronization device [160, 161]. Indications are comparable with those concerning CAD.

7.3.2.3 Hypertrophic Cardiomyopathy

Hypertrophic cardiomyopathy (HCM) is generally diagnosed in young and apparently healthy subjects, some of whom may practice sport at a high level, which may explain some of the sudden deaths in this group [162]. Some investigators [106] reported an incidence of 66% of severe ventricular arrhythmias and 19% of sustained VT in a series of 99 patients with hypertrophic cardiomyopathy. During a three-year follow-up period, six cases of cardiac arrest were observed, two of which were the result of ventricular fibrillation. The annual mortality of patients with VT was 8.6% compared to only 1% in patients without this arrhythmia. Arrhythmias were more commonly observed at night time, perhaps because of nocturnal sinus bradycardia. Another form of hypertrophic cardiopathy has been described [163] involving only the apex of the ventricle, characterized by deeply inverted T waves in the left precordial leads (see ❷ Chap. 8 of Electrocardiology: Comprehensive Clinical ECG). The diagnosis is confirmed by angiography which shows characteristic obliteration of the apex of the left ventricle. Although ventricular arrhythmias were reported for a long time in patients with HCM, the magnitude of ventricular arrhythmias and their relation with SCD have become more fully understood following a larger use of ICDs [164].

Current indications from both the American College of Cardiology and the European Society of Cardiology [110] for ICD implantation are listed below:

- Cardiac arrest
- Spontaneous sustained VT
- Family history of SCD and HCM
- Unexplained syncope
- Extreme LV hypertrophy with septal wall thickness ≥ 30 mm
- Hypotensive blood pressure response to exercise
- Nonsustained VT (Holter).

The significance of LV outflow tract obstruction has been demonstrated after many small studies had previously reported conflicting results. In 2003, Maron et al published a large study of 1101 patients followed for a mean of 6.3 ± 6.2 years [165]. Patients with obstruction (defined as a basal gradient of at least 30 mm Hg) have an increased risk of SCD (RR = 1.9; p = 0.01), but the low annual rate of death (1.5% vs 0.9%) gives a poor predictive value to this criterion beside risk stratification and is not sufficient alone to justify an ICD implantation.

Management of HCM may also change in the next few years in terms of risk stratification with the contribution of genetics and in terms of treatment due to a more widespread use of percutaneous alcohol septal ablation. However, the impact of this recent technique on the general course of the disease is unknown.

7.3.2.4 Mitral Valve Prolapse

Mitral valve prolapse (Barlow syndrome) is commonly complicated by ventricular arrhythmias. Ventricular extrasystoles are observed in almost 50% of cases [117]. Salvos of extrasystoles and sustained VT may also be recorded. However, although mitral valve prolapse is a relatively common condition, ventricular arrhythmias leading to VT are rare. Nevertheless, 25 cases of sudden death were reported in one review in 1979 [166]. The typical presentation is a woman of about 40 years of age with polymorphic VES and VT with a right bundle branch block configuration. The ECG shows characteristic ST-segment changes with inversion of the T wave in the left precordial leads. These forms of mitral valve prolapse are usually associated with mitral regurgitation.

No clinical or electrocardiographic criterion appears to be valuable in determining patients with a high-risk of SCD. The only indication for an ICD implantation is in secondary prevention [167].

7.3.2.5 Arrhythmogenic Right Ventricular Dysplasia

Arrhythmogenic right ventricular dysplasia [168–170] arises from an abnormality in the development of a part of the right ventricular myocardium. There is a progressive alteration of the subendocardial and mediomural fibers leading to fibroadipose degeneration. The general structure of the myocardium is usually preserved but the adipose cells seem, progressively, to replace the myocardial fibers. The disease progresses very slowly in most cases with preservation of strands of healthy or partially degenerated myocardial fibers within the adipose tissue, interconnecting with some strands in the subendocardial layers. The network of fibers may be the site of delayed conduction and the origin of delayed potentials favoring the initiation of VT by reentry (❷ Fig. 7.17). Major complications are ventricular arrhythmias, mainly VT, with the risk of sudden cardiac death, and congestive heart failure. This appears when right ventricular enlargement impairs left ventricle filling or when left ventricle itself is directly affected by the disease, masquerading as a dilated cardiomyopathy. Factors defining the prognosis have been clearly described by Hulot [171]: 130 patients were followed during 8.1 ± 7.8 years - 24 deaths occurred of which 21 were of a cardiovascular origin (progressive heart failure for 14 patients, sudden death for the remaining 7 patients). Multivariate analysis showed that right ventricular failure, left ventricular dysfunction and ventricular tachycardia identified high-risk subjects. Treatment strategy remains unclear in the absence of large prospective studies and a combined therapy is generally required, based on anti-arrhythmic drugs and catheter ablation [172], sometimes coupled with an ICD. Indications for defibrillator implantation are still debated except in cases of secondary prevention [167]. Two retrospective, non randomized studies have recently been published which demonstrated a better outcome in high risk patients implanted with an ICD [173, 174]. In case of frequent episodes of VT requiring external or post ICD implantation defibrillation shocks, radiofrequency catheter ablation or DC ablation remains the therapy of choice [172]. At the time of symptomatic congestive heart failure, heart transplantation or right ventricular cardiomyoplasty [175] has to be planned.

7.3.2.6 Uhl's Anomaly

Uhl's anomaly [176] is an anatomically similar condition to arrhythmogenic right ventricular dysplasia, but is associated with severe dilatation of the right heart and characteristic thinning of certain zones of the free wall of the right ventricle. The latter occurs to such a degree that, in some cases, no myocardium is observed between the epicardial and endocardial layers. Severe forms of this condition have been described as "parchment heart" and are associated with a very poor prognosis, with death intervening in the first days or weeks of life. However, there are some rare adult forms which may, like arrhythmogenic right ventricular dysplasia, lead to attacks of VT and sudden death.

7.3.2.7 Brugada Syndrome

Brugada syndrome, recently described in 1992, is characterized by a "coved" ST segment elevation in right precordial leads in generally young patients with structurally normal hearts. It is correlated with a high incidence of sudden arrhythmic deaths related to ventricular fibrillation [177]. This specific ECG pattern is the consequence of a mutation on a gene encoding for the sodium channel, leading to an imbalance between the outward potassium current and the inward sodium channel generating an electric gradient between epicardial and endocardial layers during ventricular repolarization. Sudden cardiac death risk is predicted by personal and familial presentation and by the onset of ventricular fibrillation during programmed ventricular stimulation. Screening parents and siblings is mandatory due to the autosomal dominant transmission of mutations described. In high-risk patients and in secondary prevention, an ICD implantation is required [177].

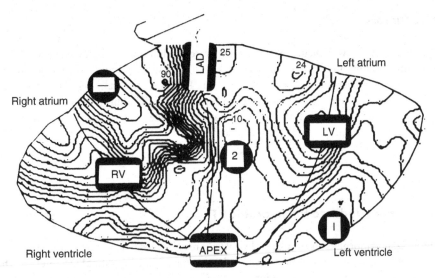

⬛ Fig. 7.17

Epicardial map showing the activation pattern in a patient with arrhythmogenic right ventricular dysplasia. The first activated area (1) is situated on the posterodiaphragmatic aspect of the left ventricle. The second area (2) of excitation appears also abnormally on the anterior aspect of the left ventricle. The right ventricle shows major delay of conduction as indicated by tightly packed isochrones. The latest activated area is located near the AV groove in the area indicated by the minus sign. This place was also the area where the VT originated. LAD indicates the left anterior descending artery

7.3.2.8 Idiopathic VT

Idiopathic VT is observed in clinically normal hearts and is generally the only symptom present. The arrhythmia starts as VES which become progressively more frequent, leading to sustained VT of the same configuration. These VES and VT mainly arise from:

- the right ventricular outflow tract (RVOT), giving a pattern of LBBB with a normal QRS axis [178] and less frequently from the left ventricular outflow tract (LVOT) or the aortic root with a RBBB pattern [56]. These are the most common type of VES or VT, occurring generally in young patients in the absence of overt cardiac disease, especially after having excluded an arrhythmogenic right ventricular cardiomyopathy which gives VES with the same morphology. Long term prognosis is generally good, except for the risk of developing a tachyarrhythmia cardiomyopathy, but medical treatment including class I or class II anti-arrhythmic drugs is required in symptomatic patients or in case of repetitive VES. These forms of VT are frequently very difficult to initiate and impossible to terminate by programmed pacing but are sensitive to isoprenaline infusion. Radiofrequency catheter ablation is performed when drugs are ineffective or badly tolerated, with a high level of success [179].
- the left Purkinje network system, also called "fascicular VT", usually seen in young patients with clinically normal hearts experiencing episodes of VT with a particular ECG pattern showing right bundle branch block with left axis deviation. This arrhythmia is frequently misleading suggesting at first sight a supraventricular tachycardia with functional aberration. Electrophysiological studies, however, demonstrate a typical VT. This arrhythmia could in many cases be triggered by ventricular or even atrial pacing. Endocardial mapping shows that the origin of the VT is located in the left inferior paraseptal area, with a presystolic potential recorded on the Purkinje system [180]. It is surprising that this arrhythmia can be reproducibly stopped by an IV verapamil (10 mg) injection. Radiofrequency catheter ablation is required in case of drug refractory VT.

7.3.2.9   Cardiac Tumors

Cardiac tumors [181] may present with recurrent VT. They are rare in adults but should be suspected in cases of childhood VT. The tumors are more commonly primary than secondary. They usually give rise to polymorphic forms of VT, the clinical characteristics of which depend on the site of the lesion. Prognosis is usually very poor except in rhabdomyoma in which some cases of spontaneous regression have been reported. Cardiac fibromas are basically benign tumors but local extension of the lesion may lead to death. Surgery may be possible in some cases, but it may be very difficult or impossible to resect the tumor from the interventricular septum.

7.3.2.10   Catecholamine-Induced Polymorphic VT

Catecholamine-induced polymorphic ventricular tachycardia is usually seen in childhood [182]. This is a rare form of VT which occurs in clinically normal hearts, almost exclusively on effort, despite a normal QT interval. These arrhythmias always occur in identical conditions after acceleration of the sinus rhythm owing to exercise or emotion. Sinus tachycardia leads to a junctional tachycardia and then VES or bigeminy which trigger polymorphic and often bidirectional VT. This finally degenerates to rapid polymorphic VT at a rate of about 300 beats/min accompanied by syncope. The arrhythmia may be reproduced during an exercise-stress test or isoproterenol infusion, and can cause sudden death. The treatment of choice seems to be beta blockade and amiodarone. Nevertheless, further studies are required to assess long-term results of this treatment.

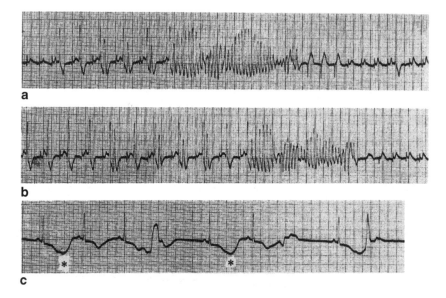

◻ Fig. 7.18

Two episodes of Torsades de pointes recorded at a very slow speed which shows the crescendo type of ventricular arrhythmias. First, in (a), there are two single extrasystoles, and then two extrasystoles following each sinus beat. Thereafter, the typical features of Torsades de pointes, which ends spontaneously, can be seen. Note the giant T wave on the last three beats before the re-establishment of the basic rhythm. The same pattern is also observed on tracing (b) recorded in the same patient. Tracing (c) is from a different patient. Note the huge deformation of the last part of the T wave, denoted by an asterisk, sometimes leading to an extrasystole. These giant waves are the harbingers of Torsades de pointes

7.3.2.11 Torsade de pointes (TdP)

The term Torsade de pointes (TdP), chosen by Dessertenne, corresponds with a continuously changing morphology of the QRS (❯ Fig. 7.18) during a VT run, with a cyclic decrease in the amplitude of the ventriculograms with a periodic rotation of QRS axis [183]. Such a polymorphic VT occurs in patients with long QT syndromes, induced by drugs or genetically inherited, with the risk of syncope during the episode and the possibility of conversion into ventricular fibrillation. Endocardial recordings show fragmented potential during QRS complexes initiating TdP, then followed by twisting electrograms with a pattern of double spikes at the time of QRS axis rotation [184]. The first hypothesis reported was the presence of two foci of activation firing simultaneously with varying degrees of fusion, but subsequently the spiral wave activity theory was confirmed following the in vitro experiments led by Davidenko [185]. Using high resolution optical mapping, he demonstrated that the core position of the arrhythmia was moving at every beat in a single direction, giving a pattern of TdP, or in various directions, leading to VF. Good results have been reported with IV injection of magnesium sulphate to prevent recurrence. It appears to be as effective as isoproterenol but without the undesirable side effects of the latter [186]. "Quinidine-like" (class I) antiarrhythmics are contraindicated in torsades de pointes with long QT intervals. Similarly, defibrillation is indicated only when torsades de pointes degenerates into VF.

7.3.2.12 Congenital Long-QT Syndrome

The congenital long-QT syndrome is a rare condition which may lead to attacks of polymorphic VT described as torsade de pointes, preceded by a very abnormal lengthening of the corrected QT (QTc) interval (calculated from Bazett's formula), associated with a U wave leading to a dimpled appearance at the end of the T wave.

Two subgroups have been defined:

- The Lange-Nielsen syndrome, described in 1957, which associates ventricular arrhythmias and ST changes with deafness, transmitted in the autosomal recessive mode; and
- The Romano-Ward syndrome, in which deafness is absent and which is transmitted in the autosomal dominant mode.

These congenital long QT syndromes correspond with mutations involving sodium or potassium channels and are classified into seven types from LQT1 to LQT7 [187]. However, sporadic cases do occur without a familial context. Syncope occurs during exercise or emotion. The QT interval is prolonged during the appearance of VES at the end of the repolarization associated with alternating changes in amplitude of the ST segment. This leads to very rapid bursts of tachycardia with cardiovascular collapse and loss of consciousness. Electrophysiological studies show prolongation of the refractory period with a large variation in its value from one point to another in the ventricle. The prognosis, conditioned by the symptoms, the QTc duration and the mutation identified, varies from less than 5% of major cardiac event at 5 years under treatment to more than 50% in high risk patients [188]. Treatment strategy is based on beta-blocker therapy for every patient with a long ST syndrome, avoiding QT prolonging drugs and sports. ICD implantation is required in secondary prevention or in case of bad observance or poor efficacy of beta-blockers [167]. Permanent cardiac pacing has limited indications, and is mostly used for rate support in cases of symptomatic bradycardia under treatment. Parents and siblings should be screened by ECG and genotypic analysis is mandatory.

7.3.2.13 Bouveret VT

"Bouveret ventricular tachycardia" (Parkinson-Papp) affects young patients without obvious myocardial disease [189]. It comprises runs of monomorphic VT, suggesting a point of origin in the upper part of the interventricular septum, as has been shown by epicardial mapping performed in a few cases. This diagnosis can only be retained after a complete cardiological checkup to exclude any other cardiac disease, remembering that sometimes VT may be the only presenting symptom of a cardiac disease for many years.

The classification of some idiopathic right ventricular tachycardias with left bundle branch block configuration and a normal or right axis, is imprecise. The prognosis is usually good [178]. However, some patients may be very disabled by these episodes of tachycardia.

7.3.3   Treatment Of Ventricular Tachycardia

All forms of VT should be treated to restore sinus rhythm. The clinical tolerance of VT depends, above all, on the underlying myocardial condition, a factor which partially determines the urgency of treatment and therapeutic choice.

7.3.3.1   Termination Methods

Pharmacodynamic Methods
The most widely used intravenous antiarrhythmic agents (❷ Tables 7.3 and ❷ 7.4) are beta blockers, procainamide, disopyramide and amiodarone (if VT is well tolerated). Lidocaine and mexiletine are mainly used to prevent VT in the acute phase of myocardial infarction, suppressing, or at least decreasing, the frequency of VES.

Endocavitary pacing
Ventricular tachycardia may rarely be terminated by atrial extrastimuli but one, two or three right ventricular extrastimuli are usually more effective. This is an elegant method of terminating VT and has the advantage that it can be used to predict the efficacy of antiarrhythmic therapy (no negative inotropic effect).

Defibrillation and cardioversion
External DC shock is normally used when the patient has lost consciousness or after a short-lasting general anaesthetic. The electrical energy delivered ranges from 80 to 300 J [190]. When VT has a tendency to recur, during transport or in the operating theatre, adhesive defibrillation electrodes may be used which reduce the discomfort and increase the margin of safety. Repetitive shocks must be used with caution in patients with a low ejection fraction, especially in dilated cardiomyopathy and acute myocardial infarction. In all cases, the lowest amount of electrical energy possible should be used, to avoid local changes in ionic concentration and cellular damage.

7.3.3.2   Termination Strategy

The strategy used to terminate attacks of VT depends mainly on the condition of the patient on admission to hospital. If VT is very rapid, and poorly tolerated with cardiovascular collapse and syncope, immediate direct current shock is required, with or without anaesthetic, depending on whether or not the patient is conscious.

When VT is better tolerated, with the risk of cardiac failure in the short term, an antiarrhythmic agent with a rapid onset of action has to be used, despite the possibility of a negative inotropic effect and the need for cardiovascular resuscitation.

When VT is well tolerated, the drug of choice is amiodarone which has the great advantage of having no negative inotropic effects, providing that it is injected over a 5–10 min period at a dose of 300–400 mg. However, if VT is well tolerated and an electrophysiological laboratory is available, electrical stimulation techniques are to be preferred to drug therapy. Endocavitary catheters can be used to confirm the diagnosis of VT and then terminate the majority of attacks by programmed pacing techniques. A catheter left at the apex of the ventricle allows better control if VT occurs.

7.3.3.3   Prevention of Recurrence

Once an attack has been terminated, measures must be taken to prevent a recurrence and to assess the effectiveness of antiarrhythmic therapy. A distinction should be drawn between VT in the acute phase of myocardial infarction

◻ Table 7.3

Properties of administration of the most widely used intravenous antiarrhythmic agents

Class	Antiarrhythmic Effects	Properties	Drug	Effect On MI[b] Ch	Effect On MI[b] In	Side effects	Dosage[c] iv	PO per 24 h (mg)	Interval Between Successive doses (h)	Antiarrhythmic effectiveness
Ia	Membrane Stabilizer	Quinidine-like	Quinidine	+	−	Cardiac GI		600 Q base	6–12	2.5 g ml⁻¹
			Procainamide	+	−	Cardiac GI	50–100 mg min⁻¹ 600 mg 24h⁻¹	4 at 8g	4	4–10 g ml⁻¹
			Disopyramide	+	−	Anticholenergic cardiac	1.5 mg kg⁻¹ in 5 min	400–600	6	3–8 ml⁻¹
			Ajmaline	−	−	Cardiac	1 mg kg⁻¹ min⁻¹			
Ib		Lidocaine-like	Lidocaine	0	−	Neurologic, GI cardiac in case of rapid injection	50 mg iv 2000 mg J ES			
			Mexiletine	0	−	Neurologic GI, cardiac in case of rapid injection	250 mg in 10 min 1200 mg J ES	600–800	8	0.5 at 2g ml⁻¹
			Aprindine	0	−	Neurologic, GI, hepatitis, hematologic	rarely used	100	12	1 at 2 μ g ml⁻¹
			Tocainide	0	−	GI, neurologic	0.5–0.75 mg kg min⁻¹ for 15 min	1200–1800	8	6 at 12 μ g ml⁻¹
Ic			Encainide	0	−	Cardiac, occular, GI	0.75–1 mg kg⁻¹ in 15 min	75–225	8	14 mg ml-1 per os
			Flecainide	0	−	Cardiac, neurologic, occular, GI	1–2 mg kg⁻¹ for 5 min then 1.5–2 mg kg⁻¹	300–400	12	0.2–1 g ml⁻¹
			Propafenone	−	−	Cardiac, GI	1 mg kg⁻¹ in 2 min	300–1200	8	0.5–2 g ml⁻¹

Table 7.3 (Continued)

Class	Antiarrhythmic Effects	Properties	Drug	Effect On MI[b] Ch	Effect On MI[b] In	Side effects	Dosage[c] iv	PO per 24 h (mg)	Interval Between Successive doses (h)	Antiarrhythmic effectiveness
II	Beta inhibiting action	ISA +	Propanolol	–	–	Cardiac, arterial, sexual		80–480	6–8	
		ISA +	Acebutolol	–	–	bronchiectatic		400–800	8	
		ISA –	Nadolol	–	–			80–240	24	
			Atenolol	–	–			50–100	12	
III	Anti thyroid like effect And Prolongation of the repolarization phase of the action potential duration		Amiodarone	–	–	Photo-sensitization corneal deposits, cardiac, GI, thyroid, neurologic pulmonary fibrosis	150 mg in 10 min 900 mg J^{-1}	200–600	24	
			Bretylium	–	–	Hypotension, GI	5 mg kg^{-1} iv then 1–2 mg min^{-1}	600	6	0.5–1.5 µ ml^{-1}
	Beta effect ISA[a]		Sotalol	–	–/0	Cardiac peripheral vascular obstructive pulmonary	0.5mg kg-1	160–480	24	
IV	Calcium blockers		Verapamil	–	–	Cardiac, GI neurologic cutaneous	10 mg in 1 min	120–480	8	
			Diltiazem	–	–	Cardiac, cutaneous GI, hepatic		180–360	6–8	
			Bepridil	–	–	GI, cutaneous cardiac	3 mg kg^{-1}	400–1000	8	
I+			Cibenzoline	–	–	Cardiac, GI	1 mg kg^{-1} in 2 min	260–390	6	200–400 mg ml^{-1}
III+										
IV										

a. ISA, intrinsic sympathomimetic activity. b. Ch., chronotropic; In., inotropic c iv, intravenous route; PO, per os; ES, electrical seringua.

◖ **Table 7.4**

Properties and administration of beta-blocking agents

ISA[a]	ESA[b] (quinidine-like)	Drug	Proteic binding (%)	Daily dosage (mg)	Interval between successive doses (h)
0	+ + +	Propranolol	90	120–480	8
+	+	Acebutolol	30	200–1200	12
++	+	Alprenolol	85	150–600	6
++	+	Oxprenolol	80	160–320	6
0	±	Timolol	30	10–60	8
0	0	Atenolol	5	100–300	12
0	0	Metoprolol	12	100–400	6–8
0	0	Nadolol	30	80–160	24
+ + +	0	Pindolol	45	15–45	6–8
0	0	Sotalol	0	160–480	> 24
0	0	Labetalol			

[a] ISA, intrinsic sympathomimetric activity. [b] ESA, extrinsic sympathomimetric activity.

◖ **Table 7.5**

Classification of antiarrhythmic drugs [191]

Class	Mechanism	Example
Ia	Sodium channel blockade	quinidine, ajmaline, procainamide
Ib	Sodium channel blockade	lidocaine, mexiletine, tocainide
Ic	Sodium channel blockade	flecainide, propafenone
II	Beta blockade	propranolo, metorprolol
III		amiodarone, sotalol
IV	Calcium channel blockade	verapamil, diltiazem

and chronic VT which occurs usually after the first week following infarction, but which may also be observed in cardiomyopathy, ventricular dysplasia, idiopathic aneurysm, mitral valve prolapse, tumors of the heart, and so forth.

Palliative methods

Cellular electrophysiological techniques have been used to classify the different antiarrhythmic drugs into four main groups [191], as shown in ❷ Table 7.5. A full discussion on the drug therapy for the treatment of VT is beyond the scope of this book. However, commonly used drugs are outlined below and further references to the advantages and disadvantages (side effects) of each are provided.

Amiodarone is widely used [192] having some advantages, such as a long half-life, but with commonly occurring side effects [193–204].

Although beta blockers do not have a direct antiarrhythmic effect, apart from sotalol, they may prevent extrasystoles induced by the autonomic nervous system by decreasing the heart rate; for example, VES occurring on waking or during exercise have a reduced frequency when treated with beta-blocking agents [205].

Verapamil [206] is a calcium antagonist which has no effect on VT except in the special case described above where VT occurs in young patients with right bundle branch block and left axis deviation.

7.3.3.4   Strategy for the Use of Palliative Methods for the Treatment of Chronic Recurrent VT

Ventricular tachycardia is a potentially dangerous arrhythmia which has to be controlled by antiarrhythmic therapy. Patients may be divided into two groups. The first group are those considered as low-risk cases, in whom the arrhythmia is perceived, is not too rapid, is infrequent and monomorphic. In these moderately symptomatic cases, amiodarone may be given at a moderate dose from 400–600 mg daily, before reducing to the maintenance dosage. The common class I antiarrhythmic drugs are selected by successive therapeutic trials. Treatment is prescribed orally and its effectiveness confirmed by Holter monitoring.

When VT is life-threatening, that is, there are frequent attacks of rapid polymorphic VT, degenerating to VF and associated with syncope or functional angina, the patient should not be discharged from hospital until the arrhythmia is well controlled. As the frequency of attacks may be greatly variable, it is not practical to wait for spontaneous recurrence of the arrhythmia and, therefore, provocative methods are used to trigger an attack, essentially by programmed pacing maneuvers.

Electrophysiological provocation tests are performed under the same conditions as those in which VT could be induced initially [49, 131, 136, 206–210], bearing in mind that these are not the usual conditions in which the patient lives. The choice of the most effective drug is made on the results of repeated provocative-pacing tests during drug therapy, which implies that VT can be inducible. Different criteria are used by different groups of workers which makes comparison of results difficult. First of all, there is no agreed definition in a recurrent tachycardia of its sustained or nonsustained character. Different protocols for electrical stimulation are used, stimulating different zones and cardiac chambers (❷ Fig. 7.19).

Nevertheless, in the subgroup of patients at high risk, programmed pacing methods seem to have made an important contribution to their treatment. However, the pacing protocol must be performed under clearly defined conditions. Some groups have based their results on studies performed in the electrophysiological laboratory with antiarrhythmic drugs administered parenterally. A judicious selection of these drugs allows assessment of two or three of them at each investigation. However, the eventual effectiveness of the same drug administered orally may be different. Therefore, it may be preferable to test antiarrhythmic drugs given only orally, which implies retesting the patient after each therapeutic trial, when the concentration of the drug has reached therapeutic levels. This is time consuming and expensive.

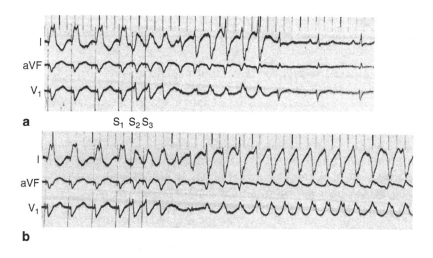

❏ Fig. 7.19

Part (a) shows the induction of nonsustained ventricular tachycardia by two premature stimuli S_2 and S_3, following a regular driven cycle. The tachycardia stops after 3 s. On tracing (b), recorded in the same patient, the same protocol induces a sustained episode of ventricular tachycardia. This suggests that each procedure has to be repeated several times, taking into consideration only the highest-grade arrhythmia obtained

In addition to electrophysiological investigation, the authors' policy is to perform exercise-stress testing. This allows an evaluation of the antiarrhythmic effect on remaining VES and, above all, aims to confirm the absence of VT during exercise.

The absence of VT on repeated 24-h Holter recordings during antiarrhythmic therapy seems to be a reliable prognostic factor [211]. This is an important investigation as the patient is assessed under everyday living conditions [212].

Whatever the results with the different antiarrhythmic drugs used, there seem to be two major factors which influence the risk of sudden or cardiac death as follows:

- Myocardial function, which may be assessed by the New York Heart Association functional classification – patients in stage IV have a higher risk of sudden and cardiac death [213, 214];
- The ability to trigger VT despite antiarrhythmic therapy [207, 215].

However, several points must be remembered. First, all antiarrhythmic drugs may aggravate or even provoke ventricular arrhythmias. This has been reported with quinidine, procainamide [216], amiodarone [217], disopyramide, propranolol, pendolol, mexiletine, tocainide, aprindine, propafenone [218, 219], encainide [220] and flecainide [221, 222]. Secondly, most antiarrhythmic agents have potentially dangerous hemodynamic effects, especially in severe cardiac disease. The risk is even higher when several antiarrhythmics are used in association [223]. Finally, any exacerbation of a stable arrhythmia should alert the physician to an aggravation of myocardial function.

Inefficacy of antiarrhythmic therapy

A number of precautions must be observed before confirming that an antiarrhythmic drug is inefficient. Sufficient time must be allowed for the plasma concentrations to reach therapeutic levels. When drug dosage is not readily available, this interval is estimated to be about five times the drug's half-life. In the case of amiodarone, which has a very long half-life compared to other antiarrhythmic drugs, the delay would be unacceptably long and so measures are taken to shorten it by using loading doses (up to 1,200 mg of amiodarone per day). When an antiarrhythmic agent is judged to be ineffective, drugs of a different group should be tried if necessary in association with drugs of another group or subgroup (e.g., quinidine, mexiletine or beta blocker, flecainide, etc.) [224].

The implantable defibrillator

The implantable defibrillator is a considerable technological achievement. It was originally designed to prevent sudden death due to ventricular fibrillation, but it is now often used to treat rapid resistant VT [226, 227]. This device is capable of storing energy of 25–30 J in a capacitor which charges when the arrhythmia occurs. An internal electric shock is delivered after an interval of less than 30 s following the onset of the arrhythmia. The theoretical total capacity is 100 shocks. Several improvements have been made to the original design. Defibrillation was initially performed using a spring electrode positioned in the superior vena cava and another patch-shaped metallic electrode positioned at the apex of the left ventricle. This design has been replaced by two epicardial patches, and since 1991, by an intracardiac coil-shaped electrode, including bipolar sensing and pacing distal electrodes for tachycardia interruption and bradycardia prevention. A microcomputer stores the number of shocks delivered, the electrograms of each arrhythmia detected, and the amount of energy remaining. The use of this device is indicated for patients with ventricular arrhythmias which start as VF, and for VT interruption.

When the patients cannot be treated by antiarrhythmic drugs, surgical ablation of the arrhythmogenic substrate, the first radical treatment, is seldom used nowadays, due to its risks of complications. It has been superseded by transcutaneous catheter ablation techniques [228, 229].

7.3.3.5 Radical Treatment

There are two radical methods of treating VT: surgery and by definitive medical treatment, namely, catheter ablation using radiofrequency methods, or sometimes fulguration.

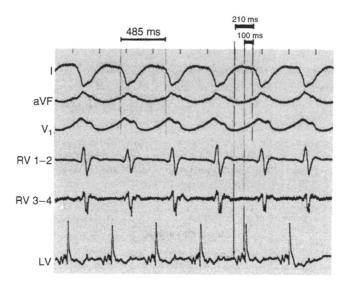

⬚ Fig. 7.20
Endocardial mapping during ventricular tachycardia using a bipolar catheter located inside the left ventricle. Fragmented activity is seen on this lead (LV). A large potential is observed 100 ms before the onset of the surface QRS complex. Note also that fragmented activity is also obtained 210 ms before QRS complexes. The right ventricle is activated later, confirming that the tachycardia originates on the left side of the heart. RV 1–2 and RV 3–4 are two bipolar tracings from a bipolar right ventricular lead

Surgery

The surgical treatment of VT is reviewed by Fontaine et al. [230]. The classical treatment of VT complicating coronary artery disease involved two main techniques: aneurysmectomy based on the perioperative findings and myocardial revascularization by coronary bypass grafting (saphenous vein or mammary artery). However, these two methods were not always effective as VT recurred in 30 – 40% of operated patients. New surgical techniques have been developed in the late seventies, based on the result of preoperative endocardial and perioperative epicardial mapping (simple ventriculotomy, encircling endocardial ventriculotomy, subendocardial excision, cryosurgery, and perioperative laser).

The site of origin of VT is determined either preoperatively or perioperatively. The former uses an endocardial recording catheter. The results depend on the thorough manipulation of the catheter within the left ventricle, usually around a myocardial scar. This method involves the following processes:

- the recording of fragmented low-amplitude diastolic potentials usually detected in the zone of the aneurysm [129, 231] which indicate areas of abnormal conduction but which do not actually determine the site of origin,
- the recording of the earliest potential during induced VT (❷ Fig. 7.20), and
- the reproduction of the morphology of the documented VT by stimulation at different points within the ventricle.

The perioperative method involves endocardial mapping and, above all, endocavitary recording during induced VT to determine the earliest potential during the arrhythmia (❷ Fig. 7.9) (during normothermia). The point of breakthrough of VT can thereby be determined with more accuracy in order to guide the surgical action (❷ Figs. 7.4 and ❷ 7.12).

The use of techniques based on electrophysiology should be adapted to the type of anatomopathological lesion. An important case is the ventricular aneurysm [232]. After opening the aneurysm, endocavitary mapping is performed. This may be followed by various alternatives as follows:

- Encircling endocardial ventriculotomy [233, 234] with the aim of interrupting the reentrant phenomenon without too much damage to the healthy myocardium;

- Subendocardial resection;
- Cryosurgery aimed at destroying or excluding the zone of abnormal conduction by freezing; and later,
- The use of preoperative laser treatment with the same objective as cryosurgery, but whose action is more rapid and less traumatic;
- Cardiomyoplasty.

These techniques may be associated with excision of the fibrous wall of the ventricular aneurysm, which gives an improved ventricular ejection fraction by remodelling the left ventricle. In addition, myocardial revascularization may be indicated [235, 236].

Other pathologies [237] and their treatments include the following:

- Arrhythmogenic right ventricular dysplasia which can be treated by simple ventriculotomy or resection of the dysplasic zones if not too extensive [238–240];
- Dilated cardiomyopathy with ventricular arrhythmias which can be treated by simple ventriculotomy when the patient's condition permits;
- Ventricular arrhythmias complicating cardiac tumors which can sometimes be cured when the tumor is resectable, although benign primary cardiac tumors are rare in adults; and
- Idiopathic VT, which can be treated by simple ventriculotomy or subendocardial excision;
- Catheter ablation.

After localizing the point of origin of VT by endocardial mapping with a mapping catheter, the arrhythmia may then be treated by applying a destructive energy at the distal electrode of the same catheter. Fulguration was the first to be applied, using the energy of an external cardiac defibrillator. It has been substituted by the thermal energy of radiofrequency ablation in the early 90's for safety reasons and for improved accuracy. The acute efficacy of this technique is tested by using the usual protocols of provocative pacing to try to reinitiate clinical VT immediately after the ablation and then ten days later. This later investigation seems to have a better predictive value.

The fulguration technique proved to be a very successful method in an evaluation of a series of 38 consecutive cases [241, 242]. It has the advantage of being applicable to patients for whom surgery has been refused because of their poor general condition and the extent of myocardial damage [243]. Owing to its excellent results, this technique has been extended to less critical cases. However, the method is long and difficult, and several sessions are necessary in half of the cases. It is also necessary to use antiarrhythmic drugs in 50% of the patients. Nevertheless, improvements should be possible in order to produce optimal results.

In practice, radical forms of treatment of VT are indicated in the following situations [244]: cases of VT with proven resistance to different antiarrhythmic agents and documented spontaneous recurrences, and cases of VT treated effectively by antiarrhythmic drugs but in which there is a surgical indication for myocardial revascularization. Ventriculotomy, plication of an aneurysm, or cryosurgery may be the associated methods in the latter situation.

References

1. Vassale, M., Physiological basis of normal and abnormal automaticity. In: Rosenbaum MB, Elizari MV, eds. Frontiers of Cardiac Electrophysiology. The Hague: Nijhoff, 1983:120–43.
2. Josephson, M.E., L.N. Horowitz, A. Farshidi, et al., Recurrent sustained ventricular tachycardia. 1. Mechanisms. *Circulation*, 1978;**57**: 431–40.
3. Cranefield, P.F., Ventricular fibrillation. *N. Engl. J. Med.*, 1973;**289**: 732–6.
4. Bozler, E., The initiation of impulses in cardiac muscle. *Am. J. Physiol.*, 1943;**138**: 273–82.
5. Segers, M., Le role des potentiels tardifs du coeur. Mem. Acad. R. Med. Belg, 1941;**1**: 1–30.
6. Cranefield, P.F., Action potentials, afterpotentials, and arrhythmias. *Circ. Res.*, 1977;**41**: 415–23.
7. Cranefield, P.F. and R.S. Aronson, Initiation of sustained rhythmic activity by single propagated action potentials in canine cardiac Purkinje fibers exposed to sodium-free solution or to ouabain. *Circ. Res.*, 1974;**34**: 477–81.
8. Cranefield, P.F., Triggered arrhythmias. In: Rosenbaum MB, Elizari MV, eds. *Frontiers of Cardiac Electrophysiology*. The Hague: Nijhoff, 1983:182–94.
9. Wit, A.L., P.A. Boyden, D.C. Gadsby, et al., Triggered activity as a cause of atrial arrhythmias. In: Narula OS, ed. *Cardiac*

Arrhythmias: Electrophysiology, Diagnosis and Management. Baltimore, Maryland: Williams and Wilkins, 1979:14–31.

10. Coraboeuf, E., E. Deroubaix, and A. Coulombe, Acidosis-induced abnormal repolarization and repetitive activity in isolated dog Purkinje fibres. *J. Physiol.*, (Paris) 1980;**76**: 97–106.

11. Coulombe, A., E. Coraboeuf, C. Malecot, et al., Role of the "Na window" current and other ionic currents in triggering early after-depolarizations and resulting re-excitations in Purkinje fibers. In: Zipes DP, Jalife J, eds. *Cardiac Electrophysiology and Arrhythmias.* Orlando: Grune & Stratton, 1985:43–49.

12. Pinet, C., B. Le Grand, G.W. John, et al., Thrombin facilitation of voltage-gated sodium channel activation in human cardiomyocytes: Implications for ischemic sodium loading. *Circulation*, 2002;**106**: 2098–2103.

13. Abriel, H., C. Cabo, X.H. Wehrens, et al., Novel arrhythmogenic mechanism revealed by a long-QT syndrome mutation in the cardiac $Na(+)$ channel. *Circ. Res.*, 2001;**88**: 740–745.

14. January, C.T. and H.A. Fozzard, Delayed afterdepolarizations in heart muscle: mechanisms and relevance. *Pharmacol. Rev.*, 1988;**40**: 219–227.

15. Wit, A.L. and M.R. Rosen, Afterdepolarizations and triggered activity: distinction from automaticity as an arrhythmogenic mechanism. In: Fozzard HA, Habert E, Jennings RB, Katz AM, Morgan HE, eds. *The Heart and Cardiovascular System: Scientific Foundations 2nd ed.* New York, NY: Raven Press, 1992:2113–2163.

16. Colquhoun, D., Neher, E., Reuter, H., et al., Inward current channels activated by intracellular Ca in cultured cardiac cells. *Nature*, 1981;**294**: 752–754.

17. Zygmunt, A.C., R.J. Goodrow, and C.M. Weigel, INaCa and ICl(Ca) contribute to isoproterenol-induced delayed after depolarizations in midmyocardial cells. *Am. J. Physiol.*, 1998;**275**: H1979–H1992.

18. Lipp, P. and L. Pott, Transient inward current in guinea-pig atrial myocytes reflects a change of sodium-calcium exchange current. *J. Physiol.*, 1988;**397**: 601–630.

19. Benardeau, A., S.N. Hatem, C. Rucker-Martin, et al., Contribution of Na + /Ca2+ exchange to action potential of human atrial myocytes. *Am. J. Physiol.*, 1996;**271**: H1151–H1161.

20. Pogwizd, S.M., K. Schlotthauer, L. Li, et al., Arrhythmogenesis and contractile dysfunction in heart failure: Roles of sodium-calcium exchange, inward rectifier potassium current, and residual beta-adrenergic responsiveness. *Circ. Res.*, 2001;**88**: 1159–1167.

21. Moe, G.K. and C. Mendez, The physiologic basis of reciprocal rhythm. *Prog. Cardiovasc. Dis.*, 1966;**8**: 461–482.

22. Wellens, H.J., D.R. Duren, and K.I. Lie., Observations on mechanisms of ventricular tachycardia in man. *Circulation*, 1976;**54**: 237–244.

23. Richards, D.A., G.J. Blake, J.F. Spear, et al., Electrophysiologic substrate for ventricular tachycardia: correlation of properties in vivo and in vitro. *Circulation*, 1984;**69**: 369–381.

24. Welch, W.J., B. Strasberg, A. Coelho, et al., Sustained macroreentrant ventricular tachycardia. *Am. Heart. J.*, 1982;**104**: 166–169.

25. Lloyd, E.A., D.P. Zipes, J.J. Heger, et al., Sustained ventricular tachycardia due to bundle branch reentry. *Am. Heart. J.*, 1982;**104**: 1095–1097.

26. Rosen, M.R. and P.J. Danilo, The electrophysiological basis for cardiac arrhythmias. In: Narula OS, ed. *Cardiac Arrhythmias: Electrophysiology, Diagnosis and Management.* Baltimore, Maryland: Williams and Wilkins, 1979:3–13.

27. Boineau, J.P. and J.L. Cox, Slow ventricular activation in acute myocardial infarction. A source of re-entrant premature ventricular contractions. *Circulation*, 1973;**48**: 702–713.

28. El-Sherif, N., B.J. Scherlag, R. Lazzara, et al., Re-entrant ventricular arrhythmias in the late myocardial infarction period. 1. Conduction characteristics in the infarction zone. *Circulation*, 1977;**55**: 686–702.

29. El-Sherif, N., R.R. Hope, B.J. Scherlag, et al., Re-entrant ventricular arrhythmias in the late myocardial infarction period. 2. Patterns of initiation and termination of re-entry. *Circulation*, 1977;**55**: 702–719.

30. Fontaine, G., G. Guiraudon, and R. Frank, Intramyocardial conduction defects in patients prone to chronic ventricular tachycardia. I. The post-excitation syndrome in sinus rhythm. In: Sandoe E, Julian DG, Bell JW, eds. *Management of Ventricular Tachycardia.* Role of Mexiletine. Amsterdam: *Excerpta. Medica.*, 1978:39–55.

31. Fontaine, G., G. Guiraudon, and R. Frank, Intramyocardial conduction defects in patients prone to ventricular tachycardia. II. A dynamic study of the post-excitation syndrome. In: Sandoe E, Julian DG, Bell JW, eds. Management of Ventricular Tachycardia. Role of Mexiletine. Amsterdam: *Excerpta. Medica.*, 1978:56–66.

32. Fontaine, G., G. Guiraudon, and R. Frank, The pathophysiology of chronic disturbances of ventricular rhythm. In: Masoni A, Alboni E, eds. Cardiac Electrophysiology Today. London: Academic Press, 1982:251–71.

33. Fontaine, G., G. Guiraudon, and R. Frank, Intramyocardial conduction defects in patients prone to ventricular tachycardia. In: Sandoe E, Julian DG, Bell JW, eds. Management of Ventricular Tachycardia. Role of Mexiletine. Amsterdam: *Excerpta. Medica.*, 1978:67–79.

34. Wit, A.L., M.A. Allessie, F.M. Bonke, et al., Excitation of the infarcted canine heart during initiation of ventricular tachycardia by premature impulses. *Circulation*, 1980;**62** (Suppl. 3): 195.

35. Janse, M.J., F.J. van Capelle, H. Morsink, et al., Flow of "injury" current and patterns of excitation during early ventricular arrhythmias in acute regional myocardial ischemia in isolated porcine and canine hearts. Evidence for two different arrhythmogenic mechanisms. *Circ. Res.*, 1980;**47**: 151–165.

36. Motte, G., Digitalis-induced ventricular arrhythmias. Apropos of oscillating post-potentials. *Arch. Mal. Coeur. Vaiss.*, 1979;**72**: 311–316.

37. de Bakker, J.M., F.J. van Capelle, M.J. Janse, et al. Slow conduction in the infarcted human heart. 'Zigzag' course of activation. *Circulation*, 1993;**88**: 915–926.

38. Brugada, P., H.J.J. Wellens, The role of triggered activity in clinical arrhythmias. In: Rosenbaum MB, Elizari MV, eds. *Frontiers of Cardiac Electrophysiology.* The Hague: Nijhoff, 1983: 195–216.

39. Haissaguerre, M., D.C. Shah, P. Jais, et al., Role of Purkinje conducting system in triggering of idiopathic ventricular fibrillation. *Lancet*, 2002;**359**: 677–678.

40. Schamroth, L., *The Disorders of Cardiac Rhythm.* Oxford: Blackwell, 1971.

41. Zipes, D.P., Specific arrhythmias: Diagnosis and treatment. In: Braunwald E, ed. Heart Disease: A Textbook of Cardiovascular Medicine. Philadelphia: Saunders, 1984:683–743.

42. Rosenbaum, M.B., Classification of ventricular extrasystoles according to form. *J. Electrocardiol.*, 1969;**2**: 289–297.

43. Josephson, M.E., L.N. Horowitz, A. Farshidi, et al., Recurrent sustained ventricular tachycardia. 4. Pleomorphism. *Circulation*, 1979;59: 459–468.

44. Krishnaswami, V. and A.R. Geraci, Permanent pacing in disorders of sinus node function. *Am. Heart. J.*, 1975;89: 579–585.

45. Josephson, M.E., L.N. Horowitz, A. Farshidi, et al., Recurrent sustained ventricular tachycardia. 2. Endocardial mapping. *Circulation*, 1978;57: 440–447.

46. Josephson, M.E., H.L. Waxman, F.E. Marchlinski, et al., Electrocardiographic features of ectopic impulse formation. Specificity of ventricular activation patterns. In: Josephson ME, Wellens HJJ, eds. *Tachycardias: Mechanisms, Diagnosis, Treatment*. Philadelphia, Pennsylvania: Lea and Febiger, 1984: 363–386.

47. Coumel, P., When should ventricular extrasystole be treated?. *Presse Med* 1983;12: 2663–2665.

48. Brodsky, M., D. Wu, P. Denes, et al., Arrhythmias documented by 24 hour continuous electrocardiographic monitoring in 50 male medical students without apparent heart disease. *Am. J. Cardiol.*, 1977;39: 390–395.

49. Rodstein, M., L. Wolloch, and R.S. Gubner, Mortality study of the significance of extrasystoles in an insured population. *Circulation*, 1971;44: 617–625.

50. Hinkle, L.E., Jr., S.T. Carver, and M. Stevens, The frequency of asymptomatic disturbances of cardiac rhythm and conduction in middle-aged men. *Am. J. Cardiol*, 1969;24: 629–650.

51. Medvedowsky, J.L., C. Barnay, C. Massat, Evolution des arythmies ventriculaires après infarctus du myocarde. Intérêt des enregistrements électrocardiographiques de longue durée. Résultats préliminaires. *Arch. Mal. Coeur. Vaiss.*, 1981;74: 809–819.

52. Kennedy, H.L. and S.J. Underhill, Frequent or complex ventricular ectopy in apparently healthy subjects: a clinical study of 25 cases. *Am. J. Cardiol.*, 1976;38: 141–148.

53. Lown, B., Sudden cardiac death: the major challenge confronting contemporary cardiology. *Am. J. Cardiol.*, 1979;43: 313–328.

54. Rodriguez, L.M., J.L. Smeets, C. Timmermans, et al., Predictors for successful ablation of right- and left-sided idiopathic ventricular tachycardia. *Am. J. Cardiol.*, 1997;79: 309–314.

55. Tanner, H., G. Hindricks, P. Schirdewahn, et al., Outflow tract tachycardia with R/S transition in lead V3: six different anatomic approaches for successful ablation. *J. Am. Coll. Cardiol.*, 2005;45: 418–423.

56. Ouyang, F., P. Fotuhi, S.Y. Ho, et al., Repetitive monomorphic ventricular tachycardia originating from the aortic sinus cusp: electrocardiographic characterization for guiding catheter ablation. *J. Am. Coll. Cardiol.*, 2002;39: 500–508.

57. Faris, J.V., P.L. McHenry, J.W. Jordan, et al., Prevalence and reproducibility of exercise-induced ventricular arrhythmias during maximal exercise testing in normal men. *Am. J. Cardiol.*, 1976;37: 617–622.

58. Udall, J.A. and M.H. Ellestad, Predictive implications of ventricular premature contractions associated with treadmill stress testing. *Circulation*, 1977;56: 985–989.

59. McHenry, P.L., S.N. Morris, M. Kavalier, et al., Comparative study of exercise-induced ventricular arrhythmias in normal subjects and patients with documented coronary artery disease. *Am. J. Cardiol.*, 1976;37: 609–616.

60. Crow, R., R. Prineas, and H. Blackburn, The prognostic significance of ventricular ectopic beats among the apparently healthy. *Am. Heart. J.*, 1981;101: 244–248.

61. Viskin, S., R. Rosso, O. Rogowski, et al., The "Short-Coupled" Variant of Right Ventricular Outflow Ventricular Tachycardia: A Not-So-Benign Form of Benign Ventricular Tachycardia? *Journal of Cardiovascular Electrophysiology*, 2005;16: 1–5.

62. Fontaine, G.H., P. Fornes, J.L. Hebert, et al., Ventricular tachycardia in arrhythmogenic right ventricular cardiomyopathies. In: Zipes DP, Jalife J, eds. *Cardiac electrophysiology: from cell to bedside*. Syracuse, New York: Saunders, 2004:588–600.

63. Hinkle, L.E., S.T. Carver, D.C. Argyros, The prognostic significance of ventricular premature contractions in healthy people and in people with coronary heart disease. *Acta. Cardiol.*, 1974;18 Suppl: 5–32.

64. Rabkin, S.W., F.A. Mathewson, and R.B. Tate, Relationship of ventricular ectopy in men without apparent heart disease to occurrence of ischemic heart disease and sudden death. *Am. Heart. J.*, 1981;101: 135–142.

65. The coronary drug project: Post-infarction electrocardiographic findings and prognosis. *Circulation*, 1971; 44 (Suppl. 2):154.

66. Kennedy, H.L., J.E. Pescarmona, R.J. Bouchard, et al., Coronary artery status of apparently healthy subjects with frequent and complex ventricular ectopy. *Ann. Intern. Med.*, 1980;92: 179–185.

67. Chiang, B.N., L.V. Perlman, M. Fulton, et al., Predisposing factors in sudden cardiac death in Tecumseh, Michigan. A prospective study. *Circulation*, 1970;41: 31–37.

68. de Soyza, N., J.K. Bissett, J.J. Kane, et al., Ectopic ventricular prematurity and its relationship to ventricular tachycardia in acute myocardial infarction in man. *Circulation*, 1974;50: 529–33.

69. Campbell, R.W., A. Murray, and D.G. Julian, Ventricular arrhythmias in first 12 hours of acute myocardial infarction. Natural history study. *Br. Heart. J.*, 1981;46: 351–357.

70. Vismaria, L.A., A.N. DeMaria, J.L. Hughes, et al., Evaluation of arrhythmias in the late hospital phase of acute myocardial infarction compared to coronary care unit ectopy. *Br. Heart. J.*, 1975;37: 598–603.

71. Lown, B. and M. Wolf, Approaches to sudden death from coronary heart disease. *Circulation*, 1971;44: 130–142.

72. Roberts, R., H.D. Ambos, C.W. Loh, et al., Initiation of repetitive ventricular depolarizations by relatively late premature complexes in patients with acute myocardial infarction. *Am. J. Cardiol.*, 1978;41: 678–683.

73. von Olshausen, K., F. Schwarz, J. Apfelbach, et al., Determinants of the incidence and severity of ventricular arrhythmias in aortic valve disease. *Am. J. Cardiol.*, 1983;51: 1103–1109.

74. Juillard, A., A. Bouajina, B. Frechon, et al., Significance of repetitive ventricular extrasystoles in the acute phase of myocardial infarction. *Arch. Mal. Coeur. Vaiss.*, 1984;77: 121–127.

75. Roberts, R., A. Husain, H.D. Ambos, et al., Relation between infarct size and ventricular arrhythmia. *Br. Heart. J.*, 1975;37: 1169–1175.

76. de Soyza, N., Bennett, F.A., Murphy, M.L., et al., The relationship of paroxysmal ventricular tachycardia complicating the acute phase and ventricular arrhythmia during the late hospital phase of myocardial infarction to long-term survival. *Am. J. Med.*, 1978;64: 377–381.

77. Fazzini, P.F., F. Marchi, and P. Pucci, Effects of verapamil in ventricular premature beats of acute myocardial infarction. *Acta. Cardiol.*, 1978;33: 25–29.

78. Wyman, M.G., Prevention of primary ventricular fibrillation in acute myocardial infarction. *Am. J. Cardiol.*, 1972; 29:298.

79. Tonet, J.L., P. Lechat, R. Frank, et al., Electrocardiographic effects and antiarrhythmic action of 1200 mg of oral amiodarone per day. *Ann. Cardiol. Angeiol.*, (Paris) 1984; **33**:309–315.

80. DeBusk, R.F., D.M. Davidson, N. Houston, et al., Serial ambulatory electrocardiography and treadmill exercise testing after uncomplicated myocardial infarction. *Am. J. Cardiol.*, 1980;**45**: 547–554.

81. Moss, A.J., J.J. DeCamilla, H.P. Davis, et al., Clinical significance of ventricular ectopic beats in the early posthospital phase of myocardial infarction. *Am. J. Cardiol.*, 1977;**39**: 635–640.

82. Vismara, L.A., E.A. Amsterdam, D.T. Mason, Relation of ventricular arrhythmias in the late hospital phase of acute myocardial infarction to sudden death after hospital discharge. *Am. J. Med.*, 1975;**59**: 6–12.

83. The coronary drug project: Prognostic importance of premature beats following myocardial infarction. Experience in the coronary drug project. *JAMA*, 1973;**223**: 1116–1124.

84. Califf, R.M., J.M. Burks, and V.S. Behar, et al., Relationships among ventricular arrhythmias, coronary artery disease, and angiographic and electrocardiographic indicators of myocardial fibrosis. *Circulation*, 1978;**57**: 725–732.

85. Ruberman, W., E. Weinblatt, C.W. Frank, et al., Ventricular premature beats and mortality of men with coronary heart disease. *Circulation*, 1975;**52**: III 199–203.

86. Horowitz, L.N. and J. Morganroth, Can we prevent sudden cardiac death? *Am. J. Cardiol.*, 1982;**50**: 535–538.

87. Moss, A.J., H.T. Davis, J. DeCamilla, et al., Ventricular ectopic beats and their relation to sudden and nonsudden cardiac death after myocardial infarction. *Circulation*, 1979;**60**: 998–1003.

88. Laurent, M., B. Miane, C. Almange, et al., Comparison of data from exercise tests and continuous electrocardiographic recording in patients with ventricular extrasystole. Apropos of 131 cases. *Arch. Mal. Coeur. Vaiss.*, 1982;**75**: 653–662.

89. Davis, H.T., J. DeCamilla, L.W. Bayer, et al., Survivorship patterns in the posthospital phase of myocardial infarction. *Circulation*, 1979;**60**: 1252–1258.

90. Schulze, R.A., Jr., H.W. Strauss, and B. Pitt, Sudden death in the year following myocardial infarction. Relation to ventricular premature contractions in the late hospitals phase and left ventricular ejection fraction. *Am. J. Med.*, 1977;**62**: 192–199.

91. Greene, H.L., P.R. Reid, and A.H. Schaeffer, The repetitive ventricular response in man. A predictor of sudden death. *N. Engl. J. Med.*, 1978;**299**: 729–734.

92. Calvert, A., B. Lown, and R. Gorlin, Ventricular premature beats and anatomically defined coronary heart disease. *Am. J. Cardiol.*, 1977;**39**: 627–634.

93. Uretz, E.F., P. Denes, N. Ruggie, et al., Relation of ventricular premature beats to underlying heart disease. *Am. J. Cardiol.*, 1984; **53**:774–80.

94. Bigger, J.T., Jr., F.M. Weld, and L.M. Rolnitzky, Which postinfarction ventricular arrhythmias should be treated? *Am. Heart. J.*, 1982;**103**: 660–666.

95. Winkle, R.A., The relationship between ventricular ectopic beat frequency and heart rate. *Circulation*, 1982;**66**: 439–46.

96. Helfant, R.H., R. Pine, V. Kabde, et al., Exercise-related ventricular premature complexes in coronary heart disease. Correlations with ischemia and angiographic severity. *Ann. Intern. Med.*, 1974;**80**: 589–592.

97. Schulze, R.A., Jr., J. Rouleau, P. Rigo, et al., Ventricular arrhythmias in the late hospital phase of acute myocardial infarction.

Relation to left ventricular function detected by gated cardiac blood pool scanning. *Circulation*, 1975;**52**: 1006–1011.

98. Ruberman, W., E. Weinblatt, and J.D. Goldberg, et al., Ventricular premature beats and mortality after myocardial infarction. *N. Engl. J. Med.*, 1977;**297**: 750–757.

99. Moss, A.J., J. DeCamilla, F. Engstrom, et al., The posthospital phase of myocardial infarction: identification of patients with increased mortality risk. *Circulation*, 1974;**49**: 460–466.

100. Moss, A.J., Update of postinfarction-risk stratification: physiologic variables. *Ann. N. Y. Acad. Sci.*, 1984;**427**: 280–285.

101. Graboys, T.B., Premature ventricular contractions. In: Harrison DC, ed. *Cardiac Arrhythmias: A Decade of Progress*. Boston, Massachusetts: Hall, 1981:567.

102. Zaret, B.L. and C.R.J Conti, Exercise-induced ventricular irritability: Hemodynamic and angiographic correlations. *Am. J. Cardiol.*, 1972;**29**: 298.

103. Bjarnason, I., T. Hardarson, and S. Jonsson, Cardiac arrhythmias in hypertrophic cardiomyopathy. *Br. Heart. J.*, 1982;**48**: 198–203.

104. Savage, D.D., S.F. Seides, B.J. Maron, et al., Prevalence of arrhythmias during 24-hour electrocardiographic monitoring and exercise testing in patients with obstructive and nonobstructive hypertrophic cardiomyopathy. *Circulation*, 1979;**59**: 866–875.

105. Ingham, R.E., Rossen, R.M., Goodman, D.J., et al., Ambulatory electrocardiographic monitoring in idiopathic hypertrophic subaortic stenosis. *Circulation*, 1975;**52** (Suppl. 2): 93.

106. Maron, B.J., Savage, D.D., Wolfson, J.K., et al., Prognostic significance of 24 hour ambulatory electrocardiographic monitoring in patients with hypertrophic cardiomyopathy: a prospective study. *Am. J. Cardiol.*, 1981;**48**: 252–257.

107. Maron, B.J., W.C. Roberts, and S.E. Epstein, Sudden death in hypertrophic cardiomyopathy: a profile of 78 patients. *Circulation*, 1982;**65**: 1388–1394.

108. Weiss, A.N., C.L. Jobe, T. Gordon, et al., Relationship of premature ventricular contractions and left ventricular hypertrophy to sudden cardiac death. *Circulation*, 1969;**40** (Suppl. 3): 213.

109. Doi, Y.L., W.J. McKenna, S. Chetty, et al., Prediction of mortality and serious ventricular arrhythmia in hypertrophic cardiomyopathy. An echocardiographic study. *Br. Heart. J.*, 1980;**44**: 150–157.

110. Maron, B.J., W.J. McKenna, G.K. Danielson, et al., American College of Cardiology/European Society of Cardiology Clinical Expert Consensus Document on Hypertrophic Cardiomyopathy. A report of the American College of Cardiology Foundation Task Force on Clinical Expert Consensus Documents and the European Society of Cardiology Committee for Practice Guidelines. *Eur. Heart. J.*, 2003;**24**: 1965–1991.

111. McKenna, W.J., S. Chetty, C.M. Oakley, et al., Exercise electrocardiographic and 48 hour ambulatory electrocardiographic monitor assessment of arrhythmia and off beta blocker therapy in hypertrophic cardiomyopathy. *Am. J. Cardiol.*, 1979;**43**: 420.

112. Bonow, R.O., T.M. Frederick, S.L. Bacharach, et al., Atrial systole and left ventricular filling in hypertrophic cardiomyopathy: effect of verapamil. *Am. J. Cardiol.*, 1983;**51**: 1386–1391.

113. Huang, S.K., J. Jones, and P. Denes, Significance of ventricular tachycardia in primary congestive cardiomyopathy. *Am. J. Cardiol.*, 1982;**49**: 1006.

114. Fuster, V., B.J. Gersh, E.R. Giuliani, et al., The natural history of idiopathic dilated cardiomyopathy. *Am. J. Cardiol.*, 1981;**47**: 525–531.

115. Silverman, K.J., G.M. Hutchins, and B.H. Bulkley, Cardiac sarcoid: a clinicopathologic study of 84 unselected patients with systemic sarcoidosis. *Circulation*, 1978;**58**: 1204–1211.

116. Charron, P., J.F. Forissier, M.E. Amara, et al., Accuracy of European diagnostic criteria for familial hypertrophic cardiomyopathy in a genotyped population. *Int. J. Cardiol.*, 2003;**90**: 33–38; discussion 38–40.

117. Winkle, R.A., M.G. Lopes, J.W. Fitzgerald, et al., Arrhythmias in patients with mitral valve prolapse. *Circulation*, 1975;**52**: 73–81.

118. DeMaria, A.N. The syndrome of mitral valve prolapse: problems and perspectives. *Ann. Intern. Med.*, 1976;**85**: 525–526.

119. Leclercq, J.F., M.C. Malergue, D. Milosevic, et al., Ventricular arrhythmias and mitral valve prolapse. A study of 35 cases. *Arch. Mal. Coeur. Vaiss.*, 1980;**73**: 276–287.

120. Campbell, R.W., M.G. Godman, G.I. Fiddler, et al., Ventricular arrhythmias in syndrome of balloon deformity of mitral valve. Definition of possible high risk group. *Br. Heart. J.*, 1976;**38**: 1053–1057.

121. Rakowski, H., M.B. Waxman, R.W. Wald, et al., Mitral valve prolapse and ventricular fibrillation. *Circulation*, 1975;**52** (Suppl. 2): 93.

122. Boudoulas, H., S.F. Schaal, J.M. Stang, et al., Mitral valve prolapse: cardiac arrest with long-term survival. *Int. J. Cardiol.*, 1990;**26**: 37–44.

123. Kligfield, P., C. Hochreiter, H. Kramer, et al., Complex arrhythmias in mitral regurgitation with and without mitral valve prolapse: contrast to arrhythmias in mitral valve prolapse without mitral regurgitation. *Am. J. Cardiol.*, 1985;**55**(13 Pt 1): 1545–1549.

124. Kennedy, H.L., S.J. Underhill, P.F. Poblete, et al., Ventricular ectopic beats in patients with aortic valve disease. *Circulation*, 1975;**52** (Suppl. 2): 202.

125. Khaja, F., A. Rastogi, J.F. Brymer, et al., Coronary anatomy and left ventricular size: Determinants of ventricular arrhythmias in aortic valve disease. *Circulation*, 1982;**66** (Suppl. 2): 355.

126. Schilling, G., T. Finkbeiner, P. Elberskirch, et al., Incidence of ventricular arrhythmias in patients with aortic valve replacement. *Am. J. Cardiol.*, 1982;**49**: 894.

127. Guerot, C., P.E. Valere, A. Castillo-Fenoy, et al., Tachycardia by branch-to-branch reentry. *Arch. Mal. Coeur. Vaiss.*, 1974;**67**: 1–11.

128. Motte, G. and R. Slama, Les Tachycardies Ventriculaires. Paris: Lab. Servier, 1979.

129. Kastor, J.A., L.N. Horowitz, A.H. Harken, et al., Clinical electrophysiology of ventricular tachycardia. *N. Engl. J. Med.*, 1981;**304**: 1004–1019.

130. Fillette, F., G. Fontaine, and Y. Grosgogeat, Ventricular tachycardia. Study methods and status of current knowledge. *Arch. Mal. Coeur. Vaiss.*, 1982;**75**: 501–505.

131. Perrot, B., B. Thiel, F. Cherrier, et al., Results of the systematic application of ventricular stimulation methods. *Arch. Mal. Coeur. Vaiss.*, 1984;**77**: 262–272.

132. Fisher, J.D., Ventricular tachycardia–practical and provocative electrophysiology. *Circulation*, 1978;**58**: 1000–1007.

133. Scheinman, M.M., Induction of ventricular tachycardia: a promising new technique or clinical electrophysiology gone awry? *Circulation*, 1978; **58**:998–999.

134. Mason, J.W. and R.A. Winkle, Electrode-catheter arrhythmia induction in the selection and assessment of antiarrhythmic drug therapy for recurrent ventricular tachycardia. *Circulation*, 1978;**58**: 971–985.

135. Mann, D.E., J.C. Luck, J.C. Griffin, et al., Induction of clinical ventricular tachycardia using programmed stimulation: value of third and fourth extrastimuli. *Am. J. Cardiol.*, 1983;**52**: 501–506.

136. Doherty, J.U., M.E. Josephson, Role of electrophysiologic testing in the therapy of ventricular arrhythmias. *Pacing Clin. Electrophysiol.*, 1983;**6**: 1070–1083.

137. Ruskin, J.N., J.P. DiMarco, and H. Garan, Out-of-hospital cardiac arrest: electrophysiologic observations and selection of long-term antiarrhythmic therapy. *N. Engl. J. Med.*, 1980;**303**: 607–613.

138. Vandepol, C.J., A. Farshidi, S.R. Spielman, et al., Incidence and clinical significance of induced ventricular tachycardia. *Am. J. Cardiol.*, 1980;**45**: 725–731.

139. Livelli, F.D., Jr. J.T. Bigger, J.A. Reiffel, et al., Response to programmed ventricular stimulation: sensitivity, specificity and relation to heart disease. *Am. J. Cardiol.*, 1982;**50**: 452–458.

140. Brugada, P., J. Brugada, L. Mont, et al., A new approach to the differential diagnosis of a regular tachycardia with a wide QRS complex. *Circulation*, 1991;**83**: 1649–1659.

141. Wellens, H.J., F.W. Bar, and K.I. Lie, The value of the electrocardiogram in the differential diagnosis of a tachycardia with a widened QRS complex. *Am. J. Med.*, 1978;**64**: 27–33.

142. Kindwall, K.E., J. Brown, and M.E. Josephson, Electrocardiographic criteria for ventricular tachycardia in wide complex left bundle branch block morphology tachycardias. *Am. J. Cardiol.*, 1988;**61**: 1279–1283.

143. Reddy, C.P. and L.S. Gettes, Use of isoproterenol as an aid to electric induction of chronic recurrent ventricular tachycardia. *Am. J. Cardiol.*, 1979;**44**: 705–713.

144. Doherty, J.U., Kienzle, M.G., Waxman, H.L., et al., Programmed ventricular stimulation at a second right ventricular site: an analysis of 100 patients, with special reference to sensitivity, specificity and characteristics of patients with induced ventricular tachycardia. *Am. J. Cardiol.*, 1983;**52**: 1184–1189.

145. Morady, F., D. Hess, and M.M. Scheinman, Electrophysiologic drug testing in patients with malignant ventricular arrhythmias: importance of stimulation at more than one ventricular site. *Am. J. Cardiol.*, 1982;**50**: 1055–1060.

146. Swerdlow, C.D., J. Blum, R.A. Winkle, et al., Decreased incidence of antiarrhythmic drug efficacy at electrophysiologic study associated with the use of a third extrastimulus. *Am. Heart. J.*, 1982;**104**: 1004–1011.

147. Graboys, T.B., The stampede to stimulation–numerators and denominators revisited relative to electrophysiologic study of ventricular arrhythmias. *Am. Heart. J.*, 1982;**103**: 1089–1090.

148. Akhtar, M., The clinical significance of the repetitive ventricular response. *Circulation*, 1981;**63**: 773–775.

149. Grenadier, E., Alpan, G., Maor, N., et al., Polymorphous ventricular tachycardia in acute myocardial infarction. *Am. J. Cardiol.*, 1984;**53**: 1280–1283.

150. Cohen, M., I. Wiener, A. Pichard, et al., Determinants of ventricular tachycardia in patients with coronary artery disease and ventricular aneurysm. Clinical, hemodynamic, and angiographic factors. *Am. J. Cardiol.*, 1983;**51**: 61–64.

151. Medvedowsky, J.L., C. Barnay, C. Arnaud, et al., Course of ventricular arrhythmias following myocardial infarction. Results of a 2-year follow-up. *Arch. Mal. Coeur. Vaiss.*, 1984;**77**: 754–765.

152. A comparison of antiarrhythmic-drug therapy with implantable defibrillators in patients resuscitated from near-fatal ventricular

arrhythmias. The Antiarrhythmics versus Implantable Defibrillators (AVID) Investigators. *N. Engl. J. Med.*, 1997;**337**: 1576–1583.

153. Kuck, K.H., R. Cappato, J. Siebels, et al., Randomized comparison of antiarrhythmic drug therapy with implantable defibrillators in patients resuscitated from cardiac arrest: the Cardiac Arrest Study Hamburg (CASH). *Circulation*, 2000;**102**: 748–754.

154. Connolly, S.J., M. Gent, R.S. Roberts, et al., Canadian implantable defibrillator study (CIDS): a randomized trial of the implantable cardioverter defibrillator against amiodarone. *Circulation*, 2000;**101**: 1297–1302.

155. Buxton, A.E., K.L. Lee, J.D. Fisher, et al., A randomized study of the prevention of sudden death in patients with coronary artery disease. Multicenter Unsustained Tachycardia Trial Investigators. *N. Engl. J. Med.*, 1999;**341**: 1882–1890.

156. Moss, A.J., W. Zareba, W.J. Hall, et al., Prophylactic implantation of a defibrillator in patients with myocardial infarction and reduced ejection fraction. *N. Engl. J. Med.*, 2002;**346**: 877–883.

157. Moss, A.J., W.J. Hall, D.S. Cannom, et al., Improved survival with an implanted defibrillator in patients with coronary disease at high risk for ventricular arrhythmia. Multicenter Automatic Defibrillator Implantation Trial Investigators. *N. Engl. J. Med.*, 1996;**335**: 1933–1940.

158. Leclerq, J.F., P. Maisonblanche, B. Cauchemez, et al., Ventricular rhythm disorders in congestive myocardiopathy. *Arch. Mal. Coeur. Vaiss.*, 1984;**77**: 937–945.

159. Johnson, R.A., I. Palacios, Dilated cardiomyopathies of the adult (first of two parts). *N. Engl. J. Med.*, 1982;**307**: 1051–1058.

160. Bardy, G.H., K.L. Lee, D.B. Mark, et al., Amiodarone or an implantable cardioverter-defibrillator for congestive heart failure. *N. Engl. J. Med.*, 2005;**352**: 225–237.

161. Bristow, M.R., Saxon, L.A., Boehmer, J., et al., Cardiac-resynchronization therapy with or without an implantable defibrillator in advanced chronic heart failure. *N. Engl. J. Med.*, 2004;**350**: 2140–2150.

162. Maron, B.J., J. Shirani, L.C. Poliac, et al., Sudden death in young competitive athletes. Clinical, demographic, and pathological profiles. *JAMA*, 1996;**276**: 199–204.

163. Yamaguchi, H., T. Ishimura, S. Nishiyama, et al., Hypertrophic nonobstructive cardiomyopathy with giant negative T waves (apical hypertrophy): ventriculographic and echocardiographic features in 30 patients. *Am. J. Cardiol.*, 1979;**44**: 401–412.

164. Maron, B.J., W.K. Shen, M.S. Link, et al., Efficacy of implantable cardioverter-defibrillators for the prevention of sudden death in patients with hypertrophic cardiomyopathy. *N. Engl. J. Med.*, 2000;**342**: 365–373.

165. Maron, M.S., I. Olivotto, S. Betocchi, et al., Effect of left ventricular outflow tract obstruction on clinical outcome in hypertrophic cardiomyopathy. *N. Engl. J. Med.*, 2003;**348**: 295–303.

166. Jeresaty, R.M. *Mitral Valve Prolapse*. New York: Raven, 1979.

167. Gregoratos, G., J. Abrams, A.E. Epstein, et al. ACC/AHA/NASPE 2002 Guideline update for implantation of cardiac pacemakers and antiarrhythmia devices: summary article: a report of the American College of Cardiology/American Heart Association Task Force on Practice Guidelines (ACC/AHA/NASPE Committee to Update the 1998 Pacemaker Guidelines). *Circulation*, 2002;**106**: 2145–2161.

168. Marcus, F.I., G.H. Fontaine, G. Guiraudon, et al., Right ventricular dysplasia: a report of 24 adult cases. *Circulation*, 1982;**65**: 384–398.

169. Fontaine, G., G. Guiraudon, R. Frank, et al., The arrhythmogenic right ventricular dysplasia syndrome. In: Hayase S, Murao S, MacArthur C, eds. *Cardiology*. Amsterdam: Excerpta Medica, 1979: 955–958.

170. Vedel, J., R. Frank, G. Fontaine, et al., Recurrent ventricular tachycardia and parchment right ventricle in the adult. Anatomical and clinical report of 2 cases. *Arch. Mal. Coeur. Vaiss.*, 1978;**71**: 973–981.

171. Hulot, J.S., X. Jouven, J.P. Empana, et al., Natural history and risk stratification of arrhythmogenic right ventricular dysplasia/cardiomyopathy. *Circulation*, 2004;**110**: 1879–1884.

172. Fontaine, G., J. Tonet, Y. Gallais, et al., Ventricular tachycardia catheter ablation in arrhythmogenic right ventricular dysplasia: a 16-year experience. *Curr. Cardiol. Rep.*, 2000;**2**: 498–506.

173. Corrado, D., L. Leoni, M.S. Link, et al., Implantable cardioverter-defibrillator therapy for prevention of sudden death in patients with arrhythmogenic right ventricular cardiomyopathy/dysplasia. *Circulation*, 2003;**108**: 3084–3091.

174. Wichter, T., M. Paul, C. Wollmann, et al., Implantable cardioverter/defibrillator therapy in arrhythmogenic right ventricular cardiomyopathy: single-center experience of long-term follow-up and complications in 60 patients. *Circulation*, 2004;**109**: 1503–1508.

175. Chachques, J.C., P.G. Argyriadis, G. Fontaine, et al., Right ventricular cardiomyoplasty: 10-year follow-up. *Ann. Thorac. Surg.*, 2003;**75**: 1464–1468.

176. Uhl, H.S. A previously undescribed congenital malformation of the heart: almost total absence of the myocardium of the right ventricle. *Bull. Johns. Hopkins Hosp.*, 1952;**91**: 197–209.

177. Antzelevitch, C., P. Brugada, M. Borggrefe, et al., Brugada syndrome: report of the second consensus conference: endorsed by the Heart Rhythm Society and the European Heart Rhythm Association. *Circulation*, 2005;**111**: 659–670.

178. Buxton, A.E., H.L. Waxman, F.E. Marchlinski, et al., Right ventricular tachycardia: clinical and electrophysiologic characteristics. *Circulation*, 1983;**68**: 917–927.

179. Wen, M.S., Y. Taniguchi, S.J. Yeh, et al., Determinants of tachycardia recurrences after radiofrequency ablation of idiopathic ventricular tachycardia. *Am. J. Cardiol.*, 1998; **81**: 500–503.

180. Tsuchiya, T., K. Okumura, T. Honda, et al., Significance of late diastolic potential preceding Purkinje potential in verapamil-sensitive idiopathic left ventricular tachycardia. *Circulation*, 1999;**99**: 2408–2413.

181. McAllister, H.A. and J.J. Fenoglio, *Tumors of Cardiovascular System*. A.F.I.P: Bethesda, Maryland, 1978.

182. Lucet, V., J. Fidelle, D. Do N'Goc, et al., Catecholaminergic polymorphic ventricular tachycardia in children. Differential diagnosis of epilepsy. *Presse. Med.*, 1983;**12**: 102.

183. Dessertenne, F., Ventricular tachycardia with 2 variable opposing foci. *Arch. Mal. Coeur. Vaiss.*, 1966; **59**: 263–272.

184. Fontaine, G., A new look at torsades de pointes. *Ann. N. Y. Acad. Sci.*, 1992;**644**: 157–177.

185. Davidenko, J.M., Spiral wave activity: a possible common mechanism for polymorphic and monomorphic ventricular tachycardias. *J. Cardiovasc. Electrophysiol.*, 1993;**4**: 730–746.

186. Tzivoni, D., A. Keren, A.M. Cohen, et al., Magnesium therapy for torsades de pointes. *Am. J. Cardiol.*, 1984; **53**:528–30.

187. Chiang, C.E. and D.M. Roden, The long QT syndromes: genetic basis and clinical implications. *J. Am. Coll. Cardiol.*, 2000;**36**: 1–12.

188. Priori, S.G., P.J. Schwartz, C. Napolitano, et al., Risk stratification in the long-QT syndrome. *N. Engl. J. Med.*, 2003;**348**: 1866–1874.

189. Sebastien, P., M. Waynberger, P. Beaufils, et al., Isolated ventricular tachycardia without patent cardiopathy. *Arch. Mal. Coeur. Vaiss.*, 1976;**69**: 919–928.

190. Weaver, W.D., L.A. Cobb, M.K. Copass, et al., Ventricular defibrillation - a comparative trial using 175-J and 320-J shocks. *N. Engl. J. Med.*, 1982;**307**: 1101–116.

191. Vaughan-Williams, E.M., Interet des etudes experimentales d'anti-arythmiques et leur application clinique. *Coeur. Med. Interne.*, 1978;**17**: 471–489.

192. Borggrefe, M., L. Seipel, G. Breithardt, Effect of amiodarone on ventricular tachycardia. In: Breithardt G, Loogen F, eds. *New Aspects in the Medical Treatment of Tachyarrhythmias*. Munich: Urban and Schwarzenberg, 1983: 177–185.

193. Fogoros, R.N., K.P. Anderson, R.A. Winkle, et al., Amiodarone: clinical efficacy and toxicity in 96 patients with recurrent, drug-refractory arrhythmias. *Circulation*, 1983;**68**: 88–94.

194. Finerman, W.B., Jr., A. Hamer, T. Peter, et al., Electrophysiologic effects of chronic amiodarone therapy in patients with ventricular arrhythmias. *Am. Heart. J.*, 1982;**104**: 987–996.

195. Frank, R., G. Fontaine, P. Blanc, Les methodes provocatives dans l'etude de l'amiodarone per os dans les tachycardies ventriculaires et celles du syndrome de Wolff-Parkinson-White. *Colloque sur L'amiodarone*. Paris: Lab. Labaz, 1977: 35–42.

196. Morady, F., M.M. Scheinman, D.S. Hess, Amiodarone in the management of patients with ventricular tachycardia and ventricular fibrillation. *Pacing Clin. Electrophysiol.*, 1983;**6**: 609–615.

197. Morady, F., M.M. Scheinman, E. Shen, et al., Intravenous amiodarone in the acute treatment of recurrent symptomatic ventricular tachycardia. *Am. J. Cardiol.*, 1983;**51**: 156–159.

198. Waxman, H.L., W.C. Groh, F.E. Marchlinski, et al., Amiodarone for control of sustained ventricular tachyarrhythmia: clinical and electrophysiologic effects in 51 patients. *Am. J. Cardiol.*, 1982;**50**: 1066–1074.

199. Rakita, L. and S.M. Sobol, Amiodarone in the treatment of refractory ventricular arrhythmias: Importance and safety of initial high-dose therapy. *JAMA*, 1983;**250**: 1293–1295.

200. Nademanee, K., B.N. Singh, J. Hendrickson, et al., Amiodarone in refractory life-threatening ventricular arrhythmias. *Ann. Intern. Med.*, 1983;**98**: 577–584.

201. Heger, J.J., E.N. Prystowsky, W.M. Jackman, et al., Clinical efficacy and electrophysiology during long-term therapy for recurrent ventricular tachycardia or ventricular fibrillation. *N. Engl. J. Med.*, 1981;**305**: 539–545.

202. Morady, F., M.J. Sauve, P. Malone, et al., Long-term efficacy and toxicity of high-dose amiodarone therapy for ventricular tachycardia or ventricular fibrillation. *Am. J. Cardiol.*, 1983;**52**: 975–979.

203. Marcus, F.I., G.H. Fontaine, R. Frank, et al., Clinical pharmacology and therapeutic applications of the antiarrhythmic agent amiodarone. *Am. Heart. J.*, 1981;**101**: 480–493.

204. Kosinski, E.J., J.B. Albin, E. Young, et al., Hemodynamic effects of intravenous amiodarone. *J Am. Coll. Cardiol.*, 1984;**4**: 565–570.

205. Glasser, S.P., P.I. Clark, A.R. Laddu, Comparison of the antiarrhythmic effects of acebutolol and propranolol in the treatment of ventricular arrhythmias. *Am. J. Cardiol.*, 1983;**52**: 992–995.

206. Belhassen, B., H.H. Rotmensch, S. Laniado, Response of recurrent sustained ventricular tachycardia to verapamil. *Br. Heart. J.*, 1981;**46**: 679–682.

207. Frank, R., G. Fontaine, R. Coutte, et al., Reproducibilité des arythmies ventriculaires déclenchées avant et après imprégnation médicamenteuse. Valeur prédictive de l'effet anti-arythmique. *Arch. Mal. Coeur. Vaiss.*, 1981;**74**: 79–86.

208. Horowitz, L.N., M.E. Josephson, A. Farshidi, et al., Recurrent sustained ventricular tachycardia 3. Role of the electrophysiologic study in selection of antiarrhythmic regimens. *Circulation*, 1978;**58**: 986–997.

209. Mason, J.W., C.D. Swerdlow, R.A. Winkle, et al., Programmed ventricular stimulation in predicting vulnerability to ventricular arrhythmias and their response to antiarrhythmic therapy. *Am. Heart. J.*, 1982;**103**: 633–639.

210. Swerdlow, C.D., G. Gong, D.S. Echt, et al. Clinical factors predicting successful electrophysiologic-pharmacologic study in patients with ventricular tachycardia. *J. Am. Coll. Cardiol.*, 1983;**1**: 409–416.

211. Vlay, S.C., C.H. Kallman, and P.R. Reid, Prognostic assessment of survivors of ventricular tachycardia and ventricular fibrillation with ambulatory monitoring. *Am. J. Cardiol.*, 1984;**54**: 87–90.

212. Platia, E.V., S.C. Vlay, P.R. Reid, A comparison of the predictive value of programmed electrical stimulation and the Holter monitoring in patients with malignant ventricular arrhythmias. *Am. J. Cardiol.*, 1982;**49**: 928.

213. Swerdlow, C.D., R.A. Winkle, J.W. Mason, Determinants of survival in patients with ventricular tachyarrhythmias. *N. Engl. J. Med.*, 1983;**308**: 1436–1442.

214. Buxton, A.E., F.E. Marchlinski, H.L. Waxman, et al., Prognostic factors in nonsustained ventricular tachycardia. *Am. J. Cardiol.*, 1984;**53**: 1275–1279.

215. Breithardt, G., Seipel, L., R.R. Abendroth, et al., Serial electrophysiological testing of antiarrhythmic drug efficacy in patients with recurrent ventricular tachycardia. *Eur. Heart. J.*, 1980;**1**: 11–24.

216. Kang, P.S., J.A. Gomes, and N. El-Sherif, Procainamide in the induction and perpetuation of ventricular tachycardia in man. *Pacing Clin. Electrophysiol.*, 1982;**5**: 311–322.

217. Sclarovsky, S., R.F. Lewin, O. Kracoff, et al., Amiodarone-induced polymorphous ventricular tachycardia. *Am. Heart. J.*, 1983;**105**: 6–12.

218. Connolly, S.J., R.E. Kates, C.S. Lebsack, et al., Clinical pharmacology of propafenone. *Circulation*, 1983;**68**: 589–596.

219. Connolly, S.J., R.E. Kates, C.S. Lebsack, et al., Clinical efficacy and electrophysiology of oral propafenone for ventricular tachycardia. *Am. J. Cardiol.*, 1983;**52**: 1208–1213.

220. Seipel, L. and G. Breithardt, Propafenone–a new antiarrhythmic drug. *Eur. Heart. J.*, 1980;**1**: 309–313.

221. Kulbertus, H.E., The arrhythmogenic effects of antiarrhythmic agents. In: Befeler B, ed. *Selected Topics in Cardiac Arrhythmias*. Mount Kisco, New York: Futura, 1980: 113–119.

222. Velebit, V., P. Podrid, B, Lown, et al., Aggravation and provocation of ventricular arrhythmias by antiarrhythmic drugs. *Circulation*, 1982;**65**: 886–894.

223. Block, P.J. and R.A. Winkle, Hemodynamic effects of antiarrhythmic drugs. *Am. J. Cardiol.*, 1983;**52**: 14C–23C.

224. Leclercq, J.F. and P. Coumel, Les indications cliniques des différentes drogues dans les arythmies rebelles. *Ther. Umsch.*, 1982;**39**: 128–136.

225. Zipes, D.P., J.J. Heger, W.M. Miles, et al., Synchronous intracardiac cardioversion. *Pacing Clin. Electrophysiol.*, 1984;7: 522–533.

226. Mirowski, M., P.R. Reid, M.M. Mower, et al., The automatic implantable cardioverter-defibrillator. *Pacing Clin. Electrophysiol.*, 1984;7: 534–540.

227. Mirowski, M., P.R. Reid, R.A. Winkle, et al., Mortality in patients with implanted automatic defibrillators. *Ann. Intern. Med.*, 1983;98: 585–588.

228. Fisher, J.D., S.G. Kim, S. Furman, et al., Role of implantable pacemakers in control of recurrent ventricular tachycardia. *Am. J. Cardiol.*, 1982;49: 194–206.

229. Hartzler, G.O., Electrode catheter ablation of focal ventricular tachycardia. *J. Am. Coll. Cardiol.*, 1983;1: 595.

230. Fontaine, G., G. Guiraudon, R. Frank, et al., The surgical treatment of cardiac arrhythmias. In: Befeler B, ed. *The Management of Cardiac Arrhythmias*, 1979.

231. Josephson, M.E., L.N. Horowitz, A. Farshidi, Continuous local electrical activity. A mechanism of recurrent ventricular tachycardia. *Circulation*, 1978;57: 659–665.

232. Harken, A.H., L.N. Horowitz, M.E. Josephson, Comparison of standard aneurysmectomy and aneurysmectomy with directed endocardial resection for the treatment of recurrent sustained ventricular tachycardia. *J. Thorac. Cardiovasc. Surg.*, 1980;80: 527–534.

233. Guiraudon, G., G. Fontaine, R. Frank, et al., Circular exclusion ventriculotomy. Surgical treatment of ventricular tachycardia following myocardial infarction. *Arch. Mal. Coeur. Vaiss.*, 1978;71: 1255–1262.

234. Guiraudon, G., G. Fontaine, R. Frank, et al., Surgical treatment of chronic ventricular tachycardias. The concept of arrhythmogenic area. In: Masoni A, Alboni P, eds. *Cardiac Electrophysiology Today*. London: Academic Press, 1982: 325–347.

235. Horowitz, L.N., A.H. Harken, J.A. Kastor, et al., Ventricular resection guided by epicardial and endocardial mapping for treatment of recurrent ventricular tachycardia. *N. Engl. J. Med.*, 1980;302: 589–593.

236. Cohen, M., M. Packer, and R. Gorlin, Indications for left ventricular aneurysmectomy. *Circulation*, 1983;67: 717–722.

237. Fontaine, G., G. Guiraudon, and R. Frank, Surgical management of ventricular tachycardia not related to myocardial ischemia. In: Josephson ME, Wellens HJJ, eds. *Tachycardias: Mechanisms, Diagnosis and Treatment*. Philadelphia, Pennsylvania: Lea and Febiger, 1984: 451–473.

238. Fontaine, G., R. Frank, J.L. Tonet, et al., Arrhythmogenic right ventricular dysplasia: a clinical model for the study of chronic ventricular tachycardia. *Jpn. Circ. J.*, 1984;48: 515–538.

239. Trigano, J.A., H. Nasta, J.L. Michaud, et al., Resistant ventricular tachycardia caused by right ventricular dysplasia. A case of surgical recovery reported 6 years after intervention. *Arch. Mal. Coeur. Vaiss.*, 1983;76: 852–857.

240. Guiraudon, G.M., G.J. Klein, S.S. Gulamhusein, et al., Total disconnection of the right ventricular free wall: surgical treatment of right ventricular tachycardia associated with right ventricular dysplasia. *Circulation*, 1983;67: 463–470.

241. Scheinman, M.M. and F. Morady, E.N. Shen, Interventional electrophysiology: Catheter ablation techniques. *Clin. Prog. Pacing. Electrophysiol.*, 1983;1: 375–381.

242. Fontaine, G., R. Frank, J.L. Tonet, et al., Treatment of resistant ventricular tachycardia with endocavitary fulguration and antiarrhythmic therapy, compared to antiarrhythmic therapy alone: experience in 111 consecutive cases with a mean follow-up of 18 months. *Tex. Heart. Inst. J.*, 1986;13: 401–418.

243. Josephson, M.E. Catheter ablation of arrhythmias. *Ann. Intern. Med.*, 1984;101: 234–237.

244. Fontaine, G., G. Guiraudon, R. Frank, et al., When is surgery of ventricular tachycardia indicated? *Nouv. Presse. Med.*, 1981;10: 3539–3540.

8 Atrial Tachycardias in Infants, Children, and Young Adults with Congenital Heart Disease

Parvin C. Dorostkar · Jerome Liebman

P. W. Macfarlane et al. (eds.), *Cardiac Arrhythmias and Mapping Techniques*, DOI 10.1007/978-0-85729-877-5_8,
© Springer-Verlag London Limited 2012

8.1   Introduction

Atrial tachycardias comprise a minority of all supraventricular tachycardias in pediatric patients. Mechanistically, these tachycardias present a multiple of different types of tachycardias that originate and sustain in the atria and often express themselves as tachycardias in association with a rapid ventricular response in the younger patient. Atrial tachycardias can be categorized into three basic mechanistic universes: those that are automatic in nature, those that are triggered in nature, and those that are reentrant in nature.

Differentiation of the three different types of atrial tachycardias is important and can sometimes be difficult. In general, abnormalities of impulse formation, that is, atrial automatic tachycardia and/or atrial triggered tachycardia, tend to express beat-to-beat variability and have been associated with a "warm-up, cool-down phenomenon." In contrast, abnormalities of impulse propagation include atrial tachycardias that are reentrant in nature and tend to have a fixed atrial rate with either a fixed or variable ventricular response. These individuals usually present with an inappropriately fast heart rate with little heart rate variability.

In contrast to atrial tachycardias that are associated with abnormalities of impulse formation, abnormalities of impulse propagation, as stated above, use a reentrant circuit within the atrium as their primary mechanism. This tachycardia usually occurs in patients with congenital heart disease, especially those who have had surgery for either repair or palliation of the underlying heart defect. The tachycardia responds transiently to atrial pacing and cardioversion and can sometimes be suppressed with antiarrhythmic medications. In most recent years, this tachycardia has proven to be responsive to ablative therapies and has been the subject of much study.

The first part of this chapter will focus on the clinical evaluation and treatment of automatic atrial tachycardia, while the second part dwells on atrial reentrant tachycardias. Representative electrophysiologic tracings and maps are interspersed.

8.1.1   Automatic/Triggered Atrial Tachycardias

Automatic or ectopic atrial tachycardias are caused by abnormal impulse formation where one or a few closely associated cells generate an atrial impulse faster than that of the sinus node. The arrhythmia has unique clinical features in that it usually occurs in a structurally normal heart. It classically expresses some degree of heart rate variability, and is often incessant. Because of its persistent nature, this tachycardia can be associated with a cardiomyopathy [1–3]. Automatic tachycardias rare also difficult to treat, because they are often resistant to medications and/or chemical or electrical cardioversion.

Automatic atrial tachycardias are thought to be focal in nature, depolarizing the atrium in a spreading fashion originating from the rapidly firing, abnormal focus. The exact underlying pathophysiology of automatic activity is not well understood. It is thought that the cells express abnormally rapid depolarization resulting in a faster pacemaker rate than that the sinus node. This tachycardia comprises approximately 15% of newly diagnosed supraventricular tachycardias in the pediatric population and comprises only 5% of all supraventricular tachycardias in the adult age group. Because the atrial rate is variable and sometimes only marginally above the sinus tachycardia rate, patients with this type of tachycardia may go undiagnosed for several years until they present with ventricular dysfunction associated with cardiomyopathy. Cardiomyopathy is more likely to occur in patients with higher heart rates (150–176 beats per minute), but may occasionally occur in patients with lower heart rates (90–136 beats per minute) [4]. When this happens, it is possible that the tachycardia is misdiagnosed as sinus tachycardia before a final diagnoses can be made. Myocardial dysfunction is noted to be present in about 50% of patients with ectopic atrial tachycardia. Automatic activity tends to be associated with either spontaneous diastolic Phase IV depolarization or abnormalities in repolarization of Phase III of the action potential. The location of the focus can be discerned by critical evaluation of the P-wave morphology suggesting direction of depolarization. Ectopic atrial tachycardias arising from the right atrium or the right atrial appendage are directed to the left and, usually, inferior, so that there are positive P-waves in leads I, II, III, and aVF, very similar to those in sinus rhythm. However, the P-wave morphology is usually distinctly different from that in sinus rhythm, although the non-electrophysiology physician may call it "sinus like." In contrast, ectopic atrial tachycardias from the left-sided atrium express a P-wave morphology very different from those seen in sinus rhythm. The P-wave is directed to the right and

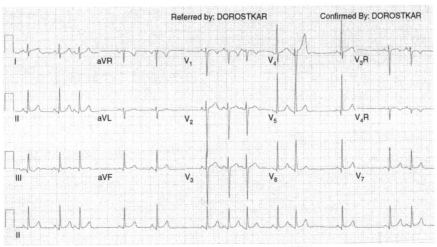

🔲 Fig. 8.1

Eight-year-old male referred for evaluation of an irregular heartbeat. Note that the ECG shows episodic salvos of a triggered atrial tachycardia arising from the right atrium as evidenced by P-waves that are positive in I, II, III, and aVF

inferior so that the P-waves of ectopic atrial tachycardia arising from the left atrium express negative P-waves in I and aVL and usually positive P-waves in II, III, and aVF.

Electrocardiographic and monitored rhythm recordings characteristic of automatic atrial tachycardia are highly variable. Heart rates range from just above the sinus rate to as fast as 300 beats per minute. In addition, this tachycardia exhibits multiple varied behaviors including the classic warm-up and cool-down behavior; expressed salvoes of beats anywhere from three beats to several seconds in duration; as well as variable atrioventricular relationships with transmission of conduction to the ventricles varying from one to one conduction to first-degree, second-degree, and "apparent" third-degree atrioventricular block or multilevel block through the atrioventricular node. Atrial tachycardia rates associated with automatic atrial tachycardia vary highly; in addition, the tachycardia heart rate, as stated above, can vary in association with the degree of atrioventricular node transmission to the ventricle (❷ Fig. 8.2). There may also be a wide complex QRS owing to aberrant ventricular conduction. As these tachycardias, typically, have "a mind of their own," they tend to express themselves with variable rates in a persistent fashion. Higher levels of atrioventricular conduction block can usually be seen while the patient is sleeping and, therefore, a Holter monitor of the heptum of such patients might be helpful in elucidating the diagnostic expression and behavior of the automatic atrial tachycardia (❷ Fig. 8.2). Adenosine can be used as a tool to diagnose automatic atrial tachycardia, as it causes transient atrioventricular node block. In the majority of cases, the tachycardia itself is not sensitive to adenosine and, therefore, P-waves can be dissociated from the ventricles unmasking the atrial tachycardia during transient atrioventricular node block with P-waves, lone-standing. A minority of automatic atrial tachycardias are sensitive and responsive to adenosine and will terminate, usually inscribing a QRS complex as the last expressed electrogram before they resume their activities a few seconds later. Electrical or chemical cardioversion may be transiently effective, but the tachycardia usually resumes. Automatic tachycardias tend to be variably initiated and are not responsive to extra-stimulation techniques or overdrive pacing in regards to initiation or termination of the tachycardia. Triggered activity is thought to be associated with delayed afterdepolarization; these tachycardias express their own behavior independent of pacing maneuvers and are difficult to induce and/or terminate with traditional electrophysiologically mediated pacing techniques.

As stated above, ectopic atrial tachycardia may arise either from the right or the left atrium. Although the origin of ectopic atrial tachycardia appears to be widely distributed throughout both atria, there is some suggestion that automaticity or increased triggered activity may have a propensity to arise near atrial appendages, or in and around atrial extensions into pulmonary veins. The reasons for this distribution are unclear, but there appears to be some association with the expression of HNK-1 antigen, which has become known as a marker for specialized conduction tissues during cardiac development [5, 6]. In a study by Blom-Gitinberger, investigators demonstrated an association between the

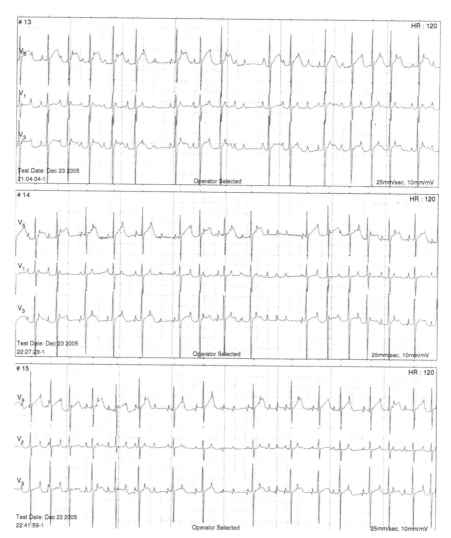

Fig. 8.2

Newborn infant with a virtually incessant atrial tachycardia that showed multilevel block on the 24 h Holter recordings

HNK-1 antigen expression and a propensity to develop automaticity [6]. However, the stimulus for automaticity expression and, therefore, tachycardia expression remains poorly understood.

Electrophysiologic testing can be performed to confirm the diagnosis of a suspected ectopic atrial tachycardia and can be especially meaningful if the patient has an associated myopathy, as it offers a potential cure if a successful ablation can be achieved [6, 7]. Activation sequence mapping can be done with newer mapping technologies, which delineate detailed localization of the automatic focus so that ablation can be successful (❯ Fig. 8.4). Should a successful ablation occur, echocardiography can then be used to follow ventricular function, which will often return to normal. Both systolic and diastolic dysfunction improve over time if successful ablation is achieved. As stated above, usually cardiomyopathy is observed in patients with higher heart rates as compared to those with lower heart rates [4].

Pharmacologic management of patients with atrial ectopic tachycardias is often quite challenging. An initial approach with rate control should be tried to maximize optimal hemodynamics. Though desirable, rhythm control is difficult and often fraught with challenging side effects from antiarrhythmic medications. Since medications, that provide rate control,

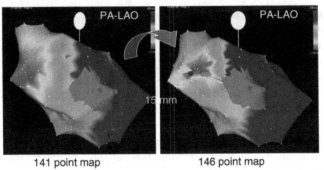

◘ Fig. 8.3

Eleven-year-old male with incessant atrial tachycardia mapped to the posterolateral left atrium and successfully ablated; bright red color denotes areas of earliest atrial activation as noted by the color bar; gray denotes absent atrial signals consistent with the orifice of the left atrial appendage; note that centric activation of the left atrium away from the mapped dominant tachycardia pacemaker

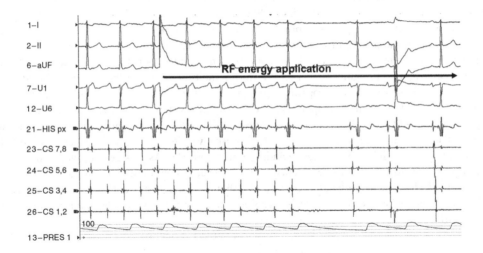

◘ Fig. 8.4

Successful radiofrequency energy application in an 11-year-old male with incessant atrial tachycardia, mapped in the left atrium

including beta-blockers and digoxin, seem to be well tolerated in the pediatric population, these drugs are chosen as a first-line option. In addition to rate control, by suppressing automaticity, beta blockers appear to control ectopic atrial tachycardia in about 20% of cases. Ultimately, successful suppression of tachycardia occurs in about 50% of cases, often utilizing multiple medications. Class IC (Flecainide and/or Propafenone) and/or Class III (Sotalol) agents are favorably used for atrial ectopic tachycardias that present a challenge in regards to control. Verapamil has been commonly cited for rate control in the adult literature, but is less commonly used in pediatrics. This drug is thought to suppress triggered activity. Thus, verapamil may offer both rate control and rhythm control. However, calcium channel blockers are contraindicated in the infant, as they are associated with asystole, probably related to the infant's poorly differentiated endoplasmic reticulum and therefore, inability to benefit form the drug's actions.

The natural history of ectopic atrial tachycardia is variable. When it occurs in younger neonates and infants, the tachycardia seems to regress spontaneously in about 50% of cases. However, when the patients are older and present with cardiomyopathy, the tachycardia tends to be more persistent and requires more aggressive intervention.

Though surgical techniques were employed effectively for drug-resistant ectopic atrial tachycardia throughout the 1980s, the advent of radiofrequency energy application changed the outcomes. The earliest attempts to ablate ectopic atrial tachycardia using transvenous methods occurred in 1984 using direct DC energy. Further developments in technology introduced the application of radiofrequency energy as an intervention. When used appropriately, this intervention tends to underscore the relatively benign course and good outcomes in association with high success rates for ablation of this type of tachycardia. The success rate with currently available technology for the ablation of ectopic atrial tachycardia is now greater than 90% with a relatively low complication rate. Nowadays, patients who present with ventricular failure due to an atrial tachycardia are promptly managed with electrophysiologic study and catheter ablation using either radiofrequency or cryoablative energy. This otherwise malignant arrhythmia can now, be often-cured (❷ Figs. 8.3 and ❷ 8.4).

Multifocal atrial tachycardia, also known as chaotic atrial tachycardia, is a rare form of automatic atrial tachycardia, where there is more than one focus firing rapidly [8]. Multifocal atrial tachycardia is mostly a condition seen in adults, particularly with cor pulmonale or chronic obstructive pulmonary disease [10]. Multifocal atrial tachycardia is frequently idiopathic in nature, although it has been associated, in rare cases, with Macrocephaly-Cutis Marmorata Telangiectatica Congenita [9] and other rare diseases. When it occurs in the postoperative period, it is often very difficult to control and may require aggressive therapy including early consideration of radiofrequency ablation of the atrioventricular node for rate control. Classic ECG (electrocardiogram) findings include P-waves that are irregularly inscribed at heart rates greater than 100 beats per minute. There may be three or more different P-wave morphologies. The ventricular response to such a tachycardia can be quite varied. Rate-related bundle branch block can be seen after short–long or after long–short ventricular responses due to variable ventricular transmission of the rapid impulses in the atrium.

The clinical course of multifocal atrial tachycardia in children includes spontaneous resolution of the tachycardia in 50–80% of the cases by 12–18 months of age. Rarely, during the time in which the multifocal atrial tachycardia is expressed, there may be progressive cardiomyopathy and sudden cardiac death, presumably associated with rapid ventricular conduction [11, 12]. Multifocal atrial tachycardia tends to be quite resistant to medical management, even aggressive pharmacologic therapy. Traditionally, beta-blockers or digoxin can be used for rate control and, sometimes, can suppress atrial and ventricular irritability. However, rhythm control is usually quite difficult in these patients. Combinations of medications have been used with limited success, including amiodarone [13]. As a last resort, ablation of the atrioventricular node can be performed to control the rate in patients who are severely symptomatic. In this case, careful consideration of the aggressive approach to the hemodynamic compromise should be weighed as the patient will most likely require a pacemaker for the rest of his/her life. Most telling is that once the tachycardia has resolved, the recurrence risk is quite low as the tachycardia does not reoccur during later life.

Regardless, short of ablation therapy, medical management of both rhythm control and rate control appears to be challenging in patients with a triggered and/or automatic atrial tachycardia. With the advent of radiofrequency energy application and/or (now) cryo-ablation, the cure rate for atrial tachycardia remains high and especially hopeful for those patients suffering from associated myocardial dysfunction.

8.1.2   Reentrant Atrial Tachycardias

As stated above, in contrast to atrial tachycardias associated with abnormalities of impulse formation, abnormalities of impulse propagation use a reentrant circuit within the atrium as their primary mechanism. The history related to the development of understanding of atrial reentrant tachycardias is of particular interest. The traditional term for atrial reentrant tachycardia is atrial flutter. The term "flutter" originates from the Anglo-Saxon word "floterian," meaning to move or flap wings rapidly without flying or to move with quick vibrations or undulations. This descriptive term was fist used by a British physiologist, MacWilliams, in 1887 while looking at a dog atrium [14]. In 1905, there was a first recording of atrial flutter by William Richie using an ink-polygraph recorder in a patient with complete atrioventricular block [15], which was followed in 1910 by a first-time recording of atrial flutter in the same patient using an electrocardiograph [16]. Einthoven in 1906 had reported a similar phenomenon in his laboratory from a patient 1.5 km away [17]. The most clear electrocardiographic recordings of atrial flutter were made in 1913 by Sir Thomas Lewis who described a classic saw-toothed pattern with negative deflections in leads II and III [18]. Once this arrhythmia was acknowledged, many investigators began to hypothesize and study its mechanism with two basic schools of thought predominating: Is the primary mechanism one of automaticity (abnormal impulse formation, as believed by Lewis) or reentry (abnormal impulse propagation)? Works by Mayer with the Scyphomedusae (1906), Mines (1913), and Garrey (1914) suggested reentry as a primary mechanism. In 1921, after a series of canine experiments, Lewis changed his mind and supported the notion that atrial flutter was supported by reentry [19]. Since mapping techniques were crude at the time, controversy continued to exist. Clinically, different ECG patterns of flutter were noted raising further questions in regards to the underlying mechanism. Telling work by Cabrera and Sodi-Pallares in 1947 showed that atrial flutter was a result of consecutive regular activation fronts oriented in the sagittal plane using data obtained from ECG and VCG recordings [20]. Despite these experiments, several clinical observations suggested that atrial flutter may be arising from a single focus firing rapidly. In a classic paper by Puech et al. in 1970, the authors identified two types of flutter: the common type, where P-waves were negative in II, III, and aVF; and the "rare" type, where flutter waves were best expressed in leads I and aVL [21]. Even though these studies showed that activation of the right atrium during common flutter preceded cranially along the interatrial septum and then caudally along the free wall of the right atrium, with the left atrium being activated at the same time as during septal activation, the question of reentry versus automaticity was not clearly answered from these studies. Finally, several ongoing studies by Waldo et al. in 1977 both in the canine sterile pericarditis model and in postoperative patients demonstrated that the mechanism for atrial flutter was reentrant and, thus, an abnormality of impulse propagation. These investigators used entrainment techniques to support the notion of reentry as opposed to automaticity as the underlying mechanism for flutter. Using epicardial electrode recordings, four electrophysiological criteria were identified with each of them sufficient to demonstrate circuit movement tachycardia incorporating an excitable gap [22–32]. Waldo also made a distinction between the two types of atrial flutter: Type 1, easily influenced by programmed pacing, and Type 2, which was infrequently seen, faster, and not easily influenced by rapid atrial pacing. In 1978, Wyndham was the first to report that atrial flutter could be interrupted using a self-activated radiofrequency generator [33]. Once identified as reentrant in mechanism, the quest to understand a more detailed mechanism continued. Pastelin et al. were able to identify that cutting the medial and posterior bundles in the atrium interrupted atrial flutter [34]. The role of anatomic and functional barriers was investigated including the proposed role of an area of slow conduction [35, 36]. Other investigators looked at the type of atrial reentry demonstrating that it was macroreentrant [37] and dependent on myocyte interconnections [38]. Another experimental model suggested that atrial reentry was possible without an area of slow conduction [39]. In the same year (1986), Guy Fontaine used radiofrequency energy in two patients to treat atrial flutter [40]. Further work demonstrated that the expression of atrial flutter was related to the time course of postoperative pericarditis. At the same time, the role of double potentials and fractionated atrial signals was interrogated by Cosio et al. suggesting that these signals were associated with areas of slow conduction [41] and that they provided an opportunity to study the reentrant mechanism further. Finally, after electrical fulguration was shown to be effective in the late 1980s [42], Feld et al. showed that atrial flutter was amenable to radiofrequency ablation in 1992 [43], targeting areas of slow conduction. As the quest to understand more complex types of atrial reentrant tachycardia continues, technology supports and parallels better understanding of the underlying mechanisms that can, therefore, support better outcomes in patients.

The observation that atrial tachycardias are more common in the postoperative patient with congenital heart disease has resulted in several investigators focusing on the role of surgical incisions in the expression of atrial reentrant tachycardia. It was thought that atrial reentry in these patients was also subeustachian isthmus dependent, although subsequently this observation has been scrutinized further to show that there are a variety of complex reentrant rhythms present in the patient with postoperative congenital heart disease.

8.1.3 Atrial Anatomy: Lessons from Atrial Flutter in Animal Models and Adult Patients with Heart Disease

Anatomic studies evaluated the role of the crista terminalis of the right atrium, which is located in the sulcus terminalis located in the right atrium inferior to the superior caval vein. The sinus node rests within the crista terminalis and supports the initiation of the sinus impulse. The origination of the impulse that initiates atrial flutter was thought to be the sinus node [35], but it is now accepted that any premature beat originating anywhere in the myocardium can serve as the initiator of atrial reentry as long as a supportive substrate is present. There is also a school of thought that atrial flutter is a later manifestation of atrial fibrillation once given the opportunity to organize. In general, right atrial pacemaker activity is thought to originate from along the sulcus terminalis, whereas premature atrial beats from the left atrium are thought to originate from the pulmonary veins. The right atrium is largely smooth-walled and derived from the embryologic sinus venosus. In contrast, the left atrium is formed from the anlage of the pulmonary veins. There is a fold between the right pulmonary veins and the superior vena cava known as the "Waterston groove." The orifice of the inferior vena cava (IVC) and coronary sinus have fibrous continuity with only variable amounts of myocardial tissue bridging the right and the left atrium superficially [44]. Posteriorly, the right and the left atrium are separated by a groove that is filled with fibro-fatty tissue; only anteriorly, there is a distinct band of muscle that passes from the anteromedial aspect of the right atrium and superior vena cava to the left atrium, known as Bachman's bundle [45]. In the right atrium, the pectinate muscles run obliquely toward the right atrial appendage. In contrast, in the left atrium, myocardial fibers encircle the pulmonary veins and to some degree the mitral valve annuals. Several natural orifices exist in the right atrium including the superior vena cava, inferior vena cava, atrial septum, tricuspid valve, coronary sinus, and right atrial appendage orifice. This geometry plays a crucial role during activation sequences involved while atrial reentry occurs, like posing selective lines of block or activating conduction pathways during expression of atrial reentrant tachycardias.

Atrial reentrant tachycardias, classically referred to as atrial flutter, have now been accepted to involve abnormalities of impulse propagation that occur within either atria. Although primarily thought to be associated with right atrial disease, atrial reentrant arrhythmias can occur involving the right, the left, or both atria. Even though atrial flutter/atrial reentrant tachycardia is a common arrhythmia seen in the adult population, this arrhythmia is much more rare in the pediatric population and usually occurs in patients with underlying cardiac abnormalities, especially those who have undergone surgery for correction or palliation of congenital heart disease. In patients with underlying cardiac abnormalities, this arrhythmia, though rare, poses a challenge with regards to diagnosis, management, and therapy. In addition, this arrhythmia is often associated with significant morbidity and mortality in young patients with structural or functional heart disease.

Improved understanding of atrial reentrant tachycardias has allowed for differentiation of different types of atrial reentry in most recent years. Both clinical and experimental studies and observations over the last 10–15 years have been able to delineate the electrophysiologic circuit(s) that support macroreentry in atrial reentrant tachycardias. It has been shown that atrial reentry most commonly occurs in the right atrium. It is a self-sustaining circuit, and usually occurs in patients with either structural or functional heart disease. Continued study of atrial reentry defined the role of the crista terminalis as an anisotropic barrier to conduction during the common forms of atrial flutter. It has also been shown that the tricuspid valve annulus serves as an anterior anatomic barrier, supporting this "classic" reentrant loop. Finally, abnormal automaticity of the crista terminalis, the remnants of the cardinal veins, the sinus venosus and pulmonary veins have been shown to serve as triggers to express premature electrical activity that subsequently serves as the initiating factor for the expression of atrial reentry. Further research has demonstrated that intrinsic anisotropic properties of the right atrial wall related to the trabeculations of the right atrium and the number and distribution of gap junctions or connexin proteins support expression of atrial reentry. There is no doubt that the expression of atrial reentry is multifactorial, but the tachycardia seems to be more present in the right atrium, especially in patients who have either functional or congenital abnormalities of the right atrium.

The debate in regards to the underlying mechanism of atrial flutter continued for several decades until a variety of experimental animal models of atrial reentrant tachycardia were developed and demonstrated that, indeed, atrial flutter and/or atrial reentrant tachycardia is an abnormality of impulse propagation supporting reentry inside the atria (mostly the right atrium). In addition to delineating the underlying mechanism for atrial reentry tachycardia, these models supported a better understanding of the exact reentrant loop and conduction behavior during atrial tachycardia. Evaluation of a variety of anatomic structures in association with the expression of the atrial reentrant tachycardia became the next subject of intensive study. Most recently, with the advent of catheter-based mapping and ablation techniques, atrial reentrant tachycardias have been further characterized and studied in regards to distribution, expression, reentrant loop and insight into the roles of specific anatomic structures and/or surgical incisions.

In 1947, Rosenblueth and Garcia-Ramos developed a model of intercaval crush injury to study atrial flutter [46]. This model served to support the notion that nonconductive barriers were necessary for the induction and sustenance of intra-atrial reentrant tachycardias. The observation that the extension of the injury to the tricuspid valve annulus terminated the arrhythmia was essential to understanding that this particular arrhythmia was reentrant in nature and required an isthmus. A second surgical model developed by Frame et al. [39] used a posterior intercaval incision that was y-shaped and demonstrated that the reentry was around the tricuspid ring sustaining flutter. In this model, it was demonstrated that the tricuspid valve annulus forced activation in a circular manner around the tricuspid valve annulus. A model of acetylcholine-induced tachycardia developed by Allessie et al. described the refractoriness of atrial tissue and its role in the support of atrial reentry in the right atrium [37]. It was thought that functional refractoriness played a critical role in determining propagation of reentrant wavefronts in the right atrium. Secondly, the sterile pericarditis model of atrial flutter assessed and proved the relative importance of anatomic boundaries, functional refractoriness, and the role of anatomic barriers in the expression of atrial reentry [22, 28, 30–32]. It appeared that in several of these models, nonconductive barriers were crucial for the expression of reentry and that some of these barriers were functional in nature. Several other models then undiscovered the importance of endocardial structures, both anatomically and functionally.

Finally, in a canine model, Boineau [35] demonstrated that the crista terminalis was crucial in regards to expression of the common type of atrial flutter in adults. This model demonstrated the interaction between anisotropic conduction and the complex geometry of the right atrium with regards to common atrial slutter expression. In addition, this model was extended by several investigators who further elucidated the role of anisotropy and conduction velocity change along the crista terminalis. It was, therefore, thought that the cellular basis for observed directional preferences for longitudinal conduction in the crista terminalis may very well be associated with the role of gap junctions and cell-to-cell interactions favoring conduction in one direction and, therefore, suggesting that anisotropy plays a critical role in the expression of atrial reentry [47–54].

8.1.4 Intra-Atrial Reentry in the Postoperative Patient with Congenital Heart Disease

Intra-atrial tachycardia has carried many names in the past, including the traditional name of atrial flutter [49, 50]. Reentrant in nature, this tachycardia uses a variety of reentrant loops, in contrast to common atrial flutter, which uses the subeustachian isthmus as a critical component of its reentrant loop. Common atrial flutter usually depicts a tachycardia cycle length of around 200 ms and inscribes P-waves that are negative in II, III, and aVF. In contrast, intra-atrial tachycardia, which typically occurs in the post-operative patient, expresses a broad range of tachycardia cycle lengths and P-wave morphologies [55]. This tachycardia has been denoted as such because the reentrant tachycardia may use reentrant circuits that are not similar to that found in common atrial flutter. Even though the tricuspid valve subeustachian isthmus can be involved in the expression of postoperative intra-atrial reentrant tachycardia in the patient with congenital heart disease, there appear to be other reentrant pathways or loops, sometimes involving the atriotomy, or other anatomic boundaries. About one third to one fourth of patients with congenital heart disease, especially those who have had either surgery or palliation for congenital heart disease, will develop or have a propensity to develop sustained atrial tachycardia that can be demonstrated using programmed stimulation [56–58]. Only about 8% of patients who develop atrial reentrant tachycardias have anatomically and functionally normal hearts, with over 80% having associated repaired or unrepaired congenital heart disease [56] (❷ Table 8.1).

In regards to intra-atrial reentry tachycardia in the postoperative patient, two key surgical models have served to improve our understanding of the atrial reentrant tachycardia in the postoperative patient with pediatric heart disease.

❑ Table 8.1

Atrial tachycardia incidence in pediatric patients

Repaired congenital heart disease	60
Palliated congenital heart disease	13
Unoperated congenital heart disease	8
Normal heart	8
Cardiomyopathy	6
Rheumatic heart disease	4
Others	2

From Garson et al. (1985)

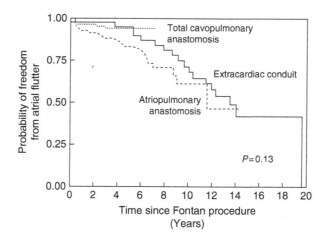

○ Fig. 8.5

The Kaplan–Meier curve depicts probability of experiencing no atrial tachycardias after Fontan operation with respect to time and type of Fontan operation performed

The first of these models was one developed by Cronin et al. [59, 60], which involved a sham Mustard operation. Rodefeld et al. [61–65] also developed a sham model of a lateral tunnel variety of the Fontan procedure (○ Fig. 8.5). In both of these models, it was felt that a common pathway for most of the observed tachycardias was in the free wall of the right atrium and that the tachycardia resolved when connecting the atriotomy to either the tricuspid valve annulus or the superior vena cava. These studies also found that the inclusion of the crista terminalis in the suture line aggravated the propensity of atrial tachycardia expression.

8.2   Epidemiology

In general, intra-atrial reentrant tachycardia in patients with congenital heart disease occurs in patients who have had significant manipulation or alterations of the right atrium, most often associated with surgery for heart disease [56]. Most of these surgeries include surgery for either atrial septal defect or ventricular septal defect repair, Mustard or Senning operations for the transposition of the great arteries (TGA), and those surgeries involving palliative procedures for single-ventricle physiology. In addition, there is a significant incidence of atrial tachycardia in association with lesions such as Tetralogy of Fallot and/or Ebstein's Anomaly. Of particular challenge is atrial tachycardia in the postoperative patient after a Fontan operation. Because of single-ventricle physiology and an often underlying myopathy, atrial tachycardia in these patients is hemodynamically poorly tolerated. Gelatt showed that 14–29% of patients after Fontan operation had atrial tachycardia at a mean follow-up of 4 years [57, 58]. One of the primary predictors of atrial tachycardia expression was the presence of atrial tachycardia in the immediate postoperative period. Another study showed that 16% of patients had atrial tachycardia at 5-year follow-up and appeared to correlate the expression of atrial tachycardia to the presence of extensive atrial baffling, and co-related the type of repair with arrhythmia expression [66]. Finally, a study from the Mayo Clinic demonstrated a prevalence of 17% at a 5-year follow-up with associated risk factors including perioperative arrhythmia, age at operation, and atrioventricular valve dysfunction [67]. It appears that about 40% of Fontan survivors have atrial tachycardia at a 10-year follow-up (○ Fig. 8.5). Although the overall prevalence of atrial tachycardia is lower in those patients undergoing total cavopulmonary connection, these patients are not completely free of the atrial arrhythmias. The incidence of atrial arrhythmias seems higher in patients with complex heart disease, there is a documented incidence of 14% in patients undergoing atrial septal defect repair. In addition, atrial arrhythmias may be associated with sinus node dysfunction as a cofactor [68–70]. The Mustard procedure has been quoted to have an incidence of 43% of atrial tachycardia with 16% having recurrent atrial arrhythmias. Patients who have undergone the Mustard procedure have an increased risk of atrial tachycardia with an incidence of 27% at 20 years, and have an increased risk of sudden death of 6.5% at a mean follow-up period of 11.6 years [57, 58]. It appears that atrial tachycardia may be associated with concordant sinus node dysfunction, as shown by a study of patients with atrial flutter after Tetralogy of Fallot [71] or atrial septal defect repair [69], superimposed on a genetic propensity.

8.3 Clinical Symptoms

Symptoms associated with intra-atrial reentry tachycardia in patients with postoperative heart disease are quite varied, ranging from no symptoms, to palpitations, to hemodynamic collapse, to sudden cardiac death thought to be associated with concomitant rapid conduction and ventricular dysfunction. From clinical observations, it is obvious that the presence of atrial tachycardia adds significant morbidity and mortality to postoperative patients. Especially in patients with single-ventricle physiology, the added burden of atrial arrhythmias is significant. In these patients, early postoperative arrhythmias were poorly tolerated, particularly atrial fibrillation and junctional ectopic tachycardia. Peters et al. observed that more than half of all patients who died in the perioperative period had atrial tachycardias [72].

Late postoperative arrhythmias are associated with higher right atrial pressures measured both early and late after the operation and worse ventricular function. Late arrhythmias may be the first manifestation of anatomic obstruction, which should be investigated promptly. In these patients with atrial arrhythmias, atrial thrombi can also be frequently noted, requiring aggressive anticoagulation.

8.4 Treatment of Atrial Tachycardia

The treatment of atrial tachycardias is challenging in patients with postoperative congenital heart disease [71, 73–80]. The acute treatment of atrial tachycardias depends on the clinical symptoms and associated cardiac defect(s). Once suspected, the patient should undergo full evaluation including documentation and definition of the arrhythmia with a 12-lead electrocardiogram and interrogation of intracardiac structures for thrombus formation and cardiac function [81]. Depending on the clinical arrhythmia, patients will often have associated cardiomyopathy. Patients with underlying complex congenital heart disease have an increased risk of intracardiac thrombus formation, especially during expression of the atrial tachycardia. Careful evaluation of intracardiac stasis or thrombus is essential prior to proceeding with plans for either chemical or electrical cardioversion to normal sinus rhythm. Acute conversion of an atrial tachycardia can be achieved in most cases where the mechanism of the tachycardia is supported by reentry. In these cases, either chemical cardioversion with Ibutilide (0.01 mg/kg/dose repeated 2 times after 5–10 min) can be tried. In these patients, it is of prime importance that the patient's electrolytes are evaluated for hypomagnesemia or hypokalemia. A defibrillator should be available with experienced staff, since Ibutilide can cause Torsades de Pointe in association with QTc prolongation, which can be exacerbated in the presence of hypokalemia or hypomagnesemia and/or concomitant myopathy.

Chronic treatment of atrial tachycardias can be achieved with Class IA, IIC, or III antiarrhythmic agents, antitachycardia pacing devices, or with a more promising and more permanent approach of electrophysiologic study with ablation. Medical management of these arrhythmias is additionally hampered, because most antiarrhythmic medications affect myocardial function, which is often depressed in patients after cardiac surgery. It appears that Sotalol may have a beneficial effect on both acute and chronic tachycardia control [82, 83]. Antitachycardia pacing has also proven to be promising, though not always successful. Often patients exhibit multiple tachycardias or are unresponsive to pacing maneuvers perhaps due to the relative small excitable gap of the reentrant loop [78, 84–86]. Antitachycardia pacing has been reported to be associated with lethal pro-arrhythmias in selected patients, so that patient selection is critical. If there is significant myopathy and a normal atrioventricular node, rapid conduction with cardiovascular compromise is more likely [85, 87–89].

Ablation procedures offer the potential for cure for patients with postoperative atrial tachycardias. Initial evaluation and outcome of electrophysiologic study with ablation was less than optimal because traditional mapping techniques were hampered by poor definition of the underlying anatomic defect(s), associated postoperative distortions and scars that are not visualized with current fluoroscopic techniques, and poor understanding of the tachycardia mechanism. In addition, traditional techniques are limited in their in-ability to outline and display impulse propagation. These limitations hindered the clinician's understanding of the complexity of the tachycardia mechanism and the identification of critical areas

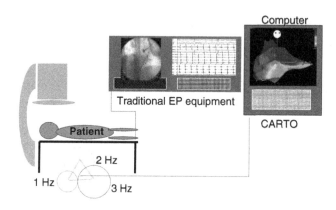

◘ Fig. 8.6

An artistic representation of the technical setup in the cardiac catheterization laboratory involving traditional electrophysiologic mapping and ablation equipment, complimented by a computer-based three-dimensional mapping system allowing study and ablation of complex arrhythmias

for successful ablative therapy [76, 80, 90–97]. Newer mapping techniques (❯ Fig. 8.6) supported by better understanding of the tachycardia mechanism and improved electrophysiologic techniques, including entrainment mapping promise improved outcomes. Therefore, newer approaches offer hope for cure of these reentrant tachycardias [98, 99].

8.4.1   Mechanisms of Postoperative Atrial Reentrant Tachycardias

In a small cohort of 21 consecutive patients with congenital heart disease, who were admitted to the University of California between 6/97 and 12/98 and to Rainbow Babies and Children's Hospital at Case Western Reserve University between 6/99 and 12/2000, a total of 33 atrial tachycardias were studied in the electrophysiology laboratory using advanced mapping techniques. All patients had documented clinical atrial tachycardia in association with postoperative congenital heart disease. Patients underwent electrophysiologic study under sedation, and in addition to the traditional electrophysiologic approach, patients underwent mapping of the clinical tachycardia using the non-fluoroscopic electroanatomic mapping (EAM) system (using CARTO) [98, 99]. Atrial tachycardia was induced using atrial overdrive pacing, atrial extrastimulation techniques, and/or isoproterenol infusion, when needed. The electroanatomic map was carefully interrogated for (1) activation sequences; (2) areas of low voltage (<0.03 mV), to identify areas that could be associated with diseased tissue and/or scar, supporting a barrier(s) for intra-atrial reentry tachycardia; (3) double potentials, which may reflect areas of slow conduction or functional and/or structural lines of conduction block. Entrainment techniques were used to define the mechanism and to identify a critical tachycardia isthmus.

Traditional electrophysiologic catheters were used to perform fluoroscopic mapping followed by electroanatomic mapping. The superior vena cava to (systemic venous) atrial junction and the inferior vena cava (IVC) to (systemic venous) atrial junction were mapped and marked with a three-dimensional ring or a tag. When possible, the His position was also tagged. In five of six patients with D-transposition of the great arteries (TGA) status post atrial switch operation, the pulmonary venous atrium was mapped from the arterial side as well. When present, double potentials and areas of scar were tagged during mapping and data acquisition.

Entrainment mapping was used to characterize each tachycardia circuit. After consistent capture was ensured, the intracardiac electrograms and the surface 12-lead ECG (electrocardiogram) were carefully interrogated to evaluate activation sequences compared to the native tachycardia. If the post-pacing interval (PPI) equaled the tachycardia cycle length and was associated with changes in either intracardiac activation sequences or surface P-wave morphology, the paced location was considered to demonstrate fusion and, therefore, labeled as manifest entrainment. These areas were considered less optimal for ablation. Concealed entrainment was present when (a) the post-pacing interval, defined as the stimulus artifact to the onset of the next atrial electrogram recorded from the pacing bipoles, was ≤30 ms of the tachycardia cycle length, (b) the intracardiac activation sequences were identical during pacing as compared to those during spontaneous tachycardia, and (c) the surface P-wave morphology was identical to the paced P-wave morphology. Areas of manifest and concealed entrainment were marked on the constructed three-dimensional image created by the EAM. Only areas with concealed entrainment were targeted for the radiofrequency energy application. Patients were subdivided into two cohorts: those with simple atriotomies (such as those seen after ASD [atrial septal defect], VSD [ventricular septal defect], AVSD [atrioventricular septal defect], or TOF [tetralogy of fallot] repair) and those with more complex atriotomies, as found in patients after Mustard or Senning operation and/or surgery for single-ventricle physiology.

8.4.2 Intra-Atrial Tachycardias Associated with a *Simple Atriotomy*

In patients with simple atriotomies (N = 12), one underwent correction of an atrial septal defect(s) (ASD), five underwent correction of an ASD and ventricular septal defect(s) (VSD), and one underwent complete atrioventricular septal defect (AVSD) repair. Five of these had a single tachycardia that was mapped and ablated. The sixth patient (with an ASD and VSD) had two separate tachycardias, of which both were mapped and ablated. Of these seven tachycardias, four had tachycardias involving the cavotricuspid isthmus and all were successfully ablated in the subeustachian isthmus. The other three tachycardias were successfully ablated by creating lesions from either anterior double potentials to the IVC (N = 2), where the tachycardia was revolving around an anterior barrier, or from the posterolateral right atrial wall double potentials to the IVC, where the tachycardia was found to revolve around a posterolateral barrier (❷ Fig. 8.7).

There were three patients with Tetralogy of Fallot. Two of these three patients had a single tachycardia. These tachycardias were successfully ablated by creating lesions from anterior double potentials to the IVC in one and from the posterolateral right atrial wall to the IVC in another, which recurred 18 months later. Repeat mapping of the same tachycardia revealed a "Figure-of-8" (previously missed) and was successfully ablated between a suspected atriotomy (mapped double potentials) and the posterolateral wall, and the posterolateral wall and the IVC. The third patient had three different tachycardias, all of which were successfully ablated; ablative lesions were successful in the subeustachian isthmus for a subeustachian-dependent tachycardia, between anterior double potentials and the IVC for an incisional tachycardia and between the posterolateral wall and the IVC for a free wall atrial tachycardia.

The remaining three patients had simple atriotomies for Ebstein's anomaly of the tricuspid valve, Marfan's syndrome, and L-TGA with a VSD; all patients had a single atrial tachycardia. Two of these tachycardias were successfully ablated in the subeustachian isthmus. The patient with Ebstein's anomaly received multiple ablative lesions in the subeustachian isthmus, which did not result in tachycardia termination. Retrospective evaluation revealed a "Figure-of-8" tachycardia with a common isthmus between an anterior atriotomy and posterolateral double potentials. This complex mechanism was not recognized at the time of the study (❷ Fig. 8.8).

In those patients where the posterolateral right atrial free wall provided a pivot area for the tachycardia (5 of 16 tachycardias), the EAM revealed a reentrant circuit that was distinctly different from classic clockwise or counterclockwise flutter around the tricuspid valve. Impulse propagation occurred around the valve, but these activation sequences were driven by a circuit that was primarily located laterally and posteriorly and almost perpendicular to the frontal plane. In these patients, entrainment from the subeustachian isthmus exhibited manifest entrainment, confirming that the subeustachian isthmus was not critical to the reentrant loop. Successful ablation of these tachycardias was achieved by ablation of an area that bridged the posterolateral right atrial free wall (behind the crista terminalis) to the IVC in all five patients (❷ Fig. 8.7).

Three other tachycardias were noted to propagate around an anterior barrier. In one patient, the tachycardia was thought to be isthmus dependent, but unsuccessful ablation of the subeustachian isthmus was thought to be due to the inability to achieve a transmural lesion or due to poor understanding of the underlying mechanism. Only a traditional ablation catheter was used.

In summary, patients with a simple atriotomy demonstrated four different tachycardia mechanisms: subeustachian isthmus dependent (7/16 or 44%), reentry around posterolateral double potentials (4/16 or 25%), reentry around anterior double potentials (3/16 or 19%), and "Figure-of-8" tachycardia (2/16 or 12%) with a common isthmus located between mapped double potentials either laterally or anteriorly and another anatomic barrier such as the tricuspid valve.

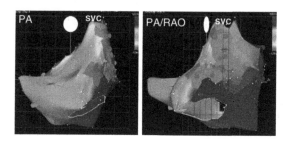

▣ Fig. 8.7

These activation maps of the right atrium in a 37-year-old male after atrial septal defect repair confirm non-isthmus-dependent atrial tachycardia. Shown are PA (posteroanterior) and RAO (right anterior oblique) projections displaying that the atrial tachycardia was mapped to revolve around a lateral scar within the right atrium in a counterclockwise fashion

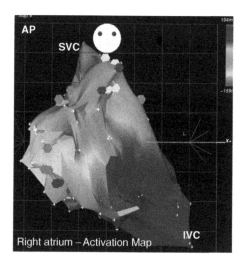

▣ Fig. 8.8

Figure-of-8 loop atrial tachycardia in a patient after simple atriotomy for tricuspid valve surgery for Ebstein's anomaly

8.4.3   Intra-Atrial Tachycardias Associated with *Complex Atriotomies*

8.4.3.1   Patients After Atrial Switch Operation

Thirteen of the 17 tachycardias were mapped in six patients after an atrial switch operation. Two of these patients had a single tachycardia that was successfully ablated in the subeustachian isthmus on the pulmonary venous side. This tachycardia traversed the isthmus arising posteroseptally on the pulmonary venous side, inscribing a clockwise propagation pattern moving anteriorly and superiorly, and then descending to the posteroseptal area. The systemic venous atrial side was passively activated by the reentrant wavefront as it traversed the upper and mid-septal portions (❷ Fig. 8.9). A third patient had two tachycardias. One of these tachycardias appeared to be focal in nature. The EAM of this tachycardia revealed passive activation of the systemic venous atrium from the posteroseptal area, where the post-pacing interval was identical to the tachycardia cycle length. Because of patient size (5 years old), the pulmonary venous atrium was not accessed. However, the patient had recurrent tachycardia with a different cycle length and surface ECG morphology

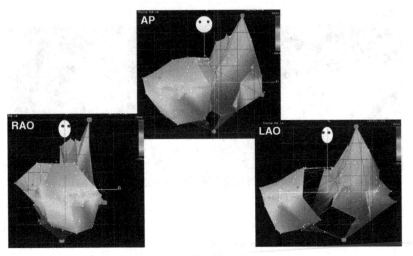

◻ Fig. 8.9
These activation maps of the systemic and pulmonary venous atrium of a 26-year-old female with transposition after atrial switch operation confirm that the atrial reentrant tachycardia is primarily confined to the pulmonary venous atrium (earliest activation is in red) with passive activation of the systemic venous atrium. Some areas of the atria could not be mapped due to technical difficulties

about 8 months later. This tachycardia was then successfully ablated with lesions in the posteroseptal area of the anatomic right atrium on the pulmonary venous side; there has been no recurrence in over 4 years.

The remaining three patients had multiple tachycardias (one patient each had two, three, and four different atrial tachycardias, respectively). The subeustachian isthmus served as the successful ablation site in only one of these tachycardias. Of the remaining tachycardias ($N = 8$), six were successfully ablated either in the systemic venous atrium ($N = 4$), or the posterolateral wall of the pulmonary venous atrium ($N = 1$), or between the posterolateral systemic venous atrial free wall and the IVC ($N = 1$). Two tachycardias were not ablated due to procedure length and/or poor understanding of the mechanism of tachycardia.

8.4.3.2 Patients After Fontan Operation

Four of 17 tachycardias were mapped in three patients' status after a Fontan operation. All of these patients had an atriopulmonary connection ("classic" Fontan connection for tricuspid atresia, $N = 2$, and for double inlet left ventricle, $N = 1$). In two patients, a single intra-atrial reentry tachycardia was addressed. Successful ablation occurred in the area between a suspected atriotomy and an atrial septal defect patch in one patient and in the area between posterolateral double potentials and the IVC in the other. The third patient had at least two tachycardias; neither could be successfully ablated.

8.4.4 "Figure-of-8" Intra-Atrial Tachycardias

"Figure-of-8" tachycardias were noted to occur more often (25%) in patients with complex atriotomies. "Figure-of-8" tachycardia with a common isthmus in the systemic venous atrium (❷ Fig. 8.10) involved clockwise propagation around a scar and/or double potentials in the right lateral free wall and counterclockwise propagation around anterior atrial

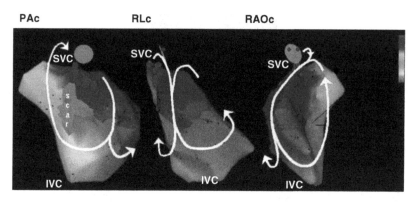

◩ Fig. 8.10

Figure-of-8 loop atrial tachycardia in a 13-year-old male patient after complex atriotomy for transposition of the great arteries and atrial switch operation (Mustard operation at 2 years of age)

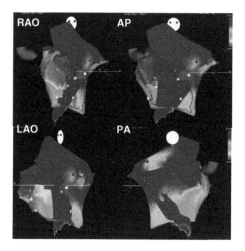

◩ Fig. 8.11

Figure-of-8 loop atrial tachycardia in an 18-year-old male patient after complex atriotomy for transposition of the great arteries and atrial switch operation (Mustard operation at 2 years of age). Shown is the electroanatomic map of both atria

incisions (lower pant leg). A long ablative lesion bridging the superior and inferior pant leg resulted in successful ablation with no recurrence in more than 4 years.

"Figure-of-8" tachycardia in the pulmonary venous side involved counterclockwise propagation around the mitral valve annulus and clockwise around double potentials recorded on the lateral right free wall of the pulmonary venous atrium. Successful ablation was achieved from the posterolateral right free wall of the pulmonary venous atrium to the mitral valve (❷ Fig. 8.11).

Another two "Figure-of-8" tachycardias were noted in patients after the Fontan operation. One of these demonstrated a common isthmus between an anterior atriotomy and an ASD patch and was successfully ablated. The second "Figure-of-8" tachycardia could not be ablated presumably because a transmural lesion could not be achieved. Ablative lesions from the right atrial posterolateral wall to both the IVC and the tricuspid valve dimple did not result in successful ablation of the tachycardia. This patient has had no clinical recurrence, however, after 8 months of follow-up.

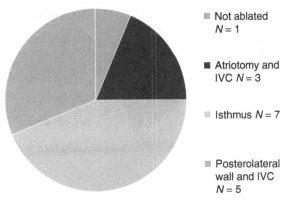

Not ablated
$N = 1$

Atriotomy and
IVC $N = 3$

Isthmus $N = 7$

Posterolateral
wall and IVC
$N = 5$

◙ Fig. 8.12
Summary of locations of successful ablation of atrial reentrant tachycardias in patients after a simple atriotomy. Atriotomies included those for ASD repair, VSD repair, TOF repair, AVSD repair, Ebstein's anomaly, and ventricular inversion. Note that the subeustachian isthmus was critical in supporting reentry in 44% of atrial tachycardias

8.4.5   Role of the Subeustachian Area (Classic Flutter Isthmus)

In patients with postoperative atrial tachycardia, only 33% of reentry tachycardias involved the subeustachian isthmus as a critical part of the reentrant loop (❯ Fig. 8.12). These findings are in contrast to those of Chan et al. [52]. This discrepancy in observation can be explained by several factors. Our patient population included patients with complex atrial surgery; the Chan study included patients with a simple atriotomy only. We used EAM in our study, allowing for more precise evaluation of the reentrant circuit. Our findings also differ somewhat from those of Collins et al. [100] and Love et al. [99], who noted that the subeustachian isthmus was critical to 57% of patients after atrial switch operation, whereas we noted that only 24% of these tachycardias involved the subeustachian isthmus. Regardless, our study confirms that intra-atrial reentry tachycardia in postoperative patients more often involves other crucial areas, such as the posterolateral right atrial wall [7, 9, 18]. We believe that the observed differences are due to the inclusion of a wider spectrum of congenital heart diseases and perhaps, more intensive evaluation of the tachycardia.

Another isthmus frequently mapped and successfully targeted for ablation was between posterolateral double potentials and the IVC. This isthmus is also recognized in adult patients with unusual types of atrial reentry tachycardia. Our study demonstrates that this reentrant atrial tachycardia is fairly common in patients after repair for congenital heart disease, involving an atriotomy that supports this unique reentrant substrate. Finally, a less common isthmus was between an anterior atriotomy and the IVC, and is in congruence with other studies. The implications of these findings for mapping and ablation suggest that subeustachian ablation may be more successful in patients after simple, rather than complex, atriotomy for congenital heart disease, and that other isthmuses could be crucially involved in postoperative reentry tachycardia and may even coexist.

The type and complexity of the reentry tachycardia varied with the type and complexity of the surgical repair. For simple atriotomies, multiple circuit tachycardias were less common than in patients with complex atriotomies (❯ Figs. 8.12 and ❯ 8.13).

8.5   Long-Term Follow-Up of Patients with Atrial Tachycardia

Even with the use of advanced imaging techniques, the long-term success rate for our patients is 71% at a mean follow-up of 29 ± 17 months and at least 25% of patients (5/21) required repeat procedures. Failures may be due to inability to create transmural lesions (especially in patients after the Fontan operation), limited ability to reach critical areas (i.e., pulmonary venous atrium), or other limiting factors (i.e., procedure time and patient tolerance).

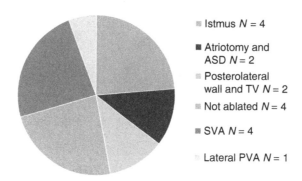

- Istmus *N* = 4
- Atriotomy and ASD *N* = 2
- Posterolateral wall and TV *N* = 2
- Not ablated *N* = 4
- SVA *N* = 4
- Lateral PVA *N* = 1

◘ Fig. 8.13

Summary of locations of successful ablation of atrial reentrant tachycardias in patients after a complex atriotomy. Atriotomies included those for Senning operation, Mustard operation, Bidirectional Glenn operation, and Fontan surgery. Note that the subeustachian isthmus was critical in supporting reentry in 24% of atrial tachycardias

In summary, there are variety of different mechanisms of tachycardias in postoperative patients, some inscribing complicated reentrant loops such as "Figure-of-8" atrial reentry tachycardia. Because patients with congenital heart disease encompass a heterogeneous population and because surgical techniques are variable and the anatomy of the expressed disease so complicated, we found the use of multiple complementary approaches to be of great benefit to successful treatment of these postoperative tachycardias.

References

1. Garson, A. Jr. and P.C. Gillette, Junctional ectopic tachycardia in children: electrocardiography, electrophysiology and pharmacologic response. *Am. J. Cardiol.*, 1979;**44**: 298–302.

2. Gillette, P.C. and A. Garson Jr., Electrophysiologic and pharmacologic characteristics of automatic ectopic atrial tachycardia. *Circulation*, 1977;**56**: 571–575.

3. Garson, A. Jr., P.C. Gillette, and D.G. McNamara, Supraventricular tachycardia in children: clinical features, response to treatment, and long-term follow-up in 217 patients. *J. Pediatr.*, 1981;**98**: 875–882.

4. Fishberger, S.B., S.D. Colan, J.P. Saul, J.E. Mayer Jr., and E.P. Walsh, Myocardial mechanics before and after ablation of chronic tachycardia. *Pacing Clin. Electrophysiol.*, 1996;**19**: 42–49.

5. Blom, N.A., J. Ottenkamp, M.C. Deruiter, A.C. Wenink, and A.C. Gittenberger-de Groot, Development of the cardiac conduction system in atrioventricular septal defect in human trisomy 21. *Pediatr. Res.*, 2005;**58**: 516–520.

6. Blom, N.A., A.C. Gittenberger-de Groot, M.C. DeRuiter, R.E. Poelmann, M.M. Mentink, and J. Ottenkamp, Development of the cardiac conduction tissue in human embryos using HNK-1 antigen expression: possible relevance for understanding of abnormal atrial automaticity. *Circulation*, 1999;**99**: 800–806.

7. Walsh, E., Ablation of ectopic atrial tachycardia in children, in *Radiofrequency Catheter Ablation of Cardiac Arrhythmias*, 2nd edn., S.K.S. Huang and D.J. Wilber, Editor. Armonk, NY: Futura, 2000, pp. 115–138.

8. Liberthson, R.R. and S.D. Colan, Multifocal or chaotic atrial rhythm: report of nine infants, delineation of clinical course and management, and review of the literature. *Pediatr. Cardiol.*, 1982;**2**: 179–184.

9. Garavelli, L., K. Leask, C. Zanacca, S. Pedori, G. Albertini, E. Della Giustina, G.F. Croci, C. Magnani, G. Banchini, J. Clayton-Smith, M. Bocian, H. Firth, J.A. Gold, and J. Hurst, MRI and neurological findings in macrocephaly-cutis marmorata telangiectatica congenita syndrome: report of ten cases and review of the literature. *Genet. Couns.*, 2005;**16**: 117–128.

10. Shine, K.I., J.A. Kastor, and P.M. Yurchak, Multifocal atrial tachycardia. Clinical and electrocardiographic features in 32 patients. *N. Engl. J. Med.*, 1968;**279**: 344–349.

11. Salim, M.A., C.L. Case, and P.C. Gillette, Chaotic atrial tachycardia in children. *Am. Heart J.*, 1995;**129**: 831–833.

12. Dodo, H., R.M. Gow, R.M. Hamilton, and R.M. Freedom, Chaotic atrial rhythm in children. *Am. Heart J.*, 1995;**129**: 990–995.

13. Zeevi, B., M. Berant, S. Sclarovsky, and L.C. Blieden, Treatment of multifocal atrial tachycardia with amiodarone in a child with congenital heart disease. *Am. J. Cardiol.*, 1986;**57**: 344–345.

14. MacWilliams, J., Fibrillar contraction of the heart. *J. Physiol.*, 1887;**8**: 296.

15. Ritchie, W., Complete heart block with dissociation of the action of the auricles and ventricles. *Proc. R. Soc. Edinburgh.*, 1905;**25**: 1085.

16. Jolly, W.A. and W.T. Ritchie, Auricular flutter and fibrillation. 1911. *Ann. Noninvasive Electrocardiol.*, 2003;**8**: 92–96.

17. Einthoven, W., Le telecardiogramme. *Arch. Int. Physiol.*, 1906;**4**: 132.

18. Lewis, T., Observations upon a curious and not uncommon form of extreme acceleration of the auricle: auricular flutter. *Heart*, 1913;**4**: 171.

19. Lewis, T.D.D. and T.T. Iliescu. A demonstration of circus movement in clinical flutter of the auricles. *Heart*, 1921;**8**: 341.

20. Cabrera, E.S.-P.D., Discusion del movimiento circular y prueba directa de su existencia en el flutter auricular clinico. *Arch. Inst. Cardiol. Mex.*, 1947;**17**: 850.

21. Puech, P., H. Latour, and R. Grolleau, Flutter and his limits. *Arch. Mal. Coeur Vaiss.*, 1970;**63**: 116–144.

22. Waldo, A.L., Atrial flutter. New directions in management and mechanism. *Circulation*, 1990;**81**: 1142–1143.

23. Olshansky, B., K. Okumura, P.G. Hess, and A.L. Waldo, Demonstration of an area of slow conduction in human atrial flutter. *J. Am. Coll. Cardiol.*, 1990;**16**: 1639–1648.

24. Waldo, A.L., Clinical evaluation in therapy of patients with atrial fibrillation or flutter. *Cardiol. Clin.*, 1990;**8**: 479–490.

25. Henthorn, R.W., Y. Rudy, and A.L. Waldo, Evolving concepts regarding the role of tissue structure in arrhythmogenesis in the infarcted human heart. *J. Am. Coll. Cardiol.*, 1990;**15**: 1608–1609.

26. Henthorn, R.W., K. Okumura, B. Olshansky, V.J. Plumb, P.G. Hess, and A.L. Waldo, A fourth criterion for transient entrainment: the electrogram equivalent of progressive fusion. *Circulation*, 1988;**77**: 1003–1112.

27. Waldo, A.L., W.A. MacLean, T.B. Cooper, N.T. Kouchoukos, and R.B. Karp, Use of temporarily placed epicardial atrial wire electrodes for the diagnosis and treatment of cardiac arrhythmias following open-heart surgery. *J. Thorac. Cardiovasc. Surg.*, 1978;**76**: 500–505.

28. Waldo, A.L., W.A. MacLean, R.B. Karp, N.T. Kouchoukos, and T.N. James, Entrainment and interruption of atrial flutter with atrial pacing: studies in man following open heart surgery. *Circulation*, 1977;**56**: 737–745.

29. Olshansky, B., K. Okumura, R.W. Henthorn, and A.L. Waldo, Characterization of double potentials in human atrial flutter: studies during transient entrainment. *J. Am. Coll. Cardiol.*, 1990;**15**: 833–841.

30. Waldo, A.L., R.W. Henthorn, A.E. Epstein, and V.J. Plumb, Significance of transient entrainment in pacing treatment of tachyarrhythmias. *Arch. Mal. Coeur Vaiss.*, 1985;**78** Spec No: 23–28.

31. Waldo, A.L., R.W. Henthorn, A.E. Epstein, and V.J. Plumb, Diagnosis and treatment of arrhythmias during and following open heart surgery. *Med. Clin. North Am.*, 1984;**68**: 1153–1169.

32. Waldo, A.L., Mechanisms of atrial fibrillation, atrial flutter, and ectopic atrial tachycardia—a brief review. *Circulation*, 1987;**75**: III37–III40.

33. Wyndham, C.R., D. Wu, P. Denes, D. Sugarman, S. Levitsky, and K.M. Rosen, Self-initiated conversion of paroxysmal atrial flutter utilizing a radio-frequency pacemaker. *Am. J. Cardiol.*, 1978;**41**: 1119–1122.

34. Pastelin, G., R. Mendez, and G.K. Moe, Participation of atrial specialized conduction pathways in atrial flutter. *Circ. Res.*, 1978;**42**: 386–393.

35. Boineau, J.P., R.B. Schuessler, C.R. Mooney, C.B. Miller, A.C. Wylds, R.D. Hudson, J.M. Borremans, and C.W. Brockus, Natural and evoked atrial flutter due to circus movement in dogs. Role of abnormal atrial pathways, slow conduction, nonuniform refractory period distribution and premature beats. *Am. J. Cardiol.*, 1980;**45**: 1167–1181.

36. Inoue, H., H. Matsuo, K. Takayanagi, and S. Murao, Clinical and experimental studies of the effects of atrial extrastimulation and rapid pacing on atrial flutter cycle. Evidence of macro-reentry with an excitable gap. *Am. J. Cardiol.*, 1981;**48**: 623–631.

37. Allessie, M.A., W.J. Lammers, I.M. Bonke, and J. Hollen, Intra-atrial reentry as a mechanism for atrial flutter induced by acetylcholine and rapid pacing in the dog. *Circulation*, 1984;**70**: 123–135.

38. Spach, M.S., W.T. Miller III, P.C. Dolber, J.M. Kootsey, J.R. Sommer, C.E. Mosher Jr., The functional role of structural complexities in the propagation of depolarization in the atrium of the dog. Cardiac conduction disturbances due to discontinuities of effective axial resistivity. *Circ. Res.*, 1982;**50**: 175–191.

39. Frame, L.H., R.L. Page, and B.F. Hoffman, Atrial reentry around an anatomic barrier with a partially refractory excitable gap. A canine model of atrial flutter. *Circ. Res.*, 1986;**58**: 495–511.

40. Fontaine, G., C. Moro-Serrano, L. Menezes-Falcao, M. Todorova, R. Frank, J.L. Tonet, and Y. Grosgogeat, Anti-tachycardia radiofrequency pacemakers. Experience with 44 cases. *Arch. Mal. Coeur Vaiss.*, 1986;**79**: 1696–1702.

41. Cosio, F.G., F. Arribas, J. Palacios, J. Tascon, and M. Lopez-Gil, Fragmented electrograms and continuous electrical activity in atrial flutter. *Am. J. Cardiol.*, 1986;**57**: 1309–1314.

42. Saoudi, N., G. Atallah, G. Kirkorian, and P. Touboul, Catheter ablation of the atrial myocardium in human type I atrial flutter. *Circulation*, 1990;**81**: 762–771.

43. Feld, G.K., R.P. Fleck, P.S. Chen, K. Boyce, T.D. Bahnson, J.B. Stein, C.M. Calisi, and M. Ibarra, Radiofrequency catheter ablation for the treatment of human type 1 atrial flutter. Identification of a critical zone in the reentrant circuit by endocardial mapping techniques. *Circulation*, 1992;**86**: 1233–1240.

44. Anderson, R.H. and A.E. Becker, *Cardiac Anatomy: An Integrated Text and Colour Atlas*: London: Gower Medical Publishing; 1980.

45. Bachmann, G., The interauricular time interval. *Am. J. Physiol.*, 1916;**41**: 309.

46. Rosenblueth, A. and J. Garcia-Ramos, Studies on flutter and fibrillation. II. The influence of artificial obstacles on experimental auricular flutter. *Am. Heart J.*, 1947;**33**: 677–684.

47. Waldo, A.L., The interrelationship between atrial fibrillation and atrial flutter. *Prog. Cardiovasc. Dis.*, 2005;**48**: 41–56.

48. Waldo, A.L., Mechanisms of atrial flutter and atrial fibrillation: distinct entities or two sides of a coin? *Cardiovasc. Res.*, 2002;**54**: 217–229.

49. Saoudi, N., F. Cosio, A. Waldo, S.A. Chen, Y. Iesaka, M. Lesh, S. Saksena, J. Salerno, and W. Schoels, Classification of atrial flutter and regular atrial tachycardia according to electrophysiologic mechanism and anatomic bases: a statement from a joint expert group from the Working Group of Arrhythmias of the European Society of Cardiology and the North American Society of Pacing and Electrophysiology. *J. Cardiovasc. Electrophysiol.*, 2001;**12**: 852–866.

50. Saoudi, N., F. Cosio, A. Waldo, S.A. Chen, Y. Iesaka, M. Lesh, S. Saksena, J. Salerno, and W. Schoels, A classification of atrial flutter and regular atrial tachycardia according to electrophysiological mechanisms and anatomical bases; a Statement from a Joint Expert Group from The Working Group of Arrhythmias of the European Society of Cardiology and the North American Society of Pacing and Electrophysiology. *Eur. Heart J.*, 2001;**22**: 1162–1182.

51. Tomita, Y., K. Matsuo, J. Sahadevan, C.M. Khrestian, and A.L. Waldo, Role of functional block extension in lesion-related atrial flutter. *Circulation*, 2001;**103**: 1025–1130.

52. Chan, D.P., G.F. Van Hare, J.A. Mackall, M.D. Carlson, and A.L. Waldo, Importance of atrial flutter isthmus in postoperative intra-atrial reentrant tachycardia. *Circulation*, 2000;**102**: 1283–1289.

53. Waldo, A.L., Treatment of atrial flutter. *Heart*, 2000;**84**: 227–232.

54. Uno, K., K. Kumagai, C.M. Khrestian, and A.L. Waldo, New insights regarding the atrial flutter reentrant circuit: studies in the canine sterile pericarditis model. *Circulation*, 1999;**100**: 1354–1360.

55. Muller, G.I., B.J. Deal, J.F. Strasburger, and D.W. Benson Jr., Electrocardiographic features of atrial tachycardias after operation for congenital heart disease. *Am. J. Cardiol.*, 1993;**71**: 122–124.

56. Garson, A. Jr., M. Bink-Boelkens, P.S. Hesslein, A.J. Hordof, J.F. Keane, W.H. Neches, and C.J. Porter, Atrial flutter in the young: a collaborative study of 380 cases. *J. Am. Coll. Cardiol.*, 1985;**6**: 871–878.

57. Gelatt, M., R.M. Hamilton, B.W. McCrindle, R.M. Gow, W.G. Williams, G.A. Trusler, and R.M. Freedom, Risk factors for atrial tachyarrhythmias after the Fontan operation. *J. Am. Coll. Cardiol.*, 1994;**24**: 1735–1741.

58. Gelatt, M., R.M. Hamilton, B.W. McCrindle, M. Connelly, A. Davis, L. Harris, R.M. Gow, W.G. Williams, G.A. Trusler, and R.M. Freedom, Arrhythmia and mortality after the Mustard procedure: a 30-year single-center experience. *J. Am. Coll. Cardiol.*, 1997;**29**: 194–201.

59. Cronin, C.S., T. Nitta, M. Mitsuno, F. Isobe, R.B. Schuessler, J.P. Boineau, and J.L. Cox, Characterization and surgical ablation of acute atrial flutter following the Mustard procedure. A canine model. *Circulation*, 1993;**88**: II461–II471.

60. Nitta, T., R.B. Schuessler, M. Mitsuno, C.K. Rokkas, F. Isobe, C.S. Cronin, J.L. Cox, and J.P. Boineau, Return cycle mapping after entrainment of ventricular tachycardia. *Circulation*, 1998;**97**: 1164–1175.

61. Bromberg, B.I., R.B. Schuessler, S.K. Gandhi, M.D. Rodefeld, J.P. Boineau, and C.B. Huddleston, A canine model of atrial flutter following the intra-atrial lateral tunnel Fontan operation. *J. Electrocardiol.*, 1998;**30**(Suppl. 1): 85–93.

62. Gandhi, S.K., B.I. Bromberg, M.D. Rodefeld, R.B. Schuessler, J.P. Boineau, J.L. Cox, and C.B. Huddleston, Spontaneous atrial flutter in a chronic canine model of the modified Fontan operation. *J. Am. Coll. Cardiol.*, 1997;**30**: 1095–1103.

63. Rodefeld, M.D., S.K. Gandhi, C.B. Huddleston, B.J. Turken, R.B. Schuessler, J.P. Boineau, J.L. Cox, and B.I. Bromberg, Anatomically based ablation of atrial flutter in an acute canine model of the modified Fontan operation. *J. Thorac. Cardiovasc. Surg.*, 1996;**112**: 898–907.

64. Gandhi, S.K., B.I. Bromberg, M.D. Rodefeld, R.B. Schuessler, J.P. Boineau, J.L. Cox, and C.B. Huddleston, Lateral tunnel suture line variation reduces atrial flutter after the modified Fontan operation. *Ann. Thorac. Surg.*, 1996;**61**: 1299–1309.

65. Rodefeld, M.D., B.I. Bromberg, R.B. Schuessler, J.P. Boineau, J.L. Cox, and C.B. Huddleston, Atrial flutter after lateral tunnel construction in the modified Fontan operation: a canine model. *J. Thorac. Cardiovasc. Surg.*, 1996;**111**: 514–526.

66. Fishberger, S.B., G. Wernovsky, T.L. Gentles, K. Gauvreau, J. Burnett, J.E. Mayer Jr., and E.P. Walsh, Factors that influence the development of atrial flutter after the Fontan operation. *J. Thorac. Cardiovasc. Surg.*, 1997;**113**: 80–86.

67. Durongpisitkul, K., C.J. Porter, F. Cetta, K.P. Offord, J.M. Slezak, F.J. Puga, H.V. Schaff, G.K. Danielson, and D.J. Driscoll, Predictors of early- and late-onset supraventricular tachyarrhythmias after Fontan operation. *Circulation*, 1998;**98**: 1099–1107.

68. Bink-Boelkens, M.T., A. Bergstra, A.H. Cromme-Dijkhuis, A. Eygelaar, M.J. Landsman, and E.L. Mooyaart, The asymptomatic child a long time after the Mustard operation for transposition of the great arteries. *Ann. Thorac. Surg.*, 1989;**47**: 45–50.

69. Bink-Boelkens, M.T., K.J. Meuzelaar, and A. Eygelaar, Arrhythmias after repair of secundum atrial septal defect: the influence of surgical modification. *Am. Heart J.*, 1988;**115**: 629–633.

70. Bink-Boelkens, M.T., H. Velvis, J.J. van der Heide, A. Eygelaar, and R.A. Hardjowijono, Dysrhythmias after atrial surgery in children. *Am. Heart J.*, 1983;**106**: 125–130.

71. Roos-Hesselink, J., M.G. Perlroth, J. McGhie, and S. Spitaels, Atrial arrhythmias in adults after repair of tetralogy of Fallot. Correlations with clinical, exercise, and echocardiographic findings. *Circulation*, 1995;**91**: 2214–2219.

72. Peters, N.S. and J. Somerville, Arrhythmias after the Fontan procedure. *Br. Heart J.*, 1992;**68**: 199–204.

73. Douglas, D.E., C.L. Case, C.O. Shuler, and P.C. Gillette, Successful radiofrequency catheter ablation of atrial muscle reentry tachycardia in a young adult. *Clin. Cardiol.*, 1995;**18**: 51–53.

74. Balaji, S., C.L. Case, R.M. Sade, and P.C. Gillette, Arrhythmias and electrocardiographic changes after the hemi-Fontan procedure. *Am. J. Cardiol.*, 1994;**73**: 828–829.

75. Balaji, S., T.B. Johnson, R.M. Sade, C.L. Case, and P.C. Gillette, Management of atrial flutter after the Fontan procedure. *J. Am. Coll. Cardiol.*, 1994;**23**: 1209–1215.

76. Case, C.L., P.C. Gillette, D.E. Douglas, and R.A. Liebermann, Radiofrequency catheter ablation of atrial flutter in a patient with postoperative congenital heart disease. *Am. Heart J.*, 1993;**126**: 715–716.

77. Flinn, C.J., G.S. Wolff, M. Dick II, R.M. Campbell, G. Borkat, A. Casta, A. Hordof, T.J. Hougen, R.E. Kavey, J. Kugler, et al., Cardiac rhythm after the Mustard operation for complete transposition of the great arteries. *N. Engl. J. Med.*, 1984;**310**: 1635–1638.

78. Porter, C.B., J. Fukushige, D.L. Hayes, M.D. McGoon, M.J. Osborn, and F.J. Puga, Permanent antitachycardia pacing for chronic atrial tachyarrhythmias in postoperative pediatric patients. *Pacing Clin. Electrophysiol.*, 1991;**14**: 2056–2057.

79. Porter, C.J. and A. Garson, Incidence and management of dysrhythmias after Fontan procedure. *Herz*, 1993;**18**: 318–327.

80. Baker, B.M., B.D. Lindsay, B.I. Bromberg, D.W. Frazier, M.E. Cain, and J.M. Smith, Catheter ablation of clinical intraatrial reentrant tachycardias resulting from previous atrial surgery: localizing and transecting the critical isthmus. *J. Am. Coll. Cardiol.*, 1996;**28**: 411–417.

81. Feltes, T.F. and R.A. Friedman, Transesophageal echocardiographic detection of atrial thrombi in patients with nonfibrillation atrial tachyarrhythmias and congenital heart disease. *J. Am. Coll. Cardiol.*, 1994;**24**: 1365–1370.

82. Beaufort-Krol, G.C. and M.T. Bink-Boelkens, Sotalol for atrial tachycardias after surgery for congenital heart disease. *Pacing Clin. Electrophysiol.*, 1997;**20**: 2125–2129.

83. Beaufort-Krol, G.C. and M.T. Bink-Boelkens, Effectiveness of sotalol for atrial flutter in children after surgery for congenital heart disease. *Am. J. Cardiol.*, 1997;**79**: 92–94.

84. Fukushige, J., C.B. Porter, D.L. Hayes, M.D. McGoon, M.J. Osborn, and R.E. Vlietstra, Antitachycardia pacemaker treatment of postoperative arrhythmias in pediatric patients. *Pacing Clin. Electrophysiol.*, 1991;**14**: 546–556.

85. Rhodes, L.A., E.P. Walsh, W.J. Gamble, J.K. Triedman, and J.P. Saul, Benefits and potential risks of atrial antitachycardia pacing after repair of congenital heart disease. *Pacing Clin. Electrophysiol.*, 1995;**18**: 1005–1016.

86. Rhodes, L.A., E.P. Walsh, and J.P. Saul, Conversion of atrial flutter in pediatric patients by transesophageal atrial pacing: a safe, effective, minimally invasive procedure. *Am. Heart J.*, 1995;**130**: 323–327.

87. Gillette, P.C., D.G. Wampler, C. Shannon, and D. Ott, Use of cardiac pacing after the Mustard operation for transposition of the great arteries. *J. Am. Coll. Cardiol.*, 1986;**7**: 138–141.

88. Duster, M.C., M.T. Bink-Boelkens, D. Wampler, P.C. Gillette, D.G. McNamara, and D.A. Cooley, Long-term follow-up of dysrhythmias following the Mustard procedure. *Am. Heart J.*, 1985;**109**: 1323–1326.

89. Gillette, P.C., D.G. Wampler, C. Shannon, and D. Ott, Use of atrial pacing in a young population. *Pacing Clin. Electrophysiol.*, 1985;**8**: 94–100.

90. Lesh, M.D., J.M. Kalman, and M.R. Karch, Use of intracardiac echocardiography during electrophysiologic evaluation and therapy of atrial arrhythmias. *J. Cardiovasc. Electrophysiol.*, 1998;**9**: S40–S47.

91. Kalman, J.M., J.E. Olgin, M.R. Karch, M. Hamdan, R.J. Lee, and M.D. Lesh, "Cristal tachycardias": origin of right atrial tachycardias from the crista terminalis identified by intracardiac echocardiography. *J. Am. Coll. Cardiol.*, 1998;**31**: 451–459.

92. Olgin, J.E., J.M. Kalman, M. Chin, C. Stillson, M. Maguire, P. Ursel, and M.D. Lesh, Electrophysiological effects of long, linear atrial lesions placed under intracardiac ultrasound guidance. *Circulation*, 1997;**96**: 2715–2721.

93. Lesh, M.D., J.M. Kalman, L.A. Saxon, and P.C. Dorostkar, Electrophysiology of "incisional" reentrant atrial tachycardia

complicating surgery for congenital heart disease. *Pacing Clin. Electrophysiol.*, 1997;**20**: 2107–2111.

94. Kalman, J.M., J.E. Olgin, L.A. Saxon, R.J. Lee, M.M. Scheinman, and M.D. Lesh, Electrocardiographic and electrophysiologic characterization of atypical atrial flutter in man: use of activation and entrainment mapping and implications for catheter ablation. *J. Cardiovasc. Electrophysiol.*, 1997;**8**: 121–144.

95. Kalman, J.M., J.E. Olgin, L.A. Saxon, W.G. Fisher, R.J. Lee, and M.D. Lesh, Activation and entrainment mapping defines the tricuspid annulus as the anterior barrier in typical atrial flutter. *Circulation*, 1996;**94**: 398–406.

96. Kalman, J.M., G.F. VanHare, J.E. Olgin, L.A. Saxon, S.I. Stark, and M.D. Lesh, Ablation of 'incisional' reentrant atrial tachycardia complicating surgery for congenital heart disease. Use of entrainment to define a critical isthmus of conduction. *Circulation*, 1996;**93**: 502–512.

97. Olgin, J.E., J.M. Kalman, A.P. Fitzpatrick, and M.D. Lesh, Role of right atrial endocardial structures as barriers to conduction during human type I atrial flutter. Activation and entrainment mapping guided by intracardiac echocardiography. *Circulation*, 1995;**92**: 1839–1848.

98. Dorostkar, P.C., J. Cheng, and M.M. Scheinman, Electroanatomical mapping and ablation of the substrate supporting intraatrial reentrant tachycardia after palliation for complex congenital heart disease. *Pacing Clin. Electrophysiol.*, 1998;**21**: 1810–1819.

99. Love, B.A., K.K. Collins, E.P. Walsh, and J.K. Triedman, Electroanatomic characterization of conduction barriers in sinus/atrially paced rhythm and association with intra-atrial reentrant tachycardia circuits following congenital heart disease surgery. *J. Cardiovasc. Electrophysiol.*, 2001;**12**: 17–25.

100. Collins, K.K., B.A. Love, E.P. Walsh, J.P. Saul, M.R. Epstein, and J.K. Triedman, Location of acutely successful radiofrequency catheter ablation of intraatrial reentrant tachycardia in patients with congenital heart disease. *Am. J. Cardiol.*, 2000;**86**: 969–974.

Part II

Body-Surface
Isopotential Mapping

9 Body Surface Potential Mapping Techniques

Robert L. Lux

P. W. Macfarlane et al. (eds.), *Cardiac Arrhythmias and Mapping Techniques*, DOI 10.1007/978-0-85729-877-5_9,

© Springer-Verlag London Limited 2012

9.1   Introduction – History and Technology

Body surface potential mapping is an extension of conventional electrocardiography that acknowledges the fact that cardiac electrical fields – the voltage distributions and current flow patterns arising from cardiac currents – exist everywhere within and on the body surface. Waller, Einthoven, Wilson, and many of the early electrocardiographers recognized that the electrocardiogram could be measured from any body surface site and that the measured signals were different at each site, but because of limitations in recording technology, they could measure only one or at best a few sites at a time. The evolution of electronic amplifiers and the advent and access of laboratory computers during the late 1960s made possible the recording of many ECGs at a time, thus allowing the *mapping* of spatial distributions of potential. The sequence of these distributions defines what has come to be known as the body surface potential map. Unlike *scalar* electrocardiography which relies on interpretation of waveform features including amplitudes, durations, and morphologies of the different electrocardiographic waves, body surface potential mapping focuses on the magnitude, location, and migration of potential extrema as well as the shape and dynamics of isopotential contours throughout the cardiac cycle.

Body surface potential mapping (BSPM) is a subset of the more general field of cardiac mapping that includes the *direct* study of cardiac fields measured in the intracavitary space, intramurally within the myocardium, and on epicardial and endocardial surfaces. While body surface mapping is completely noninvasive and makes use of passive or active electrodes placed on the body surface, direct cardiac mapping techniques are invasive and require insertion of catheter mounted arrays (balloons, baskets) in the cavities, multipolar catheters placed in the coronary veins, multipolar needles inserted directly into the myocardium, or "sock" or patch mounted arrays of electrodes for use on the epicardium at the time of open chest surgery. In all cases, the objective is to assess the 2D and 3D distributions of potential or current on and within the myocardium, thus the more the recording sites, the greater the resolution and ability to characterize the underlying cardiac electrical sources. In this chapter, we shall focus exclusively on BSPM.

The original rationale for BSPM was that the ability to visualize the dynamic patterns of cardiac generated potentials was hypothesized to provide a more complete picture of the underlying electrical sources of the heart than that provided by the limited view of six "unipolar" precordial leads and the six limb/augmented leads of which only two are independent. This, in turn, would provide better means to detect and characterize the underlying disease, namely infarction, ischemia, abnormalities of conduction, hypertrophy, and cardiomyopathy. A secondary, more powerful rationale was that the rapidly developing methodology of inverse electrocardiography offered an opportunity for body surface map data to be used to calculate, estimate, characterize, or localize the electrical sources within the heart. In fact, the work of Ramanathan et al. and others in recent years has shown the feasibility of generating reliable estimates of cardiac electrograms and extracted information such as depolarization (activation) sequence and repolarization (recovery) sequence derived from measured body surface maps and measured torso and organ geometries and resistivities [1].

In point of fact, largely because of the expense of custom recording equipment and the consideration that computing power needed for processing and display was available only as expensive, laboratory computing systems, the early mapping efforts in the 1970s and early 1980s were relegated almost exclusively to the laboratory. Additionally, the rapid evolution of ultrasonic imaging of the heart began to provide inexpensive, noninvasive means of detecting cardiac abnormalities, including wall motion abnormalities (infarction and ischemia), valve dysfunction, wall thickness (hypertrophy), and conduction defects (bundle branch block). This new technology siphoned energy and rationale for body surface mapping, leaving electrophysiology and arrhythmias as the major remaining areas of study. Nevertheless, BSPM continues to be used, particularly as a means to better characterize heart disease and, more recently, as a means to facilitate localization key circuits in arrhythmias.

9.2   Recording Techniques

Body surface mapping systems include an electrode array, electronics for amplification, and recording of the ECG data, computing resources for preprocessing the recorded ECGs, displaying them in a variety of formats, and for analyzing the signals for purposes of detection, classification, or monitoring changes in cardiac electrophysiological state.

9.2.1 Electrode Arrays

Most early mapping was done using regular arrays (fixed numbers of columns and rows) of passive metal electrodes, typically chlorided silver, attached to individual strips of nylon, rubber, or other substrate material. Conventional electrode paste was routinely used to enhance electrical contact with the skin and double-sided adhesive strips or "doughnuts" were used to hold the electrodes in place. At least one group used polished insect pins attached to individual wires to record signals and another group devised a vest embedded with active dry electrodes – electrodes that have preamplifiers mounted directly on the metal. The objective of these designs was to obtain high quality and low noise signals while minimizing the time needed to apply the electrode arrays.

In the early days of mapping, little was known about redundancy of electrocardiographic information in the sense of correlation between sites, and hence mappers used large numbers of electrodes (242, 192, 128, 64, etc.). As body surface potential map databases grew and as experience and understanding of distributions demonstrated that there was considerable redundancy in these signals, several groups focused on "limited" or "reduced" lead systems to maximize capture of information while reducing the costs associated with large numbers of leads and the associated electronics and computing needed to manage the data. This topic will be addressed later in this chapter.

Several techniques have been developed to facilitate and speed up the process of applying the electrodes to patients. These include the use of strips of electrodes with double sided adhesive, inflatable vests in which electrodes are embedded on the inner surfaces, arrays of electrodes supported by a mechanical shell and adjustable to fit each torso, and strips of electrodes attached to the patient via suction. Most electrode systems use and require use of electrode gel for purposes of ensuring good electrode–skin contact, but others have reported success using active dry electrodes that eliminate the need for electrode gel.

9.2.2 Electronics

Mapping systems require the need for amplification of the small (~2 mV magnitude) signals, analog-to-digital (A/D) converters to convert the amplified voltages into numerical representation for later processing, and a means to store these samples from each of the electrodes. The basis of all electrocardiographic recording is the electronic amplifier tailored for bioelectric signals having maximum amplitudes of 2 mV. During the late 1960s and early 1970s, such amplifiers were readily available, but not configured in size and cost to permit assemblies of the hundreds needed for the "simultaneous" recording, essential for mapping. Several groups developed their own custom amplifier systems using low noise, high performance integrated circuits that allowed packaging of tens of individual amplifiers on each circuit board. The addition of individual *sample and hold* circuits made possible the "simultaneous" sampling of data from all amplifiers, important for maintaining temporal integrity of the data. Another important contribution to the technology was the use of analog *multiplexers*, integrated circuits that allowed signals from multiple amplifiers to be switched into one data stream that could then be fed to one A/D converter. This innovation drastically reduced the system cost by eliminating the need for expensive A/D converters for each channel. The stream of digital samples was then stored in computer memory or directly to disk using double buffering techniques and finally to digital tape. Early systems were limited to short recording times, typically just a few seconds, a consequence of the limits of available computing technologies and storage media. Present systems, both custom laboratory systems and the few commercially available, can record continuously to memory or disk for long periods of time.

9.2.3 Computer Processing and Display

The advent of laboratory computers and later, the availability of personal computers, made possible the extensive processing, analysis, and display of body surface potential map data. For each multichannel recording, individual signals had to be calibrated, adjusted for baseline drift, filtered if there were excessive noise, or estimated or interpolated from other signals if the signal were excessively noisy or "missing", often a problem when hundreds of leads and connectors were considered. The signature presentation of body surface potential data is the isopotential contour map, in which potentials for each sample time are displayed as contour maps on geometric representations of the torso. Data in ❷ Fig. 9.1 show

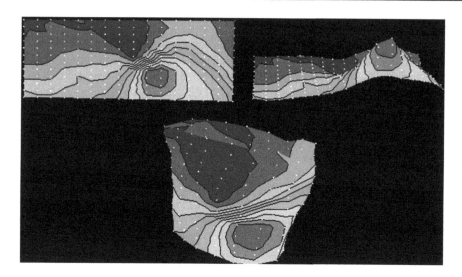

Fig. 9.1

Examples of isopotential contour map displays from the early QRS of a normal subject. On the upper left panel is a stylized 2D contour plot showing an array of 12 rows by 16 columns (192 sites) that represent a torso surface. The *top* and *bottom* edges of the rectangle correspond to the levels of the sternal notch and umbilicus, respectively. The *vertical midline* of the array corresponds to the vertical anterior thoracic midline and the *left* and *right* edges of the display correspond to the spine. On the upper right panel is the same data as displayed in the left panel except with vertical modulation of the potential, thus showing positive and negative extrema as "mountain peaks" and "valleys". The bottom panel shows the same data now presented on a 3D torso model. Contours are colored from blue (*negative*) to red (*positive*)

the same "frame" (sample) early in the QRS of a normal subject using a flat 2D array (upper left) as well as a 3D torso array (bottom). A third presentation of the same data (upper right), the orthographic projection, shows the potential distributions as "mountains and valleys" and is useful in enhancing magnitude differences and changes at the expense of extrema localization. An example of early, mid, and late "frames" within the sequence of QRS maps of a normal subject is shown in ❷ Fig. 9.2. The features of these maps used to describe them include the location and movement of the positive and negative extrema (trajectories) and the shape, steepness (gradient), and levels of isopotential contours. A variety of scaling techniques is used including *linear*, in which contours are spaced at fixed intervals, *normalized* in which a fixed number of contours is drawn for each map and which is useful for displaying data having low amplitude or widely varying amplitude, and *logarithmic* spacing for widely varying amplitudes. Additionally, since positive and negative potentials may be quite disparate in magnitude, it is often helpful to use *separate scaling* for positive and negative potentials. Such scaling options offer flexibility in assessing pattern and/or amplitude differences or changes.

9.3 Lead Systems for Recording and Estimating Body Surface Potential Maps

Since the objectives of electrocardiographic body surface potential mapping are measurement, analysis, and the use of **distributions**, measurement explicitly requires extensive spatial sampling. In contrast to the conventional 12 lead ECG and VCG techniques, which were developed from empirical considerations as well as representations of the electrical activity of the heart as a simple dipole, mapping lead systems were designed to measure "all" available ECG information.

Lead systems have been characterized as "complete" or "limited" (also referred to as "reduced lead systems"), the former implying the actual sampling of "all" data and the latter implying the sampling of a small number of sites for approximating or estimating complete distributions to a prespecified level of accuracy. Since mapping has been relegated primarily to research laboratories, there have never been standards for lead systems. Thus, there is a great variety in the

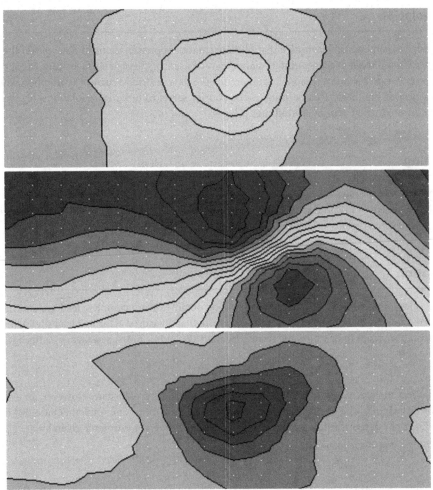

◘ Fig. 9.2
Three QRS "frames" (isopotential distributions) from a normal subject showing early, mid, and late distributions

number and placement of recording sites. "Complete" sampling lead systems published in the literature include provision to measure 64, 120, 128, 192, and 242 body surface sites. Since the purpose of extensive sampling is to define the spatial character of the cardiac generated potentials, these systems are designed to sample most of the thoracic surface. In most systems, electrodes are placed in evenly separated rows and columns over the thorax. Modifications to this basic arrangement include increased spatial sampling density in the precordial region (doubling the number of rows and columns in this region) and reduced sampling density on the posterior surface (halving the number of rows and/or columns) and placement of leads lower on the torso and higher, including the shoulders. It is important to note that the rationale for a particular lead system is dictated by the presumption that all ECG information will be sampled. Also, however, lead systems may be tied to the type of displays used. Complete lead systems were used initially because of the lack of knowledge concerning the detailed spatial character of ECG distributions or the extent of redundancy. By measuring data at all sites, direct display of the distributions and later analysis demonstrated that, for practical purposes, complete sampling was not necessary. This led to the development of a variety of "limited lead" systems for estimating complete maps [2–4]. The mechanisms by which complete ECG distributions may be "derived" from such limited lead sets include interpolation, modeling, and estimation.

9.3.1 Interpolation

Interpolation relies on mathematical formulae that provide smooth approximations to data within the regions between measurement sites. Simple linear or bilinear interpolation may be used, or curve or surface fitting may be applied. Another interpolation approach is to assume a periodic structure for the data, a strictly correct assumption when applied to the circumferential aspect of the torso. This permits use of Fourier series to build interpolation polynomials from which potentials may be approximated at unmeasured sites [5].

9.3.2 Modeling

Modeling approaches rely on physical characteristics of measurement sites – geometric location, conductivity of the torso, and its inhomogeneity – in conjunction with the field equations that *model* the problem to predict aspects of the distributions in unmeasured regions.

9.3.3 Estimation

Estimation techniques, on the other hand, utilize information obtained from complete lead systems in order to develop statistical transformations for estimating unmeasured data from that measured at limited lead sites. Ultimately, potentials Φ_u at N_u unmeasured sites, are to be estimated from potentials Φ_m at N_m measured sites, by a linear transformation, T, such that

$$\Phi_u = T\Phi_m$$

Theoretically, a perfect transformation exists for each subject and each cardiac state. However, an average transformation may function sufficiently well to permit its use in a practical system. In one implementation of this approach, the transformation, T, may be determined as the linear, least mean squared error estimator given by

$$T = K_{um}K_{mm}^{-1}$$

where, K_{um} is the cross covariance matrix between unmeasured and measured sites and K_{mm} is the covariance matrix of measured sites defined using the expectation operator, E, as

$$K_{um} = E[(\Phi_u - \overline{\Phi_u})(\Phi_m - \overline{\Phi_m})^T]$$

and

$$K_{mm} = E[(\Phi_m - \overline{\Phi_m})(\Phi_m - \overline{\Phi_m})^T]$$

where

$$K = \begin{bmatrix} K_{mm} & K_{mu} \\ K_{um} & K_{mm} \end{bmatrix}$$

In general, the covariance between any two sites i and j, k_{ij} is given by

$$k_{ij} = E[(p_i - \overline{p_i})(p_j - \overline{p_j})] = \rho_{ij}\sigma_i\sigma_j$$

in which ρ_{ij} is the correlation coefficient between potentials at sites i and j, σ_i and σ_j are the potential standard deviations at sites i and j. Regardless of the method for assigning potentials to the unmeasured sites, a variety of error criteria for assessing the adequacy of lead systems have been developed which permit selection of lead systems to suit one's needs. These criteria include root-mean-square (rms) error, correlation coefficient, peak error, and others, all of which compare estimated data with that obtained from a complete lead system. Depending on the number and placement of leads, estimation errors approaching the system and recording noise levels are possible. This approach has formed the basis for estimating BSPMs and even the 12 lead ECG from small numbers of leads.

9.4   Utilization of Body Surface Potential Map Information

There are two primary uses of map data, both ultimately aimed at understanding and characterizing normal and abnormal cardiac electrophysiology. The first and original use relates to the characterization of cardiac state, specifically with respect to disease, by direct correlation of map features with independent documentation of cardiac physiology and pathology. With regard to this use, emphasis is placed on practical application of measurements for improved, noninvasive diagnosis as compared to the 12 lead ECG. The second use of map data relates to the validation and assessment of forward and inverse models and concentrates on estimation of myocardial current distributions from which underlying physiology can be inferred. The latter is discussed elsewhere in this text and will not be described here. Regarding the former, utilization of map information is accomplished through visual assessment and/or quantitative approaches that permit rigorous analyses, particularly those involving statistical methods. Examples of these now follow.

Since the first maps were recorded, simple observation of the potential distributions has been the primary means of analysis. The sequence of distributions, including dynamics, relative magnitudes and trajectories of positive and negative extrema, and morphology of contours provide a rich characterization of each heart cycle. Classical features of maps on patients with old infarcts, bundle branch blocks, ectopic activation, WPW, etc., provide sufficient information for simple, "eyeball" classification which is often not as clear using the 12 lead ECG alone. For example, cardiac events leading to a marginally abnormal Q wave in a 12 lead examination would likely have a more definitive representation in maps, namely a negative extremum with signature temporal and spatial characteristics. In WPW, a delta wave – small deflection preceding and merging with the QRS – in the 12 lead, is transformed to an early negative extremum, whose location indirectly points to the location of the accessory pathway on the A-V ring. Ectopic ventricular beats and VT exhibit map patterns that consistently identify the location of early depolarization. The latter two illustrations characterize the "atlas" approach to map analysis in which map patterns originating from known cardiac location, whether epicardial, endocardial, or septal and both atrial and ventricular, are catalogued and then used for comparison to patterns from unknown activations [6–8]. Maps obtained from patients having a variety of cardiac pathologies are described in the following chapter. However, a brief introduction to the methods of qualitatively interpreting map distributions might be useful.

9.4.1   Qualitative Analysis

The elementary interpretation of potential distributions follows that of conventional ECGs. During the QRS, a positive wave in a unipolar lead is indicative of an approaching activation front and a negative wave reflects a receding front. Hence, Q or S waves signify receding wave fronts as viewed from the measurement site, whereas R or R′ waves are indicative of wave fronts approaching the site. In isopotential contour maps obtained during depolarization, body surface regions that are negative primarily reflect the perspective of receding depolarization surfaces, whereas regions that are positive are those which "see" approaching depolarization surfaces. During repolarization, the polarity is reversed, as is the interpretation.

In order to illustrate interpretation of map distributions, two examples are presented. The map in ❷ Fig. 9.3 shows data *early* in the QRS of a patient with an old anterior wall myocardial infarct. The dominant anterior negative extremum and left, posterolateral positive extremum, result from a depolarization surface oriented along a dominant anterior to posterior axis. This pattern persists throughout much of the QRS and the lack of anterior positivity is consistent with the loss of active, anterior wall myocardium.

The sequence of map frames shown in ❷ Fig. 9.4 shows potential distributions, *early*, mid, and late in the QRS of a patient with right bundle branch block. *The early (top) left to right axis (blue to yellow) of the potential distribution is indicative of a depolarization surface oriented in a left to right direction and would signify early left ventricular depolarization. The mid QRS transitional distribution shows a posterior-to-anterior distribution, likely dominated by LV endocardial-to-epicardial depolarization. The late QRS pattern (bottom) shows a right inferior to left superior axis and suggests a right ventricular depolarization pattern.*

Similar interpretations can be applied to ECGs and body surface maps during *repolarization*, with the exception that polarity reversal must be taken into account. In unipolar ECGs, positive T waves are measured at sites that, on the average, observe recovery receding from them. Contrariwise, negative T waves are detected at sites which observe recovery

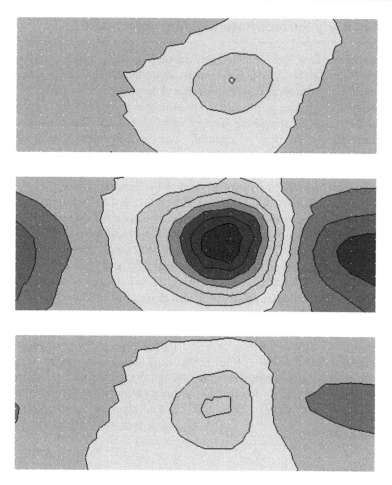

◘ Fig. 9.3
Three QRS frames from a patient with old anterior myocardial infarction

approaching them. In maps, positive regions are indicative of sites which, on average, observe repolarization receding and negative regions occur where recovery is approaching. A potential distribution during recovery of a normal subject is shown in ❷ Fig. 9.5. This distribution, which is quite static in pattern, shows a dominant right superior to left inferior axis on the anterior thoracic surface. This is consistent with the predominant epicardial to endocardial distribution of recovery observed in the normal heart following supraventricular activation.

It should be stressed at this point that the qualitative interpretation of potential distributions is correct in a general sense, although it is far from exact. The potential observed at any site results from a complex superposition of the effects of all active cardiac currents. The complexity of both the cardiac generator as well as the body volume conductor make exact interpretation difficult, if not impossible. The anisotropic, inhomogeneous, time varying nature of the active and passive tissue underscores the difficulty of carrying out unambiguous interpretation of map data from a qualitative approach.

9.4.2   Quantitative Analyses of Body Surface Maps

The simplest quantitative approaches to map analysis are those that assign numerical values to visually observable features. Thus, the *trajectories* of positive and/or negative extrema may be parameterized into x, y coordinates varying with time.

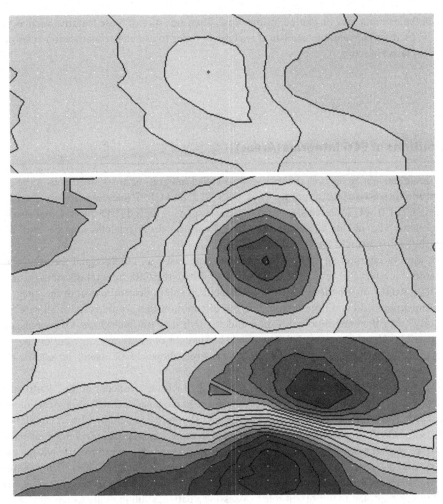

⬛ Fig. 9.4
Three QRS frames from a patient with old right bundle branch block

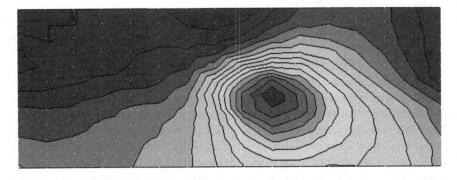

⬛ Fig. 9.5
A T wave isopotential map from a normal subject

The magnitudes of the extrema may be plotted against time. Then statistics of these features, such as the mean or peak values may then be used for conventional statistical analysis in order to establish classification rules or to demonstrate differences between classes of maps.

9.4.3   Distributions of ECG Integrals (Areas)

Another class of quantitative map features makes use of so-called integrals or areas. Segments of the sequence of maps may be integrated and displayed as distributions. Thus, QRS, STT, and QRST integral maps are obtained by integrating all ECGs over the QRS, STT, or QT intervals, respectively, and displaying their distributions. Other specialized areas have been used, including the ST_{60} in which integration is carried out over the 80 ms following the "end" of QRS, or the "Q zone" map in which the first 30 ms of the QRS is integrated.

There are two ways of interpreting integral distributions, one based on purely signal theoretic considerations and one based on theoretical aspects of cardiac electrophysiology. Thus, the QRS integral distribution may be thought of as the average QRS potential distribution, which it would be if all values determined from the integration are divided by the interval of integration. In addition, it would be the distribution that would result if all cardiac fibers depolarized "simultaneously" with the same dipole direction and strength they normally have. Of course, such an activation sequence is not possible. All other area distributions may be thought of as average distributions for the interval over which the integration was performed. These integrals have been shown to be useful in assessing cardiac state or its change.

The more powerful, theoretic interpretation of areas originated with the concept of the "ventricular gradient" first proposed by Frank Wilson [9]. He argued that in the presence of a homogeneous distribution of action potentials, that is, identical recovery properties, the integral of any ECG over the QT interval should be zero. A corollary to this, suggests that since the measured QRST area distribution is not zero, and, moreover, almost independent of activation sequence, it reflects disparity of recovery properties, that is, action potential shape and duration. Though the exact relationship between QRST area and disparity of recovery properties has not been established, it is clear that a significant one exists. Since the distribution of recovery properties is known to play an important role in some mechanisms of arrhythmogenesis, QRST area distributions may play an important role in assessing a patient's vulnerability to ventricular arrhythmias. This has been explored by several groups that relate QRST integral distributions to vulnerability [10–13]. Moreover, Plonsey and Geselowitz have provided a theoretical justification for Wilson's original work [14, 15].

The same theory that predicts that the QRST area should reflect the distribution of recovery properties suggests that the QRS area distribution should reflect the distribution of activation sequence. Experimental support for this hypothesis has been documented and the measurement may prove useful in diagnosing abnormalities of conduction. As a consequence of the relationships of QRS area to activation sequence and QRST area to recovery properties, it follows that the STT area should reflect recovery sequence.

The body surface distributions of QRS, STT, and QRST integrals obtained from a normal subject are illustrated in ❷ Fig. 9.6. Interpretation of these distributions in terms of average activation sequence, recovery sequence, and recovery properties follows along lines similar to those used for interpreting isopotential maps. The superior-right to inferior-left anterior axis of the QRS area distribution is consistent with the dominant direction of depolarization of the left ventricle, namely endocardium to epicardium that presents itself, on average, along a base to apex axis. The facts that the distribution of the STT areas is similar to that of the QRS and that the polarity associated with recovery is reversed compared to depolarization provide evidence that recovery sequence is opposite to that of activation. This epicardial to endocardial sequence of recovery in a normal heart following supraventricular activation is well documented. Finally, the distribution of QRST areas is supportive of the previously observed epicardial to endocardial gradient of recovery properties. In summary, the distributions of deflection integrals provide important information concerning the underlying electrophysiological processes in the heart. These indices and analyses of their spatial character are being examined for utility in providing insight into arrhythmia vulnerability, the extent and nature of conduction defects, as well as other abnormalities of activation and recovery.

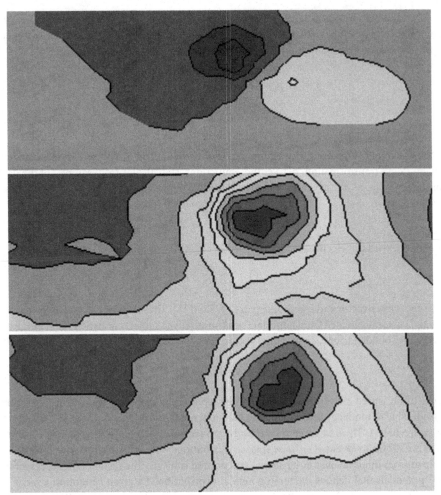

⬚ Fig. 9.6
QRS, STT, and QRST integral maps from a normal subject

9.5 Statistical Representation of Body Surface Maps

Another approach to quantitative characterization of maps is the use of mathematical or statistical representation [16, 17]. In this technique, maps are characterized using mathematical or statistically derived basis functions. All the data from a patients map, the complete sequence of potential distributions, may be represented as an n-dimensional vector that can be used to reconstruct the original maps within a prespecified error. The advantage of this technique over other, quantitative characterizations, is that the representation features are independent and common to all maps and all patients. The vector of representing parameters may be used to compare maps on a beat-to-beat basis within one patient, between patients, or between classes of patients. Furthermore, independence of the parameters greatly simplifies the statistical analysis. The technique has been particularly useful in the non-invasive diagnosis of a variety of classes of heart disease for which diagnostic performance of the 12 lead ECG is ineffective.

In this approach, each map frame (potential distribution) is represented as a linear combination (weighted sum) of 12 *independent*, normalized basis functions. Specifically, if $\mathbf{P}(k)$ is the kth sample in time of an N dimensional potential vector (map frame), then such a representation is expressed as

$$P(k) = \sum_{i=1}^{N} \alpha_i(k)\Phi_i$$

$$\Phi_i \bullet \Phi_i = \delta_{ij} = \left\{ \begin{array}{l} 0, i \neq j \\ 1, i = j \end{array} \right\}$$

where the set of basis vectors $\{\Phi\}$ can be any N dimensional mathematical functions. An efficient representation, the so-called Karhunen–Loeve transformation, derives these functions, statistically, from samples of the data that one wants to represent. For the above maps, the covariance matrix, K, can be defined as

$$K = E[(P - \overline{P})(P - \overline{P})^T]$$

while the solution of the classical "eigenvalue equation"

$$|\lambda_i I - K\Phi_i| = 0$$

leads to solutions of sets eigenvector and eigenvalue pairs, $\{\Theta\}$ and $\{\lambda\}$. These can be calculated from covariance matrices and average potential vectors estimated from large data sets (hundreds of subjects or patients and hundreds of map frames from each subject). Once obtained, for each potential vector, $P(k)$, the coefficient "wave forms" $\alpha_i(k)$ can be obtained from

$$\alpha_i(k) = P(k) \bullet \Phi_i$$

Thus, the sequence of measured map frames, $\{\mathbf{P}(k)\}$ can be replaced by the set of coefficient "wave forms," $\{\alpha_i(k)\}$ and since there is considerable redundancy in body surface potential maps, only a few, N≈10 or 15 basis functions are needed to represent the entire BSPM. The first three *spatial* body surface eigenvectors for a large set of normal and abnormal body surface maps are shown in ❷ Fig. 9.7. These spatial distributions were statistically derived from a set of over 20,000 map frames obtained from maps on over 400 patients and normal subjects. The result of the representation is to convert each frame of 192 potentials that defines the torso potential distribution at a given instant, to a set of 12 numbers. This 16:1 reduction in data removes spatial dependence or redundancy in the distributions. Importantly, the representation process is reversible in the sense that the 12 representation variables, in combination with the 12 feature distributions, may be used to reconstruct the original, measured distribution to an error of only .044 mV rms. The effect of this spatial representation procedure is to replace the sequence of map frames of a complete BSPM with a set of 12 waveforms that are the time varying weights of each of the feature frames. The process of representation can be continued for the time domain, that is, the coefficient waveforms can be represented by basis functions derived from the coefficient waveforms, $\{\alpha_i(k)\}$. The overall effect of first spatial and then temporal representation is to replace the original BSPM (100,000 potential measurements/QRST) with an equivalent set of 216 independent variables. This "vector" of 216 parameters represents the original BSPM in the sense that from it, the original BSPM may be reconstructed to a high level of accuracy. This vector of representation parameters may then be used in classical statistical strategies for classifying or comparing map data, whether beat-to-beat within one patient, patient-to-patient, or class-to-class.

9.6   Summary

The long history of body surface potential mapping, will likely continue. The rapid developments in anatomic imaging, inverse technologies, and computing speed and power will almost certainly lead to practical systems for rapid, non-invasive, or minimally invasive assessment of cardiac electrophysiology. BSPM will play a critical role in that it is the body surface potentials that ultimately are transformed into estimates of myocardial depolarization and repolarization sequences that form the basis for understanding and characterizing regional cardiac electrophysiology, arrhythmias, and disease.

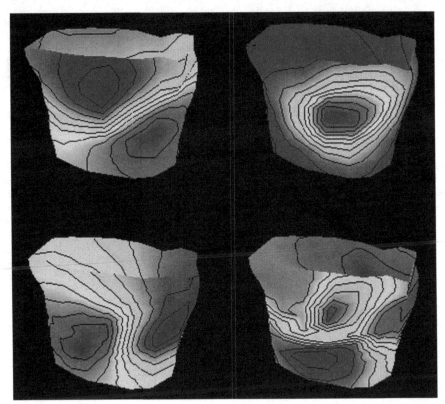

■ Fig. 9.7

First four *normalized* spatial eigenvectors calculated from a covariance matrix estimated using data from normal subjects and patients with a variety of cardiac diseases

Acknowledgement

The author wishes to acknowledge Dr. Robert S. MacLeod of the University of Utah who developed the Map3D program used to display the BSPM data that are illustrated in this chapter.

References

1. Ramanathan, C., R.N. Ghanem, P. Jia, et al., Noninvasive electrocardiographic imaging for cardiac electrophysiology and arrhythmia. *Nat. Med.*, Apr 2004;**10**(4): 422–428.

2. Barr, R.C., M.S. Spach, and G.S. Herman-Giddens, Selection of the number and positions of measuring locations for electrocardiography. *IEEE Trans. Biomed. Eng.*, Mar 1971;**18**(2): 125–138.

3. Lux, R.L., M.J. Burgess, R.F. Wyatt, et al., Clinically practical lead systems for improved electrocardiography: comparison with precordial grids and conventional lead systems. *Circulation*, Feb 1979;**59**(2): 356–363.

4. Lux, R.L., C.R. Smith, R.F. Wyatt, et al., Limited lead selection for estimation of body surface potential maps in electrocardiography. *IEEE Trans. Biomed. Eng.*, May 1978;**25**(3): 270–276.

5. Monro, D.M., Interpolation methods for surface mapping. *Comput. Programs Biomed.*, Apr 1980;**11**(2): 145–157.

6. SippensGroenewegen, A., R.N. Hauer, N.M. van Hemel, et al., Atlas of paced body surface QRS integral maps for localization of the site of origin of postinfarction ventricular tachycardia. *J. Electrocardiol.*, 1994;**27**(Suppl): 105–112.

7. SippensGroenewegen, A., H.A. Peeters, E.R. Jessurun, et al., Body surface mapping during pacing at multiple sites in the human atrium: P-wave morphology of ectopic right atrial activation. *Circulation*, Feb 3 1998;**97**(4): 369–380.

8. SippensGroenewegen, A., F.X. Roithinger, H.A. Peeters, et al., Body surface mapping of atrial arrhythmias: atlas of paced P wave integral maps to localize the focal origin of right atrial tachycardia. *J Electrocardiol.*, 1998;**31**(Suppl): 85–91.

9. Wilson, F.N., A.G. MacLeod, P.S. Barker, et al., The determination and significance of the areas of the ventricular deflections of the electrocardiogram. *Am. Heart J.*, 1934;**10**: 46.

10. Urie, P.M., M.J. Burgess, R.L. Lux, et al., The electrocardiographic recognition of cardiac states at high risk of ventricular arrhythmias. An experimental study in dogs. *Circ. Res.*, March 1978;**42**(3): 350–358.

11. Lux, R.L., P.M. Urie, M.J. Burgess, et al., Variability of the body surface distributions of QRS, ST-T and QRST deflection areas with varied activation sequence in dogs. *Cardiovasc. Res.*, Oct 1980;**14**(10): 607–612.

12. Abildskov, J.A., QRST area maps and cardiac arrhythmias. *J. Am. Coll. Cardiol.*, Nov 15 1989;**14**(6): 1537–1538.

13. Hubley-Kozey, C.L., L.B. Mitchell, M.J. Gardner, et al., Spatial features in body-surface potential maps can identify patients with a history of sustained ventricular tachycardia. *Circulation*, Oct 1 1995; **92**(7): 1825–1838.

14. Plonsey, R., A contemporary view of the ventricular gradient of Wilson. *J. Electrocardiol.*, Oct 1979;**12**(4): 337–341.

15. Geselowitz, D.B., The ventricular gradient revisited: relation to the area under the action potential. *IEEE Trans. Biomed. Eng.*, Jan 1983;**30**(1): 76–77.

16. Evans, A.K., R.L. Lux, M.J. Burgess, et al., Redundancy reduction for improved display and analysis of body surface potential maps. II. Temporal compression. *Circ. Res.*, July 1981;**49**(1): 197–203.

17. Lux, R.L., A.K. Evans, M.J. Burgess, et al., Redundancy reduction for improved display and analysis of body surface potential maps. I. Spatial compression. *Circ. Res.*, July 1981;**49**(1): 186–196.

10 Body Surface Potential Mapping

Luigi de Ambroggi · Alexandru D. Corlan

P. W. Macfarlane et al. (eds.), *Cardiac Arrhythmias and Mapping Techniques*, DOI 10.1007/978-0-85729-877-5_10,

10.1   Introduction

Body-surface potential maps (BSPMs) present the distribution of cardiac potentials on the chest surface during the cardiac cycle. They provide the spatial as well as the temporal and amplitude components of cardiac electrical activity, whereas the ECG scalar waveforms present only the time–voltage variation in a given lead point.

When an excitation wavefront spreads through atrial or ventricular heart muscle, it generates bioelectric currents, which distribute themselves to all conducting tissues in the body. This wavefront is a thin layer of heart muscle separating resting from excited areas. For the sake of simplicity, reference is made to the "classical" electrical model [1], according to which an excitation front is considered to be equivalent to a uniform dipole layer, where the dipole axis is everywhere orthogonal to the front; moreover, the tissue resistivity is supposed to be homogeneous. According to this model, currents arise from the anterior aspect of the front, flow through the thorax, and finally point to the posterior aspect of the front. ❯ Figure 10.1 illustrates the distributions of the currents and potentials, in a horizontal thoracic section, arising from an excitation wavefront in the ventricular septum. The locations of the potential maximum and minimum on the thoracic surface are correlated with the topography and orientation of the wavefront. According to the traditional solid angle theory, a potential maximum in a given area on the chest surface indicates that an excitation wave is pointing toward that area; a potential minimum indicates that the posterior or negative aspect of the wavefront is seen from the area where the minimum is present.

However, the relationship between surface potential distribution and wavefront shape is sometimes very complex. In fact, the potential distribution at the surface depends on the location, number, and geometry of the wavefronts in the thorax, the geometry of the torso, and the inhomogeneities of the conducting medium (cardiac and extracardiac tissues). For example, several excitation waves may be travelling simultaneously through the right and left ventricle, giving rise to a complex distribution of currents and potentials. Also, when an excitation wave spreading from the endocardium reaches the epicardial surface, a hole appears in the advancing wavefront. Through this hole or "window," the currents reenter the heart. If a window is close to the chest wall, a new potential minimum appears on the thoracic surface, in addition to those already present. A similar hole appears in the excitation wavefront when a portion of ventricular wall cannot be activated, because of a local myocardial infarction. In this case too, a potential minimum appears on the chest surface in the region facing the infarcted area. A further cause of complexity arises from the fact that the dipole density is not uniform on the surface of the wavefront, in that a wavefront spreading along fibers generates more current per unit area than a wavefront spreading across fibers [2, 3].

During repolarization, currents proportional to transmembrane potential gradient from the M-cell region flow toward the epicardium and endocardium, the former being of higher amplitude [4, 5]. This amounts to numerous small dipoles distributed in the whole mass of the myocardium. The orientation of these dipoles remains mostly unchanged during repolarization, and their amplitudes change relatively synchronously. Localized repolarization changes further add to the complexity of the body-surface potentials in heart disease.

Every excitation wave and every portion of repolarizing tissue in the heart influence the potential distribution on the entire body surface. It follows that information on the electrical activity of the heart can be recorded not only from the points commonly explored by conventional ECG and VCG leads, but also from the entire body surface. BSPMs provide all the information available on the entire chest surface.

10.2   History

The first example of a potential map was published by A. Waller in 1889 [6], on the basis of 10–20 ECG recordings from the surface of the human body; the potential distribution resembled that which would have appeared if a dipole had been located in the heart. Later, a few attempts to determine surface potential distributions were made by several authors with rudimentary techniques.

In 1951, Nahum et al. [7] published the first description of isopotential line distribution on the thoracic surface at successive instants during the cardiac cycle in man. They did not detect the simultaneous presence of several maxima and minima but observed that the surface potential distribution was much more complicated than that likely to result from an equivalent dipolar generator. In the 1960s, Taccardi [8, 9] described the instantaneous distribution of heart potentials during ventricular activation in dogs and in normal human subjects. These investigations clearly showed that several potential

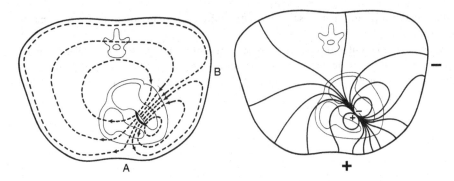

Fig. 10.1

Left: Schematic drawing of a horizontal section of the human thorax illustrating the pathway of the currents, which arise from an excitation wavefront (solid line in septum) spreading through the septum in a left-to-right direction. A indicates the area where the current lines reach the surface; B indicates the area from which the currents dip into the thorax pointing to the posterior aspect of the wavefront. *Right*: Potential distribution in the same thoracic section and at the same instant. The plus sign indicates the location of the potential maximum on the surface (corresponding to point A); the minus sign indicates the location of the potential minimum (corresponding to point B)

maxima and minima may be simultaneously present on the body surface during part of the QRS interval; moreover, an attempt was made to correlate the location of surface maxima and minima with the probable location of excitation wavefronts in the ventricles. The complexity of surface potential patterns, although not physically incompatible with a dipolar source, strongly suggested that a more complex electrical model of the heart should be adopted in order to account for the potential distributions found on the human and canine trunk.

Since then, BSPMs have been recorded from normal subjects (newborns and adults), cardiac patients, and experimental animals by many investigators in different countries.

10.3 Methods

Many lead systems have been used to record BSPMs throughout the world differing in the number of leads as well as in electrode location on the thorax. In theory, the optimal lead system should have a number of leads large enough to detect all details of the potential distribution on the torso surface. However, transformation methods have been proposed to estimate BSPM in a particular lead system from the BSPM data measured by using another lead system [10].

Techniques for recording, processing, and displaying the potential maps are illustrated in ❷ Chap. 9.

Different methods of analysis of BSPMs have been used to extract relevant information. These are described below.

10.3.1 Instantaneous BSPMs

The distribution of chest potentials in each instant of the cardiac cycle can be analyzed qualitatively, by visual inspection, or quantitatively by considering a number of numerical parameters relating to location, amplitude, and migration of potential maxima and minima.

10.3.2 Integral Maps

Since differences between maps of normal subjects and patients cannot easily be quantified by inspection of the sequence of instantaneous potential distributions, the potential–time integral maps have been considered. This approach has been proved to allow a reduction in the amount of data to be analyzed without substantial loss of information [11]. With this method, only a few maps are required to represent a cardiac cycle (QRS, ST-T, QRST, or other intervals for particular purposes). In addition, this technique permits the calculation of average maps for groups of subjects without the need for time-phase alignment.

An approximation of the potential time integral, relating to a given interval of the cardiac cycle, is obtained by computing, at each lead point, the algebraic sum of all the instantaneous potential values throughout the interval considered, multiplied by the sampling interval. The values, expressed in mVms, are transferred to a diagram representing the thoracic surface explored, and isointegral contour lines can be drawn (❂ Fig. 10.2).

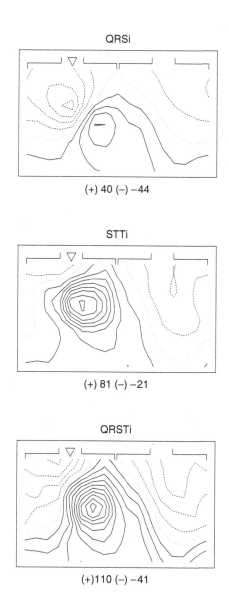

QRSi

(+) 40 (−) −44

STTi

(+) 81 (−) −21

QRSTi

(+)110 (−) −41

◘ Fig. 10.2

Integral maps in a normal subject during the QRS interval (*top*) ST-T interval (*middle*) and QRST interval (*bottom*). The left half of each map represents the anterior face of the thorax, the right half represents the posterior face. Continuous dark lines represent positive isointegrals, dashed lines represent negative isointegrals. The grey continuous line represents the zero integral line. The legend under each map indicates by (+) the maximum integral value on the respective map, by (−) the minimum integral value and (:) the gradient between isointegral lines, in 10 mVms

10.3.3 Principal Component Analysis

Reduction of the information in body-surface ECG recordings can be achieved by decomposing individual integral maps or population-wide sets of recordings or the matrix of potentials in time over an interval (such as the ST-T) into components, which are independent of (noncorrelated to) each other. For example, singular value decomposition of the matrix of instantaneous repolarization potentials in time can be written as a sum of components each consisting of a potential distribution on the body surface, changing in time. The relative spatial distribution of the potentials of each component is constant, and the only thing that changes in time is the general amplitude of the component.

❯ Figure 10.3 shows the first four components of the ST-T potentials in a normal subject. The first component contains normally over 75% of the potential amplitude, and is probably due to the general transmural gradient of the ventricular action potential. The second component is usually opposed (inversely correlated) to the QRS integral and likely corresponds to the repolarization gradient secondary to the depolarization sequence. The relative contribution of the first or

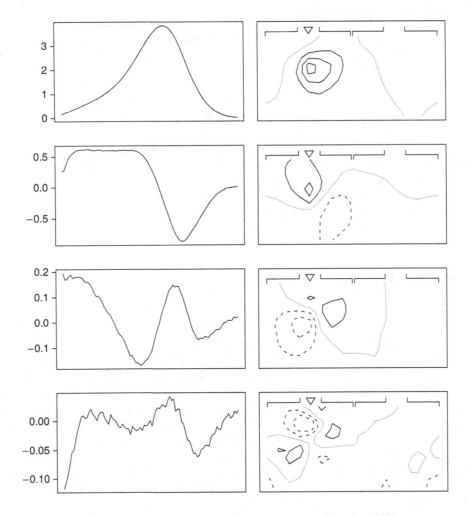

◼ Fig. 10.3

The first four components resulting from singular value decomposition of the matrix of instantaneous repolarization potentials versus time in a normal recording. Each component is represented by the body-surface potential distribution (*right*) (distance between isopotential lines is arbitrary) and the variation of its amplitude in time (*left*) (time on *x*-axis and relative amplitude on *y*-axis). The first component is at the *top*, the fourth at the *bottom*

first two components to the repolarization potentials is decreased in most pathological states and may be indicative of the presence of arrhythmogenic repolarization heterogeneity.

Reduction of the information in body-surface ECG recordings to a few numerical indices can be achieved by analysing individual recordings or population-wide sets of recordings into components that are independent of (not correlated to) each other. One method is principal component analysis in which a set of signals, either instantaneous body-surface distributions at different instants in time, or time-based signals from different leads, or integral maps in a group of individuals are decomposed into eigenvectors (components, usually sets of potentials) and eigenvalues (numbers which quantify the contribution of each eigenvector to the general variability of the overall data). Ventricular repolarization is particularly suitable to this type of analysis, as most of the variability of normal repolarization potentials in most instants over the ST-T interval can be described by a single component.

10.3.4 Autocorrelation Maps

Autocorrelation (AC) maps are square matrices of values between −1.0 and 1.0, which represent the correlation coefficients of every pair of instantaneous potential distributions from a set of successive instants in time [12]. The same time interval appears on both coordinates of the map and the matrix is symmetrical with respect to the first diagonal. Values on the first diagonal are always 1.0, representing correlations of each instantaneous map with itself.

Autocorrelation maps reflect only phenomena taking place in the ECG source (myocardium) and are very little influenced by the geometry of the volume conductor (thorax) that connects it to the lead system [13]. AC maps are very sensitive to variations in the activation sequence. For example, ❷ Figs. 10.4 and ❷ 10.5 show recordings in two healthy individuals in whom the 12 lead ECGs and QRS integral maps look very much alike, but differences in the activation sequence are evident in the instantaneous potential maps, especially in the AC maps.

The AC map of the ST-T interval is normally quite close to 1 as the normal repolarization pattern shows little change, apart from the amplitude. The extent of change can be quantified by choosing the map at the peak of T (on the root mean square signal) as a reference map and calculating the average difference from one of the lines that goes through that instant on the AC map over the S-T peak and T peak-end intervals. We call these average differences the early and late repolarization deviation indices (ERDI and LRDI), respectively.

10.4 Normal Maps

10.4.1 Atrial Excitation and Recovery

At the onset of atrial excitation, a potential minimum is generally observed near the right sterno-clavicular joint, in the right supraclavicular region, or in the right mammary area (❷ Fig. 10.6a) [14, 15]. The potential maximum or minimum is here defined as a point on the thoracic surface where the potential value is higher or lower in relation to all the surrounding points. Mirvis [16] did not observe a clear-cut minimum, but only a broad area of negative low-level potentials over the upper back and the right chest during the initial phase of atrial excitation. A potential maximum is initially located either in the right submammary area or in the lower sternal region (❷ Fig. 10.6b). During the subsequent stages of atrial activation, the maximum moves leftward, gradually reaching the left mammary region, the left lateral chest wall and, in some cases, the dorsal region (❷ Fig. 10.6c). The minimum moves slightly downward. During the leftward migration of the maximum, a secondary potential maximum sometimes appears on the left lateral wall of the thorax. The movement of the potential maximum from right to left is most likely correlated with the spread of the excitation wavefronts from the right to the left atrium.

During atrial recovery (❷ Fig. 10.6d), surface potential maps resemble those recorded in the early stages of atrial excitation, but with reverse polarity [15–17]. A potential minimum is generally located on the sternal and left mammary region and a maximum on the right shoulder both in adults and infants. This finding suggests that repolarization advances through the atrial walls in approximately the same order as does excitation. This is in agreement with experimental data, demonstrating that the atrial regions that depolarize first are also the first to recover [18].

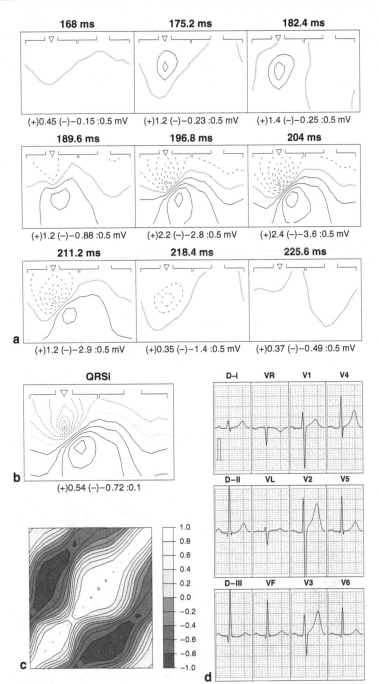

◼ Fig. 10.4

Different representations of depolarization potentials of the same cardiac cycle in a normal subject. (**a**) Successive, instantaneous potential maps during the QRS; conventions are as in ❷ Fig. 10.2, except that the lines are isopotential and are measured in mV; the label above each map indicates the timing of the instantaneous map. (**b**) Integral map with the same conventions as in ❷ Fig. 10.2. (**c**) Autocorrelation map of the QRS interval; the same time interval is on both *x*- and *y*-axis, and each point on the map represents the correlation coefficient between instantaneous potential distributions at the instants of its *x*- and *y*-coordinates, using shades of gray from black for −1.0 to white for 1.0, as indicated on the scale at right. (**d**) Standard ECG reconstructed from leads corresponding to the standard ECG leads, extracted from the body-surface lead system

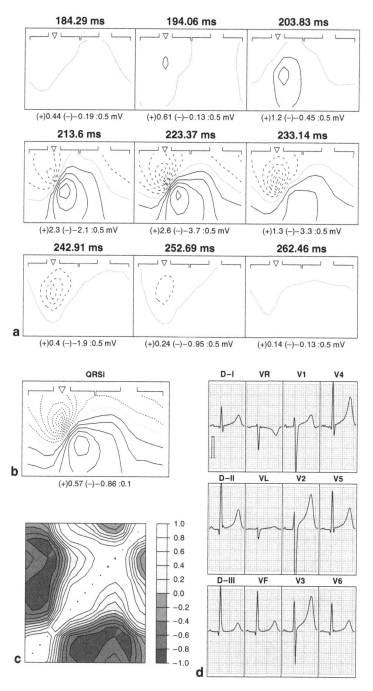

⬛ Fig. 10.5

The same representations of ventricular activation as in ❷ Fig. 10.4, for one cardiac cycle in a different healthy individual. This recording was selected from a set of 236 in healthy people as a recording with an almost identical QRS integral as that in ❷ Fig. 10.4. Note the similarity of the 12-lead ECG, the visible differences in the instantaneous potentials and the striking differences in the AC map

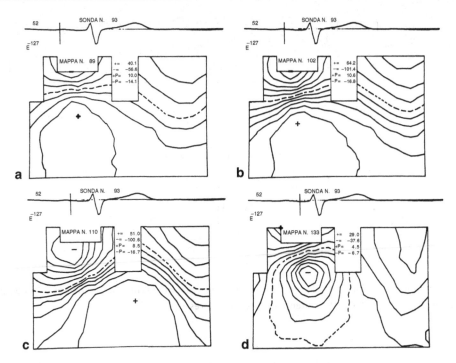

⬛ Fig. 10.6

⬛ Fig. 10.6
Averaged surface maps relating to atrial activation and recovery in a normal subject, at the instants or time indicated by the vertical line crossing the ECG at top of each figure. The time interval between the (a) and (d) is 88 ms. The zero equipotential line is dashed. The plus and minus signs indicate the value of the positive and negative peaks in microvolts; +P and −P indicate the step (in microvolts) between adjacent positive and negative equipotential lines

10.4.2 Ventricular Activation

Body-surface potential distributions during ventricular excitation have been described by many investigators in adults [9, 19–21], children [22, 23], and infants [24, 25].

The main features of maps observed in adults are as follows. At the beginning of the QRS, a potential maximum appears in the upper or mid-sternal area, and a minimum is generally located in a lower position on the left thoracic wall or on the back (❷ Fig. 10.7a). This potential pattern can be related to septal excitation, which occurs in a predominantly left-to-right direction [26, 27] and probably also to right ventricular free wall activation.

Later, the minimum migrates dorsally. In 25% of subjects, the migration is discontinuous: a separate low-amplitude dorsal minimum appears before the left lateral initial minimum has disappeared. Thus, in these subjects, two distinct minima are simultaneously present during the initial 15–20 ms of QRS [28]. The minimum then moves toward the right shoulder and finally appears in the right clavicular area (❷ Fig. 10.7a, b). In some cases, the minimum moves horizontally around the back and reaches the right axillary region. This behavior has been observed particularly in subjects with left axis deviation in the standard 12-lead ECG. Meanwhile, the maximum migrates downward to the left mammary region (❷ Fig. 10.7c). The events described above are temporally related to the spread of excitation in an endo-epicardial direction through the walls of both ventricles, with a mean direction from base to apex.

Thereafter, a new minimum often appears in the midsternal area (60% of cases in the authors' studies), at 14–44 ms after the onset of ventricular activation (❷ Fig. 10.7d). This minimum is considered to be the surface manifestation of the right ventricular breakthrough, that is, of the presence of a "window" in the advancing wavefront, through which the currents reenter the heart. In the following instants, the sternal minimum and the right clavicular minimum merge to form a single, broad anterior negative area (❷ Fig. 10.7e). In about 40% of the cases, the sternal minimum does not appear as a separate entity, and the sternal area becomes negative as a result of the migration of the main minimum.

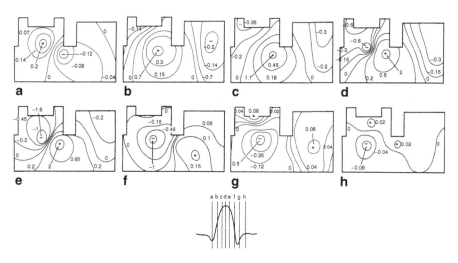

⬛ Fig. 10.7

Body-surface potential maps during normal ventricular activation. Each map refers to the instant or time indicated by the vertical line crossing the ECG (*bottom*). The potential values are expressed in millivolts

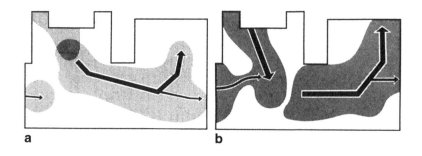

⬛ Fig. 10.8

The shaded areas encompass all locations of the potential maxima (a) and minima (b) throughout the QRS interval in 50 normal subjects. The *arrows* indicate the main direction of migration of the principal maximum (a) and minimum (b) (After Taccardi et al. [15]. © Clarendon, Oxford. Reproduced with permission)

Later, the maximum moves toward the left thoracic wall and then dorsally (❷ Fig. 10.7f). In about 55% of adults, a new maximum appears in the upper sternal area during the last 20–30 ms of the QRS interval (❷ Fig. 10.7g). In the great majority of cases, the second maximum appears while the dorsal maximum is still present, the time overlap being 10–30 ms. These potential patterns most likely indicate the presence of two separate excitation waves travelling through the heart. The dorsal maximum may be related to the activation of the posterobasal portions of the ventricles, and the upper sternal maximum to the excitation of the crista supraventricularis and pulmonary infundibulum. The time relationships between the two maxima may provide some indirect information about the time-course of excitation waves in the heart.

Green et al. [21] defined the range of normal body-surface potentials in a large population (1,113 subjects, aged 10–80 years) as a function of age, sex, and body habitus. On average, QRS potentials decreased with increasing age. Potential pattern distributions remained constant from 10 to 40 years; about 30% of the subjects older than 40 years had early negative potentials recorded more diffusely over the right thorax. This resulted in more vertically oriented zero equipotential lines. Only minor differences concerning QRS potential amplitude and distributions were noted when male and female subjects were compared within groups of similar age and body habitus.

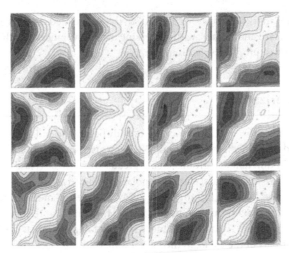

▣ Fig. 10.9

AC maps of body-surface recordings during the QRS interval in 12 healthy individuals, which are representative of the normal variability of ventricular depolarization. Same conventions as in ❷ Fig. 10.4c

Interindividual variability is due to variability of the thorax conductor [29] and source variability [30]. Normal variability of the ventricular activation may be due to the well-known variability of the conduction system.

We computed AC maps in 236 normal recordings from the dataset of Dr. F. Kornreich (Vrije University of Brussels, Belgium). We sorted them using divisive clustering analysis taking the correlation coefficient as a measure of distance between AC maps. Twelve prototype cases spanning the whole spectrum of variability of AC maps of normal activation are shown in ❷ Fig. 10.9. In each activation AC map, the size of white ($R > 0.8$) regions along the main diagonal corresponds to periods of relative stability of body-surface distribution of potentials (apart from amplitude). Sometimes, these regions are distinct, as the transition from one pattern to the next is sudden (as in types 3 and 4), while in other cases, it is less distinct, as the transition is gradual (as in type 10). Usually, three such phases can be identified, the first two being separated by the ventricular breakthrough. The dark region, which occurs symmetrically between the first two phases, corresponds to the relatively opposed disposition of potential extrema on the body surface before and after ventricular breakthrough. The third phase corresponds to activation of the basal regions of the ventricles and pulmonary infundibulum and has a very variable relationship with the first two.

The amplitudes and surface distributions of time integrals during ventricular activation were firstly reported by Montague et al. [31] in 40 men and 15 healthy women and subsequently by many other authors. The QRS integral map is characterized by a dipolar distribution with a minimum in the mid-sternal area and a maximum in the left mammary-axillary region (❷ Fig. 10.2).

In children, the main features of the maps are similar to those observed in adults. There are, however, minor differences; for instance, the sternal maximum during the last stage of QRS was present only in a small percentage of children [22], but invariably appeared during peak inspiration in the series of subjects studied by Flaherty [32]. According to Liebman et al. [23], the location of the terminal maximum can be right superior-anterior, anterior-superior, or right posterior, probably suggesting that the end of activation is in the right ventricular outflow tract, in the superior septum, or in the posterobasal left ventricle.

In newborn infants, Tazawa and Yoshimoto [24] observed that during ventricular excitation, the initial potential maximum migrated to the right instead of moving to the left and dorsally as in normal adults. This behavior of the maximum was attributed to the physiological predominance of the right ventricle in the newborn heart. Benson et al. [25] described the evolution of the surface potential during ventricular excitation and recovery in the first year of life. There was a progression of change in the body-surface QRS potential distribution: at birth. A single QRS maximum migrated to the right during the second half of QRS; at several months of age, the initial maximum evolved into two maxima: one moving to the right, and the other to the left; at 9–12 months of age, the initial maximum moved to the left lateral thorax, while the right maximum almost disappeared. Moreover, the age-related changes of the QRS maps were associated with similar changes on the repolarization maps; with increasing age, movement of both the excitation and the recovery positive potentials to the right chest progressively disappeared.

10.4.3 Ventricular Repolarization

Sizeable recovery potentials usually appear at the surface of the body before the end of the QRS interval [14] (❷ Fig. 10.7h). This finding was confirmed and quantified by Spach et al. [33], who also reported that the time overlapping of excitation and recovery potentials varied in different age groups, being greater in younger classes (8–12 and 20–29 years). In some subjects, the overlap lasted for 12–28 ms. The first signs of repolarization consist of a potential maximum, which generally appears on the sternal area, on the left precordium or, in a few cases, even more laterally, on the left axillary region (❷ Fig. 10.7h). In the latter case, the maximum soon moves toward the central anterior chest area (❷ Fig. 10.10a). During the early phase of recovery, the minimum is often ill-defined. The most negative areas can be found anywhere around the maximum, in the anterior lower part of the torso, in the lateral wall, or in the back [14].

This potential distribution is essentially in agreement with that described by Spach [33] in subjects 8–60 years old during the first 50 ms of ventricular recovery. Within 100–150 ms from the onset of ST the most negative potentials concentrate in an area covering the right scapular region, the right shoulder, the clavicular, and the upper sternal regions (❷ Fig. 10.10). In a minority of adult subjects, the most negative areas are located in the right clavicular or scapular regions from the beginning of repolarization. During the T wave the minimum is consistently found in the right clavicular or scapular areas and the maximum in the precordial region [12, 14]. Slight shifts of the potential extrema are usually observed during the entire T interval (❷ Fig. 10.10).

In a large normal population, Green et al. [21] observed that ST-T potentials decreased with age in both sexes. Moreover, in female subjects over the age of 40, there were more extensive low-level negative potentials over the precordium during the ST segment than in men. On the other hand, male subjects consistently showed greater T potential amplitudes.

The early repolarization deviation index (ERDI, see ❷ Sect. 10.3.4) is about twice as high as in females compared to males [34]. LRDI is higher in males. As the correlation coefficients between instantaneous potentials in the same subject are invariant to the features of the thorax conductor [13], it proves that gender differences in repolarization potentials are not entirely due to the systematic anatomical differences in thorax shape and conductivity between the genders, but must be due, at least in part, to differences in myocardial repolarization gradients.

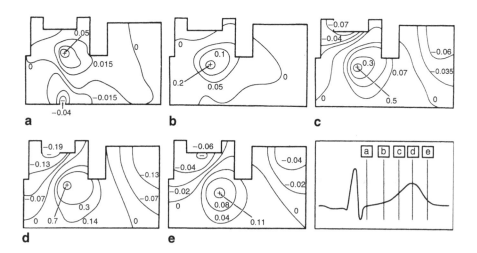

❏ Fig. 10.10

Body-surface maps during normal ventricular recovery. Each map refers to the instant or time indicated by the vertical line intersecting the ECG (After Taccardi et al. [15]. © Clarendon, Oxford. Reproduced with permission)

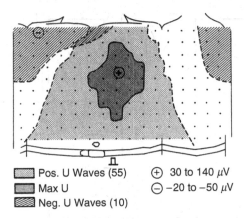

▨ Pos. U Waves (55)	⊕ 30 to 140 μV
▨ Max U	⊖ −20 to −50 μV
▨ Neg. U Waves (10)	

▣ **Fig. 10.11**

Location or potential maxima and minima during the U wave in 55 normal subjects aged 8–60 years (After Spach et al. [17].
© American Heart Association, Dallas, Texas. Reproduced with permission)

The integral maps of QRST deflections are thought to provide valuable information on the ventricular recovery process [35]. Areas of QRST deflection mainly reflect the intrinsic recovery properties and are largely independent of the ventricular excitation sequence. Actually, at the body surface, negative QRST integrals should be recorded from areas facing myocardial regions with longer recovery durations, whereas positive values are recorded from the thoracic surface facing cardiac regions with shorter recovery durations.

In normal subjects the ST-T and the QRST integral maps show a bipolar distribution of the values with a minimum on the right clavicular–upper sternal areas and a maximum on the mammary region (❯ Fig. 10.2).

A few descriptions of accurate recordings of potential distributions during the U wave have been reported [17, 36, 37]. Spach and associates [17] studied 11 children aged 1–7 years and 55 subjects aged 8–60. In the 11 children, no measurable U wave was found. In the remaining subjects, positive U-wave potentials were located within a broad area on the anterior and left lateral chest surface (❯ Fig. 10.11); the magnitude of the potential maximum varied from 30 to 140 μV. The highest U voltages were confined to the precordial area where the highest T voltages occurred. In most subjects, the specific locations of T-wave and U-wave maxima were coincident; in 17 subjects, the U-wave maximum was slightly to the right of the T-wave maximum. Clear-cut negative U waves were found in only 10 of the 55 subjects. The negative peaks varied from −20 to −50 μV and occurred on the right clavicular or scapular areas (❯ Fig. 10.11).

10.5   BSPM in Heart Disease

10.5.1   Ischemic Heart Disease

10.5.1.1   Myocardial Infarction

Descriptions of the potential distribution on the body surface in patients with anterior or inferior myocardial infarction (MI) have been published by many authors [38–53].

An attempt was made to define quantitatively the characteristic features and the range of variation of surface maps in anterior and inferior myocardial infarction during ventricular activation and recovery [38].

In patients with anterior MI (❯ Fig. 10.12), at the onset of ventricular activation, the potential minimum was located in the sternal or left mammary region. In some patients, the minimum lay outside the area where the minima were located in normal subjects. In MI patients, the minimum remained confined to a limited zone on the anterior chest wall throughout the QRS interval, whereas in normal subjects, it migrated leftward and dorsally.

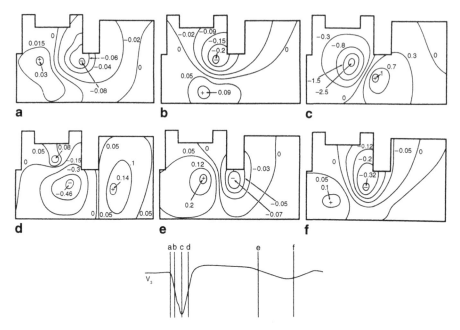

Fig. 10.12

Body-surface maps in a subject with anterior MI. Each map refers to the instant of time indicated by the vertical fine crossing the ECG. Potential values are expressed in millivolts

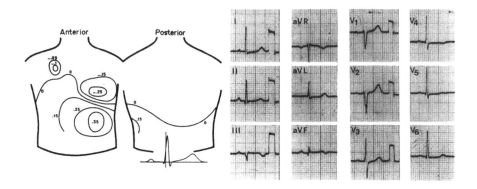

Fig. 10.13

Body-surface map of a patient with an old anterior MI not revealed by the 12-lead ECG. During the early phases of the QRS interval an abnormal potential minimum is present on the left mammary region above the area explored by the standard precordial leads

    The persistence of a negative area on the anterior chest surface could be ascribed to the presence of an infarcted region in the underlying ventricular wall. This region did not depolarize and thus acted as a current sink. Occasionally, the minimum was located above the area explored by conventional precordial leads; in these cases, as in ❷ Fig. 10.13, the 12-lead ECG did not reveal any sign of anterior MI although there are suspicious changes in the inferior leads III, aVF, and the anterolateral leads V4–V6. In 13 subjects with anterior MI, the highest absolute value of the potential minimum varied between 1.06 and 4.77 mV (mean 2.78 ± 0.3) and was significantly higher than in normal subjects ($p < 0.01$).

At the onset of ventricular activation, the location of the potential maximum was normal in the majority of cases. However, the migration of the maximum was clearly abnormal, as could be expected since the area through which the maximum should normally have passed during its migration was occupied by the potential minimum. During the first 30 ms of ventricular activation the behavior of the maximum varied. In the majority of cases, it moved superiorly toward the neck, then posteriorly toward the left scapular region, and finally reached the left axillary region; in other patients (❷ Fig. 10.12), the maximum migrated inferiorly on the anterior chest wall and reached the left axillary region; in two cases, in which the maximum was located in the left submammary region, it stayed in the same area. These various trajectories were probably related to the different extent and topography of the infarction. During the following phases of ventricular excitation the behavior of the potential maximum was within normal limits. The highest value reached by the potential maximum was significantly lower than that observed in normal subjects (mean 1.29 mV ± 0.23 standard error; $p < 0.01$). Moreover, the highest positive value was reached later than in normal subjects ($p < 0.01$), occurring between 30 and 66 ms (mean 41.8 ± 2.6).

At the beginning of the ST interval, the surface potential values were very low and the potential minimum was ill-defined, whereas the maximum was usually well developed, as occurs in normal subjects. The electronegative areas were located either on the left lateral wall of the chest, or on the lower part of the back, or both. These features are similar to those observed in normals. During the T interval, a clear-cut minimum generally appeared in the left mammary or submammary region. This location is definitely abnormal (see ❷ Fig. 10.10). In some patients, another minimum was simultaneously present in a normal area; that is, the upper sternal region. The location of the T minimum over the precordial area facing the infarction could be explained by assuming that the infarcted area did not generate recovery currents of its own and acted as a sink for repolarization currents originating in the surrounding, uninjured myocardial tissues. The highest values reached by the recovery maximum were significantly lower than in normal subjects ($p < 0.01$), whereas the highest values reached by the minimum were significantly higher ($p < 0.01$).

During the ST interval and the initial portion of the T wave, the recovery maximum was located within the normal area on the anterior chest wall (❷ Fig. 10.12e). During the second half of the T wave, in the majority of cases, the potential maxima moved away from the area where they had appeared (❷ Fig. 10.12f), and mainly scattered over the anterior lower thoracic surface. This late migration of the potential maximum was not observed in any of the normal subjects. This phenomenon is quantified by the late repolarization deviation index (LRDI, see ❷ Sect. 10.3.4), which increases in non-ischemic ventricular hypertrophy [54] as well as in old myocardial infarction compared to normal [55], even when adjusted for gender, being higher in males [34].

In the 14 cases of inferior myocardial infarction (❷ Fig. 10.14), the potential minimum was located within or near the normal area at the beginning of the QRS interval. It then moved to the inferior half of the posterior or anterior chest wall, thus passing beyond the limits of the normal scatter for the relevant instants of time. At 20 ms, the minimum was located outside the normal area in the great majority of patients. The low position of the minimum, which was observed in all patients with inferior MI at 20–30 ms, was most likely related to the presence of an infarcted area in the diaphragmatic wall of the heart. This area of non-depolarizing tissue acted as a "window" through which the depolarization currents generated by normal cardiac muscle reentered the heart.

During the following instants, the minimum migrated toward the midsternal region in some patients; in the other patients (❷ Fig. 10.14b), a new separate minimum appeared in the sternal region between 22 and 42 ms after the beginning of the QRS interval, while the first minimum was disappearing. Here, as in normal subjects, the sternal minimum was attributed to right ventricular breakthrough.

The highest absolute value of the negative potential varied between 0.45 and 1.67 mV (mean 1.3 ± 0.1) and was significantly lower than in the authors' normal subjects ($p < 0.01$). The low absolute value reached by the sternal minimum could be explained by the fact that the solid angle viewing the negative aspect of the wavefront from the sternum was smaller than in normal conditions because the wavefront did not extend over the entire diaphragmatic wall of the heart. In the authors' experience, in patients with inferior myocardial infarction, the behavior of the potential maximum during the QRS interval (❷ Fig. 10.14), its area of distribution, and its highest absolute value were within normal limits.

At the beginning of the ST interval, electronegative areas could be found on the lower half of the trunk anteriorly and posteriorly, as in normal subjects. During the T wave, the recovery minimum moved to or remained in the inferior half of the trunk (❷ Fig. 10.14e). The abnormally low location of the minimum during the T wave could be ascribed to the presence of an infarcted area in the diaphragmatic wall of the heart, which acted as a sink for recovery currents.

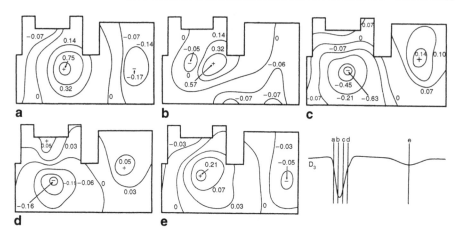

◻ Fig. 10.14

Body-surface map of a patient with inferior MI. Each map refers to the instant of time indicated by the vertical line crossing the ECG. Potential values are expressed in millivolts. The time interval between successive bars is 15 ms

The location of the recovery maximum was within the normal area, i.e., the sternal or left mammary region, during the entire recovery process (❷ Fig. 10.14e). The highest absolute values reached by the recovery maximum and minimum were not significantly different from those observed in normal subjects.

Potential patterns similar to those mentioned above were also described by Vincent and coworkers [43] in 28 subjects with inferior MI. These authors were also able to detect on BSPMs the characteristic features of inferior infarction in eight patients, whose ECGs had returned to normal or were nondiagnostic for the previous infarction. Similar findings were obtained by Osugi et al. [47].

Hirai et al. [48] described an abnormal location of the minimum at 15 ms into the QRS in 26 of the 32 cases of anterior myocardial infarction with a normal 12-lead ECG.

The possibility of detecting signs of myocardial infarction by means of body-surface mapping, even when the conventional ECG was within normal limits, was also demonstrated by Flowers et al. [41, 42]. Using departure maps, abnormalities of potential distribution were found in patients with anterior or inferior MI at the onset of ventricular excitation (corresponding to the Q wave in the conventional ECG) and during the mid-phases and late phases of the QRS interval [41].

Ohta et al. [46] compared body-surface maps with left ventriculographic findings in 24 patients with old infero-posterior MI. Using the departure-map technique as proposed by Flowers [41], they found surface potential abnormalities owing to infarction during specific phases of the QRS interval and in specific areas on the chest surface, depending on the location and extent of ventricular asynergy. In particular, some patients with inferior MI and, in addition, severe asynergy of the anterior, apical, or septal segments but without ECG or VCG signs of anterior MI, exhibited definite abnormalities of departure maps, which were different from those related to purely inferior MI.

De Ambroggi et al. [39] recorded BSPMs in 30 patients with old inferior myocardial infarction. Of these, 15 had no signs of necrosis in the conventional ECG. A number of variables relative to the instantaneous potential distribution and to integral maps were considered. The most accurate diagnostic criterion was derived from the integral values of the first 40 ms of QRS, with a sensitivity of 73% in patients without signs of necrosis in the 12-lead ECG, and of 100% in patients with pathological Q waves in the ECG, with a specificity of 83%.

In non-Q myocardial infarction of the anterolateral wall, the integral maps of the first 40 ms of QRS provided a good sensitivity (67%) in detecting signs (areas of values two standard deviations lower than normal) of the old necrosis in a group of patients with normal ECG [40].

Medvegy et al. recorded BSPM in 45 patients with documented non-Q-wave MI [52]. The main abnormality revealed by BSPM was the loss of electrical potential, but different features were characteristic for each region of the heart, so that they were suitable for the detection and localization of non-Q-wave MI, in the clinical setting of unstable coronary artery disease.

10.5.1.2 Acute Myocardial Infarction

Since the late 1970s, a simplified method of electrocardiographic mapping has been widely used in acute MI in order to obtain data on the infarct size and to assess the efficacy of various therapeutic interventions aimed at limiting myocardial injury [56].

The simplified method consists in recording 35–70 ECGs from the left hemithorax and in calculating the sum of the amplitudes of ST-segment elevations at all electrode sites, and the number of points with ST elevation. Similar procedures have also been used to evaluate the appearance of pathological Q waves and the reduction of R waves on the thoracic area explored.

The use of thoracic maps for assessing infarct size is based on experimental observations in animals demonstrating that any intervention that provokes an extension or reduction of the epicardial ischemic areas produces similar variations of the precordial areas, in which ST elevation is recorded [57, 58]. The use of these simplified methods of electrocardiographic mapping for assessing the extent of the infarction has aroused much criticism [59, 60]. In fact, there are several factors, other than the dimensions of the infarct, which can influence the ST segment elevation and, to a lesser extent, the QRS complex. These factors consist of local intraventricular conduction disturbances, electrophysiological changes in the myocardium outside the ischemic area, electrical cancellation phenomena, intra-extracellular electrolyte levels, pericarditis, heart rate, and autonomic nervous system activity. Despite the above considerations, the method does offer some definite advantages in monitoring patients with acute MI, in that it can reveal variations in the extent and severity of the ischemic process earlier than other methods, such as enzyme levels and myocardial scanning.

A description of the ST-T potential distribution on the entire chest surface in acute MI was reported by Mirvis [61], who observed a characteristic early appearance of the repolarization potentials in both anterior and inferior MI, with a longer than normal overlap between final excitation and recovery potential patterns. During the ST-T interval, the potential distributions were characterized in anterior MI by a single maximum on the left anterior chest that remained fixed in location but increased in amplitude as repolarization progressed; in inferior MI, there was a single minimum generally located on the left anterior-superior thorax, with positive potentials covering the lower thoracic portions.

The distribution of QRS and ST potentials in acute inferior myocardial infarction (mean 76 h after the onset of symptoms) has been studied by Montague et al. [62]. They computed integral maps in a group of 36 patients with acute inferior MI, and found negative areas over much of the inferior torso with extension of the positivity to the superior torso, during the first half of the QRS interval (Q zone); conversely, the ST segment integral map was characterized by abnormally positive inferior distributions and concomitant negative precordial distributions. Moreover, patients with right ventricular involvement tended to have a greater area of negative Q zone over the right anterior inferior thorax and greater inferior and rightward extension of ST segment positivity as compared with patients with exclusive left ventricular infarction. Thus, in acute inferior MI, BSPMs make it possible to detect definite abnormalities of both depolarization and repolarization potentials, which indicate right ventricular involvement.

More recently, Menown et al. [63] confirmed the ability of BSPMs (using 80 leads) to improve, with respect to conventional ECG, the classification of inferior acute MI with posterior or right ventricular wall involvement.

The same group demonstrated that the BSPM diagnostic algorithm detected acute MI with higher sensitivity than a 12-lead ECG diagnostic algorithm or a physician's interpretation, without loss of specificity [64]. They also showed the superiority of BSPM versus the 12-lead ECG in detecting acute MI in the presence of left bundle branch block (LBBB) [65].

10.5.1.3 Myocardial Ischemia

In angina patients, the resting ECG is very often normal between attacks. This can indicate that cardiac electrogenesis is normal or that there are electrical abnormalities, which are not revealed by the conventional ECG because they are too small, or because they are projected to surface areas not explored by conventional leads.

In several patients with proven angina pectoris and a normal resting ECG, surface maps exhibited an abnormal distribution of recovery potentials [66]. In these patients, the location of the potential minimum during recovery was outside the normal range during some phases of the ST segment and of the T wave, often on the lower left lateral region of the chest (❱ Fig. 10.15a).

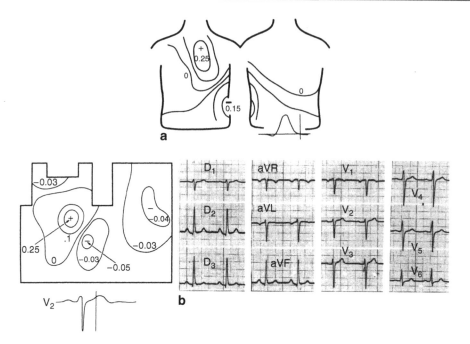

◻ Fig. 10.15

(a) BSPM of a patient with angina and normal resting ECG. The map refers to the early ST interval, as indicated by the vertical line crossing the ECG. This potential pattern lasted about 200 ms. Potential values are expressed in millivolts. (b) BSPM at the instant indicated by the vertical line crossing the ECG, in a patient with angina but normal T waves on the resting ECG. The map shows a complex potential distribution with one maximum and two minima

During the entire ST-T interval the potential maximum was located within the normal area in most patients with angina. Only in a few subjects was the location of the maximum abnormal during the final phases of ventricular recovery. In some of these patients with angina and a normal resting ECG, a complex potential distribution was observed (❯ Fig. 10.15b), with one maximum and one minimum located normally and a second minimum placed in an abnormal position.

In a study [67] performed on 14 patients with stable angina and a normal resting ECG, the analysis of BSPMs was extended to a new series of quantitative aspects; that is, temporal evolution during the ST-T interval of the highest potential on the chest, lowest potential, highest potential difference, integral of the absolute value of the potential function extended over the entire chest surface, and the percentage of the total thoracic area with positive potentials. By deriving a number of voltage-related variables from these time functions and by submitting them to multivariate analysis, it was possible to separate more than 90% of the ischemic patients from normal subjects. It has been shown [68] that, in some patients with typical angina but no evidence of MI, QRS potentials can differ from normal at some chest locations, which are not explored by the standard 12 leads.

BSPMs were also used to study the potential variations before, during, and after coronary angioplasty (PTCA). During balloon inflation in the anterior descending or right coronary artery, specific changes of QRS instantaneous and integral maps were observed, suggesting a regional conduction delay due to myocardial ischemia [69].

Shenasa et al. [70] demonstrated potential patterns 40 ms after QRS end during inflation that were specific to the three major coronary arteries dilated. The left anterior descending coronary artery was associated with the largest ST-segment shifts with a precordial maximum and negative potentials over the back; for the right coronary artery, negative potentials covered the upper left torso with a left mid-axillary minimum and positive potentials over the rest of the torso; for the left circumflex coronary artery, negative potentials covered the anterior torso with a precordial minimum and positive potentials over the back. These changes disappeared rapidly after balloon deflation. Thus, BSPMs provide a comprehensive approach for the evaluation of electrocardiographic changes and the development of optimal leads for the detection of acute occlusion of a coronary artery.

BSPMs were also used to evaluate the clinical efficacy of PTCA and were proved useful to detect restenosis [71].

10.5.1.4 Exercise Maps

Potential maps have been obtained during exercise in normal subjects and patients with angina.

Some authors [72] recorded ECGs from 16 points located on the left anterior thorax, using traditional methods. This technique should be more appropriately considered as a system of multiple precordial leads rather than surface mapping. The 16-lead system, however, has shown greater sensitivity than 12 standard leads or three orthogonal leads [73], although this has not been confirmed by other groups.

Other investigators studied the instantaneous potential distribution on the anterior thorax [74, 75] or on the entire chest [76–79]. A complete and accurate study on the QRS and ST-T wave changes induced by exercise was performed by Spach's group in healthy subjects [76]. These authors were able to obtain high-quality potential maps during exercise without averaging ECG waveforms, by using their system for calculating total body potential distributions from 24 chest leads. Exercise induced consistent changes in potential patterns. During the first 20 ms of QRS, the minimum stayed on the lower left chest, while, in the resting condition, it gradually migrated toward the upper back. In mid-QRS, the magnitude of the anterior potential maximum was approximately 60% of that observed in the map at rest while the duration of the QRS interval usually increased (2–10 ms) at peak exercise. On the basis of these findings, it was suggested that the decrease in the magnitude of the precordial potential maximum in the midportion of QRS (R wave in lead V5) might result from changes in the sequence of activation of the ventricles, rather than from blood volume variations (Brody effect).

In the early stage of ventricular repolarization (early ST segment), a potential minimum usually developed on the lower left thorax during exercise. This minimum generally decreased in magnitude in a short time after exercise. During the subsequent instants of the ST interval, the lower left precordial region became less negative and was usually positive by the early portion of the T wave. At the peak of the T wave the potential pattern showed slight changes during and after exercise with respect to the resting condition. However, the amplitude did change considerably. In particular, immediately after exercise, the magnitude of T-wave potentials increased rapidly, reaching its highest value 30–90 s after the end of exercise, before gradually decreasing; in some subjects, the potential values were still higher than resting values 10 min after exercise.

In patients with angina, Simoons and Block [77] reported some typical changes induced by exercise. The recovery minimum was located in the lower part of the left side of the chest and attained −90 μV or more 60 ms after the end of the QRS complex. This repolarization pattern was found in 21 out of 25 coronary patients, but in none of the normal subjects (sensitivity 84%, specificity 100%).

Yanowitz et al. [79] recorded BSMs before and after exercise in 25 males with documented coronary disease. By considering the integrals of the first 80 ms of the ST interval, they found abnormal negative values in 18 cases. Moreover, in 25% of the cases, BSPMs after exercise showed maximal depression of the ST-segment area at sites not sampled by the leads usually employed in exercise testing. This finding suggests that BSPMs may increase the sensitivity of the exercise testing for coronary disease.

10.5.2 Right Ventricular Hypertrophy

Hypertrophy may involve various portions of the right ventricle in different forms of heart disease. In children BSPMs were recorded in the following types of right ventricular hypertrophy (RVH) [80]: dilation of right ventricle and hypertrophy of the crista supraventricularis owing to secundum atrial septal defect; hypertrophy of the entire right ventricle, including the outflow tract, secondary to valvular pulmonic stenosis; hypertrophy of the proximal portion of the right ventricle between the tricuspid valve and the infundibular stenosis, with normal thickness of the right ventricular wall in the outflow tract, beneath the pulmonary valve (tetralogy of Fallot).

While, in normal subjects, during the second half of the QRS interval, the potential maximum moves from the precordial area toward the left axillary region and then to the back, in all patients with RVH, it migrated toward the right chest.

The movement of the maximum on the right thorax was different according to the various pathological conditions [80]. In atrial septal defect (ostium secundum) the maximum moved to the right mammary region, finally reaching the upper sternal region. In tetralogy of Fallot with infundibular stenosis, the maxima migrated toward the right lateral thoracic wall. In valvular pulmonic stenosis, the maximum migrated on the anterior right chest toward the upper central area, as in atrial septal defect; the potential values, however, were markedly higher.

These surface potential patterns were correlated with the spread of excitation through the right ventricular wall, as determined in the same patients at surgery. In all three types of RVH, the activation wavefront moved on the epicardial surface in a rightward direction. In atrial septal defect, the latest epicardial events were recorded along the atrioventricular groove and gave rise to a right-chest maximum. However, after completion of epicardial excitation on the right ventricle, a potential maximum persisted over the upper sternal area. This terminal maximum was probably related to an activation wavefront spreading through the upper part of the septum and the crista supraventricularis, which is most likely hypertrophied in right ventricular volume overload.

In valvular pulmonic stenosis, as the wavefront moved laterally across the right ventricular free wall, it produced a maximum over the right chest while a minimum was positioned over the left precordium. The terminal excitation wavefront spread superiorly through the outflow tract of the right ventricle and gave rise to the upper sternal maximum.

In tetralogy of Fallot, after right ventricular breakthrough occurred, the wavefront moved laterally toward the atrioventricular groove and produced a maximum over the lower mid-right chest with a minimum in the left precordial region. The latest portions of the right ventricle to be depolarized were along the lateral inferior part of the atrioventricular groove. The final orientation of the wavefront was such that it resulted in a maximum in the right axillary region with a minimum over the central chest. Thus, maps enable the different types of RVH to be recognized to a greater extent than does the 12-lead ECG.

Body-surface maps in adult patients with RVH owing to mild-to-moderate valvular pulmonic stenosis were obtained by Sohi et al. [81]. Using departure maps, they observed a delayed appearance of the sternal negativity, which is usually related to right ventricular breakthrough, and an abnormal positivity located in the upper anterior chest.

10.5.3   Left Ventricular Hypertrophy

Body-surface maps in patients with left ventricular hypertrophy (LVH) owing to mild-to-moderate aortic stenosis were studied by Sohi et al. [81], using the departure-map technique. They observed an abnormal delay of early negativity on the anterior right chest and a potential maximum on the upper anterior chest, which peaked later and lasted longer than normal.

An assessment of left ventricular mass in patients with LVH was attempted by Holt et al. [82] on the basis of chest-surface potential distribution. They used a mathematical model in which the ventricles and the septum were represented by 12 dipoles. The dipole activity was assumed to be proportional to the amount of viable myocardium in that region; the strength of each dipole as a function of time was determined by measuring potentials at 126 locations on the thoracic surface and by applying suitable transfer coefficients. A good correlation was found between left ventricular mass determined by angiography and that determined by surface potentials ($r = 0.85$). Moreover, the correlation coefficient was much higher using BSMs than other electrocardiographic recordings (12 standard ECG leads or VCG).

Yamaki et al. [83] used BSPMs recorded with 87 leads to determine the severity of LVH in 57 patients with concentric hypertrophy and in 30 with left ventricular dilatation. A number of parameters related to QRS voltages and ventricular activation time were measured, and some of them were proven useful in determining the severity of LVH.

Kornreich et al. [84] studied BSPMs during the entire cardiac cycle (PQRST) in 122 patients with LVH. Best classification results were achieved with ST-T features, followed by features from the P wave, QRS, and PR segment. Cumulative use of ST-T and P features yielded a specificity of 94% with a sensitivity of 88%.

Hirai et al. [85] studied QRST integral maps in patients with LVH (10 with aortic stenosis, 12 with aortic regurgitation, and 22 with hypertrophic cardiomyopathy). Abnormalities in patients with hypertrophic cardiomyopathy were manifest even in mild LVH and a greater disparity of repolarization was found in hypertrophic cardiomyopathy than in LVH due to aortic valve disease.

We reported the results on BSPMs recorded in 16 patients with LVH due to aortic stenosis, focusing on the analysis of ventricular repolarization, with the aim of searching for subtle alterations not revealed by the usual ECG processing, which are likely to reflect ventricular repolarization heterogeneities [54].

The classical signs of LVH in the standard ECG (increased QRS voltage and ST-T changes) are reflected on BSPMs as (1) increased amplitude of the QRS integral map and of the STT integral map, (2) relatively low amplitude of the QRST integral map, due to the cancellation between the depolarization and repolarization potentials, and (3) opposing aspects of the QRS and STT integral maps.

In order to detect possible minor electrical disparities of repolarization not apparent from visual inspection of the ST-T and QRST maps, we analyzed the morphology of all the recorded ST-T waves, using principal component analysis. In our patients, the "similarity index," defined as the first eigenvalue divided by the sum of all eigenvalues, was slightly but significantly lower than in control subjects (0.73 vs 0.77; $p = 0.027$), suggesting the presence of a degree of heterogeneity of repolarization higher than in the normals. The repolarization deviation indices were also computed, as described in the methods. In our LVH patients, the changes during early repolarization, as reflected by ERDI, were similar to those observed in our control group and also in the larger group of 159 normal subjects from the database of Dr. F. Kornreich (Vrije University of Brussels, Belgium). Then, we focused on the analysis of the T peak-T end period, during which possible heterogeneities of repolarization should be more likely to be detected. The LRDI was significantly higher ($p = 0.005$) in LVH patients than in normals. The values of similarity index and LRDI found in LVH patients suggest a higher than normal degree of repolarization heterogeneity, not detected by the usual electrocardiographic analysis.

10.5.4 Right Bundle Branch Block

Several types of potential patterns have been observed in patients with right bundle branch block (RBBB) [86–88]. During the initial phases of ventricular activation, the surface potential distribution was similar to that observed in normal subjects with a maximum located on the sternal or left mammary region and a minimum on the left chest wall or in the dorsal regions (❷ Fig. 10.16b). The sternal minimum, which indicates right ventricular breakthrough and which occurs in normal subjects 14–44 ms after the onset of the QRS complex, did not appear. Only at a later stage (38–70 ms after the onset of ventricular activation) did a second minimum appear, which, however, was located in an abnormal position, that is, in the left mammary region (❷ Fig. 10.16d). It should be noted that this second minimum usually occurred to the right of the potential maximum located on the left precordium. This maximum was attributed to the spread of excitation through the left ventricular wall, while the delayed minimum was interpreted as the result of excitation arriving on the surface of the left ventricle, most probably in the left paraseptal region or in the apical area.

Shortly after the appearance of the second minimum, a new potential maximum appeared on the right precordium (❷ Fig. 10.16c). This led to a complex potential distribution with two maxima (left and right) and two minima (on the right clavicular region and on the left precordial area), indicating the simultaneous presence of two excitation waves spreading into the left and right ventricles. Subsequently, the two negative areas merged, while the left maximum shifted to the back (❷ Fig. 10.16g) and eventually disappeared, as in normal subjects, about 80 ms after the onset of the QRS complex. Thus, during the final stages of the QRS interval, only the signs of delayed right ventricular activation persisted, with a maximum on the right anterior chest wall and a minimum on the left precordial area (❷ Fig. 10.17a–c). At the end of the QRS complex, early recovery potentials could often be observed before the last excitation potentials disappeared. Usually, the activation maximum and minimum shifted slightly to the right, and the recovery maximum appeared in the left mammary region, giving rise to patterns with three extrema (❷ Fig. 10.17d). Later, only two extrema remained: the recovery minimum in the sternal or right mammary region and the recovery maximum in the left mammary area (❷ Fig. 10.17e). This pattern persisted throughout the ST and T intervals (❷ Fig. 10.17f) and approximately represented a mirror image of the potential distribution observed during the last phases of ventricular activation.

In some patients, a different behavior of the potential maximum and minimum was observed during the midportion of QRS; that is, the anterior maximum, after reaching the precordial area, did not complete its leftward migration but reverted to the sternal region and then moved to the right precordium, thereby taking over the role of the second maximum observed in typical RBBB. The second minimum did not appear in the left parasternal region to the right of the maximum, as in typical cases, but to its left, in the external part of the left mammary region. The electrophysiological mechanism giving rise to this peculiar sequence of potential patterns observed could not be identified.

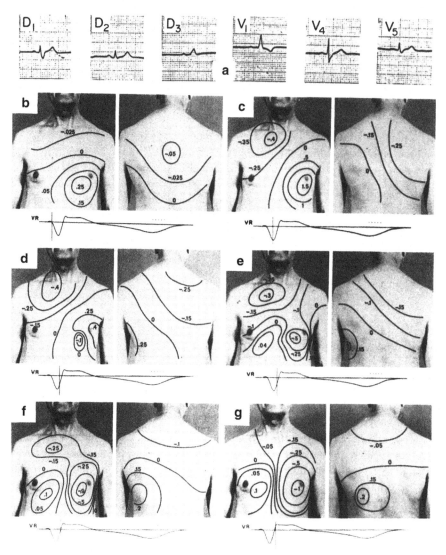

◼ Fig. 10.16

Subject with RBBB. (a) Standard ECG. (b–g) Each map refers to the instant of time indicated by the vertical line intersecting the reference ECG (VR). The values of equipotential lines are expressed in millivolts (After Taccardi et al. [86]. © Churchill Livingstone, New York. Reproduced with permission)

10.5.5   Left Bundle Branch Block

BSPMs have been described in uncomplicated left bundle branch block (LBBB), with or without left axis deviation [89–91] and in LBBB complicated by additional heart disease [90, 92].

In the uncomplicated LBBB studied by Musso et al. [90], at the onset of QRS (❷ Fig. 10.18a), the potential maximum was consistently found in the sternal area. The minimum was generally located on the right chest, anteriorly or posteriorly. A few milliseconds later a new potential distribution developed, with a minimum in the presternal area and a maximum on the left mammary region. In some patients, the minimum migrated to the sternal area from its previous location. In other cases, an independent, secondary minimum appeared in this region and subsequently increased in magnitude, while the old minimum faded away. In both cases, the minimum settled in the sternal area earlier than in

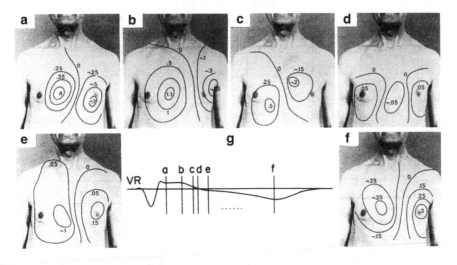

⬛ Fig. 10.17
Same subject as in ❷ Fig. 10.16. BSPMs relating to second half of ventricular activation (**a–d**) and recovery (**e, f**). At instant
d (end of QRS) recovery potentials are already present on the left side of the chest (After Taccardi et al. [86]. © Churchill
Livingstone, New York. Reproduced with permission)

normal subjects. An early appearance of this minimum, which indicates right ventricular breakthrough, was also found
by other investigators [91].

In LBBB, the initial phase of ventricular excitation differs from the normal sequence, in that the first electrical event
occurring in the normal ventricles, that is, the excitation wavefront spreading through the septum from left to right and
anteriorly, is missing. Therefore, ventricular excitation starts later than it would if the left bundle branch was functioning
normally. As a consequence, the onset of ventricular activity as a whole is delayed in relation to His-bundle excitation.

The lack of left ventricular activity may explain the differences between the maps recorded in the early stages of QRS
in LBBB patients and in normal subjects. The occurrence of the presternal minimum may be attributed, as in normal
subjects, to the excitation wavefront reaching the right ventricular surface (right ventricular breakthrough). The shorter
breakthrough time is not surprising since this time is calculated from the beginning of QRS, which is delayed in LBBB,
as indicated above.

In the subsequent stages, the maximum moved to the left axilla, while the minimum persisted in the midsternal area.
This distribution was a constant feature in the second half of QRS (❷ Fig. 10.18b). In this interval, the potential maximum
and minimum reached their peak value. However, the positive peak appeared later than the corresponding one in normal
subjects. The surface patterns mentioned above can be related to the wide excitation wavefront, which, at these stages of
the cardiac cycle, spreads through the septum from right to left and then invades the left ventricular walls.

In most cases of uncomplicated LBBB, 10–20 ms before the end of QRS a new maximum appeared in the upper sternal
area (❷ Fig. 10.18c). The maximum progressively increased in voltage and persisted throughout the ST-T interval. For this
reason it was considered to be an early manifestation of the recovery process. The recovery minimum was located in the
left axillary region (❷ Fig. 10.18d), whence it generally moved toward the dorsal area at the end of the T wave. These
events may be interpreted by inferring that (a) measurable repolarization potentials originate from the right ventricle
before left ventricular depolarization is completed because the right ventricle is the first to depolarize and (b) the left
ventricle behaves as a current sink during most of the recovery process, because of its delayed repolarization resulting
from delayed activation.

Subjects with LBBB and left axis deviation described by Sohi et al. [91] differed from those with normal axes in that
during the second half of the QRS interval, the maximum was generally located on the left shoulder and back. This pattern
was attributed to a further selective slowing of depolarization in the anterobasal portions of the left ventricle.

BSPMs in complicated LBBB have been described by two groups of investigators [90, 92]. According to Preda et al. in
LBBB associated with anterior MI, the middle third of the anterior chest wall remained negative during the final phases

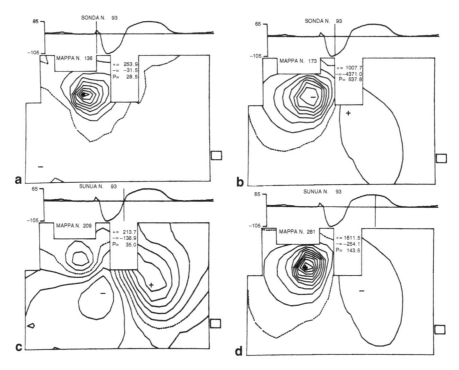

Fig. 10.18

Patient with uncomplicated LBBB. BSPMs relating to four instants of time during ventricular excitation and recovery. The zero equipotential line is dashed. The plus and minus signs indicate the value of the positive and negative peaks (in microvolts). +P and −P indicate the step (in microvolts) between adjacent positive and negative equipotential lines

of QRS. The authors attributed this finding to the lack of activation of the anterobasal region of the left ventricle, owing to the presence of the necrosis. In patients with infero-posterior MI, a persistent negativity was observed during the central portion of the QRS in the lower border of the chest, on the left lateral or posterior regions. Later, the negativity moved to the right side of the back. These findings were not confirmed by Musso et al. [90]. They studied LBBB complicated by anterior or inferior MI, LVH, myocardial ischemia, or a combination. By visually inspecting the maps, Musso et al. were unable to identify any potential pattern that could be uniquely found in a given LBBB group. However, several differences among groups were observed if the voltage values, rather than the potential patterns, were taken into account [90]. Generally, higher voltages were measured in patients with LVH and lower voltages were found in the MI groups as compared to uncomplicated cases of LBBB. These observations prompted Musso et al. to measure a set of voltage-related variables with a view to discriminating among different LBBB groups. The variables were derived by curves illustrating the behavior as a function of time during QRST of the highest instantaneous negative and positive potentials on the chest, the highest potential difference, the integral (extended to the entire chest surface) of the absolute value of the potential function, the size of the electropositive (or electronegative) thoracic areas, and so on. The statistical evaluation of the data (canonical variates analysis) permitted the classification of most complicated and uncomplicated patients into the correct group.

10.5.6 Left Anterior Fascicular Block

In left anterior fascicular block (LAFB), without MI or hypertrophy, one or more abnormal features could be detected in all patients. At the onset of QRS interval, in 8 out of 11 patients (unpublished data), the potential distribution was clearly abnormal in respect of (a) the location of the minimum, which was at a higher thoracic level with respect to the corresponding maximum, and/or (b) the anomalous position of the maximum (❷ Fig. 10.19a). This potential pattern

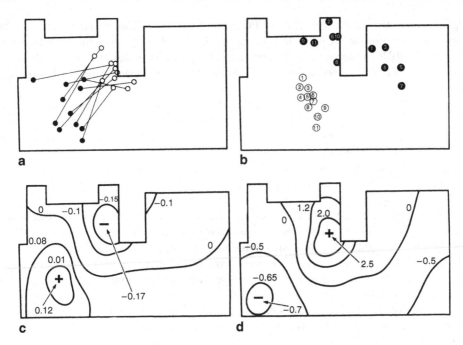

☐ **Fig. 10.19**

Top: Location of potential maxima (black circles) and minima (white circles) on the chest surface (**a**) at the onset of ventricular activation and (**b**) after 55 ms in 11 subjects with LAFB. The potential maximum and minimum relating to a given patient are indicated by the numbers inside the circles. *Bottom*: Subject with LAFB. Potential distribution at 10 ms (**c**) and at 46 ms (**d**) after the onset of ventricular activation. Potential values are expressed in millivolts

could be related to the direction of the activation wavefront, which spreads inferiorly and rightward. This anomalous direction is probably owing to the lack of early excitation of the anterosuperior portion of the left septal surface, as found in experimental studies [93].

During the mid- and late-QRS interval, a characteristic potential distribution was observed in all patients, by the authors and others [94]. After 28–30 ms from the onset of ventricular activation, the potential maximum was invariably located in the upper portion of the anterior or posterior chest surface, above the horizontal plane passing through the corresponding minimum (❷ Fig. 10.19b). The minima clustered on the lower anterior chest wall (❷ Fig. 10.19b) while the lower part of the chest was constantly electronegative. This potential distribution accounts for the left axis deviation in the standard ECG and can be attributed to the abnormal sequence of ventricular excitation in LAFB and particularly to the delayed activation of the anterosuperior part of the left ventricular wall.

The motion of the maximum to the upper thoracic areas occurred as follows. In 5 cases out of 11, the maximum did not migrate to the back, as in normal subjects, but moved directly from the left mammary region to the upper sternal or left clavicular areas. In the remaining six cases, it moved to the back and remained there (five cases) or reached the anterior left shoulder. It is suggested that in those patients where the maximum moved dorsally, a lesser degree of asynchronism existed between the activation of the posterior and anterior basal portions of the left ventricle. The variety of patterns observed may result from different degrees of delay in the anterior fascicle and/or from individual variations in the anatomical distribution of the peripheral conducting fibers.

10.5.7 Wolff–Parkinson–White Syndrome

It is well known that the Wolff–Parkinson–White (WPW) syndrome is a result of the early excitation of some portions of the ventricles through anomalous conduction pathways. These can be found at almost any location around the AV ring, including the ventricular septum. Conventional ECGs and VCGs provide useful information on the orientation and direction of propagation of the pre-excitation wavefront, but they do not enable the location of the pre-excited area to be determined reliably. A number of investigations have shown that much more information on the location of the pre-excitation focus can be gained by measuring the instantaneous potential distribution on the entire chest surface [95–102].

Yamada et al. described three types of surface maps in 22 WPW patients on the basis of QRS potential distributions [95]. Type I potential patterns were ascribed to pre-excitation of the posterior aspect of the left ventricle, type II to pre-excitation of the basal part of the right ventricle, and type III to pre-excitation in the proximity of the posterior right AV groove close to the ventricular septum.

In a group of 42 WPW patients, De Ambroggi et al. [96] were able to recognize six types of maps, on the basis of the following considerations and criteria, derived mainly from previous studies on physical, mathematical, and physiological models [1, 103, 104].

At the onset of the delta wave, the pre-excitation wavefront is small and can be approximated by a single equivalent dipole, at least as far as surface potential patterns are concerned. When the two potential extrema on the body surface have nearly equal strength, the dipole is equidistant from the surface extrema and its depth in the chest is proportional to the distance between the extrema. When one extremum is stronger than the other, the dipole is closer to the stronger extremum. The direction of the dipole is approximated by a straight line joining the two extrema. After the delta wave, the body-surface potential patterns are not clearly related to the location of the pre-excitation wavefront. However, the appearance of a sternal minimum indicating a normal right ventricular breakthrough may suggest a left or posterior localization. On the basis of these simple rules, we proposed the following classification of the patients studied.

Type 1 (❷ Figs. 10.20a, ❷ 10.21). During the delta wave, the maps of the 23 patients belonging to type 1 exhibited a potential maximum on the precordial area and a minimum on the back. It is suggested that the pre-excitation wave was located deep in the thorax, most likely in the posterobasal wall of the heart and spread in a postero-anterior direction. Between 40 and 90 ms after the onset of ventricular activation, a second minimum appeared on the sternal area in most patients, while the dorsal minimum reached the upper anterior chest wall. The second minimum was attributed to the right ventricular breakthrough. Its appearance suggested that the right anterior ventricular wall was excited through the normal pathways and was therefore not affected by pre-excitation.

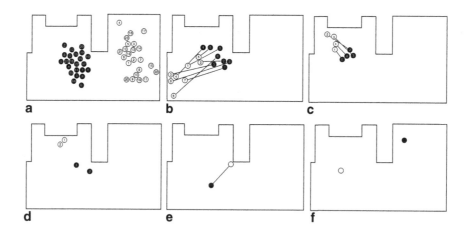

◻ Fig. 10.20

Location of potential maxima (*black circles*) and minima (*white circles*) on the chest surface during the delta wave in WPW patients belonging to type 1(a), 2(b), 3(c), 4(d), 5(e), and 6(f). The potential maximum and minimum relating to a given patient are indicated by the numbers inside the *circles* (After De Ambroggi et al. [96]. © American Heart Association, Dallas, Texas. Reproduced with permission)

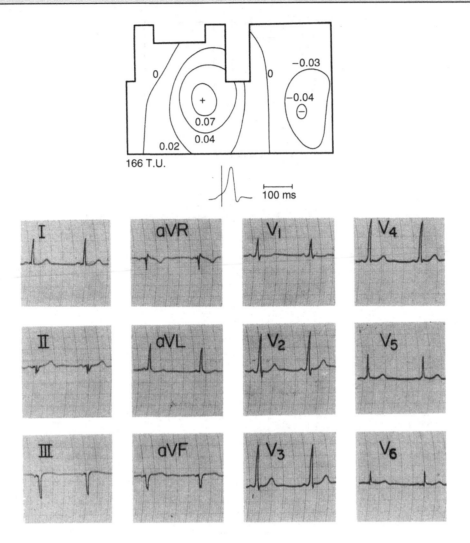

Fig. 10.21
BSPM during the delta wave, at the instant indicated by the vertical line crossing the reference ECG in a WPW subject belonging to type 1. The 12-lead ECG shows a type A WPW pattern (After De Ambroggi et al. [96]. © American Heart Association, Dallas, Texas. Reproduced with permission)

Type 2 (● Figs. 10.20b, ● 10.22). During the delta wave, in the eight patients belonging to type 2, the minimum was located on the inferior half of the right anterior chest wall and the maximum on the sternal or left mammary region. The location of the minimum and maximum suggests that the pre-excitation wave moved leftward and upward and probably spread from the lateral inferior portion of the AV groove through the right ventricular wall. In no patient of this group did a second minimum appear on the sternal area. This suggested that the right ventricular wall was not activated through the normal conducting pathways.

Type 3 (● Figs. 10.20c, ● 10.23). During the delta wave in the four type-3 patients, the minimum was initially on the back and then moved to the right subclavicular area; the maximum was located in the mid-sternal area. This potential distribution suggested that an excitation wave was spreading through the anterior wall of the right ventricle from the upper part of the right AV groove, downwards and to the left. A second minimum did not appear in the sternal area in the patients of this group, suggesting that the right ventricular wall was not excited through the normal pathways.

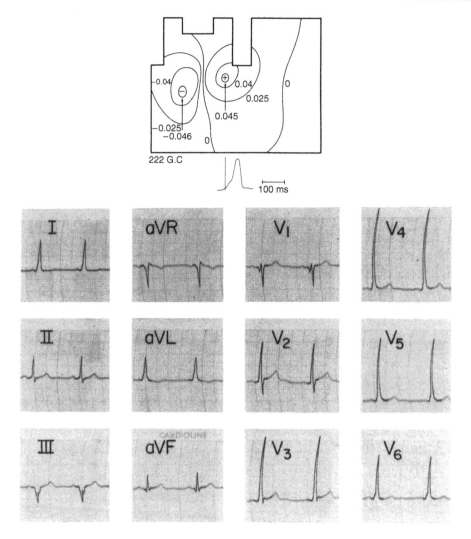

Fig. 10.22

BSPM during the delta wave in a WPW patient belonging to type 2. The ECG shows a type B WPW pattern (After De Ambroggi et al. [96]. © American Heart Association, Dallas, Texas. Reproduced with permission)

Type 4 (❯ Fig. 10.20d). Two patients were classified as type 4. During the delta wave, both the maximum and minimum were located on the left anterior chest wall, with the maximum being on the mammary region, and the minimum on the upper sternal area. This potential distribution suggested that pre-excitation probably started in the anterior portion of the left AV groove or in the anterior portion of the septal AV ring, spreading toward the apex of the left ventricle. A right-sided location was unlikely since neither extreme was on the right-chest surface. In agreement with this interpretation, a second minimum appeared on the sternal area in one patient. This minimum indicated a normal right ventricular breakthrough and showed that pre-excitation did not involve the anterior wall of the right ventricle. In the other patient, there was no second minimum; this patient, however, exhibited a sequence of surface potentials indicating right bundle branch block, which usually prevents the appearance of the sternal minimum.

Type 5 (❯ Fig. 10.20e). Type 5 was represented by a single subject. The potential minimum was located in the left axillary region and the maximum on the inferior part of the left anterior chest wall. This potential distribution indicated

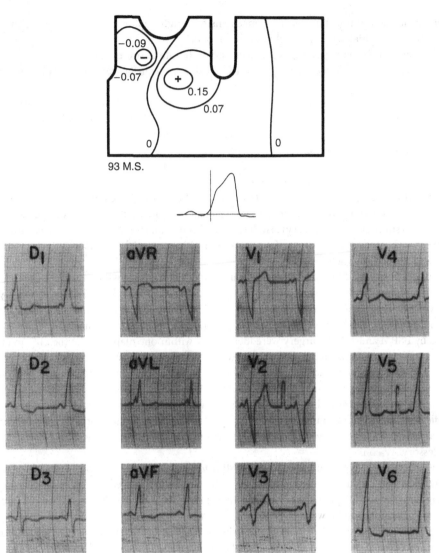

◘ Fig. 10.23
BSPM during the delta wave in a patient belonging to type 3. The ECG shows a type B WPW pattern (After De Ambroggi et al. [96]. © American Heart Association, Dallas, Texas. Reproduced with permission)

that pre-excitation most probably spreads through the left ventricular wall, starting from the anterolateral portion of the left AV groove and then moving downward and to the right.

Type 6 (❷ Fig. 10.20f). Type 6 was also represented by a single patient. The ECG showed an unusual pattern of ventricular pre-excitation. A delta wave was not clearly detectable; a small Q wave was present in V1 and the QRS duration was within normal limits. Intracardiac recordings showed a short HV interval but during ajmaline administration, the Q wave in V1 disappeared and the HV interval rose from 15 to 40 ms. At the onset of ventricular excitation, the potential distribution was characterized by a minimum at the right lower sternal border and a maximum on the left scapular area. Twenty five minutes after the onset of ventricular activation, a normal sequence of potential patterns was observed. The initial location of the minimum and maximum indicated that an excitation wave was probably spreading in an antero-posterior direction, leftward and slightly superiorly. An acceptable location for such a wavefront might be in the right side of the interventricular septum. The most likely mechanism for right septal pre-excitation would be through Mahaim fibers, stemming from the initial part of the right bundle branch.

In a number of patients belonging to types 1, 2, 3, 5, and 6, the site of pre-excitation as deduced from surface maps was in good agreement with that independently established using intracardiac recordings, epicardial maps, or surgical results [105].

Benson et al. [99] attempted to localize the site of pre-excitation in 49 WPW patients, where the location of the anomalous pathway was determined by intracardiac electrophysiological studies or surgical ablation. These authors were able to predict accurately at least seven pre-excitation sites on the basis of surface potential distribution during the QRS (at 40 ms after the onset of delta wave) and ST segment. Moreover, they found the potential distribution during early ST segment more useful than QRS maps for localizing the pre-excited area. Their classification was in reasonably good agreement with our classification previously presented.

Kamakura et al. [100] studied 41 WPW patients to determine the most reliable index for predicting the site of a single accessory pathway. They found that the location of the ventricular insertion of the accessory AV connection (determined at electrophysiological study or during surgery) is well estimated at the time the amplitude of the negative surface potential is −0.15 mV. On the basis of the chest position of the minimum with a potential of −0.15 mV, the location of the accessory AV connection was correctly predicted in 36 of 41 cases.

Liebman et al. [101] recorded BSPM in 34 patients with WPW syndrome in whom the site of ventricular insertion of the anomalous AV connection was localized by an electrophysiologic study and, in 18 cases, at surgery. Attempts were made to identify the 17 ventricular insertion sites along the AV grove described by Guiraudon et al. [106] mainly using QRS analysis (location of the initial minimum, occurrence of right ventricular breakthrough). The ventricular insertion sites determined by BSPM and EPS at surgery were identical or within one mapping site (i.e., 1.5 cm or less) in 14 of 18 cases; three of the four exceptions had more than one accessory AV connection, and the other had a very broad ventricular insertion. BSPM and EPS locations of accessory pathways correlated very well in the 34 cases despite the fact that BSPM determined the ventricular insertion and EPS the atrial insertion site of the accessory AV connection. BSPMs of QRS were very accurate in predicting the right ventricular versus left ventricular postero-septal AV connections, known to be particularly difficult at EPS in three of four surgical cases. Typical right ventricular breakthrough occurs in all patients with left ventricular free wall accessory connections, but was not observed in cases with right ventricular free wall or anteroseptal accessory AV connections.

In 1993, Dubuc et al. [102] reported on the use of BSPM to guide catheter ablation of accessory AV connection in 30 WPW patients. The catheter used for radiofrequency ablation was first placed in the vicinity of the ventricular pre-excitation site predicted by BSPMs previously recorded during the delta wave. BSPMs were then recorded during pacing with this catheter; the comparison between the pre-excited and paced BSPMs indicated whether the pacing site was too anterior or posterior with respect to the pre-excitation site, and the catheter was moved accordingly. This process was repeated until the pre-excited and paced BSPMs were almost identical, i.e., showed high correlation coefficient (>0.8) during the delta wave, and ablation was then attempted. In this way, it was possible to successfully ablate the accessory pathway in 93% of cases.

10.5.8   Arrhythmogenic Cardiopathies

10.5.8.1   Postinfarction Ventricular Tachycardias: Identification of Site of Origin of Ventricular Tachycardias

Extensive investigations were made by Sippens-Groenewegen et al. to assess the value of BSPMs in localizing the site of origin of ectopic ventricular activation in patients with a structurally normal heart and with myocardial infarction [107–109]. In patients with normal cardiac anatomy, the QRS maps allowed discrimination among 38 different LV and RV segments of ectopic endocardial impulse formation [107]. The use of 62 lead BSPMs instead of the 12-lead ECG during endocardial pace mapping technique enhanced the localization resolution of this technique and thus enabled more precise identification of the site of origin of postinfarction VT episodes [108].

In patients with previous anterior and inferior myocardial infarction, the same authors demonstrated that QRS integral maps enabled a precise localization of the origin of postinfarction ventricular tachycardia in 62% and regional approximation (identification of a segment immediately adjacent to the actual endocardial segment of origin) in 30% of tachycardias [109].

More recently, McClelland et al [110] were able to compute epicardial potentials from BSPM (80 leads) using an inverse solution method. They were able to reconstruct in 5 patients epicardial isochronal maps demonstrating the exit site and the re-entry circuit of ventricular tachycardias.

10.5.8.2   Susceptibility to Ventricular Arrhythmias

Eigenvector analysis [111] was applied to QRST integral maps of two groups of patients with old myocardial infarction (11 patients with episodes of sustained ventricular tachycardia and 62 without arrhythmias) and in a control group of healthy subjects [112]. This method makes possible the detection and quantification of nondipolar components not evident on visual inspection of the integral maps. The cumulative contribution of the eigenvectors beyond the third to an individual map, expressed as percentage contribution of the total map content, has been considered a "nondipolar content" of that map. On average, the nondipolar content was significantly greater in patients with MI than in controls (8.3 $\pm$ 6.4% vs 4.1 $\pm$ 2.2%, $p < 0.001$) and, among patients, in those with ventricular tachycardia (7.2 $\pm$ 5.3% vs 16.6 $\pm$ 8.5%, $p < 0.001$). These findings were in agreement with those reported by Abildskov et al. [113]. Thus, the high nondipolar content of QRST maps in patients with ventricular tachycardia suggests the presence of local disparities of repolarization and it may be considered a useful marker of susceptibility to malignant arrhythmias.

Hubley-Kozey et al. [114] derived 16 eigenvectors from the total set of 204 QRST maps (102 patients with ventricular tachyarrhythmias and 102 patients without) but did not find a statistically significant difference in dipolar content between the two groups (13.1 $\pm$ 9.7 vs 12.9 $\pm$ 10.2%, $p > 0.05$). Because the nondipolar content did not perform well in their study population, the authors examined how individual eigenvector patterns contribute to QRST integral maps in each group of patients. Statistically significant differences were found between the values of Karhunen-Loeve coefficients in VT and non-VT groups for the 6th, 4th, 13th, 5th, 1st, 2nd, and 11th eigenvectors, in order of significance levels. Using stepwise discriminant analysis, they selected features subsets that best discriminated between the two groups. For an optimal set of eight spatial features, the sensitivity and specificity of the classifier for detecting patients with VT in 1,000 test sets were 90 $\pm$ 4% and 78 $\pm$ 6%, respectively. The authors concluded that the multiple body-surface ECGs contain valuable spatial features that can identify the presence of an arrhythmogenic substrate in the myocardium of patients at risk of ventricular arrhythmias.

Recently, Korhonen et al. [115] studied the complexity of T-wave morphology in BSPM of patients with recent myocardial infraction and cardiac dysfunction, by applying principal component analysis. They found that the 3rd principal component derived from BSPM was a significant predictor of arrhythmic events in this population.

10.5.8.3   BSPM and Ventricular Late Potentials

Vulnerability to arrhythmias has also been related to the existence of areas of delayed conduction at the end of the ventricular activation process. Ventricular late potentials recorded on signal-averaged ECG are the expression of this phenomenon. BSPM can be applied to detect these high-frequency, low-amplitude potentials [116, 117]. Maps not only made it possible to reveal the presence of late potentials, but also to determine the spatial distribution of late potentials in patients with ventricular tachycardia. Thus, BSPM may provide additional information about the thoracic location of ventricular late potentials, which can be related to the sites of conduction delay and possibly to the sites of origin of ventricular tachycardia.

10.5.8.4   Long QT Syndrome

BSPMs in patients with idiopathic long QT syndrome were described by De Ambroggi et al. [118]. No peculiar features were observed during the QRS interval, while the ventricular repolarization presented some abnormalities in addition to QT prolongation.

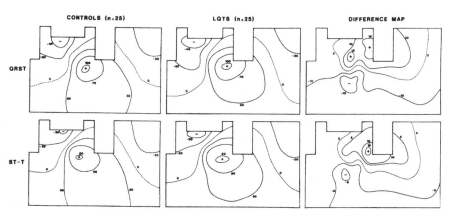

◘ Fig. 10.24

Mean integral maps of QRST and ST-T intervals in the control and LQTS groups. Difference maps are illustrated in the third column. Values are expressed in μVs (After De Ambroggi et al. [118]. © American Heart Association, Dallas, Texas. Reproduced with permission)

The visual inspection of instantaneous BSPMs revealed that the potential distributions were grossly abnormal (location of the potential extrema, presence of multiple peaks) in only a few cases. On the other hand, in most patients, BSPMs revealed less marked abnormalities in the instantaneous potential distribution. For instance, in several patients the negative potentials during the entire repolarization covered an area on the anterior thorax larger than in control subjects.

Differences between normals and LQTS patients were better quantified by analyzing ST-T and QRST integral maps. The mean integral map from the LQTS patients showed a potential distribution similar to that of the mean integral map from the control subjects. Nevertheless, the difference map (LQTS mean map minus control mean map) showed that LQTS patients had lower values on the inferior half of the trunk and on the right anterior thorax and higher values on the left anterior thorax compared with control subjects (❷ Fig. 10.24). In 13 patients, the negative values covered almost entirely the right anterior thorax. In six patients, there was a multipeak distribution of the integral values. The prominent negative area on the anterior chest in LQTS patients could result from a delayed repolarization of the underlying anterior wall so that it remains electronegative longer than other cardiac regions. Moreover, the multipolar distribution may reflect local inequalities in recovery times. ST-T integral maps were substantially similar to QRST maps, but a multipolar distribution was observed in a few more patients.

Eigenvector analysis [111] was also applied to QRST and ST-T integral maps. As already mentioned, this method makes possible the detection and quantification of nondipolar components not evident on visual inspection of the integral maps. The percent contribution of nondipolar eigenvectors (all eigenvectors beyond the third) to maps was significantly higher in LQTS patients than in normals. Moreover, eight patients who had a high nondipolar content did not show a multipeak distribution on their integral maps. This demonstrates that eigenvector analysis can detect nondipolar components not evident on integral maps.

To identify markers of dispersion of the ventricular repolarization, in a subsequent investigation on 40 patients with LQTS [119], we applied principal component analysis to all the recorded ST-T waves in each subject studied. We defined the ratio between the information content of the first principal component and the total information of the original data as "similarity index." Actually, a high value of similarity index indicates a great similarity of all waveforms to one fundamental waveform, that is, a great similarity of all waves to each other. On the contrary, a low value of similarity index indicates a large variety of ST-T waves and is considered a marker of repolarization disparities. In the 40 patients affected by congenital LQTS [119], the mean value of the similarity index was significantly lower than in healthy control subjects (49 ± 10 vs $77 \pm 8\%$, $p < 0.0001$). A value lower than 61%, corresponding to two standard deviations below the mean value for controls, was found in 35 of 40 patients and in only one control subject (sensitivity 87%, specificity 96%). In our experience, the similarity index has proved to be a more sensitive marker than multipolar distribution of QRST integral maps in revealing electrical disparities of ventricular repolarization.

10.5.8.5   Arrhythmogenic Right Ventricular Cardiomyopathy

Characteristic features of BSPMs were described in patients with arrhythmogenic right ventricular cardiomyopathy (ARVC). De Ambroggi et al. studied 22 patients affected by ARVC, nine with episodes of sustained ventricular tachycardias (VT) and 13 without [120]. The QRST integral maps showed in most ARVC patients a larger than normal area of negative values on the right anterior thorax. This abnormal pattern could be explained by a delayed repolarization of the right ventricle. Nevertheless, it was not related to the occurrence of VT in our patient population. To detect minor heterogeneities of ventricular repolarization, the principal component analysis was applied to the 62 ST-T waves recorded in each subject. We assumed that a low value of the first or of the first three components (Co 1, 2, 3) indicates a greater than normal variety of the ST-T waves, a likely expression of a more complex recovery process. The mean values of the first three components were not significantly different in ARVC patients and in control subjects. Nevertheless, considering the two subsets of patients with and without VT, the values of Co 1, of Co 1 + 2, and of Co 1 + 2 + 3 were significantly lower in the group of ARVC patients with VT. Values of Co 1 < 69% (equal to one SD below the mean value for controls) were found in six of nine VT patients and in one patient without VT (sensitivity 67%, specificity 92%). A low value of Co 1 was the only variable significantly associated with the occurrence of VT.

QRST integral maps with an abnormal negative area on the anterior thorax were also observed by Peeters et al. [121] in eight out of eight patients with ARVC, but in only two of eight patients with idiopathic right ventricular tachycardia.

10.5.8.6   Brugada Syndrome

The Brugada syndrome is a familial, "primary" electrical disease of the heart due to gene mutations encoding for the sodium channel and is characterized by a delayed activation of the right ventricle, with a QRS complex resembling that of right bundle branch block in V1, early ST elevation (J wave) in the right precordial leads, normal QT duration, inducibility of ventricular tachycardia, and a high risk of sudden cardiac death [122].

ECG changes have been quantified by 120-lead BSPMs: the QRS integrals were higher over the upper-right precordium and lower than normal over the lower left precordium; steeper negative ST gradients compared to normal were present over the upper left precordium and more positive ST gradients compared to normal over the lower left precordium [123].

Early ST elevation ($\geqslant$0.2 mV) was observed on a variable area over the right precordium. If this area is larger than 50 cm^2, it has a 92% positive and a 62% negative predictive value for inducibility of ventricular tachycardia, but similar predictive power was found for ventricular late potentials in the same patients [124].

Amplitude of maximal ST elevation was also used to differentiate Brugada syndrome patients with inducible ventricular tachycardia from asymptomatic patients [125].

10.6   Conclusions

The most general advantage of BSPMs is the fact that they record cardiac potentials from broad areas of the chest, thus enabling the detection of significant physiologic and possibly diagnostic information outside the precordial regions usually explored. Moreover, BSPMs provide the spatial as well as the temporal and amplitude components of cardiac electrical activity, whereas the ECG scalar waveforms present only the voltage variation with time in a given site.

As reported in the previous pages, investigations by different authors so far published clearly demonstrated a higher diagnostic content of BSPMs, compared with conventional ECG, in various pathological conditions.

Nevertheless, a widespread or even limited clinical application beyond the research laboratories of BSPM has not occurred up to day for several reasons: (a) the recording and processing of large numbers of leads and the displaying of maps have been complex and time-consuming, (b) a completely automated instrumentation was not commercially available, (c) use of many lead systems in different laboratories, differing in the number and placement of leads, and (d) difficulty in interpreting BSPM. The last reason is probably the most important obstacle that hampers the clinical use of BSPM.

In recent years, some of these obstacles have been overcome. BSPM recording systems, even those not widely marketed, have been (and can) relatively easily be developed and produced by several laboratories. Today's computer facilities make the recording and the data analysis easier than in the past. The time for applying electrodes and for data acquisition and analysis has been reduced considerably. Procedures, which reduce the number of leads that are necessary for reconstructing surface maps without losing too much information, have also been proposed; among these, the 32-lead system of Lux is the most commonly used [126]. Moreover, methods for converting multilead ECGs from one lead system to another have been proposed and satisfactorily applied [10].

The problem of interpreting surface maps still remains; in general, it may be approached essentially in two ways. The first approach is based on statistical methods, that is, defining the normal variability range of a number of parameters derived from maps relating to healthy subjects of different age, sex, and body shape, and then comparing these parameters by means of multivariate statistical procedures with those recorded from patients. The second approach is "deterministic"; that is, it consists of establishing the relationships between the intracardiac current sources (i.e., number, shape, location, and motion of excitation wavefronts and sequence of repolarization) and surface potential distribution (i.e., number, location, and motion of potential maxima and minima). This can be made in different ways, by using physiological or mathematical models. For instance, the distribution of currents and potentials has been determined experimentally in conducting media surrounding isolated hearts [127] thus enabling epicardial potentials to be compared with potentials recorded at a distance from the heart. Intracardiac current sources of known location have been produced by simultaneously stimulating the heart at multiple sites [128]. This allowed surface potential patterns to be correlated with known distributions of generators. The relationships between epicardial and body-surface potentials during activation and recovery were studied in intact chimpanzees [129, 130] and mathematical procedures for solving the direct and inverse problem (i.e., calculating surface potentials from internal sources and vice versa) were proposed by different authors (see ❷ Chaps. 8 and ❷ 9).

In the intact dog, Spach et al. succeeded in calculating accurately body-surface potentials from epicardial potential distributions during activation and recovery [131]. As regards the inverse problem, epicardial potentials have been calculated from potential distributions at the body surface in dogs [132–137]. In this respect, particularly important are the studies of Rudy and coworkers. They demonstrated the ability to compute noninvasively epicardial potential distribution and epicardial activation sequences from measured surface potentials. They called this new electrocardiographic modality as "ECG imaging," which, of necessity, has to utilize BSPM recording. The ECG imaging has been successfully applied in humans [138–141], using geometrical information from computed tomography and a mathematical algorithm, in different situations including the normal heart, a heart with a conduction disorder (right bundle branch block), focal activation initiated by right or left ventricular pacing, focal atrial tachycardia and flutter. A simplified method of inverse solution, which adopts a general torso model in which the same anatomic data are used irrespective of the body habitus, was applied by McClelland et al [110]. Despite these limitations they were able to reconstruct epicardial potential or isochronal maps identifying the left ventricular pacing site or indicating the exit site and the re-entry circuit of ventricular tachycardias. Very recently improvements to the inverse solution method were made by A. van Oosterom and coworkers [142]. The required computation time and the quality of the results obtained should favour the applications of this inverse procedure in a clinical setting.

In addition to all the reasons discussed above, the lack of expansion in the clinical setting of BSPM, which indeed can be considered an "advanced electrocardiographic method," is partially due to the fact that electrocardiology in recent years has lost some of its importance compared with newer sophisticated imaging techniques. The anatomic and functional information on several heart conditions (e.g., hypertrophy, location and extension of myocardial infarction, and so on) that, in the past, was obtained with varying degrees of accuracy by means of electrocardiographic techniques, can be more precisely and directly obtained today by other techniques such as echocardiography, magnetic resonance, multislice computed tomography, and nuclear imaging. On the other hand, electrocardiology still has a unique, primary role in the field of arrhythmias and conduction disturbances, into which no other technique can provide relevant insights. In particular, ECG imaging, based on the solution of the "inverse problem," which is the final aim of electrocardiography, hopefully will be able in the near future to provide, noninvasively, information on the epicardial and intramural excitation and recovery processes. This could give the possibility of identifying, with sufficient accuracy, intramural heterogeneities, transmural re-entry and intramural focal arrhythmias, and of defining ischemic or necrotic areas within the myocardium. The future of body-surface potential maps should be in that direction.

References

1. Plonsey, R., *Bioelectric Phenomena*. New York: McGraw-Hill, 1969, pp. 202.
2. Colli Franzone, P., L. Guerri, C. Viganotti, et al., Potential fields generated by oblique dipole layers modeling excitation wavefronts in the anisotropic myocardium. Comparison with potential fields elicited by paced dog hearts in a volume conductor. *Circ. Res.*, 1982;**51**: 330–346.
3. Taccardi, B., E. Macchi, R.L. Lux, et al., Effect of myocardial fiber direction on epicardial potentials. *Circulation*, 1994;**90**: 3076–3090.
4. Yan, G.X. and C. Antzelevitch, Cellular basis for the normal T wave and the electrocardiographic manifestations of the long QT syndrome. *Circulation*, 1998;**98**: 1928–1936.
5. Antzelevitch, C., W. Shimitzu, G.X. Yan, et al., The M cells: its contribution to the ECG and to normal and abnormal electrical function of the heart. *J. Electrophysiol.*, 1999;**10**: 1124–1152.
6. Waller, A.D., On the electromotive changes connected with the beat of the mammalian heart and of the human heart in particular. *Philos. Trans. R. Soc. Lond. Ser. B*, 1889;**180**: 169–194.
7. Nahum, L.H., A. Mauro, H.M. Chernoff, and R.S. Sikand, Instantaneous equipotential distribution on surface of the human body for various instants in the cardiac cycle. *J. Appl. Physiol.*, 1951;**3**: 454–464.
8. Taccardi, B., Distribution of heart potentials on dog's thoracic surface. *Circ. Res.*, 1962;**11**: 862–869.
9. Taccardi, B., Distribution of heart potentials on the thoracic surface of normal human subjects. *Circ. Res.*, 1963;**12**: 341–352.
10. Hoekema, R., G.J.H Uijen, D. Stilli, and A. van Oosterom, Lead system transformation of body surface map data. *J. Electrocardiol.*, 1998;**31**: 71–82.
11. Abildskov, J.A., M.J. Burgess, P.M. Urie, R.L. Lux, and R.F. Wyatt, The unidentified information content of the electrocardiogram. *Circ. Res.*, 1977;**40**: 3–7.
12. Abildskov, J.A., M.J. Burgess, R.L. Lux, R.F. Wyatt, and G.M. Vincent, The expression of normal ventricular repolarization in the body surface distribution of T potentials. *Circulation*, 1976;**54**: 901–906.
13. Corlan, A.D., R.S. Macleod, and L. De Ambroggi, The effect of intrathoracic heart position on ECG autocorrelation maps. *J. Electrocardiol.*, 2005;**38**: 87–94.
14. Taccardi, B., Body surface distribution of equipotential lines during atrial depolarization and ventricular repolarization. *Circ. Res.*, 1966;**19**: 865–878.
15. Taccardi, B., L. De Ambroggi, and C. Viganotti, Body-surface mapping of heart potentials, in *The Theoretical Basis of Electrocardiology*, C.V. Nelson and D.B. Geselowitz, Editors. Oxford: Clarendon, 1976, pp. 436–466.
16. Mirvis, D.M., Body surface distribution of electrical potential during atrial depolarization and repolarization. *Circulation*, 1980;**62**: 167–173.
17. Spach, M.S., R.C. Ban, R. Warrcn, D.W. Benson, A. Walston, and S.H. Edwards, Isopotential body surface mapping in subjects of all ages: emphasis on low-level potentials with analysis of the method. *Circulation*, 1979; **59**: 805–821.
18. Spach, M.S., T.D. King, R.C., O.E. Barr Boaz, M.N. Morrow, and S. Hennan-Giddens, Electrical potential distribution surrounding the atria during depolarization and repolarization in the dog. *Circ. Res.*, 1969;**24**: 857–873.
19. Eddlemon, C.O., V.J. Rucsta, L.G. Horan, and D.A. Brody, Distribution of heart potentials on the body surface in five normal young men. *Am. J. Cardiol.*, 1968;**21**: 860–870.
20. Young, B.D., P.W. Macfarlane, and T.D.V. Lawrie, Normal thoracic surface potentials. *Cardiovasc. Res.*, 1974;**8**: 187–193.
21. Green, L.S., R.L. Lux, C.W. Haws, R.R. Williams, S.C. Hunt, and M.J. Burgess, Effects of age, sex, and body habitus on QRS and ST-T potential maps of 1100 normal subjects. *Circulation*, 1985;**71**: 244–253.
22. Spach, M.S., W.P. Silberberg, J.P. Boineau, et al., Body surface isopotential maps in normal children, ages 4 to 14 years. *Am. Heart. J.*, 1966;**72**: 640–652.
23. Liebman, J., C.W. Thomas, Y. Rudy, and R. Plonsey, Electrocardiographic body surface potential maps of the QRS of normal children. *J. Electrocardiol.*, 1981: **14**: 249–260.
24. Tazawa, H and C. Yoshimoto, Electrocardiographic potential distribution in newborn infants from 12 hours to 8 days after birth. *Am. Heart. J.*, 1969;**78**: 292–305.
25. Benson, D.W. Jr. and M.S. Spach, Evolution of QRS and ST-T-wave body surface potential distributions during the first year of life. *Circulation*, 1982;**65**: 1247–1258.
26. Durrer, D., R.Th van Dam, G.E. Freud, M.J. Janse, F.L. Meijler, and R.C. Arzbaecher, Total excitation of the isolated human heart. *Circulation*, 1970;**41**: 899–912.
27. Wyndham, C.R., M.K. Meeran, T. Smith, et al., Epicardial activation of the intact human heart without conduction defect. *Circulation*, 1979;**59**: 161–168.
28. Green, L.S., R.L. Lux, D. Stilli, C.W. Haws, and B. Taccardi, Fine details in body surface potential maps: accuracy of maps using a limited lead array and spatial and temporal data representation. *J. Electrocardiol.*, 1987;**20**: 21–26.
29. Hoekema, R., G.J. Uijen, and A. Van Oosterom, Geometrical aspects of the interindividual variability of multilead ECG recordings. *IEEE Trans. Biomed. Eng.*, 2001;**48**: 551–559.
30. Kozmann G, R.L. Lux, and L.S. Green, Sources of variability in normal body surface potential maps. *Circulation*, 1989;**79**: 1077–1083.
31. Montague, T.J., E.R. Smith, D.A. Cameron, et al., Isointegral analysis of body surface maps: surface distribution and temporal variability in normal subjects. *Circulation*, 1981;**63**: 1166–1172.
32. Flaherty, J.T., S.D. Blumenschein, A.W. Alexander, et al., Influence of respiration on recording cardiac potentials. Isopotential surface-mapping and vectorcardiographic study. *Am. J. Cardiol.*, 1967;**20**: 21–28.
33. Spach, M.S., R.C. Barr, D.W. Benson, A.H. Walston, R.B. Warren, and S.B. Edwards, Body surface low-level potentials during ventricular repolarization with analysis of the ST segment. Variability in normal subjects. *Circulation*, 1979;**59**: 822–36.
34. Corlan, A.D., P.W. Macfarlane, and L. De Ambroggi, Gender differences in stability of the instantaneous patterns of body surface potentials during ventricular repolarisation. *Med. Biol. Eng. Comput.*, 2003;**41**: 536–542.
35. Abildskov, J.A., A.K. Evans, R.L. Lux, and M.J. Burgess Ventricular recovery properties and QRST deflection area in cardiac electrograms. *Am. J. Physiol.*, 1981;**239**: H227–231.

36. Sano, T., Y. Sakamoto, M. Yamamoto, and F. Suzuki, The body surface U wave potentials, in *Progress in Electrocardiology*, P.W. Macfarlane, Editor. Tunbridge Wells: Pitman Medical, 1979, pp. 227–231.

37. L. De Ambroggi, E. Locati, T. Bertoni, E. Monza, and P.J. Schwartz, Body surface potentials during T-U interval in patients with the idiopathic long QT syndrome, in *Clinical Aspects of Ventricular Repolarization*, chapter 47, G.S. Butrous and P.J. Schwartz, Editors. London: Farrand Press, 1989, pp. 433–436.

38. L. De Ambroggi, M. Besozzi, and B. Taccardi, Aspetti qualitativi e quantitativi delle elettromappe cardiache nell'infarto miocardico anteriore e inferiore. *G. Ital. Cardiol.*, 1974;**4**: 540–553.

39. L. De Ambroggi, T. Bertoni, C. Rabbia, and M. Landolina, Body surface potential maps in old inferior myocardial infarction. Assessment of diagnostic criteria. *J. Electrocardiol.*, 1986;**19**: 225–234.

40. L. De Ambroggi, T. Bertoni, M.L. Breghi, M. Marconi, and M. Mosca, Diagnostic value of body surface potential mapping in old anterior non-Q myocardial infarction. *J. Electrocardiol.*, 1988;**21**: 321–329.

41. Flowers, N.C., L.G. Horan, and J.C. Johnson, Anterior infarctional changes occurring during mid and late ventricular activation detectable by surface mapping techniques. *Circulation*, 1976;**54**: 906–913.

42. Flowers, N.C., L.G. Horan, G.S. Sohi, R.C. Hand, and J.C. Johnson, New evidence for infero-posterior myocardial infarction on surface potential maps. *Am. J. Cardiol.*, 1976;**38**: 576–581.

43. Vincent, G.M., J.A. Abildskov, M.J. Burgess, K. Millar, R.L. Lux, and R.F. Wyatt, Diagnosis of old inferior myocardial infarction by body surface isopotential mapping. *Am. J. Cardiol.*, 1977;**39**: 510–515.

44. H. Pham-Huy, R.M. Gulrajani, F.A. Roberge, R.A. Nadeau, G.E. Mailloux, and P. Savard, A comparative evaluation of three different approaches for detecting body surface isopotential map abnormalities in patients with myocardial infarction. *J. Electrocardiol.*, 1981;**14**: 43–55.

45. Toyama, S., K. Suzuki, M. Koyama, K. Yoshino, and K. Fujimolo, The body surface isopotential mapping of the QRS wave in myocardial infarction: comparative study of the scintigram with thallium-201. *J. Electrocardiol.*, 1982;**15**: 241–247.

46. Ohta, T., A. Kinoshita, J. Ohsugi, et al., Correlation between body surface isopotential maps and left ventriculograms in patients with old inferoposterior myocardial infarction. *Am. Heart J.*, 1982;**104**: 1262–1270.

47. Osugi, J. T. Ohta, J. Toyama, F. Takatsu, T. Nagaya, and K. Yamada, Body surface isopotential maps in old inferior myocardial infarction undetectable by 12 lead electrocardiogram. *J. Electrocardiol.*, 1984;**17**: 55–62.

48. Hirai, M., T. Ohta, A. Kinoshita, J. Toyama, T. Nagaya, and K. Yamada, Body surface isopotential maps in old anterior myocardial infarction undetectable by 12-lead electrocardiograms. *Am. Heart J.*, 1984;**108**: 975–982.

49. Kubota, I., M. Yamaki, K Ikeda, I. Yamaguchi, I. Tonooka, K. Tsuiki, and S. Yasui, Abnormalities of early depolarization in patients with remote anterior myocardial infarction and ventricular septal hypoperfusion. Diagnosis of septal MI BSM. *J. Electrocardiol.*, 1990;**23**: 307–313.

50. Hayashi, H., M. Hirai, A. Suzuki, et al., Correlation between various parameters derived from body surface maps and ejection fraction in patients with anterior myocardial infarction. *J. Electrocardiol.*, 1993;**26**: 17–24.

51. Suzuki, A., M. Hirai., H. Hayashi, et al. The ability of QRST isointegral maps to detect myocardial infarction in the presence of simulated left bundle branch block. *Eur. Heart J.*, 1993;**14**: 1094–1101.

52. Medvegy, M., I. Preda, P. Savard, et al., A new body surface isopotential map evaluation method to detect minor potential losses in non-Q wave myocardial infarction. *Circulation*, 2000;**101**: 1115–1121.

53. Medvegy, M., P. Savard, A. Pinter, et al., Simple, quantitative body surface potential map parameters in the diagnosis of remote Q wave and non-Q wave myocardial infarction. *Can. J. Cardiol.*, 2004;**20**: 1109–1115.

54. Corlan, A.D. and L. De Ambroggi, New quantitative methods of ventricular repolarization analysis in patients with left ventricular hypertrophy. *Ital. Heart J.*, 2000;**1**: 542–548.

55. Corlan, A.D., B.M. Horacek, and L. De Ambroggi, Prognostic value for ventricular tachicardia of indices of ventricular repolarization in patients with and without myocardial infarction. 32nd Congress of International Society of Electrocardiology. *Folia Cardiol.*, 2005;12(Suppl C): 52.

56. Muller, J.E., P.R. Maroko, and E. Braunwald, Precordial electrocardiographic mapping. A technique to assess the efficacy of interventions designed to limit infarct size. *Circulation*, 1978;**57**: 1–18.

57. Maroko, P.R., P. Libby, J.W. Covell, B.E. So bel, J. Ross Jr, and E. Braunwald, Precordial S-T segment elevation mapping. An atraumatic method for assessing alterations in the extent of myocardial ischemic injury. *Am. J. Cardiol.*, 1972;**29**: 223–230.

58. Muller, J.E., P.R. Maroko, and E. Braunwald, Evaluation of precordial electrocardiographic mapping as a means of assessing changes in myocardial ischemic injury. *Circulation*, 1975;**52**: 16–27.

59. Holland, R.P. and H. Brooks, TQ-ST segment mapping: critical review and analysis of current concepts. *Am. J. Cardiol.*, 1977;**40** 110–129.

60. Surawicz, S., The disputed S-T segment mapping: is the technique ready for wide application in practice? *Am. J. Cardiol.*, 1977;**40**: 137–140.

61. Mirvis, D.M., Body surface distributions of repolarization forces during acute myocardial infarction. I. Isopotential and isoarea mapping. *Circulation*, 1980: **62**: 878–887.

62. Montague, T.J., E.R. Smith, C.A. Spencer, et al., Body surface electrocardiographic mapping in inferior myocardial infarction. Manifestation of left and right ventricular involvement. *Circulation*, 1983: **67**: 665–673.

63. Menown, I.B.A., J. Allen, J. McC Anderson, and A.A.J. Adgey, Early diagnosis of right ventricular or posterior infarction associated with inferior wall left ventricular acute myocardial infarction. *Am. J. Cardiol.*, 2000;**85**: 934–938.

64. McClelland, A.J.J., C.G. Owens, I.B. Menown, M. Lown, and A.A. Adgey, Comparison of 80-lead body surface map to physician and to 12-lead electrocardiogram in detection of acute myocardial infarction. *Am. J. Cardiol.*, 2003;**92**: 252–257.

65. Maynard, S.J., I.B. Menown, G. Manoharan, J. Allen, J. McC Anderson, and A.A. Adgey, Body surface mapping improves early diagnosis of acute myocardial infarction in patients with chest pain and left bundle branch block. *Heart*, 2003;**89**: 998–1002.

66. De Ambroggi, L., E. Macchi, B. Brusoni, and B. Taccardi, Electromaps during ventricular recovery in angina patients with normal resting ECG. *Adv. Cardiol.*, 1977;**19**: 88–90.

67. Stilli, D., E. Musso, E. Macchi, et al., Body surface potential mapping in ischemic patients with normal resting ECG. *Can. J. Cardiol.*, 1986;Suppl A: 107–112A.

68. Kornreich, F., P. Block P, and D. Brismee, The missing waveform information in the orthogonal electrocardiogram (Frank leads). Ill. Computer diagnosis of angina pectoris from "maximal" QRS surface waveform information at rest. *Circulation*, 1974;**49**: 1212–1222.

69. Spekhorst, H., A. Sippens-Groenewegen, G.K. David, M.J. Janse, and A.J. Dunning, Body surface mapping during percutaneous transluminal coronary angioplasty. QRS changes indicating regional myocardial conduction delay. *Circulation*, 1990;**81**: 840–849.

70. Shenasa, M., D. Hamel, J. Nasmith, et al., Body surface potential mapping of ST segment shift in patient undergoing percutaneous transluminal coronary angioplasty. *J. Electrocardiol.*, 1993;**26**: 43–51.

71. Cahyadi, Y.H., N. Takekoshi, and S. Matsui, Clinical efficacy of PTCA and identification of restenosis: evaluation by serial body surface potential mapping. *Am. Heart J.*, 1991;**121**: 1080–1087.

72. Fox, K.M., A.P. Selwyn, and J.P.A. Shillingford, method for precordial surface mapping of the exercise electrocardiogram. *Br. Heart J.*, 1978: 40: 1339–1343.

73. Fox, K., A. Selwyn, and J. Shillingford, Precordial electrocardiographic mapping after exercise in the diagnosis of coronary artery disease. *Am. J. Cardiol.*, 1979;**43**: 541–546.

74. Mirvis, D.M., F.W. Keller Jr., J.W. Cox Jr., D.G. Zetlergren, R.F. Dowdie, and R.E. Ideker, Left precordial isopotential mapping during supine exercise. *Circulation*, 1977;**56**: 245–252.

75. Mirvis, D.M., Body surface distribution of exercise-induced QRS changes in normal subjects. *Am. J. Cardiol.*, 1980: **46** 988–996.

76. Miller, W.T. III, M.S. Spach, and R.B. Warren, Total body surface potential mapping during exercise: QRS- T-wave changes in normal young adults. *Circulation*, 1980;**62**: 632–645.

77. Simoons, M.L. and P. Block, Toward the optimal lead system and optimal criteria for exercise electrocardiography. *Am. J. Cardiol.*, 1981;**47**: 1366–1374.

78. Wada, M., K. Kaneko, H. Teshigawara, et al., Exercise stress body surface isopotential map in patients with coronary artery disease: comparison with coronary angiographic and stress myocardial perfusion scintigraphic findings. *Jpn. Circ. J.*, 1981;**45**: 1203–1207.

79. Yanowitz, F.G., G.M. Vincent, R.L. Lux, M. Merchant, L.S. Green, and J.A. Abildskov, Application of body surface mapping to exercise testing: S-T80 isoarea maps in patients with coronary artery disease. *Am. J. Cardiol.*, 1982;**50**: 1109–1113.

80. Blumenschein, S.D., M.S. Spach, J.P. Boineau, et al., Genesis of body surface potentials in varying types of right ventricular hypertrophy. *Circulation*, 1968;**38**: 917–932.

81. Sohi, G.S., E.W. Green, N.C. Flowers, O.F. McMartin, and R.R. Masdcn, Body surface potential maps in patients with pulmonic valvular and aortic valvular stenosis of mild to moderate severity. *Circulation*, 1979;**59**: 1277–1283.

82. Holt, J.H. Jr, A.C.L. Barnard, and J.O. Kramer Jr., Multiple dipole electrocardiography: a comparison of electrically and angiographically determined left ventricular masses. *Circulation*, 1978;**57**: 1129–1133.

83. Yamaki, M., K. Ikeda, I. Kubota, K. Nakamura, K. Hanashima, K. Tsuiki, and S. Yasui, Improved diagnostic performance on the severity of left ventricular hypertrophy with body surface mapping. *Circulation*, 1989;**79**: 312–323.

84. Kornreich, F., T.J. Montague, P.M. Rautahariu, M. Kavadias, M.B. Horacek, and B. Taccardi, Diagnostic body surface potential map patterns in left ventricular hypertrophy during PQRST. *Am. J. Cardiol.*, 1989;**63**: 610–617.

85. Hirai, M., H. Hayashi, Y. Ichihara, et al., Body surface distribution of abnormally low QRST areas in patients with left ventricular hypertrophy. An index of repolarization abnormalities. *Circulation*, 1991;**84**: 1505–1515.

86. Taccardi, B., L. De Ambroggi, and D. Riva, Chest maps of heart potentials in right bundle branch block. *J. Electrocardiol.*, 1969;**2**: 109–116.

87. Sugenoya, J., S. Sugiyama, M. Wada, N. Niimi, H. Oguri, J. Toyama, and K. Yamada, Body surface potential distribution following the production of right bundle branch block in dogs: effects of breakthrough and right ventricular excitation on the body surface potentials. *Circulation*, 1977;**55**: 49–54.

88. Sugenoya, J., Interpretation of the body surface isopotential maps of patients with right bundle branch block. Determination of the region of the delayed activation within the right ventricle. *Jpn. Heart J.*, 1978;**19**: 12–27.

89. Preda, I., I. Bukosza, G. Kozmann, Y.V. Shakin, A. Szèkely, and Z. Antalòczy, Surface potential distribution on the human thoracic surface in the left bundle branch block. *Jpn. Heart J.*, 1979;**20**: 7–21.

90. Musso, E., D. Stilli, E. Macchi, et al., Body surface maps in left bundle branch block uncomplicated or complicated by myocardial infarction, left ventricular hypertrophy or myocardial ischemia. *J. Electrocardiol.*, 1987;**20**: 1–20.

91. Sohi, G.S., N.C. Flowers, L.G. Boran, M.R. Sridharan, and J.C. Johnson, Comparison of total body surface map depolarization patterns of left bundle branch block and normal axis with left bundle branch block and left axis deviation. *Circulation*, 1983;**67**: 660–664.

92. Preda, I., Z. Antaloczy, I. Bukosza, G. Kozmann, and A. Szckely, New elcctrocardiological infarct criteria in the presence of left bundle branch block (surface mapping study), in *Progress in Electrocardiology*, P.W. Macfarlane, Editor. Tunbridge Wells: Pitman Medical, 1979, pp. 231–235.

93. Gallagher, J.J., A.R. Ticzon, A.G. Wallace, and J. Kasell, Activation studies following experimental hemiblock in the dog. *Circ. Res.*, 1974;**35**: 752–763.

94. Sohi, G.S. and N.C. Flowers, Effects of left anterior fascicular block on the depolarization process as depicted by total body surface mapping. *J. Electrocardiol.*, 1980: **13**: 143–152.

95. Yamada, K., J. Toyama, M. Wada, et al., Body surface isopotential mapping in Wolff-Parkinson-White syndrome. Noninvasive method to determine the location of the accessory atrioventricular pathway. *Am. Heart J.*, 1975;**90**: 721–734.

96. De Ambroggi, L., B. Taccardi, and E. Macchi, Body-surface maps of heart potentials. Tentative localization of pre-excited areas in forty-two Wolff-Parkinson-White patients. *Circulation*, 1976;**54**: 251–263.

97. Spach, M.S., R.C. Ban, and C.F. Lanning, Experimental basis for QRS and T wave potentials in the WPW syndrome. The relation of epicardial to body surface potential distributions in the intact chimpanzee. *Circ. Res.*, 1978;**42**: 103–118.

98. Iwa, T. and T. Magara, Correlation between localization of accessory conduction pathway and body surface maps in the Wolff-Parkinson. While syndrome. *Jpn. Circ. J.*, 1981;**45**: 1192–1198.

99. Benson, D.W. Jr., R. Sterba, J.J. Gallagher, A. Walston II, and M.S. Spach, Localization of the site of ventricular preexcitation with body surface maps in patients with Wolff-Parkinson-White: syndrome. *Circulation*, 1982;**65**: 1259–1268.

100. Kamakura, S., K. Shimomura, T. Ohe, M. Matsuhisa, and H. Yoyoshima, The role of initial minimum potential on body surface maps in predicting the site of accessory pathways in patients with Wolff-Parkinson-White syndrome. *Circulation*, 1986;**74**: 89–96.

101. Liebman, J., J.A. Zeno, B. Olshansky, et al., Electrocardiographic body surface potential mapping in the Wolff-Parkinson-White syndrome. Noninvasive determination of the ventricular insertion sites of accessory atrioventricular connections. *Circulation*, 1991;**83**: 886–901.

102. Dubuc, M., R. Nadeau, G. Tremblay, T. Kus, F. Molin, and P. Savard, Pace mapping using body surface potential maps to guide catheter ablation of accessory pathways in patients with Wolff-Parkinson-White syndrome. *Circulation*, 1993;**87**: 135–143.

103. Frank, E., Electric potential produced by two point current sources in a homogeneous conducting sphere. *J. Appl. Physiol.*, 1952;**23**: 1225–1228.

104. De Ambroggi, L. and B. Taccardi, Current and potential fields generated by two dipoles. *Circ. Res.*, 1970;**27**: 901–911.

105. Knippel, M., D. Pioselli, F. Rovelli, L. Campolo, E. Panzeri, and A. Pellegrini, Tachicardie ribelli nella sindrome da preeccitazione: trattamento chirurgico di cinque casi. *G. Ital. Cardiol.*, 1974;**4**: 657.

106. Guiraudon G.M., G.J. Klein, S. Gulamhusein, et al., Surgery for Wolff-Parkinson-White syndrome: further experience with epicardial approach. *Circulation*, 1986;**74**: 525–529.

107. Sippens-Groenewegen, A., H. Spekhorst, N.M. van Hemel, et al., Body surface mapping of ectopic left and right ventricular activation. QRS spectrum in patients without structural heart disease. *Circulation*, 1990;**82**: 879–896.

108. Sippens-Groenewegen, A., H. Spekhorst, N.M. van Hemel, et al., Localization of the site of origin of postinfarction ventricular tachycardia by endocardial pace mapping. Body surface mapping compared with the 12-lead electrocardiogram. *Circulation*, 1993;**88**: 2290–2306.

109. Sippens-Groenewegen, A, H. Spekhorst, N.M. van Hemel, et al., Value of body surface mapping in localizing the site of origin of ventricular tachycardia in patients with previous myocardial infarction. *J. Am. Coll. Cardiol.*, 1994;**24**: 1708–1724.

110. McClelland, A.J.J., C.G. Owens, C. Navarro, B. Smith, M.J.D. Roberts, J. Anderson, and A.A.J. Adgey, Usefulness of body surface maps to demonstrate ventricular activation patterns during left ventricular pacing and reentrant activation during ventricular tachycardia in men with coronary heart disease and left ventricular dysfunction. *Am J Cardiol* 2006;**98**: 591–596.

111. Lux, R.L., A.K. Evans, M.J. Burgess, R.F. Wyatt, and J.A. Abildskov, Redundancy reduction for improved display and analysis of body surface potential maps. I. Spatial compression. *Circ. Res.*, 1981;**49**: 186–196.

112. Bertoni, T., M.L. Breghi, M. Marconi, G. Bonifaccio, and L. De Ambroggi, Usefulness of the QRST integral maps to detect vulnerability to malignant arrhythmias in patients with old

myocardial infarction, in *Electrocardiology '87*, E. Schubert, Editor. Berlin: Akademie-Verlag, 1988, pp. 247–250.

113. Abildskow, J.A., L.S. Green, and R.L. Lux, Detection of disparate ventricular repolarization by means of the body surface electrocardiogram, in*Cardiac Electrophysiology and Arrhythmias*, D.P. Zipes and J. Jalife, Editors. Orlando: Grune & Stratton, 1985, pp. 495–499.

114. Hubley-Kozey, C.L., B.L. Mitchell, M.J. Gardner, J.W. Warren, C.J. Penney, E.R. Smith, and B.M. Horacek, Spatial features in body-surface potential maps can identify patients with a history of sustained ventricular tachycardia. *Circulation*, 1995;**92**: 1825–1838.

115. Korhonen, P., T. Husa, T. Konttila, I. Tierala, M. Makijarvi, H. Vaananen, and L. Toivonen, Complex T-wave morphology in body surface mapping in prediction of arrhythmic events in patients with acute myocardial infarction and cardiac dysfunction. *Europace* 2009;**11**: 514–520.

116. Faugère, G., P. Savard, R.A. Nadeau, D. Derome, M. Shenasa, P.L. Page, and R. Guardo, Characterization of the spatial distribution of late ventricular potentials by body surface mapping in patients with ventricular tachycardia. *Circulation*, 1986;**74**: 1323–1333.

117. Shibata, T., I. Kubota, K. Ikeda, K. Tsuiki, and S. Yasui, Body surface mapping of high-frequency components in the terminal portion during QRS complex for the prediction of ventricular tachycardia in patients with previous myocardial infarction. *Circulation*, 1990;**82**: 2084–2092.

118. De Ambroggi, L., T. Bertoni, E. Locati, M. Stramba-Badiale, and P.J. Schwartz, Mapping of body surface potentials in patients with the idiopathic long QT syndrome. *Circulation*, 1986;**74**: 1334–1345.

119. De Ambroggi, L., M.S. Negroni, E. Monza, T. Bertoni, and P.J. Schwartz, Dispersion of ventricular repolarization in the long QT syndrome. *Am. J. Cardiol.*, 1991;**68**: 614–620.

120. De Ambroggi, L., E. Aimè, C. Ceriotti, M. Rovida, and S. Negroni, Mapping of ventricular repolarization potentials in patients with arrhythmogenic right ventricular dysplasia: principal component analysis of the ST-T waves. *Circulation*, 1997;**96**: 4314–4318.

121. Peeters, H.A., A. SippensGroenewegen, B.A. Schoonderwoerd, E.F. Wever, C.A. Grimbergen, R.N. Hauer, and E.O. Rohles de Medina, Body-surface QRST integral mapping. Arrhythmogenic right ventricular dysplasia versus idiopathic right ventricular tachycardia. *Circulation*, 1997;**95**: 2668–2676.

122. Antzelevitch, C., P. Brugada, M. Borggrefe, et al., Brugada syndrome: report of the second consensus conference. *Circulation*, 2005;**111**: 659–670.

123. Bruns, H.J., L. Eckardt, C. Vahlhaus, E. Schulze-Bahr, W. Haverkamp, M. Borggrefe, G. Breithardt, and T. Wichter, Body surface potential mapping in patients with Brugada syndrome: right precordial ST segment variations and reverse changes in left precordial leads. *Cardiovasc. Res.*, 2002;**54**: 58–66.

124. Eckardt, L., H.J. Bruns, M. Paul, P. Kirchhof, E. Schulze-Bahr, T. Wichter, G. Breithardt, M. Borggrefe, and W. Haverkamp, Body surface area of ST elevation and the presence of late potentials correlate to the inducibility of ventricular tachyarrhythmias in Brugada syndrome. *J. Cardiovasc. Electrophysiol.*, 2002;**13**: 742–749.

125. Hisamatsu, K., K.F. Kusano, H. Morita, S. Takenaka, S. Nagase, K. Nakamura, T. Emori, H. Matsubara, and T. Ohe, Usefulness of body surface mapping to differentiate patients with Brugada

syndrome from patients with asymptomatic Brugada syndrome. *Acta Med. Okayama*, 2004;**58**: 29–35.

126. Lux, R.L., C.R. Smith, R.F. Wyatt, and J.A. Abildskov, Limited lead selection for estimation of body surface potential maps in electrocardiography. *IEEE Trans. Biomed. Eng.*, 1978;**25**: 270–276.

127. Taccardi, B., C. Viganotti, E. Macchi, and L. De Ambroggi, Relationships between the current field surrounding an isolated dog heart and the potential distribution on the surface of the body. *Adv. Cardiol.*, 1976;**16**: 72–76.

128. Abildskov, J.A., M.J. Burgess, K. Millar, G.M. Vincent, R.F. Wyatt, and R.L. Lux, Distribution of body surface potentials with experimentally-induced multiple cardiac generators. *Adv. Cardiol.*, 1974;**10**: 69–76.

129. Spach, M.S., R.C. Barr, C.F. Lanning, and P.C. Tucek, Origin of body surface QRS and T wave potentials from epicardial potential distributions in the intact chimpanzee. *Circulation*, 1977;**55**: 268–278.

130. Spach, M.S., R.C. Barr, and C.F. Lanning, Experimental basis for QRS and T wave potentials in the WPW syndrome. The relation of epicardial to body surface potential distributions in the intact chimpanzee. *Circ. Res.*, 1978;**42**: 103–118.

131. Ramsey, M. III, R.C. Barr, and M.S. Spach, Comparison of measured torso potentials with those simulated from epicardial potentials for ventricular depolarization and repolarization in the intact dog. *Circ. Res.*, 1977;41: 660–672.

132. Barr, R.C. and M.S. Spach, Inverse calculation of QRS-T epicardial potentials from body surface potential distributions for normal and ectopic beats in the intact dog. *Circ. Res.*, 1978;**42**: 661–675.

133. Colli Franzone, P., L. Guerri, B. Taccardi, and C. Viganotti, A regularization method for inverse electrocardiology applied to data from an isolated dog heart experiment, in *Modern Electrocardiology*, Z. Antaloczy, Editor. Amsterdam: Excerpta Medica, 1978, pp. 75–80.

134. Oster, H.S., B. Taccardi, R.L. Lux, P.H. Ershler, and Y. Rudy, Noninvasive electrocardiographic imaging. Reconstruction of epicardial potentials, electrograms, and isochrones and localization of single and multiple electrocardiac events. *Circulation*, 1997;**96**: 1012–1024.

135. Burnes, J.E., B. Taccardi, and Y. Rudy, A Noninvasive electrocardiographic imaging modality for cardiac arrhythmias. *Circulation*, 2000;**102**: 2151–2158.

136. Burnes, J.E., B. Taccardi, P.H. Ershler, and Y. Rudy, Noninvasive electrocardiographic imaging of substrate and intramural ventricular tachycardia in infarcted hearts. *J. Am. Coll. Cardiol.*, 2001;**38**: 2071–2078.

137. Ghanem, R.N., J.E. Burnes, A.L. Waldo, and Y. Rudy, Imaging dispersion of myocardial repolarization, II. Noninvasive reconstruction of epicardial measures. *Circulation*, 2001;**104**: 1306–1312.

138. Ramanatham, C., R.N. Ghanem, P. Jia, K. Ryu, and Y. Rudy, Noninvasive electrocardiographic imaging for cardiac electrophysiology and arrhythmias. *Nat. Med.*, 2004;**10**: 422–428.

139. Ghanem, R.N., P. Jia, C. Ramanatham, K. Ryu, A. Markowitz, and Y. Rudy, Noninvasive electrocardiographic imaging (ECGI): comparison to intraoperative mapping in patients. *Heart Rhythm*, 2005;**2**: 339–354.

140. Intini, A., R.N. Goldstein, P. Jia, C. Ramanathan, K. Ryu, B. Giannattasio, R. Gilkeson, B.S. Stambler, P. Brugada, W.G. Stevenson, Y. Rudy, and A.L. Waldo, Electrocardiographic imaging (ECGI), a novel diagnostic modality used for mapping of focal left ventricular tachycardia in a young athlete. *Heart Rhythm*. 2005;**2**: 1250–1252.

141. Wang, Y., P.S. Cuculich, P.K. Woodard, B.D. Lindsay, and Y. Rudy, Focal atrial tachycardia after pulmonary vein isolation: Noninvasive mapping with electrocardiographic imaging (ECGI). *Heart Rhythm* 2007;**4**: 1081–1084.

142. Van Dam, P.M., T.F. Oostendorp, A.C. Linnenbank, and A. van Oosterom, Non-invasive imaging of cardiac activation and recovery. *Ann Biomed Eng* 2009;**37**: 1739–1756.

Index

Note: The page numbers that appear in bold type indicates a substantive discussion of the topic.